THE PEOPLE'S MEDICAL SOCIETY

MEN'S HEALTH WELLNESS

ENCYCLOPEDIA

THE PEOPLE'S MEDICAL SOCIETY

MEN'S HEALTH AND WELLNESS

ENCYCLOPEDIA

CHARLES B. INLANDER

and the Staff of the
People's Medical Society

≡People's Medical Society.

Macmillan • USA

MACMILLAN
A Simon & Schuster Macmillan Company
1633 Broadway
New York, NY 10019-6785

Macmillan Publishing books may be purchased for business or sales promotional use. For information please write: Special Markets Department, Macmillan Publishing USA, 1633 Broadway, New York, NY 10019.

The People's Medical Society is a nonprofit consumer health organization dedicated to the principles of better, more responsive, and less expensive medical care. Organized in 1983, the People's Medical Society puts previously unavailable medical information into the hands of consumers so that they can make informed decisions about their own health care.

Membership in the People's Medical Society is $20 a year and includes a subscription to the *People's Medical Society Newsletter*. For information, write to the People's Medical Society, 462 Walnut Street, Allentown, PA 18102, or call 610-770-1670.

The information in this book is intended to help the reader make more informed choices regarding health care. It is not a substitute for expert medical advice or treatment. All matters regarding health require medical supervision.

Many of the designations used by manufacturers and sellers to distinguish their products are claimed as trademarks. Where those designations appear in this book and People's Medical Society was aware of a trademark claim, the designations have been printed in initial capital letters (e.g., Advil).

MACMILLAN is a registered trademark of Macmillan, Inc.

Book Design: A & D Howell

Library of Congress Cataloging-in-Publication Data
Inlander, Charles B.
    People's Medical Society men's health and wellness desk reference: everything a man needs to know for good health and well-being/by Charles B. Inlander and the staff of the People's Medical Society.
        p.   cm.
    "A People's Medical Society book."
    Includes bibliographical references and index.
    ISBN 0-02-862295-2
    1. Men—Health and hygiene. 2. Men—Medical care. I. People's Medical Society
(U.S.) II. Title.
RA777.75.I55 1998
613' .04234—dc21   97-40601
                                                                         CIP

Manufactured in the United States of America
10 9 8 7 6 5 4 3 2 1

CONTENTS

ACKNOWLEDGMENTS

Creating a book of this size and scope is truly a collaborative effort. We especially want to acknowledge and thank the following individuals for their invaluable contributions.

From the People's Medical Society:

As the book's editorial project manager, Janet Worsley Norwood provided insightful leadership, incredible patience, unlimited writing and editing talents, and unending dedication. This book could rightfully be called hers.

Karla Morales, vice president for editorial services and communications, oversaw all aspects of the book's development, providing her usual excellent skills and know-how, thus assuring a fine finished product.

Special thanks to these other People's Medical Society staff members, each of whom made significant contributions to the book: Michael Donio, director of projects; Jennifer Hay, managing editor; Linda Hager, editorial project manager; Karen Kemmerer, vice president for operations; Ellen Greene, publisher; Linda Swank, director of membership services; and Gayle Ebert, secretary.

Grateful appreciation to Cynthia K. Moran, who helped edit the entire manuscript, providing useful and important suggestions and direction.

This book would not have been possible without the talents of the following contributing writers: Tara Cranmer, Maureen Sangiorgio, Justine Johnson, Mark Demko, Kathleen Blease, Martha Capwell, Kim McAndrew, Andrea Monticino Riffle, and Patricia Lynch Stinner.

Thanks as well to Jerry O'Brien, who used his time and talent to provide many of the illustrations for this book.

Special acknowledgments and thanks also go to the following individuals and organizations for their assistance: Nancy Ryan, American Society of Plastic and Reconstructive Surgeons; Oldways Preservation and Exchange Trust; National Institutes of Health; Mary L. Meyer, Choice in Dying; American Cancer Society; Jon Knowles, Planned Parenthood Federation of America; National Clearinghouse for Alcohol and Drug Information; U.S. Department of Transportation National Highway Traffic Safety Administration; American Lung Association; and Linda Stalvey, Department of Veterans Affairs.

Further thanks to our colleagues at Macmillan with whom we so closely worked during the book's development. We especially acknowledge Natalie Chapman and Betsy Thorpe for their editorial suggestions and insight. Nancy Cooperman was our original editor at Macmillan. It was because of her this union between our two organizations came about. We are forever grateful.

INTRODUCTION

On my 50th birthday last year, a lot of my old high school and college buddies called to rub it in. Their mostly snide comments ranged from "How's it feel to be over the hill?" to "Have you hit male menopause yet?" But after a few minutes of conversation with each one, I started hearing health and medical issues creep in. One friend told me about his prostate problem. Another said he was going for a stress test since he'd been having chest pains. I heard about hiatal hernias and depression.

What struck me as odd was how typically unmasculine we all were to be talking about these things. I know that when my father turned age 50 almost forty years ago, he and his male friends didn't have these conversations. Oh sure, they joked around about baldness and maybe a few other problems, but men just didn't include health in their man-to-man conversations.

Because of that precedent, it's been a general misconception that men—both young and old—do not care about their health. However, while that was probably the case years ago, it's obviously much different today. And there are plenty of good reasons why.

First is the general aging of the population. Today, there are more men over the age of 40 than ever before in history. In fact, there are more men in every decade of life past 40 than ever before. On a percentage basis, the number of elderly men, aged 70 years and older, is increasing at a faster rate than that of any other male population segment.

With aging come health problems. Men are living longer than ever and are experiencing more diseases, illnesses, and injuries as a result. Therefore, their interactions with the health-care system have increased. This results in a heightened awareness and interest in one's own health and health-related information.

Men are also having to deal with many more medical issues than they once did. From AIDS to stress, conditions that were once either nonexistent or relatively minor in scope have become significant problems today. And while we have seen great breakthroughs in the treatment of heart disease and cancer, for example, we still see the incidence of these conditions increasing.

Technology has also had an impact. It was not too long ago that many conditions had few treatment options. That's not true today. A person with heart disease, for example, may be treated with medication or a variety of surgeries or both. Gallbladder disease has at least five viable treatment options. As we get more medically and technologically sophisticated, the higher the likelihood that a man will encounter the health-care system.

Add all the new medical tests to the mix. These wonders of modern medicine are able to detect problems that even ten years ago were hard to find. For example, the relatively new and controversial PSA (prostate-specific antigen) test, a blood test used to detect the possible presence of prostate cancer, has galvanized men's health care. The American Cancer Society says every man over 50 should be tested annually. It cites government figures that show prostate cancer deaths have dropped dramatically in the five years after the test went into wide use. On the other hand, the American College of Physicians issued guidelines in March of 1997 that did not recommend regular testing for men over the age of 50. They cited studies showing the uncertainties in the test's reliability. They also felt too many prostate glands were being removed unnecessarily with little benefit and many possible complications. And PSA testing is only the tip of the new, and ever growing, early medical screening of men.

And let's not forget the fitness "craze" that began in the 1980s. Men of all ages are participating in more exercise and fitness programs than ever. And they probably should, considering the startling fact that 59 percent of America's men are overweight, according to the National Center for Health Statistics.

The changing health-care delivery system has done a lot to alter the American male. Clearly, it's helped to put more men in touch with their health. Many corporations are as much interested in preventing illness and disease in their employees as they are in providing benefits for sickness. As a result, the number of annual physical examinations has increased, as has overall medical testing. Ironically, the emphasis that health maintenance organizations and other managed-care entities are placing on early detection and prevention has brought men into the health-care system at a much earlier age than in previous years.

Consequently, in just the last decade, the overall issue of men's health has moved from the back burner to the front. There are now magazines exclusively devoted to men's health issues. There are television specials concentrating on medical problems exclusive to men. But there is still a knowledge gap. Men want to know more about their health and the medical conditions that effect them.

And that's why we have written this book. As the nation's largest nonprofit consumer health advocacy organization, we hear from thousands of men every year. And if there is one resounding theme in those messages, it's give us more information about our health, our conditions, our options, and our medical rights. And that's what we have done here.

What makes this book unique and useful is it's consumer-empowering directness. This is a serious book for men of all ages who are serious about their health. No "10 Minutes to a More Muscular You" or "20 Ways to Increase Your Sexual Attraction" in these pages.

From AIDS to physical fitness, sexual dysfunction to hair loss, this book takes the health and medical subjects important to all men and presents them in a straightforward, easy-to-understand way. Our information and data come directly from medical studies and reports. Our sources are the best medical research has to offer. We give you the good news and the bad news, but most important, we give you all the news.

This is a book men told us they wanted. And we know it's a book every man needs. We are proud to have created it, and we hope that you will find it helpful and healthful.

Charles B. Inlander
President, People's Medical Society

The Systems of the Body

The body of a man is a truly complex piece of machinery, an unduplicated collection of organs and tissues that allows you to do everything from running a marathon to dreaming. Understanding how the body functions is a challenge—after all, not even science is sure of how some aspects of it work. But a good way to learn more about what's going on inside of you is to look at the systems that comprise the body. These are the systems, working together, that keep the body functioning, and you running and dreaming.

The following section breaks down the male body into ten systems (circulatory system, digestive system, immune system, lymphatic system, endocrine system, muscular system, nervous system, reproductive system, skeletal system, and urinary system) and explains their parts, how they work, and how they are interrelated. Each section mentions related conditions as well.

An understanding of the body is one of the most fundamental aspects of personal health. If you know how and why your body works, you'll have the knowledge you need to take better care of yourself. And you'll be more in charge of your own health care.

So if you're new to anatomy, this is the place to start. Even if you know your leukocytes from your macrophages and your duodenum from your ileum, you may want to browse through this section as a refresher. This section provides valuable background information that may be useful as you read about specific conditions and treatments elsewhere in this book.

CIRCULATORY SYSTEM

The circulatory system, or cardiovascular system, is responsible for nourishing all tissues of the body and removing wastes from those same tissues. The male circulatory system is comprised mainly of the blood (about five quarts), the blood vessels (sixty thousand miles of them) and the

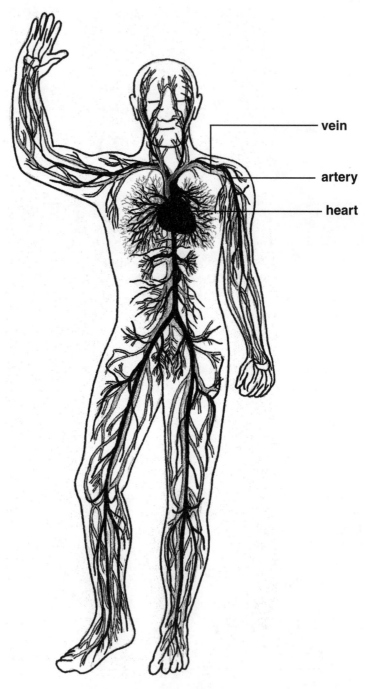

vein

artery

heart

Circulatory System

heart (which weighs on the average $10^1/_2$ ounces, about 2 ounces more than the average woman's heart). The heart, a hollow muscle, pumps the blood through the network of blood vessels. While on its trip through the body, the blood carries nutrients and oxygen to the cells it passes and collects waste.

NEED A DOCTOR?

There are several specialists who handle problems with the circulatory system. A cardiologist handles heart disease, and a thoracic surgeon performs operations on the heart, major vessels, and the lungs. A hematologist diagnoses and treats diseases of the blood and blood-forming parts of the body.

Blood consists of red blood cells, white blood cells (or leukocytes, which include granulocytes, lymphocytes, and monocytes), and platelets (the blood's clotting agents). Forty percent of blood volume is red blood cells (about thirty-five trillion red blood cells in an adult), and the white blood cells and platelets account for a total of 5 percent. The remainder of the blood is plasma, a liquid mostly comprised of water that supports cells as well as fats, proteins, and sugars found in the bloodstream. Most of the water you drink is absorbed by the blood to maintain the amount of blood in the system.

Red blood cells contain hemoglobin, a substance that helps to transport oxygen and release it when it is needed. White blood cells, as part of the immune system, protect the body from infection by destroying bacteria, viruses, and foreign bodies in the blood. Platelets collect at the site of an injury, where they become sticky and adhere to blood vessel walls to help stop bleeding. Platelets then stimulate the production of filaments that trap red and white blood cells to close the wound. The hard outer covering of this seal is a scab.

Blood vessels consist of the arteries and veins that carry the blood throughout the body. Arteries carry highly oxygenated and nutrient-rich blood away from the heart, while veins carry the deoxygenated blood back to the heart.

The heart is responsible for pumping the blood through the blood vessels. The strongest muscle in the body, the heart of an adult is 5 inches long, $3^1/_2$ inches wide, $2^1/_2$ inches thick, and it is cone-shaped. Men generally have larger hearts than women because men's bodies are usually larger (for this reason, a woman's heart must beat faster for her to reach the same level of exertion as a man). The heart is divided into a left and right side, and each side has two chambers, the atrium and the ventricle. The four chambers are separated by valves, tough flaps of tissue that act as gates to regulate blood flow through the heart. While the heart itself is fragile, it is well protected inside a sac called the pericardium, which is sheltered by the lungs and the rib cage in the front, the diaphragm muscle underneath and the spine behind.

How Does It Work?

Oxygenated, nutrient-rich blood begins its trip through the body in the left ventricle. When the ventricle contracts (an action that takes .3 seconds), the blood is pushed out of the heart through the aortic valve. It first flows through the aorta, the largest artery in the body, and is propelled through progressively smaller arteries until it reaches the capillaries, the smallest blood vessels in the body—so small, in fact, that the blood cells squeeze through in single file. Capillaries link the arteries to the veins.

While in the capillaries, oxygen and nutrients such as vitamins and minerals, fats, hormones, and amino acids are "unloaded" from the blood into the adjoining cells. At the same time, the blood collects any waste products such as carbon dioxide from the cells. Once the exchange is completed, the blood continues through the veins. Some may travel through the kidneys, where wastes are filtered out, or to the intestines, where the blood will pick up nutrients from food.

The blood returns to the heart, collecting in the right atrium. When the tricuspid valve opens, the blood flows through to the right ventricle before passing through the pulmonary valve into the lungs. Here, blood releases the carbon dioxide it has gathered as waste (which is exhaled) and takes in fresh oxygen (which has been inhaled). Once replenished, the blood flows back into the left atrium and is held there by the mitral valve. When the mitral valve opens, the blood flows back to the left ventricle where it begins its journey all over again.

It takes only thirty seconds for a drop of blood to complete a circuit of the body. The heart works hard, beating an average of seventy-two times a minute and pumping six quarts of blood every minute—meaning that a total of eight thousand quarts of blood are pumped a day. Yet that blood does not directly nourish the heart; it receives its nourishment from a subsystem of arteries known as the coronary arteries—so named for

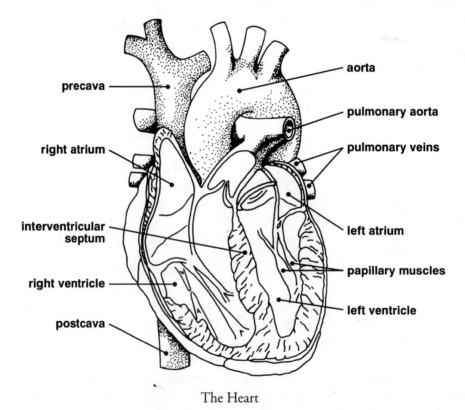

The Heart

their appearance as a thorny crown around the heart. If any of these arteries are damaged or obstructed, a condition called coronary heart disease, the heart muscle can starve.

The heart contracts and beats in response to stimulation from the sinoatrial (S-A) node, a tiny, natural pacemaker located in the wall of the right atrium. The impulse is conducted to the atrio-ventricular (A-V) node to the muscles of the ventricles, which contract. The process, which takes less than a second, produces the contraction called a heartbeat. The heart is stimulated consistently and rhythmically, and it can even adjust itself to alter the force of the contraction if needed. Even after being disconnected from all other nerves in the body, the human heart will continue to beat seventy to eighty times a minute. The "lub-dub" of the heart heard through a stethoscope is actually the sound of the valves opening and closing. The mitral and tricuspid valves opening in unison create the "lub" sound, while the pulmonary and aortic valves cause the "dub" sound.

The heartbeat has two parts. The diastole is the point in the heartbeat when the heart is at rest, and the systole is the point when the heart is contracting. The two numbers in blood pressure readings correspond to these heartbeat phases. The systolic (the top number in the blood pressure fraction) is a measurement of the blood's pressure during the contraction; the diastolic is a measurement of pressure during the heart's relaxation period. In a normal, healthy blood pressure reading of 120/80 mm Hg, read "120 over 80," the systolic pressure is indicated by the 120, the diastolic by the 80. Blood pressure readings of more than 140/90 mm Hg indicate a condition called hypertension, or high blood pressure.

THE PULSE

You can measure the number of times your heart beats a minute by taking your pulse. Place your first and second fingers of your right hand on the inside of your left wrist, below the palm, and press gently to feel the pulse. Count the beats for twenty seconds, then multiply by three to get your heart rate per minute. Compare your heart rate to the levels listed below to find your level of fitness.

50 or less	Excellent
51 to 65	Good
66 to 79	Fair
More than 80	Poor

THE LUNGS

The lungs are two organs composed of spongy tissue that sit within the rib cage. They are sometimes considered part of the cardiovascular system (also called the cardiopulmonary system) because of their role in oxygenating the blood, though they are also categorized as the respiratory system.

About a pint of air is inhaled with each breath. The air is drawn into the body with the help of a muscle called the diaphragm, which lies beneath the lungs. The air travels through the mouth and throat and into the windpipe. It continues into the two lungs through two tubes called bronchi, which branch out into smaller and smaller air passageways.

Once in the lungs, the air fills tiny air sacs known as alveoli, which are surrounded by capillaries. The oxygen in the air passes through the membrane of the air sacs into the blood in the capillaries, and the carbon dioxide waste in the bloodstream passes into the air sacs. After this exchange takes place, the diaphragm forces the air—along with the carbon dioxide—out of the lungs in an exhale.

Major Problems and Common Disorders of the Circulatory System

Blood

Anemia is a condition where the blood is deficient in red blood cells, in hemoglobin, or in total volume. Agranulocytosis, a drop in white-cell count, can be fatal if the person is not treated with antibiotics to prevent infection. Hemochromatosis is an inherited condition in which too much iron is present in the blood. Hemophilia is an inherited bleeding disorder that occurs almost exclusively in men, caused by the lack of a protein, called factor VIII, that is essential to blood clotting. Leukemia is a cancer of blood-forming organs characterized by the replacement of bone marrow with immature white blood cells and the presence of abnormal numbers and forms of immature white cells in circulation.

Blood Vessels

An aneurysm is a weak spot in an arterial wall that can be life-threatening if it causes a major artery to burst. Blood rushes out of the artery and causes blood pressure to drop quickly, resulting in death. Aneurysms may be congenital— present at birth—or they may develop as a result of arteriosclerosis.

Arteriosclerosis, also called hardening of the arteries, results when calcium deposits collect on the arterial walls and reduce the artery's elasticity. This rigidity may eventually lead to the development of an aneurysm. Atherosclerosis is the build-up of fatty deposits on the artery walls that can lead to reduced blood flow to organs and other tissue. As the deposits enlarge, they have a tendency to invade the deeper layers of the arterial wall, causing scarring. Fatty deposits may also break loose and circulate through the system, eventually clogging other arteries and causing gangrene, heart attack, or stroke.

Stroke, or cerebrovascular accident, occurs when the blood flow to the brain is disrupted, either by a blockage or a break in an artery. The incidence of stroke is about 19 percent higher for men than for women. Risk factors for stroke include high blood pressure, obesity, hardening of the arteries, diabetes, smoking, and stress.

Gangrene is a condition caused by poor circulation to any tissue, especially the extremities such as feet and hands. Normal blood flow is restricted, usually as the result of a blockage, preventing oxygen and nutrients from reaching tissue, which begins to die.

Hypertension, or high blood pressure, is a condition in which the heart is pumping blood through the circulatory system with a force greater than needed for normal blood flow. Untreated, high blood pressure can have serious negative consequences on the entire circulatory system. Men are at greater risk for hypertension than women until age 55; from age 55 to 74, the risks are equal, after which the woman's risk becomes greater.

Phlebitis is an inflammation of a vein, usually as a result of a varicose vein. Sometimes this condition can lead to the formation of clots, which may become detached and travel to another part of the circulatory system and possibly cause a blockage or death.

Varicose veins occur when valves in the blood vessels are defective or become damaged, and too much blood stays too long in one place. Veins may knot and swell four to five times their normal size. Most varicose veins develop in the legs, where blood must flow against gravity. Occasionally these fragile veins may burst and bleed. Varicose veins can be inherited, but people are also susceptible to them if they must stand for hours during the day or are obese. Women are more susceptible to varicose veins than men.

Heart

Angina pectoris is severe, suffocating chest pain caused by an insufficient blood supply to the heart muscle. This condition is often a precursor to heart attack.

Cardiomyopathy is any disease that severely affects the functioning of the heart muscle. Cardiopathy may be congenital or linked to nutritional deficiencies or alcohol consumption, or it may occur as a result of changes in the thickness of the heart wall, caused by scarring or abnormal cell changes.

Congestive heart failure is the inability of the heart to maintain adequate blood flow to the rest of the body. More specifically, it has to do with a heart muscle failure, especially defects of the valves, and affects the right or left ventricle. Water and sodium are inadequately eliminated, remain in the body, and can cause fluid overload, leading in many cases to death from total heart failure.

Constrictive pericarditis is a condition in which the pericardium becomes scarred and hard and full of calcium deposits. The movement of the heart is limited, interfering with its function. Pericarditis is an inflammation of the pericardium, leading in many cases to chest pain and fever.

Endocarditis is an inflammation of the internal lining of the heart, particularly the valves, caused by an infection.

Myocardial infarction, also called heart attack, is the damage or death of an area of the heart muscle resulting from a reduced blood supply to that area. Heart attack is the single largest killer of men in the United States.

Heart Valves

The heart valves are generally susceptible to three types of conditions: stenosis, prolapse, and regurgitation. Stenosis is a narrowing of the opening of the valve, reducing the flow of blood; prolapse occurs when the valve begins to lose its shape and sags, causing an extra clicking sound or murmur; and regurgitation occurs when a valve fails to close tightly enough and blood flows backward.

DIGESTIVE SYSTEM

The digestive system is a tubelike system that converts the three main constituents of food—carbohydrates, proteins, and fats—into substances that are used to fuel the body. From top to bottom, it is comprised of the mouth, the tongue, the teeth, the salivary glands, the esophagus, the stomach, the small and large intestines, the rectum, and the anus.

NEED A DOCTOR?

Specialists who handle problems with the digestive system include gastroenterologists, who diagnose and treat problems of the stomach and intestines. In addition, a proctologist deals with diseases of the anus, rectum, and colon.

The mouth contains the teeth, which crush and grind food, and the tongue, the muscular organ that moves food around in the mouth. The tongue is coated with tiny taste buds that allow us to taste food. The mouth also houses the salivary glands, which produce saliva, a liquid that contains enzymes that help break down the sugars in food.

The esophagus is a muscular tube about 10 inches long that contracts to move swallowed food from the throat to the stomach. The stomach is a saclike organ lined with muscle and glandular tissue that secretes digestive juices, including pepsin (an enzyme), hydrochloric acid, and other enzymes that help break down food. The average stomach can hold about 3 pints.

The small intestine is a tubelike organ about 22 feet long and $1^1/_2$ inches in diameter. The first part of the small intestine, called the duodenum, contains ducts from the gallbladder and the pancreas to receive secretions from these organs. The purpose of the small intestine is to break down foods and absorb nutrients. The large intestine is usually 6 feet long and 2 inches in diameter. It absorbs any remaining nutrients as well as any water that still remains in the digested material.

The rectum and anus make up the end of the digestive system. The rectum is a short tube in which solid waste is stored. When the rectum becomes full, the solid waste passes out of the body through the anus.

How Does It Work?

First, food is taken into the mouth, where the tongue tastes and maneuvers it so that the teeth can chew it up. In the mouth, the food is mixed with saliva, which is produced by salivary glands located at the sides of the face, below each ear. Saliva contains enzymes that help break down the sugars in the food, beginning the digestive process.

From the mouth, the food is swallowed and passed into the esophagus, which contracts with a wavelike motion to push the food to the stomach. These contractions are known as peristalsis. The stomach churns the food with rhythmic contractions and begins digestion of food with the acids it produces, turning the food into

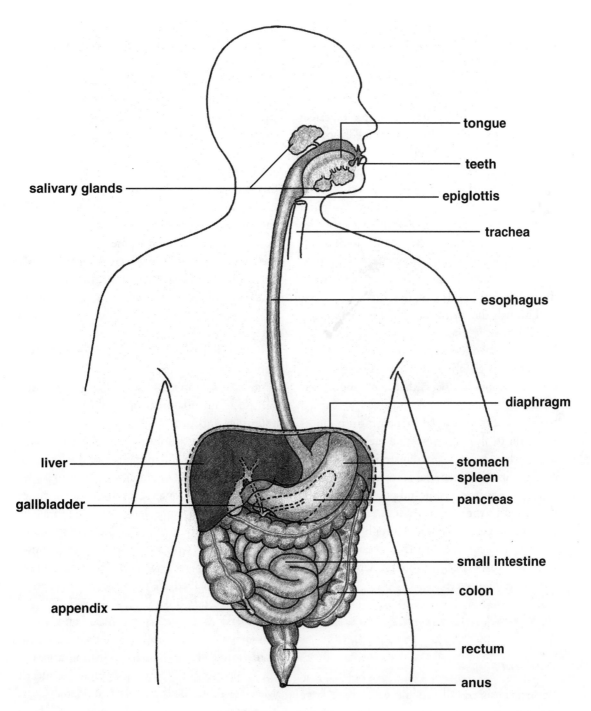

tongue

teeth

epiglottis

trachea

esophagus

salivary glands

diaphragm

liver

stomach
spleen

gallbladder

pancreas

small intestine

colon

appendix

rectum

anus

Digestive System

a thick liquid. It takes about two hours for food to pass through the stomach.

From the stomach, food enters the first 10 inches of the small intestine, called the duodenum, where digestive fluids further break down the food. Bile, a yellowish-green digestive fluid produced in the liver, is released into the duodenum by the gallbladder. The pancreas also releases enzymes into the duodenum for digestion. It is in this part of the intestine that proteins are broken down into their original building blocks, amino acids (which are used by cells to grow, heal, and fight off infection); starch and complex sugars are converted into simple sugars (used for energy); and fats are broken down into fatty acids and glycerin.

Through the next 21 feet of the small intestine (the middle section is known as the jejunum, and the final segment is known as the ileum), nutrients are absorbed through the thin lining into the blood, a process that takes about four hours. Once in the blood, nutrients are carried to the rest of the body. Any remaining substances move on to the large intestine (about 5$^{1}/_{2}$ feet long), where more digested material is absorbed. Any undigestible material is stored in the large intestine as waste: The liquid portion passes via the blood to the urinary system, and the solid portion is later eliminated through the rectum and anus. The entire digestive process typically takes five to twenty-four hours, depending on what is being digested.

Major Problems and Common Disorders of the Digestive System

Diverticulosis and diverticulitis affect the large intestine (colon) and are characterized by the formation of small pouches (called diverticula) at weak spots on the intestine wall. The condition is known as diverticulosis when the diverticula are merely present, and as diverticulitis when the diverticula become inflamed or infected. These conditions generally affect people over the age of 60; however, they have been diagnosed in people as young as age 40.

Gallstones form in the gallbladder when the liver manufactures too much cholesterol. The excess cholesterol begins to form tiny round or oval lumps of solid matter, usually less than an inch in length. Gallstones are two to three times more likely to occur in women than men, and the risk for a man greatly increases after age 65. Many people are unaware that they have gallstones until a stone becomes lodged in the bile duct, which connects the gallbladder to the small intestine.

Inflammatory bowel disease (IBD) is a general term used to describe the chronic conditions of Crohn's disease and colitis. Crohn's disease is an inflammation of the walls of the intestines and occasionally may extend to the anus, esophagus, mouth, and stomach. Colitis causes ulcers and inflammation of the lining of the large intestine, or colon.

Ulcers are raw, open sores that occur in either the lining of the stomach or the duodenum (the upper part of the small intestine). Most people associate ulcers with a high-stress lifestyle; however, many experts now believe that the cause is a bacterium called *Helicobacter pylori*. There is also a hereditary link.

Ulcers occur when stomach acid and pepsin (an enzyme) break through the protective mucous lining of the stomach (creating a gastric ulcer) or intestine (creating a duodenal ulcer). Men are more likely to suffer duodenal ulcers than women, while women are more likely to have gastric ulcers.

Constipation is the inability to move the bowels and pass stool or the infrequent passage of stool. A leading cause of constipation is a lack of sufficient fiber in the diet. Diarrhea is just the opposite of constipation and is characterized by frequent bowel movements. The probable cause of diarrhea is food or water that contains an organism (generally bacteria) that upsets the delicate balance of the large intestine. When this occurs, the normal process of passing food through the intestines is disrupted and the food passes too quickly.

Heartburn, a burning sensation in the chest, is caused by acid that moves up the esophagus from the stomach. When the acid comes into contact with the sensitive lining of the esophagus, burning—often along with excruciating pain—is felt. The pain is often mistaken for a heart attack. It often occurs after a meal of fried or fatty foods. Also contributing to heartburn are citrus fruits and juices, tomato products, chocolate, coffee, and other acidic foods.

Hiatal hernias occur where the esophagus enters the abdomen through an opening in the diaphragm (the sheet of muscles that separates the chest from the abdomen) called the hiatus. An upper portion of the stomach moves into the chest cavity through a weakness in the diaphragm. These hernias occur when pressure in the abdominal cavity increases as a result of physical exertion, coughing, or vomiting.

Other types of hernia include femoral hernia, in which intestine passes into the thigh area, and inguinal hernia, in which the intestine passes into the scrotum. Only 1 to 5 percent of femoral hernias occur in men. At least 2 percent of all men suffer inguinal hernia.

Irritable bowel syndrome (IBS), not to be confused with irritable bowel disease, or IBD, is characterized by alternate bouts of constipation and diarrhea, abdominal pain, gas, and bloating. The exact cause of these symptoms is unknown; however, it has been linked to some disturbance of the wavelike motion of the intestines. Stress is thought to contribute to this common condition.

Hemorrhoids are varicose veins located in the anus. They are caused by pressure in the anal area, usually as a result of straining during bowel movements. It is not unusual for most people over the age of 50 to have experienced hemorrhoidal problems.

ENDOCRINE SYSTEM

The male endocrine system is made up of several glands that produce hormones. These glands include the pituitary gland, pineal gland, thyroid gland, parathyroid gland, the adrenal glands, the pancreas, and the testicles. (The ovaries are the female equivalent of the testicles.) The system regulates the body's growth and sexual development and contributes to other functions through the secretion of hormones, chemicals that affect tissues. Unlike other glands that secrete substances into ducts (for example, the salivary glands), endocrine glands secrete hormones directly into the bloodstream.

NEED A DOCTOR?

An endocrinologist specializes in the diagnosis and treatment of disorders of the endocrine glands. This includes treatment of problems with the pituitary, thyroid, and parathyroid glands, located in the head and neck, as well as the testicles, thymus, and the islands of Langerhans located in the pancreas. Endocrinologists are involved in the treatment of diabetes and obesity.

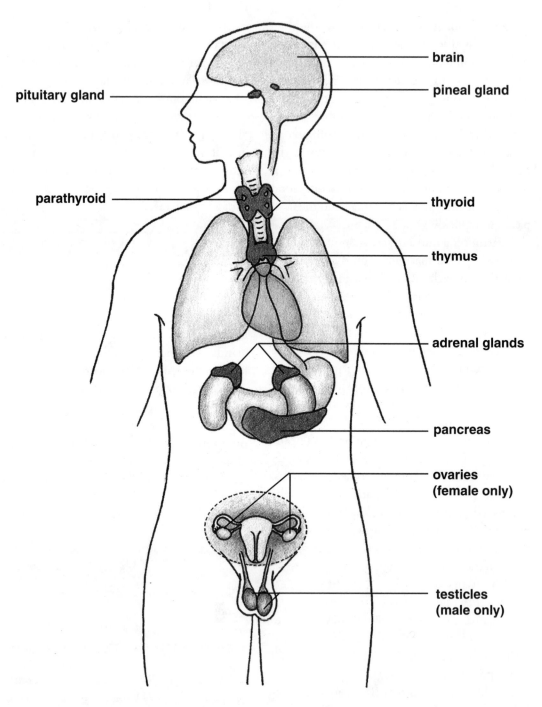

brain

pineal gland

pituitary gland

parathyroid

thyroid

thymus

adrenal glands

pancreas

ovaries
(female only)

testicles
(male only)

Male/Female Endocrine System

How Does It Work?

The endocrine system is controlled by an area of the brain called the hypothalamus. This part of the brain stimulates the adjacent pituitary gland, which in turn produces hormones that regulate the other glands in the endocrine system. The hormones secreted by the pituitary are known as trophic, or stimulating, hormones. Also located in the head is the pineal gland, a small gland that regulates the body's cycles such as the sleep/wake cycle.

The thyroid gland is located in the neck. It produces hydrocortisone, aldosterone, and androgen. These hormones regulate bone growth, metabolism, and the production of body heat. The parathyroid gland, two small glands located on either side of the thyroid gland in the neck, produces thyroxine, triiodothyronine, and calcitonin, which regulate the levels of calcium in the blood.

The adrenal glands are located on top of the kidneys. The outer region of the glands, called the adrenal cortex, produces androgens, which are sex hormones. The inner part of the gland, called the adrenal medulla, produces epinephrine and norepinephrine, hormones that speed up metabolism and respiration in response to stress.

The pancreas is located in the abdominal region below and behind the stomach. This gland secretes insulin and glucagon, hormones that control the breakdown of sugar in the blood.

The testicles, or testes, produce testosterone. This male hormone plays one of the biggest roles in the functioning of the man's reproductive system, prompting sperm production and the development of male sex characteristics such as pubic hair, a deep voice, and muscle growth. Testosterone also regulates the sex drive.

THE ROLE OF TESTOSTERONE

Testosterone is a form of the hormone androgen that is produced in the testicles. In the womb, testosterone is responsible for the development of male characteristics in a fetus genetically determined to be male. Then, at puberty, testosterone production increases in order to stimulate the development of the male sexual characteristics.

Testosterone is the hormone that is responsible for deepening of the voice, muscle growth and the growth of facial and pubic hair during puberty. It also triggers the growth of long bones—the bones in the arms and the legs—during puberty and halts their growth later. The hormone may cause the skin to produce excess oils, often the cause of acne in teenage boys. Testosterone stimulates sperm production and the sex drive, helps protect the heart by raising levels of the good HDL cholesterol, and possibly increases bone density. Testosterone is also the hormone responsible for the shrinkage of hair follicles, which leads to hair loss. Without testosterone, there would be no male pattern baldness.

The production of testosterone slows with age. By age 40, some 7 percent of men experience a drop in testosterone levels. By the age of 60, that estimate reaches 20 percent. While lower testosterone levels will not hinder the ability to have an erection, they can result in a lower sex drive.

Major Problems and Disorders of the Endocrine System

In hyperthyroidism, the thyroid gland produces an excess of the hormone thyroxine. It affects about 1 percent of the adult population and is most common in young to middle-aged women, though it does occur in men. Symptoms include weight loss, increased appetite, perspiration, and sensitivity to heat. Advanced cases may include swollen glands, hyperactivity, anxiety, and muscle degeneration.

Hyperthyroidism is often caused by Graves' disease, in which the body produces antibodies that stimulate the production of thyroxine. A symptom of Graves' disease is bulging eyes, caused by swelling of tissue behind the eyes.

Hypothyroidism occurs when not enough thyroxine is produced by the thyroid gland. Symptoms include fatigue, muscle weakness, cramps, hair loss, depression, and high cholesterol. It is usually caused by a disorder in which the body develops antibodies against its own thyroid gland, and it affects about 1 percent of the population. It is most common in elderly women, although men of all ages may get it.

Hyperparathyroidism is caused by the overproduction of hormones by the parathyroid glands. This results in thinning of the bones and stones in the urinary tract. Hypoparathyroidism is caused by underproduction of parathyroid hormones. It is rare, and symptoms include cramps, spasms, and seizures.

Diabetes, a condition in which the body cannot regulate its blood sugar levels, results when the pancreas does not produce enough of the hormone insulin or when the insulin produced malfunctions. Symptoms of diabetes include excessive hunger, thirst, and urination. About 45 percent of the sixteen million Americans with diabetes are men.

Addison's disease is a rare condition that occurs when the adrenal gland does not produce enough of the steroid hormones. Symptoms include weakness, low blood pressure, and spotty skin. Cushing's syndrome occurs when excessive amounts of steroid hormones are produced. Cushing's syndrome results in a characteristic appearance: the face becomes round and red, the upper body becomes obese with a humped upper back, and the limbs begin to waste away.

An underproduction in hormones from the testicles results in hypergonadism. Symptoms include decreased amounts of body hair, smooth skin, a high-pitched voice, underdeveloped genitalia, and a reduced sex drive. Overproduction of these hormones, hypogonadism, can cause early sexual development.

IMMUNE SYSTEM

The immune system protects against disease and illness by destroying any sort of invaders, including bacteria, viruses, toxins, foreign tissues, and germs. These invaders (those that cause disease are pathogens, while those that cause an immune response are antigens) can infect the body and cause sickness if they're allowed to spread. The properly functioning immune system has the ability to recognize and attack any foreign substances. It does this by stimulating the production of antibodies—proteins that bind to antigens to neutralize them and eliminate them from the body. The immune system can also attack invaders directly, using a special type of white blood cell.

NEED A DOCTOR?

The specialists who treat disorders of the immune system include the immunologist and the allergist. Immunologists specialize in the study and treatment of a wide range of disorders dealing with the immune system. Such disorders include allergies, infections, and life-threatening conditions such as AIDS (acquired immune deficiency syndrome). Allergists are involved only in the diagnosis and treatment of allergies and often subspecialize in a particular allergy. Allergists also treat asthma cases and skin problems such as hives and rashes.

The skin, the mucous membranes of the nose and mouth, and the stomach also act as parts of the immune system. The skin protects the body by preventing the entrance of most foreign invaders and organisms. Those organisms that are inhaled are often stopped by the mucous membranes of the nose, mouth, and throat, which are designed to filter out any foreign particles. Finally, the strong acids present in the stomach destroy any organisms that may be swallowed.

How Does It Work?

From birth, infants have some inborn protection against certain diseases; in addition, breast-feeding is thought to pass some of the mother's immunities on to the child. But immunity, for the most part, comes through adaptation. With adaptive immunity, the body comes in contact with an antigen that it cannot immediately overcome, and sickness occurs. However, once the illness has ended, the immune system "remembers" how to fight that organism—the next time that antigen appears, the immune system can immediately destroy it. This is the reason that some conditions such as chicken pox or the measles usually occur only once.

There are two types of immunity: humoral immunity and cellular immunity. In humoral immunity, a type of white blood cell called the B-lymphocyte produces antibodies that bind to invading organisms or substances to eliminate them. In cellular immunity, a type of white blood cell called a T-lymphocyte attacks the foreign cells directly. T-lymphocytes are either helper cells or killer cells; the helper cells identify invaders, while the killer cells destroy them. Both T and B cells utilize various accessory cells to destroy antigens. Macrophages in particular are used; these cells engulf antigens and present them to the T and B cells for recognition and disposal.

Humoral immunity is an important defense against bacteria, while cellular immunity is effective against viruses, parasites within the blood, and, possibly, cancer cells.

At times, the immune system responds to antigens that are not harmful such as foods, dust, and fur, in what is known as an allergic reaction. The antigens trigger the production of disease-fighting chemicals called histamines to eliminate the substances. Histamines can cause swelling of the respiratory tract, sneezing, watery eyes, and itchy skin.

There are also times when the immune system can turn against the body's own tissues. These diseases, known as autoimmune disorders, include lupus (much more prevalent in women than in men) and rheumatoid arthritis.

Roles of Lymphatic Tissue and Organs

The functioning of the immune system relies upon the lymphatic system, the system that produces, stores, and transports the lymphocytes.

The central organs of the lymphatic system—the bone marrow and the thymus gland—are responsible for production and development of the T- and B-lymphocytes. These cells develop from lymphatic stem cells in the bone marrow. The T cells first migrate to the thymus gland in order to be processed into mature T cells. The B cells are processed either in the bone marrow or in other lymphatic tissues.

After the lymphocytes reach maturity, they reside in lymphoid tissues, which include the lymph nodes, the spleen, the gastrointestinal tract, and other mucosa-associated lymphoid tissue (MALT). Lymphoid tissue is located close to areas that are particularly susceptible to infection, making it easier to intercept invading antigens. Both T and B cells remain in separate areas of the lymphoid tissue where they respond to antigens.

For more information on the disease-fighting abilities of the body, see Lymphatic System (below).

LYMPHATIC SYSTEM

The lymphatic system is a system of glands, tissues, and vessels that plays a vital role in defending the body against invading pathogens and other dangerous organisms. A partner of the immune system, the lymphatic system is involved in producing lymph and lymphocytes and includes the lymph vessels, lymph nodes, bone marrow, thymus, spleen, and tonsils. Lymph glands are one of the body's front line defenses in fighting disease.

NEED A DOCTOR?

The specialist that handles diseases of the lymphatic system is the immunologist. These practitioners handle a wide range of conditions and diseases relating to the immune and lymphatic systems.

How Does It Work?

Lymphocytes are white blood cells important to the immune system's job of fighting off infection. These cells are produced in the organs of the lymphatic system: the bone marrow (soft tissue located inside bone), the spleen (a small organ located in the upper left abdomen, behind the stomach), and the thymus gland (a butterfly-shaped gland located at the base of the neck).

Lymphocytes are circulated through the body in lymph, a yellowish fluid that contains lymphocytes and fats as well as other nutrients. Lymph is carried through the bloodstream and is released to the cells through the thin walls of the capillaries (the body's smallest blood vessels). The lymph bathes the tissues of the body, supplying them with oxygen and nutrients and picking up wastes and foreign particles that are present. Lymph also absorbs fats from the intestine, which is why lymph appears milky.

While some of the lymph returns to the bloodstream after bathing the tissues, the remainder—along with cells and foreign bodies such as bacteria—trickles gradually into small channels. These channels empty into larger ones known as lymphatics or lymphatic vessels. These vessels are independent of the circulatory system, and the lymph that flows through them is not pumped. Instead, it is drawn slowly through the vessels by internal pressure and exertion from

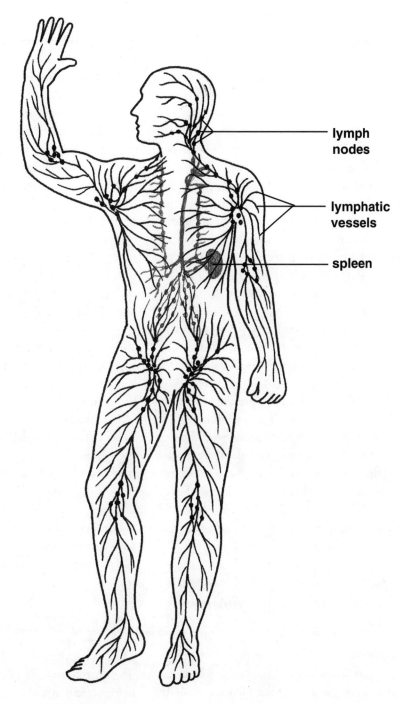

lymph nodes

lymphatic vessels

spleen

Lymphatic (Immune) System (with Spleen)

the body tissues; one-way valves keep it from flowing in the wrong direction.

Through the vessels, the lymph flows to lymph nodes, where any foreign bodies or organisms are filtered out. Lymph nodes, spongelike masses of tissue ranging from the size of a pinhead to the size of a penny, contain lymphocytes and macrophages—immune system cells that destroy any antigens. Lymph tissue also produces antibodies to destroy antigens. For example, the tonsils (located in the back of the throat) are lymph nodes, catching bacteria and other organisms that are inhaled before they can enter the body. After it has passed through the lymph nodes, the clean lymph then makes its way back into the bloodstream.

Lymph nodes help prevent the spread of infection. If there are too many invaders to destroy quickly, lymphocytes and the bacteria or viruses collect in the lymph node, sometimes causing swelling. For this reason, swelling of lymph nodes can indicate the presence of an illness such as an infection or a common cold.

If lymph nodes are bombarded with a great deal of bacteria that enter the bloodstream directly, the spleen aids in the process of filtration. The spleen, a fist-sized organ under the lower portion of the rib cage, filters all of the blood in the body. The spleen and lymph nodes also aid in the production of lymphocytes.

Major Problems and Common Disorders of the Lymphatic System

Hodgkin's disease is a cancer that develops in the lymphatic system and may spread to other organs. It is more common in men than in women, but affects only 1 percent of the population. Symptoms of Hodgkin's disease are prolonged swelling of the lymph nodes, fever, itchy skin, night sweats, tiredness, and weight loss.

Non-Hodgkin's lymphomas is the name of a group of cancers that develop in the lymphatic system and may spread throughout the body. Some 56 percent of these cancers develop in men. Symptoms of non-Hodgkin's lymphomas are swelling of the lymph nodes, fever, itching skin, night sweats, tiredness, and weight loss.

Lymphedema is an abnormal accumulation of lymph in the tissues, causing swelling of an arm or leg. The lymph is unable to drain normally because the vessels are blocked, damaged, or removed. Vessels may become blocked by cancer cells that collect in the lymph system, or they may be damaged by radiation therapy given for cancer. Lymphedema that occurs without a cause affects twice as many women as men. Some early signs of lymphedema are puffiness of an arm or leg, gradual swelling, and a feeling of heaviness in the limb.

Lymphadenopathy, or swollen glands, occurs as a result of an accumulation of white blood cells in the lymph nodes. Swollen glands are very common and occur whenever the body's immune system is fighting off an invading organism or pathogen. Lymph glands are distributed throughout the body, but the ones most people are familiar with are in the neck, underarms, and groin.

For more information, see Immune System (p. 14).

MUSCULAR SYSTEM

Muscles, working with the bones and the joints, do more than just allow the body to stand upright and move around. Muscles are also responsible for a number of involuntary functions: for example, keeping the blood flowing, generating heat, and pushing air, food, and other substances through the systems of the body. Muscle tissue has four general properties: the ability to respond to stimuli, the ability to contract, the ability to extend and stretch, and the ability to return to its original shape. Some muscles are voluntary, meaning they can be consciously controlled, while others are involuntary, not under conscious control.

Men are typically stronger than women: Studies have found women to be 43 to 63 percent weaker in upper body strength and 25 to 30 percent weaker in lower body strength. However, when the strength of men and women is compared taking into account muscle mass, this difference in strength disappears, showing that muscle tissue and motor control are the same for both genders.

NEED A DOCTOR?

An orthopedist is a specialist whose domain includes the treatment and correction, usually surgically, of deformities and damage to the musculoskeletal system. An orthopedist handles bone, muscle, and ligament problems throughout the body.

A physical therapist—a practitioner that is not a doctor—handles the rehabilitation of muscle injuries.

The three types of muscle tissue are skeletal (muscle attached to bones), smooth (found in internal structures such as the walls of the stomach, intestines, and blood vessels), and cardiac (found in the walls of the heart). Muscle is also categorized according to where it is found in the body and according to what type of function it serves. For example, an extensor muscle opens a joint and a flexor muscle closes it. An adductor muscle brings a body part inward and an abductor pulls it outward. A constrictor or sphincter muscle controls a passage or opening in the body.

Sheets of fibrous tissue known as fascia surround the muscles and organs, connecting and holding muscles together. Fascia also stores water and fat, protects and insulates the body, lines the walls of the body, separates muscles into groups, and carries nerves and blood vessels.

How Does It Work?

Muscles are made up of muscle fibers, or muscle cells, which are arranged into bundles called fasciculi or fascicles. In order to contract, muscles need to receive nerve impulses, nutrients, and oxygen from the bloodstream and, on a cellular level, a chain reaction of chemicals, including calcium ions, potassium, and sodium.

A muscle contracts by first receiving impulses from motor neurons. Nerve cells, or neurons, carry the impulse through its fibers (called axons) and deliver it to the muscle cells. The impulse stimulates a chemical reaction in the muscle fibers, and the tiny units that comprise the fiber, called myofilaments, slide over each other until they are overlapping. As a result, the muscle becomes shorter, or contracts. When the nerve impulse is over, the chemical reaction ends and the muscle fibers slide back, causing the muscle to relax.

Muscle fibers cannot partially contract; if a partial contraction of a muscle is required, the nerves stimulate only the portion of muscle fibers within a muscle needed to complete that movement. An example of partial contraction is muscle tone, essential in maintaining posture. With any contraction, energy is released as heat, which helps the body maintain its internal temperature.

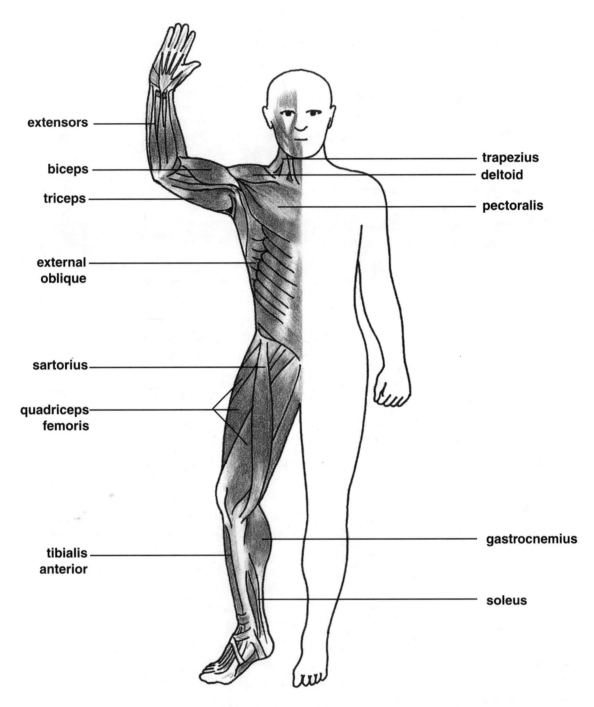

extensors —

biceps —

triceps —

external —
oblique

sartorius —

quadriceps —
femoris

tibialis —
anterior

— trapezius
— deltoid

— pectoralis

— gastrocnemius

— soleus

Muscular System (front view)

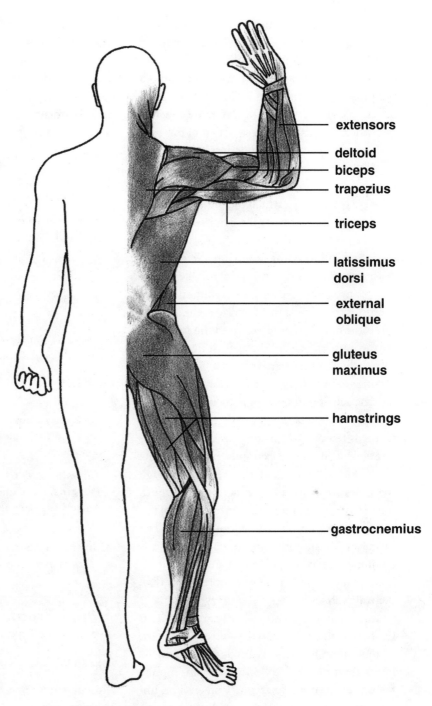

extensors

deltoid

biceps

trapezius

triceps

latissimus dorsi

external oblique

gluteus maximus

hamstrings

gastrocnemius

Muscular System (back view)

Different types of muscles work in different ways. Skeletal muscles number more than six hundred and comprise the bulk of the muscular system. These permit body movement through the process of contraction and relaxation. Skeletal muscles move voluntarily. They are attached by tendons (cords of connective tissue) to bones at a junction known as the periosteum.

When a skeletal muscle contracts, one bone moves toward another bone, which remains stationary. The point at which the tendon attaches to the stationary bone is the origin. The other point at which the tendon joins the non-stationary bone is the insertion. Within the muscular group, there are several muscles working to produce a desired movement: The agonist is the muscle that contracts, the antagonist is the muscle that relaxes, and the synergists are the muscles that aid the agonist in executing a smooth, clean movement.

Smooth muscle tissue comprises the walls of the stomach, intestines, uterus, blood vessels, and bladder. Smooth muscle tissue, or visceral tissue, is responsible for the movements of the internal organs—for example, peristalsis, the wave-like contractions that move food through the digestive system, is an action of smooth muscle. The widening and narrowing of blood vessels is also controlled by smooth muscle. The impulses for smooth muscle come from the autonomic nervous system and are involuntary. Smooth muscle fibers contract more slowly than skeletal muscles.

Cardiac muscle, also called heart muscle, is the muscle that makes up the walls of the heart. Cardiac muscle tissue is involuntary, and its fibers are stimulated collectively by an impulse from the autonomic nervous system. The impulse is conducted through the cells of the heart to contract the chambers of the heart alternately.

In fact, cardiac muscle tissue is divided into two sections: the muscle tissue comprising the atria, the upper chambers of the heart; and the muscle tissue comprising the ventricles, the lower chambers of the heart. Different from skeletal muscle tissue, cardiac muscle contracts in a rhythmic, rapid, and continuous fashion.

WELL-KNOWN MUSCLES

Biceps. Muscle on the front of upper arm that bends elbow.

Triceps. Muscle on the back of the upper arm that extends elbow.

Deltoid. Muscle of the shoulder that raises the arm.

Trapezius. Muscle on the upper back that brings shoulder backward and upward.

Obliques. Muscles that cover the abdominal area.

Quadriceps. Group of muscles on the front of the thigh that bends the thigh at the hips and straightens the knee.

Gluteus maximus. Muscle on the buttocks that extends the thigh in activities such as walking or climbing.

Gastrocnemius. Muscle on back of the calf that bends the knee in walking and extends foot in jumping.

Major Problems and Common Disorders of the Muscular System

Muscular dystrophy (MD) is the name for a group of inherited, progressive diseases that cause a weakness of muscle tissue and eventually death.

This condition strikes only males and is usually diagnosed before the age of five. Symptoms of MD are muscle weakness, lack of coordination in movement, and difficulty lifting the arms.

Though the exact cause of MD is unknown, it has been discovered that men with MD lack a protein essential to muscle function. As the disease progress, muscles are gradually replaced by fat tissue and a general body deformity is noted. Most people with MD become very susceptible to chest infections, especially pneumonia, which is responsible for many deaths associated with this disease. There is no known treatment for muscular dystrophy.

Myasthenia gravis is a rare disorder that affects the transmission of nerve impulses to the muscles. Symptoms include drooping eyelids, double vision, and problems eating, speaking, and swallowing. In some cases, mobility is affected because of a general weakness in the arms and legs. The exact cause of myasthenia gravis is unknown; however, it does appear as though some factor causes the immune system to turn against muscle tissue.

Myofascitis is inflammation of the muscles and the tissues that surround them (the fascia). It usually occurs as a result of putting strain on the muscles and connective tissue by strenuous exercise or overuse. The result is tenderness and pain around the muscle.

Tumors in muscle tissue are rare. They grow between the muscle and the layers of skin and are usually visible, appearing as a lump on the skin. Most muscle tumors are benign, or noncancerous; however, when one is malignant, or cancerous, it must be treated quickly.

A muscle pull occurs when too much of a strain is placed on a muscle and it is overstretched. Many "weekend athletes" suffer pulled muscles when they fail to adequately warm up prior to physical activity. Stretching properly can eliminate most muscle pulls. A more serious muscle pull occurs when the muscle fiber tears and internal bleeding occurs.

Sprains occur at joints where muscles, tendons, and bones meet. Because these three are interconnected, any trauma to one affects the others. A sprain is caused by an activity that causes the joint to move outside its normal range, such as when a joint is twisted or stretched.

Muscle spasms (also called cramps) are painful, involuntary contractions of muscles that occur for no apparent reason. Some cramps may be traced to over strenuous exercising or prolonged sitting or standing. Most cramps resolve themselves.

NERVOUS SYSTEM

The nervous system is responsible for receiving sensory stimuli such as lights, sounds, smells, textures, and tastes, generating and coordinating responses, and controlling bodily activities. The body is wired much like a giant electrical network, with messages being passed along the nerve cells, called neurons, through the spinal cord and finally to the brain.

The major components of the nervous system include the brain, spinal cord, nerve cells, and ganglia (concentrated masses of interconnected nerve cells). The nervous system is divided into the central nervous system (brain and spinal cord) and peripheral nervous system (nerves extending from the brain and spinal cord to other parts of the body). The central nervous system is protected by the skull and spinal vertebrae in addition to layers of membranes known as meninges.

The brain is the center of the nervous system and is responsible for processing the information received from the body. It weighs about three

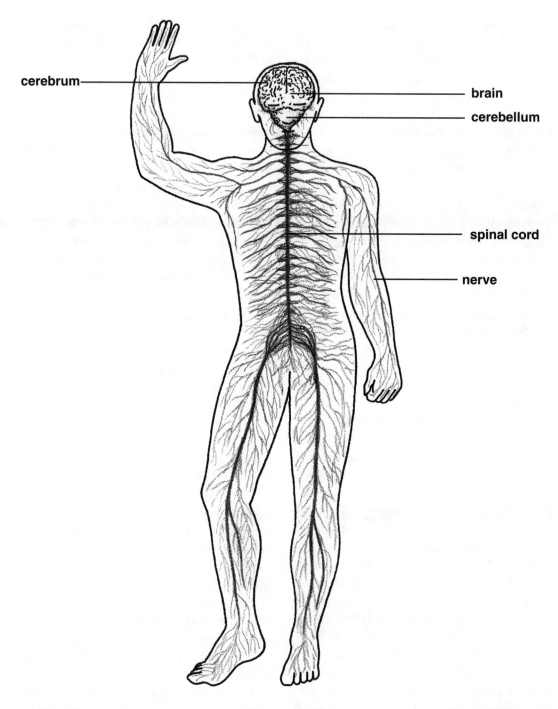

cerebrum

brain

cerebellum

spinal cord

nerve

Nervous System

pounds and is composed of cells called neurons, some 100 billion in all. Its cells are grayish - white in appearance, hence, the term "gray matter" used when referring to the brain. Like all organs, the brain must be nourished and protected from injury; it is encased in the skull and fed via a system of arteries and capillaries that supply it with blood and nourishment.

The brain is divided into three distinct parts: the brain stem, cerebellum, and cerebrum. The brain stem is what connects the brain and the spinal cord; it is also responsible for many of the involuntary functions of the body, such as blood circulation and breathing. The cerebellum is composed of nerve tissue and is also divided into the right and left hemispheres. It is responsible for many of the conscious activities of living, such as intelligence, memory, speech, and vision. These hemispheres are further subdivided into lobes known as the frontal, parietal, occipital, and temporal lobes, with each having a specific function. The cerebrum is located beneath the cerebellum and is responsible for maintaining balance, coordination, and other subconscious functions.

The trunk line of the nervous system is the spinal cord, which is encased within the bony protection of the spine. Think of it as a large cable where wires enter from near and distant parts of the body. The nerves entering the cord are named for the sections of the spine where they enter, such as the sacral nerve roots (at the bottom of the spine), lumbar (lower back), thoracic (middle back), and cervical (neck).

Nerve cells (called neurons) are the basic components and building blocks of the entire nervous system. A neuron consists of a cell body with a nucleus and branching fibers called dendrites. Neurons also have projections called axons that branch out to form terminals that connect to dendrites of other cells, muscles, or glands. The space between the axons and the receptor, or receiving, cells is called the synapse. This is where signals are passed by neurotransmitters, special chemicals that carry the messages across the gap.

Ganglia are bundles of nerve cells found outside of the central nervous system as well as within the brain or spinal cord. They help direct the reflexive actions of the sympathetic nervous system, the system that produces an involuntary reaction when the body needs to guard against being injured.

How Does It Work?

Scientists once believed that the nervous system operated much like the electrical system of a house or car, that stimuli such as light, heat, cold, and pain were transmitted from nerve cells to the brain through electrical impulses. However, neurons are not physically connected; rather, the process by which stimuli are transmitted to the brain is primarily chemical.

Cells in the body receive stimuli from the outside world. These cells are called receptor cells, or neurons, and are separated by a gap called the synapse. When a stimulus is being transmitted to the brain, the neuron produces specific chemicals called neurotransmitters that filter across this gap and stimulate neighboring neurons. This stimulation causes a charge within the neighboring neurons, resulting in their production of neurotransmitters to stimulate the next neurons, and so on in a chain, until the charge reaches the spinal cord and finally, the brain.

The brain monitors all the incoming sensations from hunger to pleasure to pain. The brain also formulates responses to these stimuli. The brain is made up of sections called lobes, which receive stimuli and formulate responses. Visual

NEED A DOCTOR?

Two specialists who deal with nervous-system disorders are neurologists and neurosurgeons. A neurologist specializes in diagnosing problems with the nerves of the spine, and relies on noninvasive therapies, such as medications, as treatment. A neurosurgeon specializes in surgery involving the nervous system.

stimuli are transmitted by nerves in the eyes and received by the occipital lobe. Nerves in the nasal passages send messages to the olfactory lobe. Sensory nerves in the skin, which produce messages of temperature and touch, send messages to the parietal lobe. Other lobes are responsible for hearing and tasting, and other portions of the brain formulate responses to these stimuli, completing the cycle of the nervous system.

When the body is in danger of being injured, such as when a hand is suddenly exposed to something very hot, reflexes take over and cause the hand to snap away quickly and involuntarily. Reflexes are the body's response to danger. They are involuntary in that the stimulus received is reacted upon before it even reaches the brain. If the message being transmitted is one of emergency, it is received by a mass of nerve cells called a ganglion in the spinal cord. An immediate response is sent back to the motor cells in the area from which the stimulus came, causing the muscles to respond by pulling away from the danger.

Reflexes are part of the autonomic nervous system, the part of the nervous system that controls involuntary, unconscious activities. These activities include the functioning of the internal organs, blood vessels, and glands. The autonomic nervous system is divided into the sympathetic nervous system (the part that heightens activity) and the parasympathetic nervous system (the part that slows bodily activity). Each part balances the other. For example, the sympathetic nervous system may increase heart rate in the event of an emergency, and the parasympathetic system would slow down the heart rate once the emergency has passed. The part of the nervous system that controls conscious activity—responding when you want to raise your arm or take a step, for example—is called the somatic nervous system.

Major Problems and Common Disorders of the Nervous System

Alzheimer's disease is a progressive degeneration of brain cells leading to loss of memory, confusion, anxiety, depression, and, eventually, death. The exact cause of Alzheimer's is not known; however, some researchers have investigated a link between the degeneration of the brain cell and the neurotransmitter called acetylcholine. There is currently no effective treatment for Alzheimer's disease, though its progress may be slowed.

Amyotrophic lateral sclerosis (ALS) also causes progressive degeneration of nerve cells in the brain and spinal cord that control muscle movement. Also known as Lou Gehrig's disease, ALS leads to a wasting away of the muscles once the nerve cells are destroyed. As the muscle tissue is destroyed, paralysis results, ultimately leading to death. Its cause is unknown and there is no effective treatment.

A brain tumor is any abnormal growth of tissue that forms in the brain. The tumor may be primary or secondary. A primary tumor is one that develops in the brain tissue; a secondary tumor is one that originates elsewhere and migrates to the brain. These tumors can be benign (noncancerous) or malignant (cancerous). Brain tumors may produce symptoms of double vision, headache, memory loss, impaired thinking, personality changes, weakness, and vomiting.

Encephalitis is an inflammation of the brain caused by a virus. Very often, the brain is affected secondarily to an existing viral infection in another part of the body. For example, the virus that causes chickenpox, measles or mumps could spread to the brain and cause encephalitis.

Huntington's disease is a fatal, inherited, progressive, degenerative disorder of brain cells, involving actual shrinkage of tissue. It has been linked to an abnormal gene found on chromosome 4; however, researchers are still searching for the exact gene. The condition produces involuntary movements of the arms, face, trunk, and feet. It also leads to dementia. If a parent is affected with this disease, each child has a 50 percent chance of developing it as well. Huntington's disease is usually diagnosed around the age of 35; however, even though it is fatal, death may not occur for ten or twenty years following diagnosis.

Meningitis is an inflammation of the membranes covering the brain and spinal cord. The symptoms usually include headache, fever, and a stiff neck. Its cause is attributed to contagious bacteria and viruses, with bacterial meningitis being the more serious illness.

Multiple sclerosis (MS) results when the insulating cover that protects nerve fibers, the myelin, is destroyed or damaged. Symptoms include impaired vision, rapid eye movement, numbness (tingling) or weakness in a limb or paralysis in one or more limbs, lack of coordination, tremor, and unsteady gait. Heredity may play a factor in who gets the disease, which tends to strike slightly more women than men. Although the exact cause of MS has not been determined, it has been linked with a defect in the immune system. Medications may be prescribed to control the immune response or muscle movements; however, they cannot cure the condition.

Narcolepsy is a neurologic condition characterized by sudden periods of sleepiness during normal daily activities. People affected by narcolepsy may suddenly fall asleep when they are engaged in other activities such as working or driving. The exact cause of narcolepsy is unknown; however, it is thought that REM (rapid eye movement) sleep patterns somehow intrude during waking hours.

Seizure disorders (at one time called epilepsy) occur when the normal electrical patterns of the brain cells become disrupted for some unknown reason. This disorganization of signals causes the body to go into spasms, called seizures. There are two classes of seizures: grand mal and petit mal. The grand mal seizure is the most serious because there are convulsions and loss of consciousness. They may come on suddenly with no warning. Once the seizure begins, the person loses consciousness, which is followed by violent movement, then a period of sleep. After these phases, the person regains consciousness, although he or she may be confused.

A *petit mal* seizure is a small seizure that lasts for only few seconds or minutes. Loss of consciousness is not accompanied by any violent body movements, and when consciousness is regained there is no confusion. These types of seizures typically begin in children who are between the ages of 6 and 12.

Spinal cord trauma is a general term that applies to anything that injures the spinal cord, possibly affecting they way it conducts nerve impulses to the brain. Injury to the spinal cord may result in weakness and loss of sensation in a part of the body to complete paralysis if the cord is severed.

Bell's palsy is a condition that results in the paralysis of facial muscles due to nerve damage. It is typically characterized by sagging muscles and a general weakness on one side of the face. While its exact cause is unknown, the condition is temporary, usually with full recovery expected within a few months, perhaps with some residual weak spots remaining.

Headache occurs when the pain-sensing structures within the head are stimulated. As a rule, women tend to suffer headaches more than men. There are three recognizable types of headaches: tension, migraine, and cluster.

Tension headaches occur when the muscles of the neck contract painfully due to stress or other psychological factors. Tension headaches tend to affect men and women equally.

Migraine headaches are caused by the dilation of blood vessels in the face, neck, or scalp, and may produce nausea, vomiting, or visual symptoms such as auras, sparkling lights, or blind spots. Migraines affect about 11 percent of the U.S. population, and an estimated 30 percent of migraine sufferers are men. Migraines also have a genetic tendency: 65 percent of those who get migraines report having a close family member who also gets them.

Cluster headaches produce a steady burning pain in and around the eyes or temple. While they affect only 1 percent of the population, 85 percent are male. During a cluster headache, the eyes may appear irritated with redness and constant watering, accompanied by sinus stuffiness. These headaches have a sudden onset with very little warning, tend to follow a pattern of occurrences, and may last for up to two hours.

REPRODUCTIVE SYSTEM

The purpose of the reproductive system is the continuation of the human race—without the all-important meeting of the sperm and the egg, there would be no future generations. While pleasure usually accompanies sexual intercourse, the act is actually part of the process of creating new life in a biological environment singularly designed for that purpose.

The reproductive system of a man is much more obvious than that of a woman, which is, for the most part, hidden inside of the body. The components of the male system include the penis, testicles, prostate gland, seminal vesicles, and vas deferens. A sperm, or spermatozoa, is a male sex cell responsible for fertilizing the female ovum, or egg. It carries twenty-three chromosomes, which join the twenty-three in the female egg at fertilization. Sperm also carries the X and Y chromosomes that determine the gender of the baby.

Penis

The penis, the external male sex organ, is cylindrical in shape and filled with spongy erectile tissue. In its relaxed state, the penis is soft and flexible. During sexual excitement, the tissue fills with blood, causing the penis to enlarge and become hard and erect. The erection makes it

NEED A DOCTOR?

The specialist who deals with problems of the reproductive system is, for men, the urologist. This doctor diagnoses and treats a wide range of disorders, including infertility, erection problems, and sexually transmitted diseases, as well as prostate and urinary disorders. The gynecologist is the reproductive health specialist for women.

possible for the penis to easily penetrate the vagina during intercourse.

When flaccid, the penis measures between 2.8 and 5.6 inches in length, and the erect penis measures between 5 and 7 inches. There is no relationship between penis size and body size, just as there is no relationship between size and sexual adequacy.

The urethra, the tube that carries both urine and semen out of the body, runs the length of the penis. A system of valves closes off the bladder during ejaculation, the release of semen from the body, to prevent urination and ejaculation at the same time.

The head of the penis, called the glans, is covered with nerve endings, making it the most sensitive part of the penis. The glans is covered with a thin layer of skin, called the foreskin. Lined with mucous membrane, the foreskin protects the sensitive glans and secretes smegma, a lubricating fluid, to prevent friction. The foreskin is often surgically removed just after birth, in a procedure called circumcision. This may be done for religious or cultural reasons or to reduce the risk of infection by preventing the accumulation of smegma under the foreskin, where bacteria can breed.

Testicles (Testes)

The testicles, also called testes, are pink-white, oval-shaped glands that weigh half an ounce each and are about $1^1/_2$ inches long. They produce sperm cells and testosterone, the male hormone that drives the libido, or sex drive, and promotes the development of male characteristics such as body hair, a deep voice, and increased muscle growth.

At birth, the testicles are in the abdomen, but shortly thereafter they descend into a fluid-filled pouch called the scrotum, which hangs outside the body. The testicles are held here because they need to be kept cooler than the rest of the body, at 94° F, in order to produce fertile sperm. To achieve this, the scrotum contains sweat glands that allow evaporation to cool the testicles. In addition, the cremaster muscles, which support the testicles in the scrotum, can contract or relax—pulling the testicles closer to the body for warmth or allowing them to fall away from the body to cool them off. This reflex is known as the cremasteric reflex.

The testicles are connected to the rest of the body by the spermatic cord, which contains blood vessels, nerves, and the vas deferens. The testicles contain seminiferous tubules (a series of canals within the testicles), which produce sperm, the male reproductive cells. Sperm cells are the smallest cells in the body and resemble tiny tadpoles. Sperm cells can swim seven inches per hour, a necessary task if they are to reach the egg of the woman and penetrate it with the help of enzymes. On average, the testicles produce about fifty million sperm cells a day, and a man can release up to 600 million sperm cells in a single ejaculation. The seminiferous tubules empty into the epididymis, a series of ducts, where sperm is stored until it is mature. Sperm are released from the epididymis through tubes

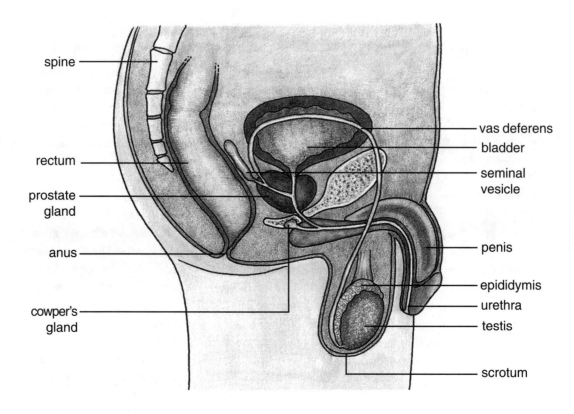

Male Reproductive System (side view)

known as the vas deferens, which connect to the urethra.

Sperm cells contain twenty-three chromosomes, including both the Y chromosomes (which result in a male child) and the X chromosomes (which result in a female child). Since the woman produces only X chromosomes, it is the chromosomes of the sperm that determine the gender of the baby.

The testicles also contain millions of Leydig cells. When a boy reaches puberty, the pituitary gland in the brain releases hormones that cause the Leydig cells to release another hormone called testosterone. Testosterone causes muscle to develop, the voice to deepen, and a beard to grow. It also stimulates a man's sex drive. However,

testosterone does not affect a man's ability to have an erection.

The highest levels of testosterone are produced when the man is between the ages of 25 and 30. After 60, the levels may drop in some men, possibly decreasing sex drive; however, there is still enough in the system to retain male characteristics.

Semen

Semen is the liquid that carries the sperm from the body. Made up of fluid from the seminal vesicles, the prostate gland and, of course, the sperm stored in the epididymis, semen contains fructose, vitamins, and amino acids to nourish the sperm, mucus for lubrication, and

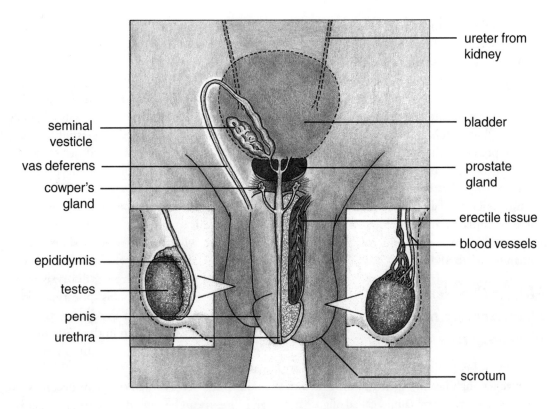

seminal vesticle

vas deferens

cowper's gland

epididymis

testes

penis

urethra

ureter from kidney

bladder

prostate gland

erectile tissue

blood vessels

scrotum

Male Reproductive System (front view)

prostaglandins. Only a tiny percentage of the semen is sperm—almost 70 percent is fluid from the seminal vesicles, while the prostate contributes almost 30 percent.

Prostate Gland

The chestnut-sized prostate gland, which lies just under the bladder, secretes a fluid that counteracts acidity in the vas deferens, the tube that leads from the epididymis to the urethra. Under the prostate are two tiny yellow glands called Cowper's glands, which secrete a cleansing fluid into the urethra just before ejaculation to prevent damage to the sperm. Also, urine and semen are kept from simultaneously exiting the urethra by nervous reflexes. This

is to protect the sperm from the urine's acidic contents.

How Does It Work?

During sexual excitement, the heart rate increases, blood pressure rises, and the testicles begin to contract rhythmically, causing sperm to move from where they are stored in the epididymis, through the vas deferens, and into the urethra. In the urethra, the sperm mixes with fluid from the prostate and the seminal vesicles, creating semen.

At the height of sexual excitement, contractions of muscles at the base of the penis cause ejaculation, a release of the semen through the urethra. Following this climax, called an orgasm, the penis returns to a flaccid state.

During intercourse, the semen is ejaculated into the woman's vagina, close to the cervix the entrance to the uterus, also called the womb. The sperm in the ejaculate swim through the uterus into the fallopian tubes. If an egg cell, called an ovum, is present in the tube, a sperm may fertilize it by breaking through its outer wall with the help of enzymes. A fertilized egg then travels back down through the fallopian tube to the uterus, where it implants and develops into a fetus. Sperm can live in the reproductive system of a woman for up to 48 hours.

Major Problems and Common Disorders of the Male Reproductive System

Infertility is the inability of the male to produce or deliver enough healthy sperm to bring about conception. A low sperm count, called oligospermia, occurs when the man does not produce enough sperm cells. The man may also produce defective sperm cells that aren't able to survive very long after ejaculation and never reach the egg.

Erection problems, sometimes called impotence, involve an inability to attain an erection adequate to complete sexual intercourse. Such problems are common and occur in many men at one time or another. The cause is usually fatigue, illness, stress, or anxiety. Other causes may be the use of drugs, neurological diseases, diabetes, arteriosclerosis, cancer, radical prostate surgery, infections, and genitourinary injuries. Treatment varies, depending on the exact cause.

Sexually transmitted diseases (STDs), once known as venereal diseases, are common in both men and women. STDs include chlamydia, gonorrhea, hepatitis B, herpes, HIV (the virus that can cause AIDS), and syphilis.

Penis

Cancer of the penis is a rare form of cancer that affects the glans or the foreskin. It is usually slow growing and can be treated successfully when it is caught early. Symptoms include a sore on the penis, unusual liquid coming from the penis (abnormal discharge), a lump in the groin, or pain or bleeding during erection or intercourse.

Chordee is a painful curvature of the penis that occurs when the urethra is shorter than the penis. It is a congenital condition that can be corrected surgically. Peyronie's disease is a condition in which the erect penis appears crooked, caused by scarring within the spongy tissue of the penis. It occurs in men in their 50s and 60s and may not require treatment unless it is painful.

Balanitis occurs when the glans becomes red and sore. It can be caused by a urinary tract infection, irritation from clothing or detergents, or a yeast infection. Treatment involves antibiotics or antifungal medications if infection is present.

Phimosis is defined as an abnormally tight foreskin that cannot be drawn back from the glans, the tip of the penis. While the condition usually disappears with age, it can make urination and erections difficult and painful. Paraphimosis usually develops as the result of phimosis. It occurs when the foreskin retracts and becomes constricted, causing swelling and pain that may cause permanent damage. Treatment is circumcision or partial circumcision to release the foreskin.

A penis fracture can occur if the cylinders of spongy tissue within the penis are broken, causing pain and swelling. Priapism is an erection that does not subside that occurs when the spongy tissue of the penis does not drain of blood. It can be caused by an injury, drugs used to treat impotence, blood disorders, and a number of other factors. Both conditions require immediate treatment. Untreated, permanent impotence could result.

In urethral stricture, a rare condition, the urethra narrows and may become blocked because of injury or infection that causes scar tissue. Symptoms include difficulty urinating and pain during urination.

Urethritis is inflammation of the urethra. It is often caused by sexually transmitted disease, though at times the cause remains unknown. Symptoms include pain during urination, an urge to urinate frequently, and discharge from the penis.

Prostate

Cancer of the prostate is the second most common cancer in men; fortunately, early detection and treatment are the keys to a full recovery. Symptoms usually include difficulty in starting urination, weak stream, and increased frequency of urination.

Prostatitis, inflammation of the prostate, can be caused by irritation to the gland or by infection. It can affect a man at any age. Symptoms include discharge of fluid from the penis, pain or itching deep within the penis, discomfort during urination, difficulty urinating, fever, aches and pains, and lower-back pain.

Benign prostatic hyperplasia (BPH) is a noncancerous enlargement of the prostate. It affects over 50 percent of men over the age of 50 and approximately 80 to 90 percent of men over the age of 80. In BPH, the prostate slowly becomes larger, squeezing the urethra and obstructing urination. BPH can lead to bladder problems,

frequent urinary tract infections, and, possibly, urinary retention, in which a man becomes unable to urinate.

Testicles

Cancer of the testicles affects about two men in 100,000 per year and is the most common cancer in men between the ages of 15 and 34. Tumors in the testicles can be discovered early by means of periodic self-examination. Fortunately, this form of cancer responds well to chemotherapy when detected early.

Epididymitis is inflammation of the epididymis, a tube that transports sperm from a testicle to the vas deferens. Symptoms include severe pain in the scrotum, fever, and a swollen area that may feel hot to the touch.

A hydrocele is a buildup of fluid within the sacs that house the testicles. This harmless swelling is soft and usually painless. Treatment—surgical removal of the fluid—is usually not required unless the swelling has become exceptionally large or uncomfortable.

Orchitis is an inflammation of the testicle. It is usually caused by the mumps, though it can also result from an infection in the prostate or epididymis. Symptoms include pain in the scrotum, swelling (usually only on one side of the scrotum), and a feeling of weight in the scrotum. Without treatment, orchitis can result in permanent damage to one or both testicles and may cause infertility.

In testicular torsion, the spermatic cord that suspends the testicles within the scrotum becomes twisted, cutting off the blood supply to a testicle. This may occur after physical activity, though often there is no known cause. Symptoms include sudden, severe pain in a testicle; one testicle higher within the scrotum; nausea and vomiting; swelling; and fever. Prompt treatment to untwist the cord is required because the testicle may die due to lack of blood.

An undescended testicle occurs when a testicle does not descend from the abdomen into the scrotum shortly before or after birth. This occurs in 1 percent of males, and usually corrects itself, though corrective surgery may be performed if necessary. If a testicle remains undescended in a child over the age of 5, infertility may result. A testicle that was previously undescended is more vulnerable to cancer than a normal testicle and is also more likely to contribute to infertility.

A varicocele is a collection of varicose veins within the scrotum, characterized by a painless swelling that usually occurs on the left side. While the varicocele itself is not harmful, the collection of blood in the testicles may cause infertility. If infertility occurs, surgery can be done to tie off the varicose vein and restore fertility.

Trauma to the testicles, caused by a blow to the area, can cause agonizing pain caused by the swelling of the testicle within its protective sac. Permanent injury to the testicles is rare. If swelling and pain persist for longer than an hour or the scrotum is bruised, quickly seek medical care. Too much pressure within the scrotum can cause tissue damage that might lead to infertility, blood clots, or even the loss of a testicle.

SKELETAL SYSTEM

The skeletal system is the framework that gives the body its shape. The adult skeleton is made up of about 206 separate bones and weighs about 20 pounds. Without the skeleton, the body would be little more than a collection of tissue without shape or definition.

The skeleton serves several important purposes. It protects the internal organs and provides the body's rigid internal structure. The bones anchor the muscular system so that movement is possible. In addition, bone marrow, the soft tissue found inside the bones, produces red blood cells that carry nutrients to the tissues of the body. Bone marrow also produces white blood cells that help protect the body from potentially harmful diseases.

Each bone is covered with a thin layer of skin called the periosteum. The periosteum contains nerves and blood vessels that supply the bones with nutrients. Beneath the periosteum lies dense, rigid, compact bone, which contains thousands of tiny holes and passageways. Through these run more nerves and blood vessels that carry nutrients into the bone. Inside the layer of compact bone lies spongy bone that encases a soft substance filled with blood vessels, called bone marrow. Bone marrow produces white blood cells (which fight infection), red blood cells (which carry oxygen), and platelets (which help blood to clot).

The skull, vertebrae (the spinal bones), and rib cage form the axial skeleton. The skull has twenty-eight bones, eight of which are fused to cover and protect the brain. The spinal cord, the collection of nerves that leads to the brain, passes through a large hole at the base of the skull and runs down the spine through a channel in the vertebrae, the bones that make up the spine. The twenty-eight vertebrae are held together by a network of muscles and ligaments, an arrangement that allows the back flexibility while providing protection for the spinal cord. Between each vertebra are spongy, fluid-filled cushions called discs. The lowest bone in the line of vertebrae is known as the coccyx, or tailbone.

Along with the thick breastbone, the twenty-four ribs anchored to the spine protect the heart and lungs.

NEED A DOCTOR?

The specialist who deals with problems of the skeletal system is the orthopedist. This doctor's domain includes the treatment and correction, usually surgically, of deformities or damage to the musculoskeletal system.

A rheumatologist is another type of specialist concerned with the treatment of arthritis and other degenerative diseases having to do with the joints and connective tissues.

The rest of the skeletal bones form the appendicular skeleton and include the bones of the shoulders, arms, hands, hips, legs, and feet. The shoulder group includes the shovel-shaped scapula (shoulder blade) and the key-shaped clavicle (collarbone). The upper arm bone is known as the humerus, which connects with the lower arm bones, the radius and ulna. From these extend the wrist bones (carpals), palm bones (metacarpals), and fingers (phalanges).

The lower half of the skeletal system begins with the pelvis and continues down to the thigh bone (femur), kneecap (patella), shin bones (tibia and fibula), ankle (talus), heel (calcaneus), feet bones (metatarsals), and toes (phalanges).

Bones are connected by joints. There are three types of joints: fixed joints, which hold bones firmly together, as in the plates of the skull; partly movable joints, which allow some mobility, as in the spine; and freely movable joints, which allow for plenty of mobility, as in major joints such as the knees and elbows.

Male and female skeletons differ slightly in that the pelvic bones of the female are spaced farther apart to allow room for carrying a baby.

Also, male bones are somewhat larger and heavier than female bones.

Major Problems and Common Disorders of the Skeletal System

Bone cancer is a relatively uncommon disease. Types of bone cancer include osteosarcoma (originating in the leg bones), chondrosarcoma (originating in cartilage), and fibrosarcoma (originating in fibrous tissue). Bone cancer has often spread to distant organs, such as the lungs, by the time it is diagnosed. Cancer may also spread to the bones from other areas of the body.

Arthritis is simply characterized as pain in the joints. Types of arthritis include osteoarthritis, caused by degeneration and wear and tear; rheumatoid arthritis, an autoimmune disease in which the immune system attacks the body's tissues; gout, a painful buildup of uric acid in the joints (usually the toes); and ankylosing spondylitis, in which the joints of the vertebrae become inflamed and may fuse. While men are less likely than women to suffer rheumatoid arthritis, they are as likely to have osteoarthritis, and more likely to have gout. Ankylosing spondylitis affects men almost exclusively. Arthritis is a chronic condition.

Osteoporosis is a disease in which the bones become thin and brittle, making them porous, weak, and more susceptible to fractures, especially of the vertebrae, thighbone, and wrist. Risk factors for men include smoking and drinking alcohol. Osteoporosis is often considered a natural effect of aging.

Scoliosis is a progressive, degenerative condition that affects the spine, causing it to rotate and become misshapen, often appearing S-shaped. This condition may be diagnosed during infancy or adolescence. Although the

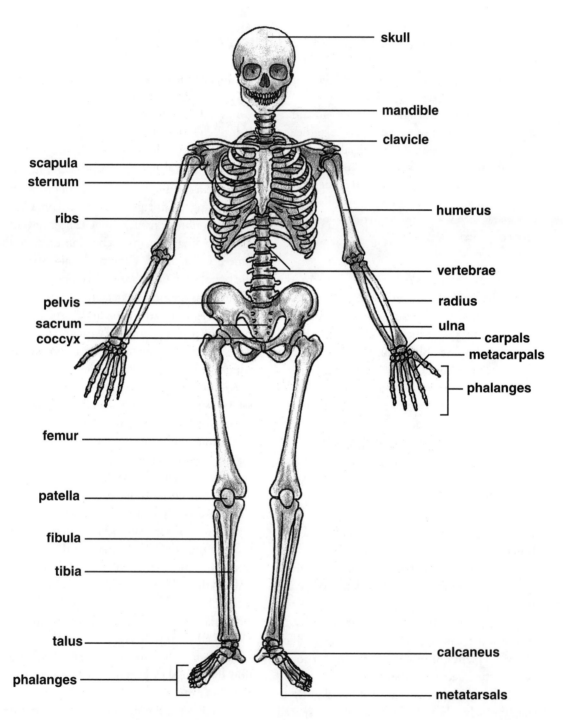

skull

mandible

clavicle

scapula
sternum

ribs

humerus

vertebrae

pelvis

radius

sacrum

ulna

coccyx

carpals

metacarpals

phalanges

femur

patella

fibula

tibia

talus

calcaneus

phalanges

metatarsals

Skeletal System

FRACTURES

Bones are very strong. However, if enough pressure is applied, they will break. A break, rupture, or discontinuity of a bone, which occurs as a result of a physical force being exerted on a bone, is called a fracture. Symptoms of a fracture are local pain, swelling or bruising over a bone, tenderness, and deformity where the injury occurred. Medical attention should be sought. A doctor may be able to tell whether a bone is fractured just by looking at it. In some instances, however, an x-ray of the bone may be necessary. Inspection of vessel and nerve damage may also be necessary.

- A compound fracture is one in which the broken bone is exposed through a wound in the skin. This is also called an open fracture.

- A simple fracture is a simple break in which the bone does not pierce the skin. It is also known as a closed fracture.

- A greenstick fracture occurs mostly in immature long bones of children, in which one side of the bone is broken and the other side is unbroken but may bend.

- A comminuted fracture is one in which a part of the damaged bone is broken into fragments or shattered.

- A pathological fracture is one that occurs in bone already weakened by an existing pathological process such as osteoporosis, metastatic cancer, or tuberculosis.

These five types of fractures can be further classified according to the angle of the break:

- A transverse fracture occurs at right angles to the long part of the involved bone.

- An oblique fracture is one that breaks at a slanting, or oblique, angle.

exact cause of scoliosis has yet to be determined, it is believed to be a genetic defect.

As the condition progresses, the space between the vertebrae increases, causing them to become thicker on one side. Eventually the person develops severe deformity such as rounded shoulders, swayback, or sunken chest. Spinal braces or surgery may be used to halt or correct the deformity.

Spondylolisthesis occurs when one of the vertebra slips over the one below it, especially in the lower back or lumbar region. When the normally bony arch of the vertebrae becomes soft, they tend to slip forward, putting pressure on spinal nerves and causing pain. This condition may also result when osteoarthritis has caused the joints between the vertebrae to become worn and unstable.

URINARY SYSTEM

The urinary system is responsible for eliminating liquid waste products from the body.

During metabolism, the process that releases energy from food and nourishes the cells of the body, waste products are created as the cells use the nutrients delivered by the bloodstream. The urinary system filters the blood and removes these waste products. The urinary system also assists in maintaining a balance of salts and other dissolved minerals in the blood.

The urinary system is composed of two kidneys, a pair of organs that filter blood; the ureters, tubes that connect the kidneys to the bladder; the bladder, a reservoir within the body for liquid waste; and the urethra, the thin tube that carries the urine out of the body.

How Does It Work?

The kidneys are a pair of bean-shaped, reddish-brown organs, about the size of a fist, located in the back of the abdomen on each side of the spine. Each kidney weighs about 5 to 6 ounces. The kidneys filter urea, uric acid, and creatinine (liquid waste) that have been collected and carried to the kidneys by the blood.

Blood passes through the kidneys continuously. The kidneys clean and filter it, ridding it of waste that, if left to accumulate, can be deadly. This is achieved by the kidney's one million tiny filtering units, called nephrons. The kidneys prevent red blood cells and protein from passing through the nephrons and return these materials to the bloodstream.

Other functions of the kidneys include the production of red blood cells and the regulation of levels of potassium, sodium chloride, and other substances. Each hour the kidneys filter the blood in the body twice, restoring it and its essential vitamins, amino acids, glucose, hormones, and so on. Kidneys slow their activity to about one-third during nighttime hours.

About two quarts of the filtered product, called urine, is produced daily. Tiny droplets of urine pass from the tubules in each kidney and collect in a reservoir at the kidney's center, which is connected to the bladder.

Urine is passed to the bladder via wavelike muscular contractions of the ureters every 10 to 30 seconds. The ureters are two narrow (about the size of pencil lead), 12-inch long tubes. The ureters empty urine into the bladder, where it is stored over several hours until urination occurs. Special valves between the bladder and ureters prevent urine from flowing back toward the kidneys.

The bladder is a punching-bag-shaped flexible, muscular reservoir, with a urine capacity of 6 to 24 ounces. As urine collects, the bladder gradually expands until it becomes full. Reflexes in the bladder help hold the urine until enough has been collected for urination, the process by which urine is excreted from the body. Worry, anxiety, and fear can increase blood pressure and increase the speed at which urine is produced. Although the bladder may not be full, these stresses may tighten the bladder wall and cause the person to feel the need to urinate.

Urination begins when the muscles of the bladder contract, allowing urine to flow out of the bladder through the urethra. The amount of fluid that passes through the urethra varies each day, from one pint to two gallons, depending on food and liquid intake and fluid losses from sweat glands and lungs. Cold weather, which prompts the body to reserve fluid, can increase frequency of urination, and warm weather, which promotes perspiration, can decrease it.

The components of urine can reveal a great deal about what is happening in the body. This analysis is done through a test called a urinalysis, defined as any physical, chemical, or microscopic

NEED A DOCTOR?

The specialist who deals with problems of the urinary system is a urologist. A urologist handles a wide range of conditions, including prostate, urinary, and reproductive health problems. A nephrologist deals with diseases of the kidneys.

examination of urine. A number of other medical conditions such as heart disease, psoriasis, and endocrine disorders can be diagnosed with the help of a urinalysis. Virtually all organs empty waste products into the bloodstream, which are then filtered through the kidneys and show up in urine. An examination of these waste products can help determine how well a particular organ or gland is functioning.

Major Problems and Common Disorders of the Urinary System

Bladder tumors, which may or may not be cancerous, develop inside the lining of the bladder and occur more often in men than in women. These tumors grow from the walls and tend to resemble small mushrooms.

Cancer of the kidneys generally falls into three categories: nephroblastoma (also called Wilms' tumor), renal cell carcinoma, and transitional cell carcinoma. Nephroblastoma affects children under the age of four and accounts for about 20 percent of all cancers in children. Renal cell carcinoma usually occurs after the age of 40 and accounts for about 75 percent of all kidney cancer. Transitional cell carcinoma affects the cells lining the renal pelvis and usually develops in smokers or in those who have taken large quantities of painkillers.

Glomerulonephritis is the name given to a serious kidney condition that affects the filtering part of the kidney. It may occur as either an acute (short-term) or chronic (long-term) infection. When it enters the chronic stage, it eventually leads to kidney failure at which point the person must rely on dialysis to artificially filter the blood.

Polycystic kidney disease is a hereditary condition that causes large quantities of cysts to grow within the kidney. As these cysts increase in size, they destroy normal kidney tissue, causing the kidney to fail. As kidney function is reduced, it is necessary to artificially cleanse blood through a process called dialysis. The only effective treatment for polycystic kidneys is a kidney transplant.

Cysts are fluid-filled sacs that grow within the kidney. It is not unusual for people over the age of 50 to have some growth of cysts in their kidneys. In most cases, these cause no problems.

Discolored urine usually indicates that the urine is very concentrated, which may be as a result of decreased fluid intake, the recent completion of strenuous exercise, certain drugs or medications being taken, or a number of other factors. Light-colored urine indicates an increase in the amount of fluids consumed and the kidneys' ability to eliminate excess water.

Hematuria, the presence of blood in the urine should be treated seriously, as this could indicate injury to the kidney and subsequent bleeding or the presence of an infection, or it could be as a result of strenuous exercise such as jogging or bicycle riding. A physician should be consulted immediately whenever blood is noticed.

Kidney stones may indicate that a high level of uric acid is present in the kidneys, ureters, or bladder. Stones are formed when the mineral content of urine becomes too concentrated due to a lack of fluid intake, chronic infections, misuse of medication, blockages, or certain metabolic disorders. Lack of exercise and loss of water through perspiration during warm weather can increase the risk of stones. These stones may vary from the size of tiny bits of gravel to extreme cases of fourteen pounds.

Urinary tract infection (UTI) is a term that may be used to describe urethritis (inflammation of the urethra), cystitis (inflammation of the bladder), or pyelonephritis (inflammation of the kidney). These infections are most often caused by bacteria that have spread from the rectum to the urethra and bladder.

Symptoms associated with urethritis and cystitis are generally a frequent need to pass urine and pain upon urination. The urine may or may not have a distinctive odor, and there may or may not be blood present. The symptoms associated with pyelonephritis are chill, fever, and lower back pain.

Women tend to experience a higher incidence of UTIs than men because of the shortness of their urethras (the tube through which urine is expelled from the body) and diaphragm use. UTIs such as nonspecific urethritis are most likely contracted as a result of sexual activity.

Health and Well-Being

As important as it is to know what can go wrong with your body, it's just as important to understand what's going on when things go right. After all, good health means much more than just not being sick—it means optimizing your body's performance so that you can reap the benefits of a longer, happier life.

In the following pages, you'll find what you need to know about how to enhance your health. Information on physical fitness and nutrition helps you understand how to keep your body's machinery running smoothly. There are valuable facts about the effects of stress, cholesterol, caffeine, and smoking on your health, as well as clear, straightforward discussions of complex issues such as cholesterol, vitamins, and the importance of screening examinations. Plus you'll find plenty of helpful tips on handling your own health care, from everyday needs such as home remedies to life-changing decisions such as long-term care and living wills. Where appropriate, resources are listed so that you can seek any additional information you may need.

DIET AND NUTRITION

Breakfast might be leftover spaghetti, lunch might be a quick bite at the corner deli, and dinner could be half a pizza consumed in front of the TV. The truth is, men are known better for their tendency to fuel up fast and satisfy hunger than they are for their careful food choices.

But proper nutrition is vital to good health for everyone, young and old. Food, after all, is what keeps the body going—providing energy, as well as necessary vitamins and minerals. With-out a balanced diet that provides for all the body's needs, the body's systems simply don't function as effectively as they could, which opens up the door for a number of health problems.

According to experts, four of the ten leading causes of death in men are directly linked to diet. A proper diet has been shown to reduce the risk of premature death from the biggest killers of men: heart disease, cancer, stroke, and diabetes. Food choices also can reduce risk factors for chronic diseases such as high blood pressure, obesity and high blood cholesterol—conditions that are more common in men than in women.

The Nutrients

Nutrients include fats, protein, carbohydrates, and vitamins and minerals. (See Vitamins and Minerals, p. 51.) In addition, the body requires water to function. Some 60 percent of a man's body weight is water, meaning that a 155-pound man contains about 87^1/$_2$ pints of water. Water is essential to the maintenance of the correct chemical balance of the body and contributes to blood volume.

Fat

Fat comes from animal and vegetable sources. In the body, it can be broken down into glucose for energy, or it can be stored within cells until its energy is needed. Less than 30 percent—some experts say less than 20 percent—of the calories you consume in one day should come from fat. A higher percentage can lead to an increased risk of heart disease and certain cancers.

Several types of fat can be found in foods. Saturated fats are solid at room temperature. They are the main component of the white marbling in meats, of the visible fat around meat, of butter and cheese, and of whole milk and ice cream. Saturated fats are also plentiful in coconut oil, palm-kernel oil and palm oil, three plant oils widely used in commercial baked goods such as cookies and crackers. You should get a minimal amount of your fat intake from saturated fats—they tend to raise the blood levels of low-density lipoproteins (LDL), an unhealthy, "bad" form of cholesterol. LDL cholesterol contributes to the development of plaque, the deposits of fatty substances that block arteries to cause heart

BUTTER VS. MARGARINE: THE GREAT DEBATE

Butter is high in saturated fat, but margarine contains trans fatty acids—molecules found in hydrogenated fats that have the same cholesterol-raising properties of saturated fats. So which is better?

For healthy people who stick to a diet with less than 30 percent of calories from fat, most experts agree that a small amount of butter shouldn't do any harm. However, if you're concerned about fat and cholesterol in your diet, choose soft-spread margarines that have water or liquid (not hydrogenated) vegetable oil listed as their first ingredient. Such margarines have fewer calories from fat and fewer trans fatty acids. And if you've been using margarine to melt in cooking, switch to olive or canola oil instead.

disease. (See Cholesterol, page 89) High-density lipoproteins (HDL) are known as "good" cholesterol because they help escort fats from the body, lowering cholesterol levels.

Trans fatty acids are fats contained in products that have hydrogenated vegetable oils (oils that have been processed with hydrogen to make them hard), for example, some types of margarine and vegetable shortening. These fats should also be avoided because they act in ways similar to saturated fats, raising LDL cholesterol levels. About half a dozen studies have found that the amount of trans fatty acids found in the typical American diet (8 to 15 grams a day) can raise LDL cholesterol levels just as much as saturated fats. Trans fatty acids also lower HDL cholesterol levels, increasing the risk of heart disease. You should get no more than 10 percent of your calories daily from saturated fat and trans fatty acids combined—about 18 to 26 grams, for most men.

Polyunsaturated fats are liquid at room temperature and are the predominant fat in common vegetable oils such as corn, safflower, sunflower, cottonseed, and soybean oils. These oils were once thought to reduce cholesterol levels. However, research now suggests that while polyunsaturated fats don't raise LDL cholesterol levels, they do lower levels of HDL cholesterol.

The main portion of your fat intake should come from monounsaturated fats, the predominant fats in olive and canola oil. These fats seem to lower levels of LDL cholesterol levels without dropping HDL cholesterol levels.

CALCULATING FAT CONTENT

In order to reduce the risk of heart disease and other adverse medical conditions, the American Heart Association and current federal guidelines recommend that Americans reduce their daily fat calories to 30 percent or less of their daily calorie intake.

You can calculate the number of calories from fat by multiplying the number of grams of fat in the food by 9, the number of calories in 1 gram of fat. To figure the percentage of calories by fat, divide the number of calories from fat by the total number of calories.

RECOMMENDED DAILY FAT CALORIES FOR MEN*

Age	Average Daily Calorie Needs	Maximum Fat Calories
11–14	2,000–3,700	600–1,100
15–18	2,100–3,900	630–1,170
19–22	2,500–3,300	750–990
23–50	2,300–3,100	810–930
51–75	2,000–2,800	600–840
over 76	1,650–2,450	495–735

*30 percent of total calorie intake

Protein

Proteins come from animal and plant sources. They are the main structural components of tissues and organs, and they regulate and maintain body growth. They also perform the critical function of bringing into the body the essential amino acids, which the body itself cannot produce, as well as a number of nonessential amino acids such as tyrosine, which the body can make.

Sources of protein include fish, beef, poultry, eggs, dairy products, nuts, and beans.

The recommended dietary allowance of protein is about 56 grams for a 150-pound man—about 0.37 grams per pound. (For reference, a 6-ounce serving of beef, poultry, or fish has about 50 grams of protein.) However, active men who exercise regularly are thought to need slightly more protein than sedentary men.

HOW TO GO LOW-FAT

Here are some tips to reduce the fat in you diet:

- Eat beans and peas rather than meats as your main source of protein.

- Limit meat portions to no more than three or four ounces daily. For reference, a portion of three to four ounces of meat is about the size of a deck of cards.

- Choose lean cuts of meat, fish, and poultry.

- Avoid all fried and sauteed foods.

- Choose milk, yogurt, cottage cheese, and cheese products that are low-fat or nonfat.

- Eat at least five servings of fruits and vegetables a day. Most vegetables are low in fat (except for avocados and olives) and high in fiber. Be sure to prepare them without adding extra butter or oils.

- Avoid baked goods high in saturated fats. This includes doughnuts, pastries, croissants, and pie crusts.

- Stay away from prepackaged foods and frozen dinners. While these may be quick, they often have twice as much fat as a home-cooked version of the same meal. Processed foods are often high in sodium, as well.

- Choose desserts low in fat such as gelatin desserts, sorbet, ice milk, angel food cake, and fruit. Be careful when choosing low-fat snacks and desserts; these often are high in calories.

For the most part, though, the average American man gets too much protein in his diet.

Carbohydrates

Carbohydrates provide the body with energy and are essential for getting vitamins and other nutrients into our bodies. Carbohydrates can be simple (glucose, fructose, and galactose) or complex (starches and fiber).

Fiber can be soluble (capable of being dissolved in water) or insoluble. Insoluble fiber is thought to perform a cleaning function by scraping the walls of the organs of the digestive system of carcinogens, cancer-causing agents

likely to build up under stress or because of exposure to various pollutants. Fiber also helps to resolve constipation. Studies show that in countries where there was a greater intake of foods high in insoluble fiber, there were fewer cases of colon and rectal cancer.

Federal Nutrition Guidelines

The latest federal *Dietary Guidelines for Americans*, published in 1995, recommend a balanced, varied diet rich in grain products, fruits, and vegetables and low in sugars and sodium. These current dietary guidelines also recommend a diet low in total fat, saturated fat, and cholesterol. If you drink alcoholic beverages, it is recommended you do so in moderation—no more than two drinks a day—with a drink defined as 12 ounces of beer, 5 ounces of wine, or 1¹/₂ ounces of liquor.

And for the first time, the guidelines recommend that men maintain their weight within a healthy range instead of allowing their weight to increase as they age. At the same time, the guidelines warn against rapid, or "crash," weight-loss programs, suggesting instead gradual weight loss of about one-half to one pound per week through exercise and healthful food choices with lower total calories. In addition, the guidelines advise thirty minutes or more of moderate physical activity on most days of the week.

Calorie needs vary by age and activity level. Older men generally need fewer calories because they are usually less active than younger males. The recommended calorie intake for an active adult male is approximately 2,800 a day.

Food Pyramids

The U.S. Government Food Guide Pyramid—which replaces the "four food groups"—translates the current dietary recommendations into a suggested eating pattern based on a

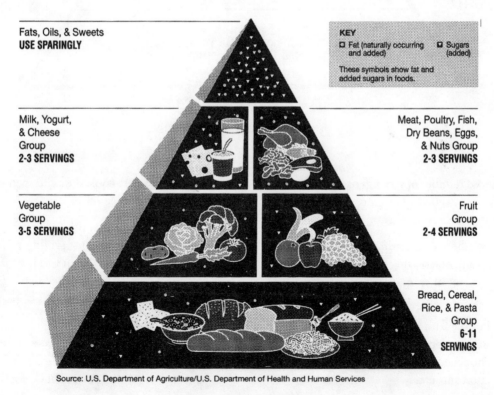

Fats, Oils, & Sweets
USE SPARINGLY

KEY
◻ Fat (naturally occurring and added)   ◼ Sugars (added)
These symbols show fat and added sugars in foods.

Milk, Yogurt, & Cheese Group
2-3 SERVINGS

Meat, Poultry, Fish, Dry Beans, Eggs, & Nuts Group
2-3 SERVINGS

Vegetable Group
3-5 SERVINGS

Fruit Group
2-4 SERVINGS

Bread, Cereal, Rice, & Pasta Group
6-11 SERVINGS

Source: U.S. Department of Agriculture/U.S. Department of Health and Human Services

Food Guide Pyramid
A Guide to Daily Food Choices

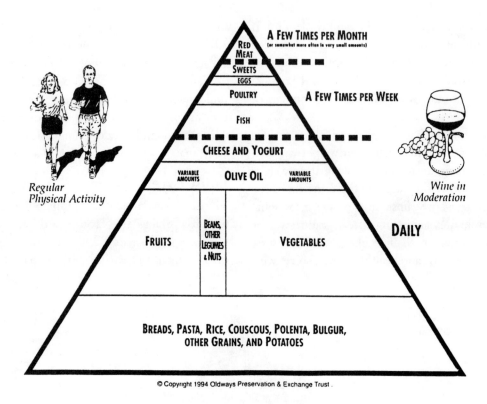

A FEW TIMES PER MONTH
(or somewhat more often in very small amounts)

RED MEAT

SWEETS

EGGS

POULTRY

A FEW TIMES PER WEEK

FISH

CHEESE AND YOGURT

VARIABLE AMOUNTS   OLIVE OIL   VARIABLE AMOUNTS

FRUITS

BEANS, OTHER LEGUMES & NUTS

VEGETABLES

DAILY

BREADS, PASTA, RICE, COUSCOUS, POLENTA, BULGUR, OTHER GRAINS, AND POTATOES

Regular Physical Activity

Wine in Moderation

© Copyright 1994 Oldways Preservation & Exchange Trust .

Mediterranean Diet Pyramid

balanced number of servings of foods from each of the six categories. The groups, along with their servings, are as follows:

- For the bread, cereal, rice, and pasta group, one serving equals: 1 slice of bread; 1 ounce of ready-to-eat cereal; or $1/2$ cup cooked cereal, rice, or pasta.

- For the fruit group, one serving equals: 1 medium apple, banana, or orange; $1/2$ cup chopped, cooked, or canned fruit; or $3/4$ cup fruit juice.

- For the vegetable group, one serving equals: 1 cup raw, leafy vegetables; $1/2$ cup other vegetables (cooked or chopped raw); or $3/4$ cup vegetable juice.

- For the meat, poultry, fish, dry beans, eggs, and nuts group, one serving equals: 2 to 3 ounces of cooked lean meat, fish, or poultry; 1 to $11/2$ cups cooked dry beans; 2 to 3 eggs; or 4 to 6 tablespoons of peanut butter.

- For the milk, yogurt, and cheese group, one serving equals: 1 cup of milk or yogurt; $11/2$ ounces of natural cheese; or 2 ounces of processed cheese.

- Fats, oils, and sweets should be used sparingly.

Two other pyramids, the Mediterranean and Asian Diet Pyramids, were developed by private interest groups and extol the traditional diets of Greek farmers and Chinese peasants, respectively. Dozens of studies over the last 30 years have shown that the simple Greek diet of whole-wheat bread, olive oil, beans, nuts, vegetables, fruits, small amounts of cheese, moderate amounts of fish and occasional consumption of meat, combined with physical activity, reduces their incidence of cancer and the risk of heart disease.

To bring this message to the public, the Harvard School of Public Health, in cooperation with the nonprofit Oldways Preservation and Exchange Trust and the World Health Organization, developed the Mediterranean Diet Pyramid. The Mediterranean model keeps saturated fats to a minimum but encourages generous amounts of olive oil, a monounsaturated fat. This type of fat raises your body's levels of HDL cholesterol, which protects against heart disease by escorting harmful LDL cholesterol out of the body. In contrast, the U.S. Food Pyramid lumps all fats together. The Mediterranean Pyramid also differentiates between healthful plant proteins (beans, other legumes, and nuts) and animal protein, which contains high levels of saturated fat.

In 1995, Cornell University joined with the Harvard School of Public Health and Oldways

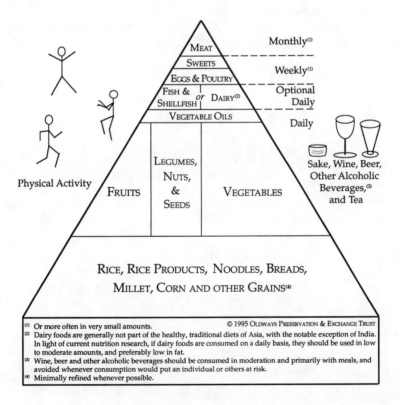

Traditional Healthy Asian Diet Pyramid

to create the Asian Diet Pyramid. The traditional Asian diet is plant-based with little or no animal foods, not even dairy products. The backbone of the diet is rice and rice products accompanied by vegetables and, occasionally, small portions of fish or meat. Soy products, which recent studies have shown are powerful cancer fighters, are also staples of the Asian diet. (Soy products, however, are high in sodium.)

Vegetarianism

For social, religious, cultural, and health reasons, many Americans have chosen vegetarian diets, which are free of most, if not all, animal products. Many scientific studies have shown that plant-based diets can lead to reductions in the risk of heart disease, cancer, obesity, and other health risks. Reflecting these findings, the most recent government guidelines state that vegetarian diets can satisfy the recommended dietary allowances for nutrients. There are several types of vegetarians.

- *Vegans* consume only plant foods. They omit all animal foods, including meat, poultry, fish, eggs, dairy products, and honey. The federal dietary guidelines suggest vegans supplement their diet with vitamin B_{12}, which occurs naturally only in animal products.

- *Lacto* vegetarians include milk and milk products along with vegetable foods in their diets. Ovo-lacto vegetarians include eggs as well as milk in their diets.

- *Pesco* vegetarians include fish along with vegetable foods in their diets.

- *Pollo* vegetarians eat poultry along with vegetable foods.

READ THE LABEL

Nutrition Facts

Serving Size 1 cup (228g)
Servings Per Container 2

Amount Per Serving

Calories 260   Calories from Fat 120

	% Daily Value*
Total Fat 13g	**20%**
Saturated Fat 5g	**25%**
Cholesterol 30mg	**10%**
Sodium 660mg	**28%**
Total Carbohydrate 31g	**10%**
Dietary Fiber 0g	**0%**
Sugars 5g	
Protein 5g	

Vitamin A 4%	•	Vitamin C 2%	
Calcium 15%	•	Iron 4%	

* Percent Daily Values are based on a 2,000 calorie diet. Your daily values may be higher or lower depending on your calorie needs:

	Calories:	2,000	2,500
Total Fat	Less than	65g	80g
Sat Fat	Less than	20g	25g
Cholesterol	Less than	300mg	300mg
Sodium	Less than	2,400mg	2,400mg
Total Carbohydrate		300g	375g
Dietary Fiber		25g	30g

Calories per gram:
Fat 9 • Carbohydrate 4 • Protein 4

Source: Food and Drug Administration, 1994

continues

To be sure your food choices are contributing to your dietary goals, you need to learn how to read food labels. Food labels became standardized in the United States in May 1994, allowing consumers to compare and compute nutritional components more easily. Important label items to check include:

- *Serving size.* In the past, manufacturers determined what a serving size was; however, today the Food and Drug Administration has researched and regulated serving sizes based on the amount of food customarily consumed by an adult. But remember a serving size is not a *recommended* amount, and it may bear no relation to your own personal serving size. Be sure to compute the amount of nutrients based on the amount of food that you eat—for example, if you eat only one half of one serving, you'll get only half of the nutrients, while if you eat twice as much, you'll get double the nutrients.

- *Percent daily value.* Percent daily value is based on a 2,000 and 2,500 calorie-per-day diet. A section on the bottom of the food label explains how much of each nutrient you should eat if you consume 2,000 calories a day. That amount is the daily value. Thus, the percent daily value tells you what percent of that daily value is contained in one serving of that food.

- *Front label claims.* Front labels of products have also changed. Food makers must now meet specific requirements to label their foods healthy, light, lean, extra lean, high or low in a nutrient, having fewer, more or less of a nutrient, or a good source of a nutrient. Here are a few description definitions based on one serving size:

- *Low fat.* 3 grams or less.

- *Low saturated fat.* 1 gram or less.

- *Low sodium.* 140 milligrams or less.

- *Low cholesterol.* 20 milligrams or less.

- *Low calorie.* 40 calories or less.

- *Light.* Containing one-third fewer calories or one-half the fat of the regular food; or containing 50 percent less sodium.

- *Reduced.* Altered to contain at least 25 percent less of something than a regular product.

- *Healthy.* Low in fat and saturated fat; limited sodium and cholesterol; and containing at least 10 percent of the daily value of a nutrient.

- *Good source.* Contains 10 to 19 percent of a particular nutrient's daily value.

For more information:

American Dietetic Association
216 W. Jackson Blvd., Suite 800
Chicago, IL 60606
800-366-1655
312-899-0040

American Society for Nutritional Sciences
9650 Rockville Pike
Bethesda, MD 20814
301-530-7050

Food and Drug Administration
5600 Fishers Ln., HFE88
Rockville, MD 20857
301-827-4420

Food and Nutrition Information Center
National Agricultural Library (USDA)
10301 Baltimore Ave., Room 304
Beltsville, MD 20705-2351
http://www.NAL.usda.gov/FNIC

Vegetarian Resource Group
P.O. Box 1463
Baltimore, MD 21203
410-366-8343
http://www.vrg.org

VITAMINS AND MINERALS

Vitamins and minerals are essential to life. These substances, found in foods and available in supplements, bolster reproductive health, contribute to growth, strengthen the immune system, and keep the body's systems functioning. If you're deficient in even one of the necessary vitamins or minerals, your body will not function properly.

Vitamins are organic substances that are used in the body to make coenzymes, which enable the body to use energy from food and produce immune cells. There are thirteen known vitamins. Vitamins A, E, K, and D are water soluble, meaning they dissolve in water, and vitamin C and the eight B vitamins—B_1 (thiamin), B_2 (riboflavin), niacin, B_6, B_{12} (cobalamin), folic acid, pantothenic acid, and biotin—are fat soluble. Fat-soluble vitamins are more likely to build up in the system and, to be most effective, need to be taken with a meal that contains some fats.

Minerals are inorganic substances. There are fifteen essential minerals: calcium, magnesium, phosphorus, sodium, potassium, sulfur, chlorine, iron, iodine, copper, manganese, zinc, molybdenum, selenium, and chromium. Minerals, like vitamins, play a role in most of the body functions, ranging from blood clotting, blood pressure regulation, and heart rate to maintenance of the thyroid gland, body temperature, and brain function.

Antioxidants are the vitamins that contain molecules that help limit oxidative reactions, chemical reactions within the body that involve oxygen. These reactions—the same ones that cause butter to turn rancid and iron to rust—result in the formation of free radicals, molecules that can damage cells within the body, in some cases leading to diseases such as cancer and heart disease. Antioxidants, which include vitamins C, E, beta-carotene (a substance that becomes vitamin A), and selenium, neutralize the free radicals, making them harmless.

Studies show that antioxidants may help lower the risk of cancer, prevent cataracts, and reduce damage to the lungs caused by pollution. While research is still being done on the benefits of antioxidants, most practitioners recommend that you eat plenty of fruits and vegetables to get your share of antioxidants from natural sources.

Getting What You Need

The Food and Nutrition Board of the National Academy of Sciences has recommended certain levels of intake, called recommended dietary allowances (RDAs), thought to meet the nutritional needs of most healthy persons. It's important to remember that these RDAs are not necessarily the ideal amounts for optimal health. Rather, they are the amounts that will prevent deficiency and related health problems in most people.

Vitamins and minerals are sometimes referred to as micronutrients, because the body requires very small quantities of them in comparison with the calorie-providing macronutrients: carbohydrates, protein, and fat. You can get most of the vitamins and minerals you need from eating a balanced diet that includes at least five servings of fruits and vegetables a day, as well as grains, dairy products, and meats or other sources of proteins. Still, chances are you won't be able to get them all. You need to eat much more than you normally would in a day, for example, to get enough vitamin E or chromium from food to match the RDA. Also, if you're dieting, it's unlikely you're getting all your vitamins and minerals from the reduced number of calories you're ingesting.

Of course, there are other ways to get your RDA of vitamins and minerals. One way is through enriched or fortified foods. Enriched foods are those that have vitamins and minerals added to them to replace those lost during processing. In general, the more a food has been processed, the fewer natural vitamins and minerals remain. Fortified foods have vitamins and minerals that would not necessarily appear naturally added to them—for example, the addition of calcium to orange juice.

Supplements can also be taken to reach your RDA. While experts agree that supplements can't make up for a poor diet, they can help provide some of the vitamins and minerals not easily obtained in a healthy diet. It is important to note, however, that boosting vitamin and mineral intake by eating nutrient-dense foods (such as vegetables, whole grains, lean meat, and fruits) is preferable to taking supplements in nearly all cases. This is because vitamins and minerals always work in concert with other nutrients, and the "partner" nutrients often occur in the same foods. So many (perhaps all) micronutrients are most effective when they are consumed as part of a balanced, varied diet.

Single-nutrient supplements, on the other hand, make it possible to easily ingest a large amount of a single vitamin or mineral. This is desirable in some cases, but at other times this may be ineffectual and simply a waste of money. At worst, large doses of single vitamins or minerals (called megadoses) can have adverse effects. These should not be taken without medical supervision.

How Much Do You Need?

The vitamin and mineral needs of men and women are similar, in many cases differing only in quantity due to different average body size. But adequate—and in some cases, extra—levels of some micronutrients may be especially important for men because of their physiology, risk profiles, and health habits. Keep in mind that the RDAs are only suggested minimum amounts—many experts recommend taking much more of certain vitamins to reap other benefits such as disease prevention. Talk with a doctor or nutritionist about what doses are appropriate for you, but also keep in mind that some vitamins such as vitamin A and niacin may be toxic in large amounts. Some vitamins may interfere with medications.

CHOOSING A SUPPLEMENT

When deciding on a supplement, keep the following points in mind:

- Try an "insurance" supplement. These multivitamins contain most of the nutrients you need to be sure you're getting enough of the essential vitamins and minerals. However, check the label to see what vitamins and minerals the supplement contains. Often, manufacturers include less of the more expensive and bulky vitamins and more of the cheaper, smaller vitamins. Be sure to choose one that includes the essential vitamins selenium and biotin. But don't worry if vitamin K, phosphorus, and iodine are missing, because most people usually get too much of these in a regular diet.

- Read the label carefully. The amount of each vitamin and mineral contained in a particular supplement is listed on the label along with the percent of daily requirements. Before you go vitamin shopping, make a list of what you're looking for and choose the supplement that most closely matches your needs. Watch out for supplements that advertise that they are specially formulated for men or for a specific age group—these often contain no more or less of various vitamins than other varieties, but they're usually more expensive.

- Check the expiration date. If the date is less than nine months away—or if there is no date at all—choose another supplement.

- Buy generic brands. Except for price and fancy packaging, there are no other differences between brand name vitamins and generic vitamins.

- Don't worry about the difference between natural and synthetic vitamins. For the most part, they're the same.

- Talk with your practitioner or get a referral. A few physicians are knowledgeable about nutrition, though studies show that the majority know little or nothing about nutrition—despite the fact that six of the ten leading causes of death are linked to nutrition. Ask your doctor what he or she knows about nutrition—some practitioners may even be certified by the American Board of Nutrition. If the answer is not very much, ask to be referred to a qualified nutritionist or knowledgeable practitioner. You can also contact the American Dietetic Association for information.

What follows is a list of the recommended daily allowance of each vitamin and mineral, plus a brief rundown of some of the more important vitamins and minerals, their benefits, and their sources.

Vitamin A and Beta-Carotene

Vitamin A helps maintain the epithelial cells, found in the eyes, skin, lining of the blood vessels, and other internal and external surfaces of

The RDAs for Men

Age	VitA	VitD	VitE	Vit K	VitC	Thiamin	Ribofl.	Niacin	VitB$_6$	VitB$_{12}$	Folate
	RE	mcg.	mg.	mcg.	mg.	mg.	mg.	mg.	mg.	mcg.	mcg.88
11–14	1,000	10	10	45	50	1.3	1.5	17	1.7	2.0	150
15–18	1,000	10	10	65	60	1.5	1.8	20	2.0	2.0	200*
19–24	1,000	10	10	70	60	1.5	1.7	19	2.0	2.0	200*
25–50	1,000	5	10	80	60	1.5	1.7	19	2.0	2.0	200*
over 51	1,000	5	10	80	60	1.2	1.4	15	2.0	2.0	200*

Age					Calcium	Phos.	Mag.	Iron	Zinc	Iodine	Sel.
					mg.	mg.	mg.	mg.	mg.	mcg.	mcg.
11–14					1,200	1,200	270	12	15	150	40
15–18					1,200	1,200	400	12	15	150	50
19–24					1,200	1,200	350	10	15	150	70
25–50					800	800	350	10	15	150	70
over 51					800	800	350	10	15	150	70

*Formerly 400 mcg.; revised 1989

Source: Food and Nutrition Board, National Academy of Sciences, 1989

Estimated Safe and Adequate Daily Dietary Intakes of Selected Vitamins and Minerals

These vitamins and minerals do not have an RDA.

biotin	pantothenic acid	copper	manganese	fluoride	chromium	molybdenum
mcg.	mg.	mg.	mg.	mg.	mcg.	mcg.
30–100	4–7	1.5–3.0	2.0–5.0	1.5–4.0	50–200	75–250

Source: Food and Nutrition Board, National Academy of Sciences, 1989

the body. Beta-carotene is a precursor to vitamin A, meaning it is turned into vitamin A once it is inside the body. Vitamin A deficiency can cause night blindness, eye disorders, poor tooth development, fertility problems, and lowered resistance to infection. Vitamin A and beta-carotene are also antioxidants, and some studies have indicated that a diet high in beta-carotene may protect smokers and smokeless tobacco users against mouth, throat, and lung cancer. Vitamin A also may be helpful in treating skin problems and ulcers.

Both are found in green and yellow fruits and vegetables as well as fish liver oils and animal livers. More than 50,000 I.U. (international units) daily of vitamin A on a long-term basis may be toxic, while beta-carotene has no known toxicity.

Vitamin B$_6$

This vitamin promotes healthy immune function and cell replication; for these reasons, it is thought to help prevent cancer. It also influences the functions of the brain and the nervous system and is thought to possibly help treat asthma and carpal tunnel syndrome. Deficiency rarely occurs, but may involve weakness, nerve problems, and a reduction of resistance to infection. Sources include chicken, fish, liver, kidney, pork, and eggs, as well as brown rice, soybeans, oats, whole-grain products, peanuts, and walnuts. Toxicity has been observed, although rarely, with doses of 100 to 200 mg. Most problems, however, have occurred at doses higher than 500 mg. a day.

Vitamin B$_{12}$

Vitamin B$_{12}$ supports the growth and function of the blood marrow, nerves, and the spinal cord. Most people get enough B$_{12}$ in their daily diets, though some have trouble absorbing the nutrient and require regular injections. A deficiency can cause nerve damage, resulting in memory loss, decreased reflexes, fatigue, tingling in the hands or feet, and impaired touch or pain sensation. However, those with a deficiency often experience an energy boost after taking B$_{12}$, and it may also help depression and anxiety. Sources include liver and organ meats, muscle meat, fish, eggs, shellfish, milk, and dairy products. Vegetarians who do not eat any animal products may need to supplement. Alcohol depletes levels of B$_{12}$ in the body. Vitamin B$_{12}$ has no known toxicity.

Folic Acid

Folic acid is essential for normal growth and reproduction. In fact, folic acid helps to prevent birth defects and reduces the risks of lung cancer in people who smoke. Symptoms of folic-acid deficiency include anemia, loss of appetite, diarrhea, and gastrointestinal problems. Sources include liver, brewer's yeast, fresh oranges, whole grains, and green, leafy vegetables. Toxicity is rare, but has occurred in some studies with doses of 8 grams or more a day.

Niacin

Niacin, or B$_3$, helps the body manufacture enzymes that provide energy and the building blocks for cell reproduction and repair. It is thought to play a role in cancer protection by contributing to a substance that helps to repair genetic damage caused by exposure to viruses or harmful drugs. It may also help to lower cholesterol levels. Symptoms of deficiency include anxiety, depression, a reddish skin rash, and a sore mouth and tongue. It is found in brewer's yeast, peanuts, wheat bran, chicken, tuna, turkey, and whole grains. Doses of several hundred milligrams can cause flushing of the skin and intense itching; doses of 1,500 to 3,000 mg. can cause jaundice and liver damage.

Thiamin

Thiamin, or B$_1$, helps the body release the energy stored in food and is essential for almost every cellular reaction in the body—for normal growth, development, reproduction, physical fitness, and good health. A deficiency results in a condition known as beriberi, characterized by numbness in the toes and feet, difficulty walking, cramping in the legs, and finally, paralysis of the legs. Sources include brewer's yeast, organ meats, beans, whole grains, and pork. Long-term toxicity produces symptoms of hyperthyroidism: headache, trembling, rapid pulse, and insomnia. Five milligrams daily is the lowest oral dose known to cause side effects.

Biotin

Biotin contributes to the body's metabolism of carbohydrates and fats and helps to make protein. It helps to keep fingernails from splitting and may also help some skin disorders. A deficiency is uncommon, but symptoms include loss of hair, a rash around the nose, depression, hallucinations, sleeplessness, and muscle pain. Sources include organ meats, brewer's yeast, egg yolks, beans, whole grains, breads, fish, nuts, meat, and dairy products. Biotin has no known toxicity.

Pantothenic Acid

This vitamin also plays a role in the body's metabolism. Studies show that pantothenic acid may boost energy and athletic ability, and some say it may help in the treatment of arthritis. Signs of deficiency include fatigue, headache, insomnia, numbness and tingling in the hands and feet, muscle cramps, and immune problems. Sources include brewer's yeast, liver, eggs, wheat germ, bran, peanuts, and peas. The risk of toxicity is low.

Riboflavin

Riboflavin, or B_2, aids the metabolism and is crucial for the development and maintenance of nerves and blood cells, for iron metabolism, for adrenal gland function, for immune function, and for the formation of connective tissues. A deficiency has been associated with an increase of throat cancers and the development of cataracts. Symptoms of deficiency include skin problems, red or swollen lips, loss of appetite, weakness, fatigue, depression, and anemia. Sources include organ meats such as liver and kidney, dark green leafy vegetables, meat and dairy products, and enriched white flour and cereal. Strenuous exercise increases the need for this vitamin. The risk of toxicity is very low.

Vitamin C

This vitamin, also called ascorbic acid, helps to produce connective tissue throughout the body (in skin, muscles, gums, blood vessels, and bone). As an antioxidant, it helps to neutralize potentially damaging free radicals in the system. It is thought to help to prevent many types of cancer as well as reduce effects of the common cold, the early stages of heart disease, cataracts, damage from pollutants, and even a common form of infertility in men in which the sperm cells clump together. Symptoms of a deficiency include easy bruising, bleeding gums, muscular weakness, nosebleeds, frequent infections, and slow wound healing. Scurvy, a condition that is a result of vitamin C deficiency, is marked by breaking of small blood vessels, bleeding of the skin and gums, loose teeth, and weakness. Scurvy can cause death.

Sources of vitamin C include citrus fruits, red bell peppers, black currant, guava, strawberries, broccoli, brussels sprouts, and papaya. Doses as low as 500 mg. a day may cause diarrhea in some people, but most people can take much larger doses with no problem. People prone to gout or kidney stones should not take large doses without medical supervision.

Vitamin D

This vitamin regulates the absorption and use of two minerals, calcium and phosphorus, which are both essential for bone growth and development. Researchers think vitamin D has little to do with cancer or immune function, but it does help to strengthen bones and prevent osteoporosis in men and women. Signs of deficiency include soft, thin bones; bone pain; and muscle weakness. Sunlight stimulates the body's production of vitamin D, which can also be found in fatty fish, liver, egg yolks, and fortified milk and cereals. Toxicity may occur at levels of more than 1,000 I.U. daily, resulting in high calcium levels in the blood and calcium deposits in soft bone tissues.

Vitamin E

The most potent antioxidant, vitamin E also works in concert with other antioxidants. It is thought to reduce the risk of heart disease by helping to keep plaque from forming on blood-vessel walls and also by keeping blood cells from clumping together. It is also thought to help prevent cancer by destroying free radicals, enhancing the body's immune system, and inhibiting the formation of carcinogens. When applied topically, it's also used to prevent scars from forming. Signs of deficiency include lethargy, inability to concentrate, loss of balance, and anemia. Sources include hazelnut oil, wheat-germ oil, sunflower oil, mayonnaise, eggs, and fortified cereals. At levels of less than 1,000 I.U. per day, there is no known risk of toxicity.

Vitamin K

This vitamin helps the blood to clot. As a result, a deficiency results in prolonged clotting time, easy bleeding and bruising, and frequent nosebleeds. However, deficiency is not common. Sources include dark green, leafy vegetables (kale, spinach, and parsley), Chinese cabbage, lettuce, carrots, olive oil, and avocados. Large amounts of vitamin K may interfere with the action of blood-thinning drugs.

Calcium

Calcium builds the bones and the teeth and is essential for nerve conduction, muscle contraction, heartbeat, blood clotting, metabolism, and the maintenance of immune function. Calcium can help prevent osteoporosis, muscle cramps and possibly colon cancer, some research says. Signs of deficiency include abnormal heartbeat, muscle pain, cramps, numbness, dementia, and stiffness in the hands and feet. Sources include milk and dairy products, kale, turnip greens, kelp, tofu, canned salmon and sardines (with the bones), and soybeans. Doses up to 2,500 mg. a day are considered safe.

Chromium

Chromium, the same metal used to make car bumpers, is used by the body to help burn sugar for energy—a function called glucose metabolism. It is thought to help treat insulin resistance and hypoglycemia, which are possible early signs of diabetes. However, it is not proven to help prevent or treat established diabetes. It may help treat high cholesterol levels. Signs of deficiency include weight loss, diabetes-like symptoms, and nerve degeneration. Sources include liver, brewer's yeast, black pepper, thyme, beef, poultry, whole grains, beer, and oysters. Little is known about the toxic effects of chromium.

Copper

Copper is necessary for the formation of red blood cells and helps to store and carry iron. There is some evidence that it may help prevent heart disease and cancer. Signs of deficiency include anemia, paleness, connective tissue disorders, impaired glucose tolerance, and increased blood pressure. It is found in beef or chicken liver, crab, chocolate, sunflower seeds, peanut butter, oysters, and beans. The dose should be kept to 2 to 3 mg. a day if it is being taken for an extended period to avoid toxicity. People with Wilson's disease (a condition marked by an overaccumulation of copper in the body) should not take copper supplements.

WHAT ABOUT IRON?

A few years ago, iron fell under a black cloud as far as men's nutrition was concerned, when several studies appeared to link excess iron storage in men's bodies with an increased risk of heart disease and cancer. However, some subsequent studies failed to support this hypothesis.

Medical researchers have also found that hemochromatosis, a hereditary disorder of iron overabsorption, is more common than once believed—over one million Americans, mostly men, suffer the joint pain, fatigue, diabetes, cirrhosis, and eventual heart disease iron overload causes. Once diagnosed, hemochromatosis can be controlled simply by donating blood several times a year. For more information on iron overload and hemochromatosis, contact the Iron Overload Diseases Association, Inc., 433 Westwind Dr., Dept. P, North Palm Beach, FL 33408-5123; 561-840-8512.

Until research resolves the question of whether or not high iron intake is risky for men, it would be prudent to get all your iron from food (lean meats, dried beans, and dried fruit such as prunes and apricots are good sources) and avoid taking supplements, including multivitamins that include iron.

Iodine

Iodine is necessary for formation of two hormones produced in the thyroid gland, which regulates metabolism. Signs of deficiency include chronic fatigue, dry skin, weight gain, and enlargement of the thyroid (a condition called goiter). However, deficiency has been rare since iodized salt was introduced. Other sources include kelp, fish, shrimp, lobster, and clams. Elemental iodine can be toxic in amounts as small as 2 grams. Several milligrams daily have been linked with thyroid problems and the enlargement of salivary glands.

Iron

Iron carries oxygen throughout the body and is involved in the production of thyroid hormones and connective tissue as well as in the maintenance of the immune system. High levels of iron in the body can contribute to the risk of heart disease and some forms of cancer. Low levels can result in anemia, irritability, and an inability to learn and concentrate. Many people do not get enough iron in their diets. However, many experts advise against supplementation without medical supervision because of the problems related to higher levels of the mineral. Sources include liver, meats, beans, nuts, poultry, fish, whole grains, and most dark green, leafy vegetables.

Magnesium

This mineral is necessary for every major biologic process in the body, including the production of energy from sugar and the manufacture of genetic material. It also plays a role in muscle contraction, nerve conduction, blood-vessel tone, and heartbeat. Low levels are associated with high blood pressure and heart disease. Signs of deficiency include weakness, nausea, muscle cramps, dizziness, depression, and irregular heartbeat. It is found in whole grains, nuts, avocados, beans, and dark green, leafy vegetables. It is relatively safe, though it is not appropriate for people with kidney problems.

Potassium

Potassium contributes to muscle contraction, nerve conduction, regulation of heartbeat, energy production, and the manufacture of genetic material and protein. Low levels are associated with high blood pressure and stroke. It can be lost in perspiration, so it is often added to sports drinks to replenish what is lost during exercise. While depletion of potassium leads to muscle weakness, muscle pain, abnormal heartbeat, and fatigue, potassium supplementation is not thought to improve athletic performance in those who are not deficient. Sources include fruits (especially bananas) and vegetables. Potato skins, yams, avocados, prunes, beet greens, and raisins all contain potassium. High doses of several grams can result in heart failure. People with kidney problems and those who take spironolactone (a diuretic) or angiotensin converting enzyme (ACE) inhibitors (a blood pressure medication) should take potassium only under medical supervision.

Selenium

This mineral acts as an antioxidant and appears to help prevent some forms of cancer and heart disease. It also boosts the body's immune system. Signs of deficiency include muscle pain, muscle wasting, and heart problems. Sources include broccoli, mushrooms, brewer's yeast, cabbage, celery, whole grains, fish, and organ meats. More than 5 mg. a day can result in damaged fingernails, garlic breath, nausea, vomiting, and nervous system problems.

Zinc

Zinc is a mineral involved in the structure and function of cell membranes as well as the production of more than two hundred enzymes. It is necessary for proper wound healing, healthy skin, normal taste, smell, vision, and sexual function. It is very important in the functioning of the immune system. Zinc may be helpful in treating male fertility problems and preventing prostate cancer, since low levels of zinc in the body are associated with a reduction in the production of testosterone. Signs of deficiency include growth retardation, poor appetite, underfunctioning sex glands, abnormalities in taste, smell, and vision, skin changes, and increased susceptibility to infection. Sources include oysters, beef, pork and beef liver, lamb, crab, and wheat germ. Zinc may interfere with amounts of copper in the system. In addition doses as low as 25 mg. have been found to decrease immune system function.

For more information:

American Dietetic Association
216 W. Jackson Blvd., Suite 800
Chicago, IL 60606
800-366-1655
312-899-0040

American Society for Nutritional Sciences
9650 Rockville Pike
Bethesda, MD 20814
301-530-7050

Society for Nutrition Education
2850 Metro Dr., Suite 416
Minneapolis, MN 55425-1412
800-235-6690
612-854-0035

PHYSICAL FITNESS

In its very basic definition, the body is a machine. It requires fuel and maintenance and produces energy. And its parts must be used regularly to keep it running smoothly. If the body receives poor-quality fuel and is used very little, it produces little energy and becomes sluggish. But exercise—along with a healthy, balanced diet—keeps the body's mechanics running smoothly and efficiently.

Exercise is simply a movement of the body intended to improve physical fitness. Exercise can take the form of a planned workout or a change of daily routine—such as riding a bike to work instead of driving—that lets the body move more. Yet, according to the Centers for Disease Control and Prevention (CDC), some 58 percent of adults get little or no exercise—and 24 percent or more are completely sedentary. In fact, only 22 percent of adults get enough exercise to meet the standards set by the CDC and the American College of Sports Medicine—thirty minutes or more of light or moderate physical activity on most or all days of the week.

Benefits of Physical Fitness

Regular exercise helps the body maintain, repair, and improve itself. Exercise involves the use of the heart, lungs, and muscles and helps to keep all these mechanisms in working order. Without exercise, the systems of the body suffer and become vulnerable to a number of conditions and diseases such as coronary heart disease, obesity, low-back pain, and stress.

Exercise can help you live longer and healthier. A 1996 study in the *American Journal of Epidemiology* reported that aerobic exercise, sustained exercise that raises heart and breathing rates and trains the heart and lungs, can prolong life while preventing disability in the later years. The study observed more than five hundred subjects over the age of 50 who ran or exercised more than four hours a week, as well as some four hundred less active people of the same age. Over a period of eight years, the exercising group had

significantly fewer disabilities and deaths than the less active group.

Exercise lowers risk of heart disease. Lack of exercise is one of eleven factors listed by the American Heart Association that predisposes a person to heart disease. Exercise helps to prevent coronary heart disease by strengthening the muscles of the heart and helping to rid the body of excess fat and calories. Exercise also helps to prevent or eliminate other factors that may lead to heart disease such as obesity, stress, high blood pressure, and high cholesterol. When it is free of disease, the heart of an older person pumps as well as that of a younger adult, according to the National Institutes of Health. In addition, the National Institute of Neurological Disorders and Stroke maintains that exercise also helps to prevent stroke, which affects 500,000 Americans every year.

Exercise combats non-insulin-dependent diabetes by increasing insulin sensitivity, thereby, improving blood-glucose levels and helping in the long-term control of the disease.

Exercise helps prevent osteoporosis, a bone-thinning disease, by supplying stress on the bones that encourages the growth of new, stronger bone.

Exercise prevents the accumulation of excess weight. Without exercise, any excess calories are stored as fat rather than burned away, eventually leading to weight gain and obesity (weighing 20 percent more than the ideal weight). Obesity increases the risk for heart disease, hernia, backache, diabetes, and certain types of cancer. It is also a suspected factor in other disorders.

Exercise protects against back pain. Lower-back pain can also be prevented with exercise, which keeps the muscles and joints of the back strong and flexible. Exercise also prevents excess weight, a contributing factor to back pain. Eighty percent of those suffering from lower-back pain can find relief from their discomfort through exercises that improve the elasticity and strength of tense, weakened muscles.

Exercise relieves stress and boosts self-esteem. One research study discovered that a fifteen-minute walk reduced neuromuscular tension in a group of men over the age of 50 more effectively than a dosage of tranquilizers. It also helps relieve depression by improving self-image and by managing stress and anxiety, according to the National Institutes of Mental Health. Research supports theories that regular exercise promotes greater self-sufficiency.

Other benefits of exercise include sounder sleep and less sexual tension.

INACTIVITY TAKES ITS TOLL

So you don't exercise, but you do watch your weight, keep tabs on your cholesterol, and don't smoke. That should be enough to stave off heart disease, right?

Actually, no. A study in a 1996 *Journal of the American Medical Association* found that inactive people who don't smoke and have normal blood pressure and cholesterol are more likely to die early than active people who do smoke and have high blood pressure and cholesterol levels. In fact, the statistics showed that low levels of fitness raises the risk of heart disease just as much as smoking does—doubling the risk of early death for both men and women.

ACTIVITIES AND THE CALORIES THEY CONSUME

Most people think of exercise as running, weight lifting, or bicycling. But everyday activities—from vacuuming the living room to working in the garden—also burn calories. (Calories expended are estimates for a man weighing approximately 150 pounds.)

Activity	Calories expended per hour
Rest and light activity	*50–200*
Lying down or sleeping	80
Sitting	100
Typing	110
Driving	120
Standing	140
Shining shoes	185

Moderate activity	*200–350*
Bicycling (5$\frac{1}{2}$ mph)	210
Walking (2$\frac{1}{2}$ mph)	210
Cleaning car	220
Gardening	220
Laundry (outside drying)	220
Canoeing (2$\frac{1}{2}$ mph)	230
Shopping	230
Golf (foursome)	250
Lawn-mowing (power mower)	250
Painting (house)	290
Fencing	300
Rowing a boat (2$\frac{1}{2}$ mph)	300
Swimming (1/4 mph)	300
Calisthenics	300
Walking (3$\frac{1}{4}$ mph)	300
Having sex	315
Badminton	350
Horseback riding (trotting)	350
Square dancing	350
Volleyball	350
Roller-skating	350
Stacking heavy objects (boxes, logs)	350

Vigorous activity	*over 350*
Baseball pitching	360
Ditch-digging (hand shovel)	400
Ice-skating (10 mph)	400
Chopping or sawing wood	400
Bowling (continuous)	400
Tennis	420
Dancing (square or folk dancing)	430
Lawn-mowing (hand mower)	430
Shoveling snow	450
Hiking	460
Waterskiing	480
Hill-climbing (100 feet per hour)	490
Aerobics (high-impact)	500
Basketball	500
Football	500

Skiing (10 mph)	600
Squash and handball	600
Dancing (rock and roll)	630
Bicycling (13 mph)	660
Rowing (machine)	720
Scull-rowing (race)	840
Running (10 mph)	900

GUIDELINES FOR EXERCISE

Before Starting an Exercise Program

For men who are healthy and for those following their doctors' advice, the benefits of exercise far outweigh any risks. But if you are over the age of 35 and have not exercised in years, it would be best to consult your doctor before starting an exercise program.

In addition, the President's Council on Physical Fitness and Sports recommends that if you currently have, or have ever had, any of the following medical conditions, you should see your doctor before starting any exercise program:

- High blood pressure

- Heart trouble

- Family history of stroke or heart attack

- Frequent dizzy spells

- Extreme breathlessness after mild exertion

- Arthritis or other joint problems

- Severe muscle, ligament, or tendon problems

- Other known or suspected diseases or medical conditions, including back problems

SAY NO TO SNOW

Snow shoveling is especially dangerous for sedentary people and for those at risk for heart disease. In fact, more than 1,200 people die each year from heart attacks or related causes after major snowstorms from shoveling snow. One 1996 study showed that shoveling snow in cold temperatures pushed the heart rate beyond the upper limits usually recommended. While physically fit people may be able to handle such a high level of exercise, it is not safe for inactive people or for those with a risk for heart disease.

The Difference Between Aerobic and Anaerobic Exercise

The word *aerobic* means "with oxygen." During aerobic exercise (walking, running, or swimming, for example), your muscles demand the use of all the oxygen that's being carried by the blood. As a result, aerobic exercise trains the heart, lungs, and cardiovascular system to process and deliver oxygen more quickly and efficiently to every muscle in the body. As the heart muscle becomes stronger and more efficient, a larger amount of blood can be pumped with each heartbeat, thus supplying a larger amount of oxygen to the muscles. The more oxygen the muscles receive, the harder they can work.

The word *anaerobic* means "without oxygen." With anaerobic exercise (strength training, for example) the muscles are working at such an intense level that the blood cannot supply them with enough oxygen to keep them working. This point of intensity is called the *anaerobic threshold*, a term coined in 1972 by California physiologist Karl Wasserman. Upon reaching the threshold, the body cannot continue at the same intensity, at least not for long. Anaerobic exercise strengthens muscles, but it does little to improve the output of the heart and the lungs. The anaerobic threshold becomes higher with training, meaning it takes a longer and more intense workout to reach it.

The anaerobic threshold can be measured by monitoring a person's respiration—specifically oxygen intake and carbon dioxide output—with special equipment during exercise. (For example, a man might run on a treadmill while breathing through a system of tubes monitored by a computer.) Scientists call this measurement VO_2max. The VO_2max can then be associated with a heart rate that can be used for training purposes. Athletes in training use their VO_2max to monitor their progress.

It is important to make aerobic conditioning a priority before attempting anaerobic activities. It is dangerous to participate in anaerobic activities if the heart is not conditioned or if high blood pressure is a factor.

The Elements of an Exercise Program

There are three elements basic to a successful exercise program. They are aerobic exercise to increase cardiorespiratory endurance (the body's ability to take in and deliver oxygen to all parts of the body), strength training to increase muscular strength and endurance (the muscles' ability to sustain repeated contractions), and flexibility.

An effective program incorporates all these elements, as well as a warm-up at the beginning and a cooldown at the end. A warm-up session consists of five to ten minutes of slow exercise that uses the large muscle groups (legs, arms, and back, for example). You may want to walk at a moderate pace or use a stair climber or stationary bike to warm up. Calisthenic exercises such as knee lifts, arm circles, and trunk rotations can also be helpful.

Warming up is very important in that it helps to prevent soreness and injury. More of a warm-up may be necessary on cold days, and older men generally need longer than five to ten minutes to warm up. Warm up until you have just started to sweat.

To cool down after a workout, do at least five minutes of slow, easy exercise such as slow walking, combined with stretching, after you've completed your workout. This helps to bring the heart rate down, lessen muscle soreness, and even boost the effectiveness of your exercise session.

TOO SICK FOR A WORKOUT?

If you're suffering from a cold, review your symptoms before heading to the gym, said one 1996 study published in the journal *Physician and Sportsmedicine*. If your symptoms lie above the neck—for example, a stuffy nose, sneezing, sore throat, or headache—exercise is probably safe. However, if you have below-the-neck symptoms—for example, muscle aches, coughing, chills, fever, or diarrhea—avoid exertion. You should also avoid exertion if you have a fever.

Choosing a Trainer

If you're going to be choosing a personal trainer or signing up for a fitness program led by an instructor, it's important to ask about qualifications. Several organizations offer highly respected instructor-certification programs. These include IDEA Foundation, Aerobics and Fitness Association of America (AFAA), and American College of Sports Medicine (ACSM). All these programs require certification in CPR. Some require a written exam in physiology and anatomy in addition to the ability to put together a sound exercise routine. The American College of Sports Medicine requires a bachelor's degree or equivalent in an allied health field as well.

You should consider some of the following questions when looking for a fitness instructor:

- Are you asked to complete a fitness questionnaire before beginning the program?

- Does the trainer regularly ask about your health—whether you're feeling sore or have had any recent injuries, for example?

- Are you instructed on how to warm up and cool down?

- Does the trainer pay attention to clients and work with them, or is he or she busy getting a workout?

- Does the trainer constantly remind you about correct techniques and posture?

- Does the trainer demonstrate each exercise for you?

A number of celebrities and exercise gurus have produced exercise videos that can be bought or rented for home use. It is best to check with your doctor before beginning a home exercise program.

FINDING TIME FOR FITNESS

If you think you can't find the time for a workout, there might be some exercise hidden in your daily routine. Recent research has found that the effects of exercise are cumulative, meaning that you don't need to get your recommended twenty minutes all at once. Consider what changes you can make that will benefit your general physical fitness.

- Instead of using the elevator, take the stairs.

- Don't waste time searching for a parking space that's close by. Park farther away and walk.

- If you take the bus to work, get off one stop before and walk the rest of the way.

- Take fifteen minutes from your lunch hour and walk, indoors or out.

Exercise Addiction

It is true that you can get too much of a good thing, and exercise is no exception. Though it may seem unlikely, it is possible to become addicted to working out. Those who are addicted feel compelled to exercise and push themselves through workouts that may harm rather than help. Exercise addiction, also known as compulsive exercise, can lead to joint problems, stress fractures, and exhaustion, and it is often associated with eating disorders.

Signs of exercise addiction include working out more than fifteen hours a week; feeling tense and aggravated before a workout; feeling extremely upset or guilty when a workout is missed; and insisting on exercising despite illness or injury. Fatigue, which occurs when the body isn't given time to rest itself, is also a symptom.

An addiction to exercise often goes hand-in-hand with an eating disorder (though it may also occur independently of it). In fact, compulsive exercise is often considered a symptom of anorexia and bulimia, conditions in which weight is obsessively controlled through periods of fasting or by purging—vomiting or taking laxatives. Often, instead of purging after a food binge, many men with eating disorders exercise—often for hours on end—to get rid of any excess weight. See Weight Reduction, (p. 80.)

For more information:

Aerobic and Fitness Association of America
15250 Ventura Blvd., Suite 200
Sherman Oaks, CA 91403-3297
800-466-2322
818-905-0040

American College of Sports Medicine
P.O. Box 1440
Indianapolis, IN 46206-1440
317-637-9200
http://www.acsm.org/sportsmed

American Running and Fitness Association
4405 East West Highway, Suite 405
Bethesda, MD 20814-4535
301-913-9517
http://www.arga.org

President's Council on Physical Fitness and Sports
701 Pennsylvania Ave., N.W., Suite 250
Washington, DC 20004
202-272-3421

AEROBIC EXERCISE

Aerobic exercise, sustained exercise that raises heart and breathing rates, helps to condition the heart and the lungs, giving you greater endurance. You'll become winded less easily, burn fat faster, and benefit from improved cardiovascular health. You should do at least three twenty-minute sessions of aerobics per week, incorporating the cardiovascular training with your strength-training and flexibility programs.

Measuring Your Maximum Heart Rate

To get the most benefit from a workout, it's important to exercise at 70 percent of your age-specific maximum heart rate (MHR) for at least ten to twenty minutes per session (it takes at least fifteen minutes to get the metabolism into the fat-burning zone), with at least three sessions per week.

MHR is the maximum number of times the heart beats in one minute. To determine your age-appropriate MHR, subtract your age from 220. Since research shows that the body burns fat best when you're working at 70 percent of your MHR, multiply the result by 0.7 to find your fat-burning zone.

Choosing a Form of Exercise

Aerobic exercise includes running, bicycling, racquetball, swimming, and walking—any type of activity that boosts heart and breathing rates and keeps them there for a period of time. Varying the type of aerobic exercise can make your workout more interesting—if your workout plan includes activities you don't enjoy, you're not likely to stick to it.

You'll need to choose an activity that suits your physical needs as well. Some forms of aerobic exercise, such as running, can strain the joints with jarring movements. Most risks can be minimized with proper training; for example, runners can avoid injury by using the correct form. Proper footwear is also essential in preventing injury.

Swimming might well be the safest form of aerobic exercise. It involves no jarring or awkward motions, and the buoyancy of the water eliminates some of the pressure on joints. For these reasons, swimming is often used in the rehabilitation of injuries.

Walking is the most popular form of exercise in the United States, and it is the only exercise in which the number of participants does not decline with their age. Almost 40 percent of all walkers are men age 65 or older. Walking briskly on a regular schedule improves the body's aerobic ability—that is, the heart and lungs become more efficient at consuming oxygen and distributing it throughout the body. By increasing the body's aerobic ability, walking helps reduce blood pressure and the risk of stroke and obesity.

Walking is probably one of the best exercises for those who are interested in getting back into shape after a long bout of inactivity. Walking is just about as effective as running, but without the risk of injuries often associated with the latter. Brisk walking one mile in fifteen minutes burns just about the same number of calories as running the same distance in eight minutes. And while this walking pace is advanced, it is achievable, and this example shows what an effective exercise it can be.

BENEFITS OF WALKING

The President's Council on Physical Fitness and Sports lists the advantages of walking. They are the following:

- Almost anyone can do it. No lessons are necessary. All you need to do to become a serious walker is to step up your pace and walk more often.

- You can do it almost anywhere. The variety of settings available to this form of exercise is one reason why it is so popular. If the weather is inclement, malls are usually available.

- You can do it almost anytime. You don't have to get a partner or a team together in order to walk.

- It doesn't cost anything. You don't need to join a health club or pay a fee to become a walker. The only equipment required is a sturdy pair of walking shoes.

- You can do it alone, with a friend or spouse, or with a group, whatever suits your taste. If you enjoy interaction, you can walk with any number of people.

THE BEST EXERCISE MACHINE

The indoor treadmill, according to a 1996 study published in the *Journal of the American Medical Association*, is better at helping you burn calories than the rowing machine, stationary bicycle, cross-country skiing simulator, stair climber, or bicycle-rowing machine (Airdyne). The study measured the heart rate and levels of exertion for thirteen healthy men and women as they used the machines and found that those using the treadmill had the highest energy expenditures at any level of exertion. Experts believe that the advantage of the treadmill lies in the fact that it works the large muscle groups used for running and walking.

STRENGTH TRAINING

Strength-training exercise is the only way to build muscles and add lean body mass. Muscles grow in response to stress, which is why an effective strength-training regimen should steadily increase your weight and strength. While aerobic exercise—running, stair climbing, cycling—and flexibility training are important parts of a complete fitness program, both do little to build muscle.

Get a minimum of three thirty-minute sessions per week that involve the major muscle groups. Each session should focus on a different muscle group to prevent overtraining—muscles generally require forty-eight hours of rest between workouts.

BODY TYPE

There are three different body types, called somatotypes, that describe the shape, build, and frame of the body. Though no one falls exactly into a single category, these general guidelines can help determine how easily you'll be able to build muscle.

1. *Endomorph*. Endomorphs have a large, strong body type and can easily build muscle bulk. However, they are prone to weight gain if they don't stay in shape. The best sports for endomorphs include bicycling, rowing, and walking.

2. *Mesomorph*. Mesomorphs have strong, well-developed bones and muscles. Mesomorphs are generally lean and muscular, though they are slightly prone to weight gain if they're not in shape. Mesomorphs excel at a variety of sports.

3. *Ectomorph*. Ectomorphs have tall, thin physiques with light bones and muscles. They also have high metabolisms, meaning they burn calories quickly and may have trouble gaining weight and putting on muscle. Long-distance running is one of the best sports for ectomorphs.

If you have never done strength training before, enlist the advice of a qualified coach or trainer at a well-run gym. He or she will discuss your goals, the demands of your sport, your available time, and your current level of conditioning with you and then tailor a program to your needs. Although it is possible to do-it-yourself, a coach will teach you proper lifting form (which prevents injuries), suggest which exercises will accomplish your goals in the least amount of time, keep you from overtraining (which breaks down muscle tissue faster than it can grow back), and give you a regimen to keep you on track.

Getting the Results You Want

The type of exercises and the number of repetitions you do depends on the results you're looking for.

- If you're interested in bulk, go for more weight and fewer reps. (A rep, short for repetition, is one exercise. A set is a specific number of reps.)

- If you're interested in a muscular look, use moderate weights for roughly eight to twelve repetitions.

- If you're interested in cardiovascular endurance, use light weights for high numbers of reps.

While these signs may occur independent of overtraining, they are an indication that you should take a few days off from your training program.

The Role of Protein

It was long thought that a high-protein intake was needed to build muscles. Not only has this proven to be false, but the traditional, high-protein diet young men used (and still use) along with a strength-training program to help build strength and bulk—plenty of ice cream, milk shakes, and red meat—is also extremely high in fat (especially saturated fat) and cholesterol. And with their greater risk of premature heart disease, men of any age should control their fat and cholesterol intake.

While it is true that athletes do need more protein than sedentary people, their requirements are not much higher: 0.6 to 0.8 grams per pound of body weight, compared with 0.37 grams per pound for inactive people. Regardless of their fitness level, most Americans eat more protein every day than even elite athletes.

Not only does protein-loading deliver too much of two nutrients no one needs an excess of—fat and protein—but recent research has also shown that adding calories in the form of carbohydrates is actually more effective for building

---

SIGNS OF OVERTRAINING

With weight training, you can't double your gains simply by doubling your workout time. Muscles need time to recover between workouts, generally about forty-eight hours. Overtraining your muscles can slow your progress and lead to injury.

Signs that you may be working too hard include the following:

- Difficulty performing your usual workout

- Slow healing of cuts or bruises

- More bouts with colds and flu

- An increase in your resting heart rate of more than 10 percent

- Dizziness

- Fatigue

- Sleep disturbances

WHAT ABOUT SUPPLEMENTS?

Athletes and bodybuilders have been looking for a magic muscle-building potion since the sport began. Unfortunately, the only substances that seem to work like magic—anabolic steroids, hormonal drugs that build muscle mass—are both illegal and extremely dangerous to your health. (See Steroids, p. 78.) The quest has brought protein powders, amino acid mixes, herbal concoctions, and all sorts of exotic brews to the market as potential "safe anabolics," but most of them are pricey and all of them are more or less ineffective. The simple truth is that there is no shortcut—eating more than you need of the right foods and exercising enough but not too much are the only ways to build muscle.

According to sports nutritionist Nancy Clark, M.S., R.D., you can make your own weight-gain formula by adding 1 cup of powdered milk and four instant breakfast packets to a quart of 2 percent milk. Mix thoroughly (a whirl in the blender will help) and store in the refrigerator. Your "powered-up" milk will deliver 1,400 calories (compared with 520 from a quart of plain 2 percent milk), a hefty dose of easily-absorbed protein and calcium, and some essential B vitamins. This is exactly what you'd get in a cannister featuring some brawny guy on the label, and it costs about 90 percent less.

lean muscle mass and gaining weight. In one study, a group of weight lifters who added 830 calories a day via a high-carbohydrate liquid supplement gained 3 1/2 pounds more than the control group, who did not take the supplement. In addition, the test group doubled their lean body mass, gained more strength, and lost some body fat, while the control group stayed pretty much the same.

FLEXIBILITY

Flexibility is just as important to a proper exercise program as strength and cardiovascular training are, yet it often falls by the wayside. Flexibility helps to prevent injury, gives you a greater range of motion, and helps fight off tension and stress in the muscles. Many athletes, eager to get to the heavy weights, skip stretching exercises. Yet saving a few minutes by skimping on stretching may lead to an injury that will definitely set you back.

Flexibility exercises can be done as part of your warm-up, but they should be considered a separate part of your workout as well. Ten minutes to twelve minutes of daily stretching should be performed slowly and without a bouncy motion. You can stretch before or after working out, or in between sets. Hold a stretch for about thirty seconds—any longer probably won't do any good.

Again, ask your trainer about stretches that will complement your workout program.

SPORTS INJURIES

Men between the ages of 17 and 44 have up to 60 percent more injuries than women, and suffer most of the three to five million sports injuries incurred each year. Athletes generally sustain two types of injuries: acute trauma and overuse syndrome. Acute trauma is a sudden, violent injury such as a broken bone or torn ligament that requires the immediate attention of a doctor. Overuse syndrome results from the repeated stress on a part of the body, perhaps because of abnormal use, and can be treated without professional care.

Preventing Sports Injuries

Athletes and nonathletes who exercise regularly need to learn to recognize the symptoms of developing injuries, to prevent injuries, to treat them, and to identify conditions that require professional care. The equipment and techniques used to treat athletic injuries have become greatly sophisticated in just the last five years. But the best treatment for most sports injuries is prevention.

1. *Stretch properly.* Athletes should know that injured muscles tighten when they heal and that stretching exercises can reduce some injuries by up to 80 percent, particularly those to the calf and hamstring muscles in the back of the legs. Ten to twelve minutes of daily stretching should be performed slowly and without a bouncy motion.

2. *Learn proper form.* Athletes should learn how to exercise—whether it be when or how much to lift or proper form for running—for the best results. Exercising incorrectly is one of the major causes of sports injuries.

3. *Balance your workouts.* Athletes should learn to identify the muscles that work together and against each other, such as the quadriceps and hamstrings of the leg and try to ensure that one does not become much stronger than the other, which heightens the risk of injury.

4. *Use the right equipment.* The correct shoes and gear for a sport can go a long way toward preventing injury. Athletes should talk to a trainer, health-care practitioner, or knowledgeable salesperson about which shoes and clothes are right for them. Also, protective pads and eyewear should be used when they're called for.

First Aid for Sports Injuries

The RICE program is recommended for those times a muscle is pulled or a bruise occurs. RICE is an acronym for *r*est, *i*ce, *c*ompression, and *e*levation.

1. *Rest.* Stop exercising. Continued motion forces more blood into damaged tissue.

2. *Ice.* Apply ice to the injury to minimize swelling. Use ice continuously for the first fifteen minutes, then apply it ten minutes on and ten minutes off during the first hour. Don't apply the ice directly to your skin. Instead, wrap the ice in a towel.

3. *Compression.* Wrap an elastic bandage over the injury to help prevent local fluid accumulation. The wrap should be snug but not so tight as to cut off circulation.

4. *Elevation.* If the injury is to one of the extremities, raise the injured area above chest level. This helps blood flow back into the heart and prevents accumulation of fluid due to gravity.

Consult a doctor after beginning RICE if you suffer traumatic injury to a joint, severe pain, extreme swelling or discoloration of an injured area that doesn't improve, infection or pain in a joint or bone that lasts for more than two weeks.

Types of Sports Injuries

Following is a list of the most common types of sports injuries, along with methods of prevention and treatment.

Foot Injuries

Containing twenty-six bones and acting as interface between body and earth, the foot is vulnerable to many injuries, especially from jogging and basketball, field hockey, tennis, and other sports that require running. Injuries include the following:

- Black toenails, common among runners and hikers, occur when a blood clot or blister forms beneath the toenails because of an injury or irritation. Blood should be drained from an injured toenail; this can be done by applying heat to the top of the nail. If the nail is torn or infection or swelling occurs, a doctor should be consulted.

- Stress fractures, also called march fractures because they often affect soldiers, are incomplete cracks in a bone caused by repeated stresses of running or jumping. Prevention includes wearing cushioned shoes and avoiding hard surfaces and rapid increases in speed or distance. Treatment includes temporary cessation of the activity that caused the fractures, especially running, while switching to a new activity such as swimming or bicycling to remain

fit. Protective padding, heel cups, and in a few cases, casts can be worn. The athlete should not resume the offending activity for four to eight weeks.

(See Foot Conditions, p. 264, for information on ingrown toenails, athlete's foot, and blisters.)

Ankle Injuries

A hinge joint composed of three bones bound together by ligaments, tendons, and connective fibers, the ankle can be pushed suddenly or gradually beyond its limits of flexibility by the forces of propulsion. Injuries include the following:

- Achilles tendon injuries, also called tendinitis, affect the tendon extending from the lower calf to the heel, especially in flatfooted athletes or those with high arches. Inflammation of the blood vessels near the tendon can cause a burning sensation; inflammation of the tendon causes shooting pain during activity. An overstressed tendon may pop or rupture. Prevention includes stretching exercises. Treatment for mild or moderate symptoms includes stretching, ice application, heel lifts, avoidance of running on hills, and wearing supportive shoes. Immobility (use of a cast) and rehabilitation with physical therapy may be required in severe cases.

- Ankle sprains, graded as mild, moderate, or severe, are acute injuries occurring usually when the foot turns under the leg, stretching or tearing the ligaments. Proper treatment is necessary to avoid a chronically unstable ankle. Mild sprains can be treated with RICE (rest, ice, compression, and elevation); activity may be resumed in several days. Moderate and severe sprains should be treated by a doctor; they require immobilization, casts, crutches, and even surgery to repair ligaments. A rehabilitation program is necessary to regain strength and range of motion.

Lower-Leg Injuries

Injuries to the portion of the leg between the ankle and knee often result from repeated stresses and from relying on the leg to absorb too much stress. Injuries include the following:

- Leg length discrepancy, or short limb syndrome, results from the body's attempt to compensate for a difference as small as $^1/_4$ inch between the lengths of the two legs. The condition can be caused by a fracture during childhood, polio, congenital abnormalities, or a greater flattening in the arch of one foot. Treatment includes shoe lifts and other orthotic devices, which serve to realign the position and structure of the limb and level the pelvis.

- Muscle pulls and tears occur when muscle fibers overstretch, tear, or even rupture, causing pain, swelling, bruising, and loss of function. Muscles prone to pulls and tears include the hamstring (in the back of the thigh) in sprinters, the groin (inner thigh) in basketball players and others who must change direction quickly, the calf (lower leg) in jumpers, and the shoulder muscles in swimmers. Inadequate warm-up, overdevelopment of some muscles (muscle imbalance), overly ambitious exercise programs, accidents,

and injuries cause pulls and tears. Minor pulls can be treated by applying heat before activity and ice afterward. A moderate tear requires RICE (rest, ice, compression, and elevation) for twenty minutes three to four times a day for two to three days, after which heat treatments should replace ice. Range-of-motion exercises, preceded by stretching, may be begun. Surgical treatment and extensive rehabilitation may be required for severe tears and ruptures.

- Shin splints are tiny tears in the muscles attached to the tibia bone, the front bone in the lower leg. Pain may be felt in the front or rear portion of the leg. Shin splints may be caused by an imbalance between the stronger posterior leg muscles and the weaker anterior muscles. Other causes include running on the toes, flattening of the arches, tight anterior muscles, and insufficient shock absorption. Prevention includes strengthening and stretching exercises. Treatment includes aspirin or nonsteroidal anti-inflammatory drugs (NSAIDs) to counter inflammation, ice massages after activity, avoiding hills and hard running surfaces, temporarily reducing activity by 50 percent, and wearing athletic shoes to overcome arch flattening.

Knee Injuries

The knee, the body's largest joint, is a hinge composed of the femur (thighbone), tibia (front bone of lower leg) and fibula (rear bone of lower leg) and the patella (kneecap). The knee is vulnerable to acute trauma when perpendicular force is applied. Injuries include the following:

- Chondromalacia patella, or runner's knee, occurs when repeated stress causes inflammation and softening of the cartilage under the kneecap. Causes include a flattened, or pronated, foot that, when running, causes the lower leg to rotate inward and the kneecap to slide from side to side and rub against the groove of the femur. Prolonged sitting, weak thigh muscles, trauma, muscle imbalance, and neglected ligament injury can also aggravate the cartilage. A doctor should be consulted. Activity that causes pain should be decreased or stopped. Rest, ice, and anti-inflammatory drugs are helpful. Exercises can be done to strengthen the thighs. Abnormal foot mechanics can be corrected with orthotic devices and physiotherapy.

- Knee sprain is an injury to the ligaments that connect the bones of the knee and provide, along with muscles, tendons, and soft tissues, the knee's stability. Knee sprains are less common in running than in contact sports and skiing, which can subject the hyperextended knee to sideways trauma. Treatment depends on severity and can include rest, ice, crutches, cast immobilization, surgery, and rehabilitation.

- Patellar tendinitis, or jumper's knee, results from overuse of the tendon connecting the kneecap to the lower leg, or tibia. Frequent jumping up and down, in an activity such as basketball or volleyball, can cause pain just below the kneecap. Difficulty kneeling may also be experienced. Treatment includes rest and heat, avoiding stressful activity, and taking anti-inflammatory drugs such as aspirin. Braces may be used. Surgery may be necessary to reattach the tendon to the kneecap. Prevention is more effective. If pain is felt, vigorous kicking and jumping should be reduced, and ice, heat, and anti-inflammatory drugs should be used.

Thigh and Hip Injuries

Groin pulls, acute tears to the muscles of the inner thigh, are common among athletes who must change directions quickly while running, run in bursts, and stop and start while running straight ahead. Sudden pain accompanies the injury. Bruising from the crotch to the knee may follow, although the injury is confined to the inner thigh. Treatment includes rest, ice, compression, and elevation and a wait of one to six weeks before resumption of activity. Injured muscles tighten while healing and must be stretched gradually during rehabilitation, which consists of stretching and strength exercises.

Hamstring injuries are common among runners and other athletes such as basketball players and sprinters who must propel their legs quickly. The three hamstring muscles extend from the base of the buttock down the back of the leg to the top of the lower leg bones, the tibia and fibula. Tears and ruptures to the hamstrings can be prevented by stretching the head to the toes along a straightened leg from a sitting or standing position before activity. Bicycling strengthens the hamstrings. Treatment of hamstring injuries ranges from rest and ice to anti-inflammatory drugs, wraps, and crutches.

Lower-Back Injuries

The lower back, or lumbar region, provides strength to the hips, thighs, and torso, and also absorbs shocks and stresses that pass through the feet and legs. Overuse or abuse of the back from bending, twisting, and poor posture can cause a sore back and impinge on nerves in the spinal vertebrae. (See Back Pain, p. 173.)

The back is vulnerable to problems caused by imbalance of muscle use. Overuse of the psoas muscle, which bends the hip, can place stress on the spinal column and increase the curvature of the lower back. Tight hamstring muscles, common among long-distance runners, also contribute to lower-back problems by causing a hesitant heelstrike and transmitting more stress to the back.

Runners, especially those with sedentary jobs, should take care to condition and strengthen those muscles such as abdominal muscles that are not greatly exercised during running. This helps avoid an imbalance between overused and underused muscles.

Other Injuries and Conditions

Bursitis, in the shoulders or the hips, occurs when a lubricating sac of fluid near the joint called the bursa is inflamed during strenuous or repeated outward motions of the arm. The bursa is located near the rotator cuff, a group of muscles that cover the top of the shoulder and help stabilize it. Treatment of bursitis requires rest and anti-inflammatory drugs, followed by gentle stretching exercises. Failure to rehabilitate properly can result in frozen shoulder.

Muscle cramps occur when muscle fibers suddenly and painfully contract, usually during exercise. Cramps can last a few seconds or several hours. Causes include injury, a deficiency in salt and other minerals, especially potassium, slowing of blood supply to the muscle by repeated muscular contractions and hyperventilation.

Treatment includes gently stretching and squeezing the affected muscle and eating fruits (bananas) and vegetables (baked potatoes) to replace potassium. Salt and minerals can be restored by drinking sports drinks such as Gatorade.

Rotator cuff injuries are common among skiers and golfer as well as among baseball players, tennis players, and other athletes who engage in throwing sports. The rotator cuff, muscles that cover the shoulder, rotate the humerus (upper arm bone) and stabilize the shoulder. As they do their work, they often rub against a small shoulder bone called the acromion. The tendon can become frayed and weakened; the muscles can then tear or rupture. Treatment is rest and anti-inflammatory drugs, followed by physical therapy. Steroids are sometimes injected to reduce inflammation, but with care, as they can wear away the rotator cuff. Surgery is performed in severe cases, but it is not always effective, in part because the blood supply to the shoulder is not always generous. Prevention, by strengthening exercises and stretching before activity, is more effective than treatment.

Tennis elbow is a tear in the tendons that attach the forearm to the elbow. Pain, which is felt when the wrist straightens or bends against resistance, can occur on the inside (forehand tennis elbow) or outside (backhand tennis elbow) of the wrist. Preventive measures include using two hands for a backhand stroke, using the entire upper arm rather than just the wrist to hit the ball, switching to a lighter racket, reducing the tension of the racket strings and avoiding playing on grass and cement. Treatment is rest and ice. When healing has begun, bending and straightening the wrist while holding small weights helps strengthen the tendon.

SPORTS INJURIES BY ACTIVITY

Based upon information collected by the National Injury Information Clearinghouse and reported to the Consumer Product Safety Commission, the following activities (or their apparel or equipment) were related to the majority of sports injuries in 1995.

Activity	Number of Injuries
Basketball	692,396
Bicycling (excluding mountain biking)	549,988
Football	389,463
Baseball	210,395
Soccer	156,960
Softball	155,669
Snow skiing	126,116
In-line skating	99,550
Volleyball	86,551
Fishing	80,515
Roller-skating	75,745
Trampoline jumping	66,174
Horseback riding	65,103
Weightlifting	56,353
Wrestling	46,592
Golf	39,247
Ice-skating	37,532
Mountain biking	36,820
Swimming	36,207
Martial arts	28,199
Tennis	25,934
Ice hockey	24,869
Bowling	22,224
Track and field	15,558
Paddleball/Squash/Racquetball	13,234
Water skiing	13,103
Mountain climbing	8,735
Boxing	6,905
Rugby	6,315
Surfing	5,175
Billiards/pool	4,484
Archery	4,267
Toy sports equipment	3,446

Handball	2,653
Horseshoes	2,379
Tetherball	1,869
Scuba diving	1,184
Fencing	275

SPORTS MEDICINE: TREATING SPORTS INJURIES

The sports medicine specialty encompasses the prevention and treatment of injuries to athletes, fitness training for nonathletes, the effect of exercise on body functions, the use of exercise for recovery from nonsports injuries, drug use by athletes, and nutrition for athletes and fitness buffs.

In 1991, the first board-certification program for sports medicine was put into place, designed to improve training in sports medicine and create a recognized standard of medical compentency in the field. Sports medicine, however, has not yet been recognized by the American Board of Medical Specialties. This board, which stamps the official brand of respectability on any medical discipline, currently recognizes twenty-four mainstream medical specialties. (See Board Certification, page 428.)

Of course, there are other health-care professionals besides sports medicine specialists who are capable of handling sports injuries. Most men may initially visit a primary-care practitioner for an injury or see a emergency room physician if the injury is severe. Another option is a physiatrist, a medical specialist who handles physicial medicine and rehabilitation for conditions involving the skeleton, muslces, nerves, and other body systems. Physiatrists use nondrug and nonsurgical therapies such as exercise, hydrotherapy, ice, and heat.

There are also several professionals who are not medical doctors. A physical therapist usually works with a physician to provide treatment after an injury. Such treatments usually focus on exercise and other nondrug therapies such as massage or hydrotherapy. Occupational therapists, who often work in conjunction with physiatrists, specialize in rehabilitation for specific parts of the body, such as the hands or feet.

STEROIDS

Glossy magazine advertisements, pervasive television images, and the worship of brawny athletic heroes leave no question about society's current standard for men's muscular development: the bigger, the better. In response to the pressure to look good, American men and teenage boys are more and more frequently turning to illegal anabolic steroids to achieve the bulk they want.

Anabolic steroids are a synthetic version of testosterone, the naturally occurring male hormone that controls secondary male characteristics (such as a deep voice and facial hair) and is largely responsible for the development of skeletal muscles and fat distribution in the body. These steroids are legally prescribed to treat hypogonadism, a condition in which the testicles do not produce enough testosterone, and there are possibilities for its use as a contraceptive or a treatment for "male menopause." (See Male Menopause, page 319.) But anabolic steroids are more often used illegally, in doses a hundred times those prescribed for a therapeutic reason. In mimicking the functions of testosterone, such doses of anabolic steroids make a person bigger, faster, and stronger, adding an average of twenty to thirty pounds of muscle to a bodybuilder in a month of regular use.

According to the National Institute on Drug Abuse (NIDA), over one million Americans (mostly men) use anabolic steroids; however, this number is admittedly low because few people want to confess to using muscle-enhancing drugs. A University of Michigan study released in December 1994 found that more than 200,000 high school males took steroids within the year. Other studies between 1988 and 1994 estimated the number of teenaged users to be as high as 500,000 per year. There have been confirmed reports of children as young as age 10 using illegal steroids. The typical steroid user is middle-class, white, and male.

Dangers of Steroids

Though, on the surface, steroids produce desirable results for bodybuilders, there's a price to be paid for their use. Anabolic steroid users repeatedly dose themselves with one hundred times the testosterone the body produces naturally. Possible side effects include severe acne, fever, lethargy, dizziness, headache, early balding, and yellowing of the skin and eyes due to liver malfunction. It may also affect sexual health, causing enlarged breasts, testicular shrinkage, decrease in libido, erection problems, and sterility. Alterations in tendons, reduction of high-density lipoprotein cholesterol (the "good" cholesterol), and increased total cholesterol are also possibilities. Steroids can also curtail the development of long bones, thereby stunting a person's growth. Furthermore, steroid users who share needles run the risk of contracting HIV and hepatitis.

In addition to the physical dangers of steroids, accumulating evidence indicates that steroids can trigger psychological side effects. Along with feelings of invincibility and euphoria, steroid users may experience irritability and sudden bursts of anger accompanied by an urge to fight. These "roid rages," as they are commonly called, can grow to include such signs of mental illness as delusions and paranoia. Many steroid abusers end up in prison for violent vandalism, assault, and even murder.

Steroids are also known to increase sexual appetites. However, there is no evidence that steroids increase sexual pleasure. In fact, more cases of sexual dysfunctions, such as erection problems and difficulty achieving climax, are reported in steroid users than in nonusers.

Steroid Use

Steroids, which come in either pill or injectable form, are taken in four- to eighteen-week cycles, with breaks in between cycles. During these breaks, muscles often get smaller, which causes many steroid users to panic and take even larger doses of the drugs. Most users take a combination of three to five types of steroids at once, a practice known as "stacking." Steroid use can create a cycle of dependency in which users who try to stop become depressed and sometimes rely on recreational drugs to boost their spirits. (See Drug Abuse, p. 250.)

HISTORY OF STEROIDS

Anabolic steroids were developed in the 1930s to treat patients malnourished as a result of disease and war. Their use as performance enhancers dates back at least to the 1950s, when weight lifters in the Eastern Bloc used them to "pump up." Steroid experts believe sports and bodybuilding sensations, such as Ben Johnson and Arnold Schwarzenegger, both of whom used steroids at one time, have contributed to the increase in steroid abuse. Even though the International Olympic Committee began testing for steroid use in 1976 and the National College Athletic Association (NCAA) followed suit in 1986, the National Football League is the only one of the four major sports leagues in the United States that requires steroid testing.

Adolescents receive mixed messages from their coaches, teachers, and even parents. A 1991 statewide study in Illinois found that 21 percent of steroid users were encouraged to start using the drugs illegally by a coach or teacher. The director of an Illinois sports-medicine clinic says he receives calls from as many as a dozen parents each year inquiring about illegal performance enhancers for their children.

Although they are illegal without a prescription, anabolic steroids are seemingly more available than ever. Federal government seizures indicate that Mexico is the primary source of steroids imported into the United States. The international steroid market generates as much as $750 million yearly. Because federal sentencing guidelines are based on the amount of drugs in a trafficker's possession and a single dose of steroids is fifty pills, the threat of incarceration is not much of a deterrent for steroid traffickers.

For more information:

American Council for Drug Education
1119 Taft St.
Rockville, MD 20850
800-488-3784
301-294-0600

Drug Abuse Information and Treatment Referral
Line
11426 Rockville Pike, Suite 410
Rockville, MD 20852
800-662-4357
800-662-9832 (Spanish)
800-228-0427 (hearing impaired)

National Clearinghouse for Alcohol and Drug
Information
Substance Abuse Prevention
P.O. Box 2345
Rockville, MD 20847
800-729-6686
301-468-6433
http://www.health.org

American College of Sports Medicine
P.O. Box 1440
Indianapolis, IN 46206-1440
317-637-9200
http://www.acsm.org/sportsmed

WEIGHT REDUCTION

In 1996, the National Center for Health Statistics announced the bad news: There are now more overweight Americans than there are Americans of a healthy weight. The survey, which was conducted between 1991 and 1994, found that 59 percent of American men and 49 percent of American women are overwieght, an alarming statistic by all accounts.

Being overweight can lead to a variety of serious medical conditions, including diabetes, high blood pressure, coronary heart disease, and stroke—especially for men. This greater risk occurs because men tend to accumulate excess fat in their abdomens and upper torsos, creating a potbelly or an "apple-shaped" body. Because the abdominal fat is in close proximity to the heart and more likely to interfere with the heart, this "apple" pattern significantly raises the risk of coronary-artery disease. Women, on the other hand, tend to accumulate fat deposits on the hips, buttocks, and thighs (creating a "pear-shaped" body), which does not increase the risk of heart disease as much.

Guidelines for a Healthy Weight

Through the years, the guidelines for a healthy weight have changed somewhat. While at one time it was thought that a reasonable amount of weight gain was natural and even healthy over the years, today's standards show that—no matter how old you are—the less you gain, the better.

The first weight recommendations were created in the 1940s. They were based on charts created by insurance companies that analyzed which policyholders lived longest. These charts received criticism because they did not include a breakdown by age or bone structure, only by height. In 1990, the "Age-Adapted Healthy Weight" chart was developed, breaking the information down by age group and height. However, critics say the data of the new charts, like that of previous ones, is based solely on statistics of people who are insured and presents an incomplete—if not inaccurate—conclusion about optimal body weight.

To estimate your ideal healthy weight, consult the chart, reading for your age and your height.

Age-Adapted Healthy Weights for Men

Years

Height	20–29	30–39	40–49	50–59	60–69
4' 10"	84–111	92–119	99–127	107–135	115–142
4' 11"	87–115	95–123	103–131	111–139	119–147
5' 0"	90–119	98–127	106–135	114–143	123–152
5' 1"	93–123	101–131	110–140	118–148	127–157
5' 2"	96–127	105–136	113–144	122–153	131–163
5' 3"	99–131	108–140	117–149	126–158	135–168
5' 4"	102–135	112–145	121–154	130–163	140–173
5' 5"	106–140	115–149	125–159	134–168	144–179
5' 6"	109–144	119–154	129–164	138–174	148–184
5' 7"	112–148	122–159	133–169	143–179	153–190
5' 8"	116–153	126–163	137–174	147–184	158–196
5' 9"	119–157	130–168	141–179	151–190	162–201
5' 10"	122–162	134–173	145–184	156–195	167–207
5' 11"	126–167	137–178	149–190	160–201	172–213
6' 0"	129–171	141–183	153–195	165–207	177–219
6' 1"	133–176	145–188	157–200	169–213	182–225
6' 2"	137–181	149–194	162–206	174–219	187–232
6' 3"	141–186	153–199	166–212	179–225	192–238
6' 4"	144–191	157–205	171–218	184–231	197–244

Source: National Institutes of Health

Another way to determine if what you weigh is a health risk is to estimate your body mass index (BMI) and waist-to-hip ratio. To find your BMI, multiply your weight in pounds by 700. Divide that figure by your height in inches. Take that figure and divide by your height in inches again to arrive at your BMI. If your BMI is 25 or less, your risk for heart disease is very low to low. If it is between 25 and 30, your risk is low to moderate. If your BMI is 30 or above, your risk is moderate to high.

To determine the waist-to-hip ratio, take a tape measure and measure the circumference of your waist at its narrowest point with your stomach relaxed. Next, measure the circumference of your hips at their widest part. Divide the waist measurement by the hip measurement. You are considered to be at low risk for heart disease if the ratio is less than 0.95. However, your risk increases the greater the ratio above 0.95.

Reasons for Weight Gain

The most common reason for being overweight is eating more calories than you expend. According to the American Heart Association, 25 percent of Americans over age 18 report no physical activity during leisure time, and 33 percent of overweight men are not physically active during leisure time.

Even though it is now generally accepted that there are genetic influences on body weight and that a relatively slow metabolism may contribute to obesity, such conditions are actually quite rare, affecting only a small number of men. Chances are, you are not one of them.

Men tend to start gaining weight in their thirties because they do not realize that they can no longer eat the way they did in their teens and twenties. A sedentary job, long commute, too many restaurant meals, too much TV watching, and too much alcohol all add up to too many calories and too little exercise. In addition, the basal metabolic rate, the rate at which the body burns fuel, begins to decline—though only about 2 percent a decade—after about age 30.

This causes the ratio of lean body tissue (that is, muscle) to adipose tissue (fat) to shift. Since muscle burns energy and fat does not, this means that the number of calories being burned drops. The cycle continues as more fat is created by eating more calories than are burned, which in turn lowers the number of calories that are burned, which makes more fat, and so on. So when a man, especially one who was lean, muscular, and active in his teens and twenties, keeps eating later in life as though neither his metabolism or lifestyle has changed, the result is middle-aged spread.

The Road to Weight Loss

The way to get rid of unwanted pounds is simple: Eat less and exercise more.

Eat Less

Eating less doesn't mean that you should drastically cut back on your food intake or switch to a diet of weight loss shakes and formulated meals. In fact, the chief reason most reducing diets fail is because they are too strict and too limited in food choices, making it hard for anyone to stick to them. Sudden, drastic weight loss—such as that achieved by liquid fasting diets—is seldom, if ever, lasting. Think of Dodgers manager Tommy Lasorda, portly again after his much publicized ultrafast weight loss, and now suffering from heart disease as well.

Gradual modification of eating patterns results in healthier, sustainable changes in food habits, as well as a slow, steady reduction in body weight. (See Diet and Nutrition, p. 41.) Aim to reduce your food intake by 200 calories a day per week until you are consuming no more calories than your basal metabolic requirements. Here are some simple ways to cut calories and build a better diet:

1. Watch for fat. Try to get less than 30 percent of your calories from fat— preferably unsaturated rather than saturated fats. Check for calories as well— some low-fat and nonfat products are extremely high in calories because manufacturers tend to include more sugars to make up for the missing flavor of the fat.

2. Measure portions. Big helpings are as much a culprit in excess weight as eating the wrong foods. To determine what makes a proper serving, use the serving size on the Nutrition Facts label as a guide or purchase a calorie-counter book. Then, measure or weigh each portion before eating. After a while, you won't need to measure—you'll be able to portion out the appropriate serving size by sight and feel.

3. Eat slowly. It takes up to 20 minutes after you've eaten enough for your mind to realize that you're not hungry anymore. If you eat quickly, you're almost sure to be eating more than you need. Begin with a small portion, then wait to see if you're satisfied before taking a second helping. You might also start a meal with a salad or low-fat appetizer that might help you feel full sooner.

4. Use cooking methods that don't add fat: broiling, steaming, baking, or microwaving. Never fry foods, and saute only in water or broth.

5. Use only nonfat milk and dairy products. Try to stick to soft-spread margarines that

list water—not hydrogenated vegetable oil—as their first ingredient. These have less fat and fewer trans fatty acids than regular margarine or butter.

6. Eat at least eight servings a day of high-fiber carbohydrate foods such as fruits, vegetables, and whole-grain breads and cereals. Complex carbohydrates aren't quickly stored within the body as fat and are thought to reduce the craving for fats.

7. Drink at least eight glasses of water a day.

8. Avoid alcohol, which not only provides a lot of empty calories, but appears to slow down the burning of calories from food.

EATING DISORDERS

If you think that eating disorders are limited to women, you should know that the first person ever diagnosed with an eating disorder was a man. Today it is estimated that 10 percent of Americans with anorexia and bulimia are men and that 40 percent of those with binge-eating disorder are men. In some 6 percent of the estimated 8 million cases of eating disorders in men and women in the United States, the disorder results in death.

Eating disorders are caused by a combination of psychological, sociological, and biological factors, including low self-esteem, depression and mood disorders, substance abuse, childhood physical and sexual abuse. Eating disorders often develop after dieting or because of intensive athletic training.

The three types of eating disorders are anorexia nervosa, bulimia, and binge-eating disorder (also called compulsive overeating). Anorexia is marked by a fear of becoming fat, severe weight loss, and a distorted body image. Those with anorexia eat very little or not at all. Bulimia, also called binge-purge disorder, involves compulsively eating large amounts of food and then purging it through forced vomiting, use of laxatives, or excessive exercise. Those with bulimia usually maintain a normal weight. A man with binge-eating disorder eats frequently and repeatedly, feeling out of control. Binge eaters are generally obese. These eating disorders can result in permanent physical damage or death. Side effects include heart, liver, and kidney damage; muscle loss; anemia; malnutrition; and reproductive and emotional problems.

continues

If an eating disorder is suspected, treatment should be sought immediately. Though men tend to avoid treatment for what's considered a "female" problem, more men are receiving help—in the way of psychotherapy and medical treatment—than ever before.

For more information:

American Anorexia/Bulimia Association
165 W. 46th St., Suite 1108
New York, NY 10036
212-575-6200
http://members.aol.com/AmAnBu

Anorexia Nervosa and Related Eating Disorders, Inc.
P.O. Box 5102
Eugene, OR 97405
541-344-1144
http://www.anred.com

Take Off Pounds Sensibly (TOPS)
4575 S. Fifth St.
Milwaukee, WI 53207
800-932-8677

Exercise More

It is necessary to exercise aerobically while cutting calories to counter the natural slow-down in metabolism that occurs when we eat less. Aerobic exercise is sustained exercise that helps to build heart and lung capacity. Not only does aerobic exercise such as walking, swimming, running, or cycling stimulate metabolism and burn calories, but it may also inhibit the appetite temporarily. Aerobic exercise also has beneficial impact on mood and helps improve cardiovascular health, bone strength, and flexibility, making for better overall health. (See Aerobic Exercise, page 66.)

Anaerobic exercises such as weight training and sprinting strengthen the muscles, but do not usually strengthen the heart or lungs or burn fat. However, stronger muscles require more energy to function on a daily basis, meaning that you'll burn more calories overall—even when you're sitting or sleeping. Recent research has demonstrated the value of weight training as an aid to weight control, particularly in middle-aged people. In addition, weight training results in muscle tone, which helps restore a more youthful figure. (See Strength Training, page 68.)

You should aim for at least twenty to thirty minutes of aerobic exercise three times a week, working up to longer, more frequent sessions as you become more comfortable. Weight-training exercises, along with flexibility exercises, should be combined with aerobic activities for a good, overall workout. (See Physical Fitness, page 59.)

Like reducing food intake, exercise becomes a lasting habit if you begin moderately—don't start out by trying to run five miles, or even one. Exercise is most effective at aiding weight loss when it is done steadily and consistently—daily for thirty minutes is far more effective than three hours on Saturday.

HOW MANY CALORIES DO YOU NEED?

The average 30-year-old man who does no exercise training needs 13 calories per pound of body weight to maintain his weight. Thus a 160 pound man that age can eat 2,080 calories a day without gaining weight. But the basal metabolic rate slows about 2 percent every decade past age 30, so a 60 year old man who weighs 160 lb. actually needs 6 percent fewer calories, or 1,955 per day. Of course, if that 60-year-old man walks two miles in an hour every day, he could eat about 250 more calories and not gain weight.

For more information:

American Dietetic Association
216 W. Jackson Blvd., Suite 800
Chicago, IL 60606
800-366-1655
312-899-0040

American Obesity Association
401 N. Michigan Ave.
Chicago, IL 60611
800-98-OBESE

Weight Watchers International
175 Crossways Park W.
Woodbury, NJ 11797
516-390-1400

Take Off Pounds Sensibly (TOPS)
4575 S. Fifth St.
Milwaukee, WI 53207
800-932-8677

Weight Control Information Network
1 WIN Way
Bethesda, MD 20892-3665
800-WIN-8098
301-951-1107
http://www.niddk.nih.gov/NutritionDocs.html

CAFFEINE

Legend has it that people have been enjoying caffeine since as early as 2700 B.C., when Chinese Emperor Shen Nungtea sipped hot brewed tea. Coffee originated in Africa around A.D. 575 but was considered "the devil's brew" by some Westerners until the late 1500s, when Pope Clement VIII declared a liking for it and gave it his blessing.

Caffeine, known chemically as 1,3, 7-trimethylxanthine, is a mild stimulant found naturally in the leaves, seeds, or fruits of more than 60 plants, including coffee and cocoa beans, kola nuts, and tea leaves, and is consequently found in coffee, colas, chocolate, and tea. It is a psychoactive drug that can improve clearheadedness, promote happiness and calmness, and decrease tension. Other possible effects of caffeine include increases in heartbeat, respiration, metabolic rate, and production of stomach acid and urine, as well as quickened reaction time and prolonged alertness.

The Benefits of Caffeine

The mood- and performance-enhancing properties of caffeine have their benefits. Research shows that athletes, for example, have more energy and stamina after drinking caffeinated coffee—the reason the international Olympic committee has banned athletes with high blood-caffeine levels from competition. Caffeine also has some medicinal effects. Aspirin combined with caffeine is thought to relieve pain more quickly than aspirin alone. Caffeine has also been shown to have a decongestant effect on those with colds, help prevent and treat asthma, and possibly relieve some of the effects of jet lag.

Caffeine may also have a positive effect on your sex life, especially in your later years. In a

Caffeine Content

Have you ever wondered how much caffeine you're really getting in that cup of coffee or can of soda? Here's a rundown of the average caffeine levels for some common items:

Product	Mg.
NoDoz (maximum strength) or Vivarin (1)	200
Coffee, brewed, (8 oz.)	135
Coffee, instant (8 oz.)	95
Espresso (2 oz.)	70
Cappuccino (16 oz.)	70
Anacin (2)	65
Cola (20 oz.)	60
Mountain Dew (12 oz.)	55
Tea, leaf or bag (8 oz.)	50
Hot chocolate (8 oz.)	5
Decaffeinated coffee (8 oz.)	5

survey of 2,000 men and women over the age of 60 published in the *Archives of Internal Medicine*, researchers found that coffee drinkers were much more likely to be sexually active than those who avoided the brewed beverage. Among men, the researchers found that 59 percent of those who didn't drink coffee admitted to occasional impotence, compared with 36 percent of coffee drinkers. (However, the caffeine-sex correlation could be nothing more than coincidence because researchers failed to ask the subjects if they drank caffeinated or decaffeinated coffee.)

Another group of studies has shown that caffeine added to sperm in laboratory dishes can give sperm cells a jolt that increases both their speed and liveliness, suggesting a way to improve chances of conception during *in vitro* fertilization.

The Down Side of Caffeine

But caffeine has as many drawbacks as it does benefits. Athletes who expect to benefit from its effects, for example, suffer from long-term use. This is because caffeine speeds you up by speeding up your heart and respiration rates, which can leave you even more tired when the drug wears off. Caffeine also has a dehydrating effect, which can be draining for athletes. Dehydration is the enemy of travelers as well, and makes it hard to adjust to new time zones, cancelling out its jet-lag benefits. And contrary to popular belief, beverages and food containing caffeine will not sober up an intoxicated person.

While it's true that a little caffeine can provide a harmless "quick fix," too much caffeine can make you ill. The diagnostic manual for psychiatrists, *DSM-IV*, defines "caffeine intoxication" as a mental disorder characterized by restlessness, insomnia, and nervousness, which causes "significant distress" in one's social and occupational functioning. Caffeine doses of more than 750 mg. can cause a panic reaction: fear, ringing ears, and flashes of light.

Caffeine can also react with certain drugs to cause harmful side effects. Antihypertensives, antidepressants, nicotine replacements, and ulcer drugs may all interact with caffeine. If you are taking any prescription or over-the-counter drugs, check with your doctor or pharmacist on the possibility of an interaction.

Some people are much more sensitive to caffeine than others and, therefore, will feel its effects more quickly. In addition, regular caffeine consumption increases one's tolerance, thereby lessening the drug's effects. Caffeine does not accumulate in the bloodstream or body; normally, it exits the body within several hours of consumption, leaving a person feeling "down" and in need of another jolt.

Although caffeine is addictive—some experts say as addictive as crack or heroin—it is very different from drugs of dependence. Caffeine is not taken in steadily increased doses, and it is not difficult to stop consuming it. People who make a sudden, substantial reduction in their daily caffeine intake may experience temporary withdrawal symptoms: headaches, depression, anxiety, fatigue, and irritability; however, they can avoid these symptoms by gradually decreasing their caffeine intake over several days. Furthermore, unlike drug abuse, caffeine consumption is not linked with antisocial behavior.

Caffeine and Your Health

Coffee consumption in the United States peaked in 1962 at 3.12 cups per person per day and has declined steadily for three decades, despite the barrage of coffee shops that now dot the nation from coast to coast. Because of its long-standing popularity—80 percent of American adults consume about 200 mg. each day (the equivalent of two five-ounce cups of regular coffee)—much scientific research has been done to determine the effects of caffeine on the body. While the results have at times been contradictory and confusing, for the most part, the findings have been good news for caffeine drinkers.

In 1987, the U.S. Food and Drug Administration (FDA) reported that, after reviewing the results of scientific research on caffeine, it "found no evidence to show that the use of caffeine in carbonated beverages would render these beverages injurious to health." In January 1994, the American Medical Association (AMA) reaffirmed the results of a 1984 AMA Council on Scientific Affairs report that stated, "Moderate tea or coffee drinkers probably need have no concern for their health relative to their caffeine consumption provided other lifestyle habits (diet, alcohol consumption) are moderate, as well."

Studies on caffeine have focused on the following health concerns:

1. *Heart disease.* Most scientific research has found no connection between moderate caffeine consumption—fewer than four or five cups a day—and heart disease. In 1989 the National Research Council on Diet and Health said evidence linking the two is "weak and inconsistent." A 1989

report from the well-respected Framingham Heart Study, the longest-running heart study in the United States, found no link between caffeine and heart attacks, and a 1990 Harvard University study confirmed this finding. However, cardiac trouble may begin at five or more five-ounce cups of coffee a day, especially in people with high blood pressure.

2. *Blood pressure.* Although both the National Institutes of Health and the American Heart Association report that increased blood pressure associated with moderate caffeine use is slight, it is important to note that men with mild hypertension (high blood pressure) who mix caffeine and exercise could induce a dangerous rise in blood pressure.

3. *Cholesterol level.* Until recently, scientists believed that caffeine could raise blood-cholesterol levels. But a team of Dutch researchers has found that although unfiltered coffee can raise blood-cholesterol levels, caffeine is not to be blamed. The culprit is cafestol, an alcohol found in suspended coffee-bean particles and in oil droplets that float on the surface of unfiltered coffee. Filtering coffee removes the cafestol. However, increasingly popular brews such as espresso, Scandinavian-style boiled coffee, and Turkish coffee are chock full of the harmful substance. If you must have your espresso, drink it only occasionally in limited amounts, or—better yet—pass it through a filter first.

A Stanford University study sponsored by the National Institutes of Health signals potentially bad news for decaffeinated coffee drinkers. Research

suggests that decaf is more likely than caffeinated brew to raise levels of artery-damaging LDL cholesterol. The study's director said stronger-flavored coffee beans, known as robusta, used to compensate for flavor lost in the decaffeinating process, may be at fault. These beans are also used in instant coffees with and without caffeine. Most brewed caffeine-rich coffee is prepared from milder arabica beans. As of yet, no other studies have confirmed this finding.

4. *Cancer.* Despite numerous scientific investigations, speculation that caffeine could be a cancer risk has not been confirmed. In 1981, a group of Harvard researchers reported that coffee (with and without caffeine) was linked to pancreatic cancer, but at least seven major studies done since then found no such correlation. After further analyzing their data, the researchers retracted their findings.

An inverse relationship has been found between coffee consumption and cancers of the colon and rectum. One study of 1,255 cancer cases and 3,883 matched patients with unrelated conditions found that those who drank at least five cups of coffee per day had a 40 percent lower risk of developing colon cancer.

An ongoing debate exists about the relationship, or lack of a relationship, between coffee consumption and bladder cancer. An initial study linked the two; however, the risk factor involved was later found to be cigarette smoking, not coffee. After extensive analysis of 35 studies, Yale University researchers concluded in 1993 that, indeed, moderate coffee consumption was not a risk factor for bladder cancer. But a subsequent study linked heavy coffee consumption to bladder cancer in nonsmokers.

Nevertheless, the American Cancer Society's position on caffeine is that "there is no indication that [it]...is a risk factor in human cancer."

A FEW COFFEE TIPS

- Practice moderation. Based on current findings of scientific research on caffeine, it's safe to say "drink up"—just don't overdo it. If you find that you're particularly sensitive to caffeine and its effects are bothersome, use common sense: avoid it.

- Don't rely on coffee for your energy. While coffee may make you feel more energetic for a short time, in the end you'll be left even more tired than usual. Get your energy instead from a balanced diet and exercise program.

- If you swear off coffee, cut back slowly. Sudden withdrawal can lead to headaches, nervousness, and depression.

- Watch the fat. While coffee is fat free, you're adding fat and calories when you ask for milk and sugar. Cappuccino, latte, and other dessert coffees may have as much fat and calories as ice cream.

CHOLESTEROL

Cholesterol is a confusing subject. You hear that it's bad for you—then you find out that certain types of it are good for you. You're told to stay away from foods high in cholesterol, but then you find out that cholesterol you eat may have little bearing on your blood levels of the stuff. And what exactly is cholesterol anyway?

For starters, cholesterol is a soft, fatlike waxy substance found in all of the body's cells. Cholesterol is not a fat, but a closely related substance that belongs to a class of compounds called sterols. The body uses cholesterol to form cell membranes, certain hormones, and other necessary substances. Cholesterol is present in the body's tissue and in the bloodstream. Serum cholesterol is the name for the level of cholesterol in the blood.

Despite the fact that the body needs cholesterol, too much can mean trouble. Most medical experts agree that high blood-cholesterol levels are linked to the formation of atherosclerosis (accumulation of fatty tissue on the inside of the arteries) and with it coronary heart disease or stroke. High cholesterol is a major risk factor of heart disease, which kills 500,000 Americans each year and is the most frequent cause of death in men over age 35. According to the American Heart Association, 53.6 percent of non-Hispanic white males, 47.1 percent of non-Hispanic black males, and 48.8 Mexican-American males have high total cholesterol levels, that is, 200 mg/dl (milligrams per deciliter of blood) or higher.

Other risk factors of heart disease include smoking, obesity, high blood pressure, diabetes, and folic acid (a B vitamin) deficiency.

Lipoproteins

Being so closely related to fat, cholesterol doesn't dissolve in water, the major component of blood, and cannot move through the blood on its own accord. Instead, it attaches to protein to travel, forming lipoproteins. (*Lipo* means "fat," and cholesterol is a fatlike substance.)

The principal lipoproteins are high-density lipoproteins (HDL) and low-density lipoproteins (LDL). The small intestine and liver manufacture and release HDL into the bloodstream. HDL then carries cholesterol back to the liver to be processed and disposed. Because this lipoprotein escorts excess cholesterol from the body and helps to excrete it, HDL is called "good" cholesterol, and therefore, a high level of HDL in the body is desirable.

Low-density lipoprotein carries cholesterol to cells in the body where it is used to form cell membranes. However, if there is more cholesterol available than cells can take up and use, LDL ends up circulating in the bloodstream until, eventually, the cholesterol sticks and accumulates on the inside of arteries, forming plaque. It is this role of artery clogger that earns LDL cholesterol the name "bad" cholesterol. A low LDL cholesterol level, therefore, is desirable.

You can remember which cholesterol is good and which is bad by associating the "H" in HDL with "healthy" and the "L" in LDL with "lousy."

Atherosclerosis

The technical name for clogged arteries is atherosclerosis. This condition is characterized by an accumulation of plaque, a substance made up of LDL cholesterol and other cellular waste products, on the artery walls. This build-up causes the arteries to become thicker, harder, less flexible, and less efficient at transporting blood. If plaque occurs in the arteries feeding the heart muscle, blood flow to the heart may be restricted, and chest pain (called angina) can result. If blood flow is drastically impaired, bleeding or the formation of a blood clot may occur. If either of these happen and completely block the flow of blood, a heart attack or stroke may result.

TRIGLYCERIDES

Triglycerides are often discussed along with cholesterol. While they're not related to cholesterol—triglycerides are also fats, but they have a different chemical structure—they can affect cholesterol levels in the blood and increase the risk of heart disease.

Triglycerides, found in animal fats and plant oils, provide your body with fats that can be burned for energy or deposited in your body's fat stores for later use. They don't stick to artery walls. However, high levels of triglycerides go hand-in-hand with low levels of the good HDL cholesterol and often with high levels of the bad LDL cholesterol. A triglyceride level of more than 500 mg. is borderline high, while levels of 200 mg. or lower are considered normal.

The Helsinki Heart Study found that people with high triglyceride levels and no other risk factors had a 50 percent increased risk for coronary-artery disease, compared with people with normal levels. In those who had high triglyceride levels and low HDL levels, a threefold risk of coronary-artery disease was found.

Cholesterol Levels

In the past, cholesterol level guidelines focused on total cholesterol levels. However, recent research suggests that it is the proportions of HDL and LDL to total cholesterol that provide a more accurate indication of risk. In other words, the problem is not how much cholesterol there is in the system, but how it circulates and whether it is in the form of HDL or LDL.

The conservative recommendation for minimum heart disease risk is a total cholesterol level under 200 mg/dl, preferably in the 160 to 180 range. But recent studies suggest that total cholesterol tests are a crude measurement and inaccurate indicator of health risks.

Most experts now favor tests that give the proportions of "good" and "bad" cholesterol to total cholesterol. The real danger does not seem to be a high total cholesterol level, but, rather, a low HDL and a high LDL level. If total cholesterol is high because of a high LDL level, then risk factors are likely. However, if total cholesterol is high because of high HDL, then there usually is not a need for concern.

Because the test that isolates LDL levels is costly, some physicians may simply test for HDL and total cholesterol, thereby determining the ratio of HDL to total cholesterol. (LDL may be calculated by subtracting HDL from total cholesterol.) Medical guidelines suggest a ratio of 3.5 (total cholesterol divided by HDL) as desirable, 3.5 to 6.9 as having a moderate risk, and anything over 7.0 as dangerous. Dropping cholesterol levels doesn't clean out existing plaque from arteries, but new studies show it appears to make the fatty build-up less likely to form the clots that cause heart attacks.

What Should Your Cholesterol Level Be?		
Risk	*LDL Cholesterol*	*Total Cholesterol*
Men with heart disease	100 mg/dl or less	160 mg/dl or less
Men with no heart disease but with two or more risk factors	under 130 mg/dl	under 200 mg/dl
Men with no heart disease and fewer than two risk factors	under 160 mg/dl	under 240 mg/dl

These are the cholesterol levels recommended by the National Cholesterol Education Program, 1993.

THE ELDERLY AND CHOLESTEROL

In June 1996 the General Accounting Office (GAO) of the U.S. federal government issued a report stating that existing research provides little or no evidence of benefits of cholesterol-lowering treatments in the elderly. The report—which was initiated to evaluate the National Heart, Lung and Blood Institute's National Cholesterol Education Program guidelines—emphasized that more studies are needed to determine if cholesterol treatment in the elderly population, as well in women and minority groups, is worthwhile. And although the GAO report acknowledges that studies have proven that cholesterol-lowering treatments benefit middle-aged white men who have high cholesterol and heart disease, it concludes that the expense of drug treatment is not justified in other cases.

In a response to a draft of the report, the National Heart, Lung and Blood Institute disputed the GAO report and insisted that there's much indirect evidence that suggests potential benefits of treatment in the elderly, women, and minorities. The institute added that the GAO report places insufficient emphasis on recent studies that show that men with high cholesterol and no symptoms of heart disease benefit from treatment as well. In conclusion, the institute contends that an extensive body of evidence "provides a sound scientific basis for the National Cholesterol Education Program and its central guidelines."

Controlling Cholesterol Levels

Diet

Many studies have shown that you can significantly lower your risk of heart disease and perhaps live longer by reducing your cholesterol level. One of the most significant ways to begin to lower your cholesterol level is through diet. (See Diet and Nutrition, p. 41.)

Most doctors believe that too much fat in the diet, especially saturated fat, plays a major role in raising cholesterol levels in the body. This is because saturated fats have been found to raise blood levels of LDL cholesterol by inhibiting the uptake of LDL by the cells. The main component of whole milk, butter, cheese, and the white marbling in meats is saturated fat.

There is some controversy over whether eating cholesterol affects the levels of cholesterol in the blood. Dietary cholesterol is found in animal products such as meat, eggs, milk, yogurt, and cheese. The American Heart Association recommends no more than 300 mg. of cholesterol a day from food, the equivalent of three to four large eggs a week. The average man gets about 450 mg. of cholesterol in his diet per day.

There have, however, been studies that show some people can eat unlimited dietary cholesterol with little or no effect on their blood-cholesterol level. Nevertheless, most practitioners tell the majority of their patients to eat a low-fat, low-cholesterol diet—just in case. (Keep in mind that many foods containing dietary cholesterol also have significant amounts of saturated fat.)

TYPES OF FATS

1. Saturated fats are solid at room temperature. They are the main component of the white marbling in meats, of the visible fat around meat, of butter and cheese, and of whole milk and ice cream. Saturated fats are also plentiful in coconut oil, palm-kernel oil, and palm oil, three plant oils widely used in commercial baked goods like cookies and crackers. These fats raise blood levels of LDL cholesterol.

2. Trans fatty acids, contained in margarine and vegetable shortening, act in ways similar to saturated fats—they raise LDL cholesterol levels.

3. Polyunsaturated fats are liquid at room temperature and are the predominant fat in common vegetable oils, such as corn, safflower, sunflower, cottonseed, soybean, and walnut oils. These oils were once thought to reduce cholesterol levels. However, research now suggests that while polyunsaturated fats don't raise "bad" (LDL) cholesterol levels, they lower "good" (HDL) cholesterol levels.

4. Monounsaturated fats, the predominant fats in olive and canola oil, seem to lower levels of "bad" (LDL) cholesterol levels without dropping "good" (HDL) cholesterol levels.

LOWER YOUR CHOLESTEROL

Here are some more tips to help lower your blood-cholesterol level:

- Eat fewer calories, because losing weight helps. It isn't as important as other risk factors, but it shouldn't be ignored.

- Limit your dietary fat intake to 30 percent or less of your daily calories.

- Eat foods rich in fiber. A word of caution here: Although there is research to support the popular—and commercially successful—notion that daily servings of oat bran can help reduce cholesterol, such findings also indicate that the amount needed to do so are somewhere around six cups a day. Furthermore, oat bran and other fibers may combine with calcium in the stomach to form a substance that your body cannot absorb.

- Eat more fruits and vegetables and replace saturated fats with monounsaturated fats.

- Get yourself a chart of foods and their dietary cholesterol content and place a ceiling of 300 mg. a day on your meals, as suggested by the American Heart Association.

Exercise

Studies indicate that physical activity can help prevent heart disease. Specifically, exercise raises blood levels of "good" HDL cholesterol. How much it goes up depends on your initial cholesterol level, age, weight, and amount of body fat, as well as the intensity of your workouts. If you begin to lose weight as you exercise, you'll also probably see a drop in LDL cholesterol, and you may reduce your risk of developing diabetes or high blood pressure—two other major risk factors for heart disease.

Cholesterol-Lowering Drugs

If diet and exercise are not enough to lower your cholesterol to recommended levels, your physician may add cholesterol-lowering medication to your regimen. In some cases, medications may be prescribed from the beginning of treatment.

Because of the findings of a recent study—the Scandinavian Simvastatin Survival Study, or "4S" study—many physicians are prescribing a new, potent class of drugs called HMG CoA reductase inhibitors.

In that study, simvastatin (Zocor), a type of reductase inhibitor, performed impressively. It reduced the overall risk of death by 30 percent and decreased the risk of death from heart attack by 42 percent. It also cut people's risk of having to undergo bypass surgery. Following these impressive findings, the Food and Drug Administration in July 1995, allowed Zocor's maker, Merck, to relabel this drug as the first anticholesterol drug that reduces deaths and prevents heart attacks in people with heart disease and high cholesterol.

Another HMG CoA reductase inhibitor, pravastatin, has been found to rapidly reduce the risk of a first-time heart attack in people with high cholesterol. The West of Scotland Coronary Prevention Study found that treatment with pravastatin lowered the risk of having a first-time heart attack by 31 percent and the risk of death by 22 percent. This study extends prior research that demonstrated that the drug significantly lowered the risk of heart attack in patients with high cholesterol and diagnosed heart disease.

HMG CoA reductase inhibitors are generally well tolerated. However, they should not be taken by people with liver disease, and it occasionally can cause muscle disease. The most common side effects are skin rashes and gastrointestinal upset. Further studies are needed to determine the effects of long-term usage.

Another group of drugs used to lower cholesterol is called bile acid binding resins. These synthetic resins come as a powder to be mixed with liquid, called cholestyramine (Questran), or as a bar, called colestipol (Cholybar), that has to be chewed thoroughly. Studies have shown that these drugs, which have fewer side effects than other cholesterol-lowering drugs, reduce the chance of developing heart disease. Because of their safety record, they are often the first choice for people with high LDL cholesterol, especially young adult men with high LDL cholesterol and no other risk factors of heart disease. Possible side effects of bile acid binding resins include constipation and hardened stools.

For many years, the consensus among experts was that only if dietary therapy and weight loss regimen have failed over the course of a year or so should drugs be used, and that except in dire emergencies, they should not be the first treatment turned to. However, new research is growing that aggressively fighting cholesterol in heart disease patients by dropping cholesterol quickly and to ultra-low levels is critical.

For more information:

American Dietetic Association
216 W. Jackson Blvd., Suite 800
Chicago, IL 60606
800-366-1655
312-899-0040

American Heart Association
7272 Greenville Ave.
Dallas, TX 75231
800-AHA-USA1
214-373-6300
http://www.amhrt.org

National Cholesterol Education Program
NHLBI Information Center
P.O. Box. 30105
Bethesda, MD 20824-0105
800-575-WELL

SMOKING

The nicotine in cigarettes is, research shows, as addictive as heroin or cocaine, and it has some startling effects on the mind. For one, nicotine increases the levels of certain brain chemicals, stimulating feelings of reward and well-being. Smoking also helps people to perform tasks more easily, reducing hunger and anxiety and improving memory while increasing a tolerance for pain.

But for all of the minor pleasures of smoking, there are more than enough serious hazards. Smoking causes lung diseases such as chronic bronchitis, which is inflammation of the airways, and emphysema, an irreversible condition in which lung tissue breaks down, making breathing difficult. Nicotine is a stimulant, meaning it can prolong stress. And, of course, smoking also causes lung cancer—in fact, it is responsible for 90 percent of lung cancer cases in men. (See Lung Cancer, p. 202.)

Then there's the risk of heart disease. Smoking speeds the development of atherosclerosis,

in which deposits of fat, cholesterol, and other substances (called plaque deposits) collect on the walls of the arteries, restricting the flow of blood. In addition, nicotine increases heart rate, raising blood pressure in the narrowed blood vessels. According to the American Heart Association, smokers are more than twice as likely to suffer from a heart attack than nonsmokers are, and are more likely to die suddenly (within an hour) from a heart attack than a nonsmoker. In addition, smoking reduces the amount of oxygen in the blood and increases its thickness, increasing the risk of blood clots and stroke.

RATES OF SMOKING

In October 1991, the National Cancer Institute and the American Cancer Society started working together on the American Stop Smoking Intervention Study, or ASSIST, a national effort to curb smoking. As part of the study, a nationwide census of smokers was undertaken. Here are some of the findings:

- The national smoking rate was 26.8 percent for adult men and 21.8 percent for adult women.

- The rate of smoking among men varies, according to the region of the country. The rate for the South is the highest, at 29.1 percent, followed by the Midwest at 28.2 percent, the West at 24.1 percent, and the Northeast at 24 percent.

- When the regions are further broken down into divisions, statistics show that men in Kentucky, Tennessee,

continues

Alabama, and Missisipi have a rate of 32.7 percent, the highest in the country.

- For the most part, women and men follow the same regional trends, with women, for the most part, showing smoking rates of only one to two percentage points lower than men in the same region.

- African-American men have the highest rate of smoking—31.3 percent—among ethnic groups. The rate was 26.4 percent for white men, 25 percent for Hispanic men, and 22.8 percent for men who are Asian/ Pacific Islanders.

- The rate of smoking among blue-collar and service workers was higher than for white-collar workers. Female white-collar workers had higher rates of smoking than male white-collar workers, though female service and blue-collar workers had lower rates than their male counterparts.

If you need some more incentive to start thinking about quitting, consider these statistics from the American Lung Association:

- Smoking is the number one cause of cancer death in men.

- Men over 35 who smoke are ten times more likely than nonsmokers to die of lung disease.

- Men over 35 who smoke are twenty-two times more likely than nonsmokers to die of lung cancer.

You might also want to consider what goes on each time you take a puff. The inhaled smoke dries out the bronchial tubes, damaging the lining and the cilia—thin hairs that catch dirt, germs, and pollutants. Without the cilia to block them, the foreign substances get into the lungs, clogging the airways with mucus and making you vulnerable to colds and other infections. Once in the bloodstream, the nicotine also constricts the blood vessels, meaning your tissues get less of the oxygen they need.

Smoking also disrupts sleep. Nicotine withdrawal kicks in three to four hours after a smoker has fallen asleep. Often, its effects are not enough to wake a smoker up, but they are enough to disrupt and fragment sleep.

Smoking is also credited with contributing to aging by causing wrinkles and weathered skin. One study showed smokers were four times as likely to have gray hair than nonsmokers, and men who smoked were twice as likely to be bald or losing their hair than men who did not smoke.

CIGARS VS. CIGARETTES

In many circles, cigars have become a new trend, even for those who don't regularly smoke. But how do they measure up to cigarettes? According to a report in the *Journal of the American Medical Association,* a single cigar may have as much tobacco as a pack of cigarettes. And though many cigar smokers don't inhale, they are inhaling the smoke that's in the air around them, in addition to absorbing the nicotine through the mucous membranes in the mouth. Though cigars are less likely to cause lung cancer than cigarettes, they are toxic and may cause cancer of the mouth, throat, and larynx.

Secondhand Smoke

Secondhand smoke—the smoke in the air that is breathed by nonsmokers—has all the same risks as inhaled smoke. The Environmental Protection Agency estimates that some 4,000 lung cancer deaths annually are caused by secondhand smoke. Studies have found that nonsmoking wives of smoking husbands have a 30 percent increased risk of lung cancer compared with women whose husbands don't smoke. And nonsmokers married to heavy smokers were found to have two to three times the risk of lung cancer compared with those married to nonsmokers. In addition to increasing the risk of lung cancer, secondhand smoke also causes heart disease, aggravates allergies and asthma, and affects circulation.

Smoking and Sexual Health

Smoking is also quite likely to harm your sex life and your reproductive life. First of all, smoking can contribute to heart disease and high blood pressure, both of which can result in erection problems. Smoking can also directly cause erection problems by damaging small arteries, such as the ones needed to fill the penis with blood to create and maintain an erection. Studies have found that the vast majority of men with erection problems are current or former smokers.

Smoking also may reduce the number of sperm your body produces, as well as the quality of what sperm you do produce—both common causes of male infertility. A man who smokes also has a much greater chance than a nonsmoking man of having a child with birth defects such as hydrocephalus or who is at increased risk for cancers such as lymphoma and leukemia.

Some evidence also shows that penile cancer is more likely to occur in smokers than in nonsmokers. Experts estimate that your risk of penile cancer rises sharply even if you smoke only ten cigarettes a day.

In addition, women who smoke (or who inhale secondhand smoke from others) have an increased risk of cervical cancer. Smoking by pregnant women can also result in birth defects in their children.

Snuffing Out the Habit

Though smoking is dangerous—even deadly—it's important to know that the damage to your body caused by smoking begins to reverse itself as soon as you quit. In fact, according to the American Cancer Society, your heart rate and blood pressure return to normal after twenty minutes of not smoking. Within twenty-four hours of quitting, your risk of heart attack drops to closer to normal, and within forty-eight hours, the nerve endings in your mouth and nose begin to regenerate, improving your sense of smell and taste. Gradually, the cilia in the lungs grows back, your circulation improves, and lung function increases by 30 percent. Within ten years of quitting, your risk of death is almost back to that of a nonsmoker.

But the first thing you need to do to reap these health benefits is to make up your mind to quit. All the stop-smoking advice in the world (and all the no smoking signs, for that matter) won't help unless you commit yourself to quitting.

The best way to do that, say groups such as the National Cancer Institute and the American Lung Association, is to think about your reasons for smoking and your reasons for wanting to quit. These reasons must be *your* reasons—you must find your own motivation. Perhaps you

ON THE DAY YOU QUIT

- Tell everyone about your goal.

- Throw away your cigarettes and lighters. Hide or give away your ashtrays.

- Take a walk.

- Give yourself a nonsmoking, noncaloric treat. Go to the movies, for example, or buy something you've wanted.

In the first smoke-free days:

- Keep telling yourself that withdrawal won't last forever. Physical symptoms should subside within two weeks.

- Take it one day at a time. Instead of thinking about never smoking again, think about not smoking today.

- Spend as much time as you can in places where smoking isn't allowed—for example, libraries, supermarkets, churches, and museums.

- Drink a lot of water and juices. Stay away from caffeine and alcohol.

- Get your teeth cleaned. Enjoy how nice they feel and resolve to keep them that way.

- Get up from the table right after eating; brush your teeth.

- Try to stay away from familiar situations where you smoked. For example, take a walk instead of having a predinner drink or spending an evening in front of the TV.

- For the first few weeks, try to avoid social situations that will make you want to smoke. If you can't, try to socialize only with the nonsmokers at the gathering.

- Get plenty of sleep.

are afraid of getting cancer, you want to be more energetic, or you don't want to expose your loved ones to secondhand smoke. Perhaps you want to the save the money you've been spending on cigarettes. Or perhaps you want to quit smelling like stale smoke, take control of your life, or even want to stop being the dupe of tobacco companies that push a dangerous, addictive product.

Once you've committed yourself to stopping, set a date to actually do it in the next seven days. Tell everyone around you that you are going to quit, and ask your family, friends, and coworkers for their help and support. In the week before your quit date, examine your smoking habits—where and when you smoke, with whom or with what (a cup of coffee, a snack), and why (to relax, to get energized). Once you've sorted out your habits, make an effort to avoid or change those situations. If you always have a cigarette with a coworker on your break, take a walk around the block instead. Make your desk, phone area, car, or TV room a smoke-free zone. Change what you drink while you're smoking. In short, change the things in your life that make it comfortable for you to smoke.

Dealing with Withdrawal

Quitting isn't easy. Don't kid yourself—you're breaking the bonds of a highly addictive drug. Surveys show that of the 15 million Americans who quit smoking each year, only 3 percent actually succeed in the long term. In fact, experts say, it often takes three or four tries for most people to quit. But remember that withdrawal symptoms usually disappear within two weeks and that the reason you feel lousy is because your body is ridding itself of a toxic substance. Here's a list of common withdrawal symptoms, along with some tips on how to handle them:

1. *Headache.* Take a warm bath or shower. Try meditation or another relaxation technique. (See Relaxation Techniques, page 124.)

2. *Insomnia.* Stay away from caffeine, especially in the evenings. Try meditation or relaxation.

3. *Fatigue.* Take a nap and get to bed early. Don't push yourself—you're healing.

4. *Increased appetite.* Drink water; eat low-calorie snacks, such as carrots and celery. Chew sugarless gum. Experts say not to worry too much about the possibility of gaining weight while quitting smoking—the average quitter gains only about two pounds (and the health risk of smoking is

much greater than the risk of those few pounds).

5. *Dry or sore mouth.* Sip cold water or fruit juices and chew sugarless gum.

6. *Constipation.* Add high-fiber fruits and vegetables to your diet (apples and carrots, for example) and drink eight 8-ounce glasses of water daily.

7. *Irritability.* Take warm baths and walks. Exercise to keep your mind off smoking and to release some of your energy. Try meditation or relaxation techniques.

8. *Coughing.* Suck on cough drops or sugarless hard candy.

Nicotine Replacement

A lot of people have stopped smoking with the help of "replacement" nicotine delivered via either gum or a transdermal patch that is worn on the skin. Both gum and the patch work by delivering a low dose of nicotine into the body. Gradually, the level of nicotine can be tapered by using patches with successively lower doses or by chewing fewer pieces of the gum. Recently, a nicotine spray delivered through an inhalant has also become available through prescription.

Nicotine gum is recommended for use in a twelve-week program. While it is generally considered less effective than the patch, it allows the user to decide when more nicotine is needed, providing more control over nicotine levels in the body. The patch is used for about six to eight weeks. It releases steady levels of nicotine into the body, preventing the sudden drops in nicotine levels that can lead to cravings. The patch works best for those who have serious physical withdrawal symptoms, who regularly smoked within thirty minutes of waking in the morning, and who smoked twenty or more cigarettes a day.

Although nicotine gum and the patch are designed for limited use, some people continue to use them in the long term. While experts agree that the goal of the therapy is to eliminate the nicotine addiction entirely, most feel that dependence on the gum or the patch is still healthier than smoking because it does not involve the carcinogens of smoke.

The most important thing to know if you choose to try nicotine replacement is that you *cannot* smoke while using the patch or chewing the gum. Doing so can drive the level of nicotine in your system dangerously high and cause high blood pressure, dizziness, severe nausea, and even unconsciousness.

Smoking cessation experts had mixed feelings when both kinds were made available without a prescription in 1996, because while that move lowered the price and made them available to people who might not go to the doctor for them, many experts feared that people wouldn't precisely follow the directions without professional guidance. Most feel people should still consult a doctor when using nicotine replacement because it can be difficult for people to discern what dose of nicotine they should be getting. In addition, both the gum and the patch can have side effects, which include headache, dizziness, nausea, weakness, and blurred vision. These can be relieved by changing the dose or, in some cases, by changing the location of the patch on the body.

Getting Help

It's also important to remember that nicotine replacement alone won't succeed in making you a nonsmoker—you need to change your behaviors as well. For many people, this takes some extra help and support. Many people say that final success came when they got into a self-help program or support group, such as Smokenders or a program from the American Lung Association. Many hospitals and large medical practices offer such programs. Check the Yellow Pages under "Smoking Treatment Programs," or call one of the organizations listed below for a referral to a group in your area.

In addition, some alternative therapies such as acupuncture and hypnosis have been shown to be effective in helping people to quit smoking. (See Complementary Therapies, p. 436.)

For more information:

Action on Smoking and Health
2013 H St., N.W.
Washington, DC 20006
202-659-4310
http://ash.org

American Cancer Society
1599 Clifton Rd., N.E.
Atlanta, GA 30329-4251
800-227-2345
404-320-3333
http://www.cancer.org

American Heart Association
7272 Greenville Ave.
Dallas, TX 75231
800-AHA-USA1
214-373-6300
http://www.amhrt.org

American Lung Association
1740 Broadway, 14th floor
New York, NY 10019-4374
800-LUNG-USA
212-315-8700
http://www.lungusa.org

National Cancer Institute
Cancer Information Service
9000 Rockville Pike
Bethesda, MD 20892
800-4-CANCER
800-638-1234 (Alaska)
800-524-1234 (Hawaii)
301-496-5583
http://cancernet.nci.nih.gov

Office on Smoking and Health Hotline
Centers for Disease Control and Prevention
4770 Buford Hwy., N.E., Mailstop K-50
Atlanta, GA 30341-3724
800-CDC-1311 (recorded message)
770-488-5705
http://www.cdc.gov/tobacco

Smokenders
4455 E. Camelback Rd., Suite D150
Phoenix, AZ 85018
602-840-7414
smokenders@aol.com

STRESS

The American Medical Association defines stress as any interference that disturbs a person's mental and physical well-being. However, most people define stress as their response to conditions and events, both routine and out of the ordinary.

Stress is not all bad. Running a race or planning a big event can be stressful, but also fun and rewarding. Stress can add color to your life and keep you on your toes. But when stress becomes long term or unmanageable, it can lead to health problems. This chronic stress brings with it physical symptoms, including headaches, indigestion, sleeplessness, sweaty palms, edginess, irritability, and lack of concentration. In addition, the systems of the body, including the circulatory system and the immune system, gradually become drained under constant stress,

opening the door for heart disease and other illness.

National Institute for Mental Health studies and other surveys show that 70 to 80 percent of all visits to the doctor are for stress-related and stress-induced illnesses. Seven of ten respondents to a national poll in 1995 said they feel stress in a typical workday, and 43 percent of those interviewed said they suffer noticeable physical and emotional symptoms of stress. In addition, people who live in a high state of anxiety are $4^{1}/_{2}$ times more likely to die of a heart attack or stroke than those who have little stress in their lives.

While men are at greater risk of stress-related illness than women, only 20 percent of those in stress-management programs are men. In the past, hard work and exercise—the staple of most men's days—served as a natural release for stress. Not true today, when most people live sedentary lifestyles (only 22 percent of adults get the minimum amount of activity recommended by the Centers for Disease Control and Prevention). In addition, the lives of men have become increasing complicated. No longer are male and female roles so clearly defined, making problems with relationships, sexual harassment, and marital fidelity more widespread. Financial futures are also not what they once were—the average man graduating from college will hold eight jobs during his lifetime and lose four of them, one survey shows. Societal problems such as crime and pollution, as well as a general lack of spiritual fulfillment, also contribute to modern-day stress.

The Causes of Stress

Stress is very individualistic. The stress and stress-related symptoms you may experience depend on your personality, outlook, life experiences, and health. What one person finds stressful (situations or factors that trigger stress are called stressors), another might actually enjoy. An executive who loves to stay busy might find that a day on the beach is an aggravating waste of time. More commonly, though, the top stressors adults list are family, finances, and work.

LIFE CHANGE INDEX

To rate how much stress you are experiencing in your life, add up the numbers listed for life events you have undergone within the last year. If you score more than 200, you have a 50 percent chance of becoming seriously ill from stress; a score of 300 or more raises your chance of illness to 80 percent.

Life Event	*Score*
Death of a spouse	100
Divorce	73
Marital separation	65
Jail term	63
Death of a close family member	63
Personal injury or illness	53
Marriage	50
Being fired	47
Marital reconciliation	45
Retirement	45
Change in health of a family member	44
Pregnancy	40
Sexual difficulties	39
Having a baby	39
Business readjustment	39
Change in financial state	38
Death of a close friend	37
Change to a different line of work	36
Change in number of arguments with spouse	35
Mortgage large in relation to income	31
Foreclosure of mortgage or loan	30
Change in responsibilities at work	29
Son or daughter leaving home	29
Trouble with in-laws	29

continues

Outstanding personal achievement	28
Spouse begins or stops work	26
Begin or end school	26
Change in living conditions	25
Change in personal habits	24
Trouble with boss	23
Change in work hours or conditions	20
Change in residence	20
Change in schools	20
Change in church activities	19
Change in recreation	19
Change in social activities	18
Small mortgage in relation to income	17
Change in sleeping habits	16
Change in number of family get-togethers	15
Change in eating habits	13
Vacation	13
Christmas	12
Minor violations of the law	11

Reprinted with permission from the *Journal of Psychosomatic Research* 11(2), Holmes and Rahe 1967:213–218. Elsevier Science Inc.

The Stress Response

When your body experiences a stressor, it reacts as though it is facing a physical threat and gears up for fight (facing the challenge) or flight (finding the strength to move out of the way). This is called the stress response.

When a threat appears, the pituitary gland in the brain stimulates the adrenal glands (which sit atop the kidneys) to release several types of hormones, including epinephrine (also called adrenalin) and cortisol. Epinephrine is sometimes called the "emergency hormone" because its primary function is to prepare the body to deal with sudden danger or stress.

The release of a large amount of epinephrine causes several changes in the body to prepare it to react to the immediate danger. The heart beats faster, the passageways in the lungs expand, and the blood vessels of the skin and digestive system narrow to increase the blood supply to the muscles. Your stomach has a sinking feeling, your breathing speeds up, your muscles tighten, your face becomes flushed, and you begin to perspire.

Ideally, the body's stress response is rewarded with one of the intended actions—fight or flight—which serves as a release. After action is taken, the heart returns to a normal pace, the lungs are not overworked, and the blood flow to the skin and digestive system is fully restored. However, many of the stressors faced today—family or marital problems and financial worries—can't be handled by fighting or fleeing. Instead, the stress response lingers, which strains the body's systems and makes you susceptible to health problems such as migraines, indigestion, high blood pressure, backaches, and insomnia.

How Stress and Illness Are Connected

Doctors don't know all of the ways that stress and illness are interrelated, but they do know that the central nervous system and the immune system influence each other during stress. A new field of medicine called psychoneuroimmunology now studies the links.

While many of the connections between stress and chronic conditions are unknown, there are some definite links. For example, during the stress response, the cortisol that is produced suppresses the immune system, increasing its susceptibility to infectious diseases, such as colds and flu and tuberculosis.

The effects of the stress response on the cardiovascular system (a quicker pulse, constricted blood vessels, and thickened blood to promote clotting, should an accident occur) make a person susceptible to heart rhythm irregularities, chest pain called angina, high blood pressure, heart disease, and stroke. People who are "hot reactors" exhibit extreme increases in heart rate and blood pressure; these surges may gradually result in injury to the heart and coronary arteries. (See Hypertension, p. 307, for more information on "hot reactors.")

Muscles tighten with the onset of stress, which can intensify pain from headaches, backaches, and conditions such as arthritis. Stress can also affect sexual health, causing testosterone levels to drop and the blood vessels in the penis to constrict, often resulting in erection problems.

If you have asthma, the rush of epinephrine caused by a stressful situation can bring on an attack. Stress also draws the blood supply away from the abdominal area and encourages the overproduction of acids in the digestive system, so if you have an ulcer or irritable bowel syndrome or if you are prone to bouts of indigestion, stress can make your symptoms worse. The effects of stress on the body can also cause indigestion, insomnia, sweaty palms, and irritability.

Managing Stress

The best ways to keep stress from getting the better of you include taking care of your body, preventing or anticipating potentially stressful situations, and—if stress occurs—by practicing a relaxation technique to counter the body's stress response.

Lifestyle Factors

When you're feeling your best, your resistance to stress and stress-related illness is increased. To bolster your health and increase concentration, stick to nutritious foods and get five servings of fruits and vegetables every day. Avoid foods high in fat, which can sap your energy, and stay away from simple sugars, which stimulate the release of epinephrine and boost the stress response. Also, limit your intake of caffeine and don't smoke. Stimulants such as nicotine and caffeine increase the heart rate and blood pressure and make your stress worse. Caffeine, nicotine, and alcohol can also hinder sleep, which is important to stress-resistance. Most adults need between seven and eight hours a night.

Exercise is also important. Physical activity serves as a release from the stress response and satisfies the "fight-or-flight" impulse. In addition, the natural decrease of epinephrine levels after exercise can counteract the stress response. You'll also be able handle stress better if you're in shape because the body can better meet and recover from the physical effects of the stress response. Try to get at least twenty minutes of exercise a day. Do whatever activity you enjoy, and take it at your own pace. You may want to listen to music while you exercise or workout in a pleasant setting to further reduce stress.

Where you work also has an effect on your health and stress levels. In a study of workers at a Volvo plant in Sweden, researchers found that those who had control over their day-to-day activities were more motivated and subject to fewer stress-related medical conditions than lower level workers with little control over their jobs. If you find that your job is producing too much stress, think about what it is that bothers you and take action to change it. You might be able to change your workload or rearrange your schedule.

TIME-SAVING TIPS

1. Set some goals. To stay in control of your time, catagorize the things you need to do, according to how important they are. Determine a deadline and a specific outcome for each item. Break larger projects down, using smaller goals to make things more manageable.

2. Make a list. Putting your thoughts on paper lessens your mental load and helps you see exactly what needs to be done. Plus, checking off tasks adds to your sense of accomplishment.

3. Use your answering machine. The phone is an invention intended for *your* convenience— don't let it take over your life. If you're having trouble getting everything done, put your phone on the answering machine or voice mail and set aside an hour or so a day to take care of those incoming calls.

4. Pick up some habits. Getting into a routine saves time and relieves stress because it becomes second nature. Choose a particular time or day to do laundry, visit the gym, pay the bills, or go through the junk mail. Plan logically—you might want to deliver your dry cleaning at a certain time because the cleaners is on the way to the gym, for example.

5. Be prepared. By padding your schedule with a few extra minutes, keeping a full tank of gas in the car, or reserving some cash for an "emergency fund," you might be able to thwart some of the obstacles life throws your way.

6. Delegate responsibility. Trying to do everything yourself is a prescription for stress. Just make sure the person you're asking knows how and when to do your project.

7. Just say no. Some people get in over their heads because they have trouble turning down a request for a favor. When someone asks you to take on a new task, think carefully before you answer, and then be honest in your response.

Relaxation Strategies

Studies show that true relaxation stimulates the release of endorphins, brain chemicals that promote feelings of well-being. You can learn to relax by using a specific relaxation strategy. Herbert Benson, M.D., introduced the idea of the relaxation response, the concept that blocking conscious thoughts results in decreased tension, lower heart and breathing rates, and slower metabolism. According to Benson, relaxation must involve four elements to invoke the response: a mental device on which to focus (a single word or phrase, known as a mantra); a calm attitude; a comfortable position; and a quiet environment.

There are several techniques such as meditation, imagery, muscle relaxation, and deep breathing that can be used to relieve stress and bring on the relaxation response. If you practice them regularly, you'll be able to relax at will—even in the face of stress. (See Relaxation Techniques, page 124.) Try setting aside time for relaxation at least three times a day, for about ten minutes a session.

Even if you don't have time for a true relaxation session, you can build time-outs into your day fairly easily. For example, take a few minutes here or there to unwind and relax. Lie awake in bed for a minute or two before getting up in the morning. Enjoy your short walk from your car to the office. Reflect and regroup for a few moments every time you hang up the phone. Or, wait in your car before going into the house after work in the evening.

For more information:

American Institute of Stress
124 Park Ave.
Yonkers, NY 10703
914-963-1200
http://www.stress.org

National Mental Health Association
1021 Prince St.
Alexandria, VA 22314-2971
703-684-7722
http://www.nmha.org

HEALTH AND HYGIENE

While, of course, taking care of your body means a longer, healthier life, it also means looking good on the outside. After all, if you're concerned with your weight or the whiteness of your teeth, you aren't thinking about long-term benefits of exercise such as improved cardiovascular health or about good dental hygiene. Instead, you're thinking of how you'll look in a bathing suit or how eye-catching your smile will be.

What you might not realize is that in addition to a boost in self-esteem, a better complexion, and shinier, healthier-looking hair, grooming and good hygiene practices boost physical health as well as mental health. In other words, you'll not only look your best, you'll feel your best, too. With that in mind, here is a brief, head-to-toe guide on some body basics.

Hair

Though your hair might seem to have a life of its own some days, it's nothing more than a collection of dead skin cells that have been pushed out of a hair follicle by new cell growth. And, even though everyone talks about having healthy hair, your hair actually has little to do with your physical health.

What you can do, however, is keep your hair *looking* healthy by washing and conditioning it daily. Be careful not to abuse your hair—too much blow drying, brushing, dyeing, or sun exposure can damage hair and leave it looking dry and strawlike. Experts recommend switching shampoos on a regular basis to avoid build-up and avoiding hair products that contain alcohol, which dries and dulls hair.

If you're dealing with dandruff, be careful not to use dandruff shampoos too often, because these can dry hair and scalp. Instead, use it only when needed and switch to a gentler shampoo on other days. Home remedies for dandruff include applying a few capfuls of apple cider vinegar to your hair after a shower, following with a small amount of castor oil rubbed into the scalp. Another option that may help is a daily dose of 100 mg. of the vitamin PABA, a B-complex vitamin, used along with a vinegar rinse.

Facial Hair

As teenagers, most boys are eager for facial hair—a sign that they've finally entered the realm of manhood. However, the thrill of whiskers wears off over time, especially when it means shaving as a daily project, one often resulting in nicks, cuts, and burning skin.

Most shaving problems can be overcome with some preparation. Before shaving, you'll want to soften your facial hair—either in a shower, by covering your face with a hot, wet towel or by soaking your face in warm water. Then, cover your face with shaving cream or gel and let it soak in for about two minutes. Softer hair is easier to remove, which means fewer bumps and nicks.

You'll want to use a sharp razor for the best shave—many men prefer using a razor with a lubricating strip and pivoting head. Shave the sides of the face first, moving the razor in the direction that your hair is growing and rinsing the blade frequently in hot water. Continue your shave with the neck, then go on to the chin and mouth area. The whiskers there are the toughest, so shaving these areas last gives the hair more time to soften. Apply only light pressure throughout your shave, and use slow strokes.

After you've finished, rinse your face thoroughly. You may want to apply aftershave or another lotion, but avoid those with alcohol because they can irritate skin. If you cut yourself, use a styptic pencil to stop the bleeding—it does a much better job than tissue paper. Hydrocortisone ointment can be used to soothe razor-burned skin.

Electric razors provide an alternative to the ordeal of shaving with a blade. An electric shave tends to be easier and faster than a traditional shave, and it may be the best option if you have sensitive skin, acne, or razor bumps (sensitive bumps caused by hair growing back into the skin) that are irritated by shaving. However, an electric shave is usually not as smooth as a shave with a blade because it doesn't cut off hairs below the skin. For the best electric shave, wash your face before shaving and allow your face to dry thoroughly. Shave with a light, smooth motion.

Of course, growing a beard is an option to shaving every day, though a beard requires daily maintenance as well. While it can be washed in the shower while shampooing the hair, a beard needs to be trimmed and shaped regularly. Electric beard trimmers and clippers can make the job easier. You may also need to shave the edges of a beard with a blade to redefine the line of the beard.

Teeth

Unlike hair, whose importance to your health is minimal, teeth play an important part in eating—one of the most crucial daily activities—and they also aid speech. While taking care of your teeth properly can boost your appearance and prevent bad breath, what is more important is that it maintains good health and good dental hygiene and prevents plaque (a mixture of sugars and bacteria that solidifies on the teeth), tooth decay, gum disease, and other painful conditions.

To keep your teeth in the best shape, follow your dentist's instructions. Brush regularly—at least twice a day—and brush for at least three minutes a session. You will want to angle the brush (preferably a soft-bristled brush) toward the gumline and brush in small circles. Finish by brushing your gums and tongue gently. This stimulates the gums and removes bacteria from the tongue, which can cause bad breath. Use a toothpaste that contains fluoride.

Flossing your teeth daily is also necessary. Slide the floss between each tooth and the gums, using an up-and-down motion rather than a sawing motion. Ideally, you'll want to floss before brushing to loosen any particles of food that may be caught between the teeth. However, it is also acceptable to floss after brushing and then rinse with a plaque-control mouthwash. If your gums bleed during flossing or brushing, this is a sign of gum inflammation, an early sign of gum disease.

To keep your teeth their whitest, don't smoke or drink too much tea or coffee—this can yellow teeth over time. Certain medications such as tetracycline can also discolor teeth. Over-the-counter teeth whiteners are available; however, these aren't usually very effective and may be too abrasive on your teeth. If you're interested in whitening your teeth, talk with your dentist about having it done professionally.

Breath

Halitosis, or bad breath, is usually the result of food that has been left in the teeth or dentures after brushing. The tongue, whose surface harbors bacteria, also contributes to bad breath. Halitosis can be easily remedied by brushing the teeth and tongue thoroughly, or by using mouthwash. However, in some cases, bad breath is a symptom of a health problem. Mouth infections, digestive disorders, sinusitis, bronchitis, and even kidney failure and cirrhosis can be the cause of bad breath. Also, some medications such as antidepressants can cause halitosis.

To keep your mouth fresh, avoid strong smelling foods and brush your teeth and tongue after eating. Floss carefully to remove food that may be trapped between the teeth. A specially designed scraper is also available to help remove odor-causing substances from the tongue. If these techniques don't do the trick, visit your practitioner to be sure your halitosis isn't a sign of a larger problem.

Skin

Your skin is your largest and most visible organ. It is also your most vulnerable—routinely exposed to chemicals, bacteria, ultraviolet rays, and other damaging factors. While you may think taking care of skin is merely a cosmetic concern, keep in mind that by keeping your skin healthy you're also bolstering your immune system, helping your body regulate its temperature, and helping in the production of vitamin D.

A healthy diet, at least eight glasses of water a day, and regular exercise can also boost skin health. Also, wash your skin daily with gentle soap. If you have dry skin, use a moisturizing soap or lotion and avoid harsh deodorant soaps and lotions that contain alcohol. If your lips are dry, try to avoid licking them to make them feel better—this only serves to dry them out more. Instead, use a lip balm or petroleum jelly for relief.

Daily care of the skin should include protection from the sun. Though most people associate a deep tan with health, ultraviolet rays damage the skin, contribute to the risk of skin cancer, and cause premature aging and wrinkles. Screen them out, using a sunscreen with a sun protection factor (SPF) of at least 15 and avoid exercising or working outdoors between 10 A.M. and 2 P.M., when the sun's rays are the strongest. While some people believe a slight tan protects the skin and lessens the need for a sunscreen, this is just a myth. More and more, dermatologists are recommending sunscreen for protection against daily exposure to the sun—meaning it's not just for the beach.

The sweat glands in the skin are designed to regulate body temperature—a noble occupation—but, of course, they're also responsible for body odor. Body occur occurs when sweat fosters the growth of bacteria, which create the foul smell. The best way to combat body odor is through regular washing (of your body and your clothes) and use of deodorants and antiperspirants. Deodorants work by reducing odor, but do not affect sweating, while antiperspirants stop sweating but do not control odor. An antiperspirant containing aluminum chloride is recommended for men who sweat heavily. (For a detailed discussion of skin and skin care, see Skin Conditions, p. 341.)

Fingernails and Toenails

Again, nails are a product of nothing more than dead skin cells. Though at times they may become infected by bacteria or a fungus (see Skin Conditions, p. 341), for the most part, they require little care other than washing them daily and keeping them properly trimmed. Cut fingernails and toenails straight across, not in an arc, to prevent ingrown nails.

To prevent problems, don't bite your fingernails (this can lead to infection) and keep your cuticles (the skin at the edge of the nails) moisturized to prevent cracking and tearing. If you work with water for long periods, wear gloves to keep your hands from getting too wet. Too much moisture can lead to infection.

PHYSICALS AND PREVENTIVE SCREENING

How long has it been since you visited the doctor for a routine physical? If you're like most men, it's been a long, long time. Men are notorious for avoiding their doctors, especially for regular examinations. Instead, many men wait until they're having a health crisis before seeking care—a dangerous gamble, considering many conditions, including high blood pressure, high cholesterol, heart disease, diabetes, and cancer, often don't cause symptoms until they have progressed to a serious stage.

Men make a reported 150 million fewer visits to physicians than women do. One recent survey of 1,500 physicians by the Men's Health Network showed that doctors believe that, compared with women, men have more trouble discussing health concerns (especially sexual concerns), are less likely to seek medical attention for complaints, are more likely to delay treatment until a condition worsens, and are less likely to stick to any prescribed treatment plans.

Many experts think that this reluctance to seek care is part of the reason that men don't live as long as women—72 years for men, compared with 79 for women. While physiology and risky behavior—men smoke and drink more than women and are more likely to die in accidents, for example—account for part of the seven-year discrepancy, a lack of preventive care is also one reason men's lives are shorter. While exercise and proper nutrition go a long way toward ensuring a long, healthy life, preventive medical care is the basis for good health.

The Doctor-Shy Patient

Women tend to become familiar with the medical system early in life, visiting a gynecologist or other practitioner for yearly examinations, birth control advice, or reproductive health concerns. Men, however, may feel that they have no reason to visit a doctor on a regular basis and may only have a physical when it's required, perhaps for a sport. Active, healthy men may feel they don't need to have regular exams, or they might believe they're too busy to waste time or money on preventive care. Unfortunately, men also tend to put off care when they have serious symptoms, shrugging off health problems as unimportant, or perhaps postponing care because they're afraid of what the diagnosis may be. They may also be afraid of what the doctor will recommend—lose weight, cut back on salt, quit smoking, quit drinking.

What You Need and When You Need It

While not all health-care practitioners and organizations agree on the recommendations for routine screening, the following is a concise listing of what many experts feel to be an appropriate screening schedule for men.

Basic Physical Examination

When: Every three years for healthy men under the age of 40, and every two years after that. After the age of 50, every year.

A physical exam should include a medical history and a head-to-toe examination. The medical history is a series of questions about lifestyle,

occupation, recent medical complaints, and personal and family history. The information is used to determine any possible health risks and to aid diagnosis of any problems. The exam involves checking the eyes, ears, and skin; listening to the heart; examining the inside of the mouth and throat; taking height and weight measurements; and tapping the knees to check the reflexes. Most of the tests described below are done at the same time as the physical.

Urinalysis

When: Every three years until the age of 40, then every two years until the age 50. After the age of 50, every year.

A urine sample is collected for analysis to screen for conditions such as diabetes, urinary tract infections, hormone imbalances, and liver and gallbladder health. (Self-test kits are available to test for urinary tract infections.)

Blood Pressure Check

When: Every year, according to the American Heart Association.

A sphygmomanometer, or blood pressure cuff, is used to measure the pressure of the blood as it travels through the arteries and veins. Routine screening is important because high blood pressure often has no symptoms, and can cause heart disease, stroke, blindness, and kidney failure if untreated. Blood pressure can be monitored at home.

Testicular Examination

When: The American Cancer Society recommends screening by a practitioner every three years after age 20, and every year after the age of 40. A testicular self-examination should be done on a monthly basis.

The testicles are examined by palpation for swelling or any sign of a hernia (the famous "turn-your-head-and-cough" test, see Testicular Cancer, page 224).

Blood Tests

When: Every three years until the age of 40, then every two years until the age of 50. After the age of 50, every year.

Blood tests include a complete blood count (CBC), SMAC blood test, cholesterol test, blood glucose test, and human immunodeficiency virus (HIV) test.

- The CBC measures the levels of each type of blood cell, a screening for anemia.

- The SMAC test looks at blood-sugar levels, blood gases, electrolytes and evaluates heart, liver, and kidney function.

- The cholesterol test measures the levels of the different kinds of cholesterol in the blood. A finger-prick home version of this test is available.

- The HIV test is recommended for all sexually active individuals, especially those at risk of HIV and AIDS. If you have had unprotected sex with someone at risk for the disease or have used intravenous drugs, you should definitely have this test done.

Tuberculosis Test

When: Every five years.

Men are twice as likely than women to get tuberculosis, an airborne bacterial infection that is beginning to make a reappearance in the United States. The test is a simple skin test in which a small amount of a substance called purified protein derivative is injected under the skin. If TB is present, there will be a reaction in the area injected within forty-eight to seventy-two hours. After the test is administered, you must return to the office in a few days so the skin can be examined for a reaction.

Chest X-Ray

When: Every year after the age of 30 for smokers.

The x-ray uses radiation to create an image of the lungs, screening for signs of cancer, tuberculosis, or other conditions.

Electrocardiogram (EKG)

When: Every three years after the age of 30 if you're at risk for heart disease; every three to four years after age 50 if you are not. Some experts recommend getting a baseline EKG at the age of 40 that can be used as a basis for comparison with future EKGs.

Electrodes are placed on the body to measure the amount of electrical activity of the heart. This test is used to diagnose certain forms of heart disease. A variation of the test, known as a stress EKG, involves measuring the heart's electrical activity during exercise on a treadmill or stationary bike.

Digital Rectal Examination (DRE)

When: Every year after the age of 40, according to the American Cancer Society.

A gloved and lubricated finger is inserted into the lower part of the rectum to check for tenderness, swelling, and other abnormalities in the area. The prostate is also felt through the wall of the rectum to check for lumps and hardening. It is done to screen for colon and rectal cancer, prostate cancer, benign prostatic hyperplasia, and other conditions.

Fecal Occult Blood Test

When: Every year after age 50, according to the American Cancer Society, though many experts recommend annual testing beginning at the age of 40.

A sample of stool is analyzed for the presence of blood. This test screens for colon and rectal cancer as well as for other abnormalities.

Prostate-Specific Antigen (PSA) Test

When: The American Cancer Society and the American Urological Association recommend screening every year after age 40 if you're at risk for prostate cancer; every year after age 50 if you are not. The American College of Physicians, the U.S. Preventive Services Task Force, and the American Academy of Family Physicians recommend against routine PSA screening, and suggest a man discuss the benefits and risks of testing with a practitioner before making a decision on whether to have the test.

This blood test measures the amount of prostate-specific antigen in the blood. High levels of PSA may indicate prostate cancer or benign prostatic hyperplasia. This test is controversial because high levels of PSA may not necessarily mean a health problem is present—PSA levels vary, according to age and race, and may be affected by a number of health conditions and medications. Some experts fear the test may lead otherwise healthy men to seek unnecessary treatment. (See Prostate Cancer, p. 214.)

Sigmoidoscopy

When: Every three to four years after age 50, according to the American Cancer Society.

A fiberoptic scope is inserted into the rectum to view the rectum and colon. It screens for colon cancer and for other digestive diseases.

Getting the Most From Your Office Visit

A trip to the doctor should involve more than a litany of recommended tests and examinations. To ensure the best of health, you'll need to form a partnership with your practitioner. This means that your physician will need to listen to your concerns, address your questions, and work with you when making any decisions on treatment. For your part, you'll have to be honest with your doctor, ask plenty of questions, and follow the treatment program you both have decided on. If you don't feel comfortable with your practitioner or if you don't feel that your practitioner is listening to you and your concerns, look for a new physician who will hold up the other end of your partnership. (See Choosing a Practitioner, p. 424.)

To help your physician help you, prepare for your visit. Before you go, make a list of any concerns or symptoms you've been having and be specific. If you're having pain, describe how it feels, when it occurs, and how long it lasts. Such details can make diagnosis easier, and writing them down ensures that you won't forget to mention any of them.

If you're visiting a new doctor, obtain your medical records before you go. Write your former physician and request copies and/or the transfer of your records, including all laboratory and x-ray reports. Jot down what you remember about your medical history: surgeries, major illnesses, hospitalizations, previous drug regimens, and allergies. Know your family history as well.

Also, know what drugs you're taking. If you're unsure of the names and dosages, check with your pharmacist and bring the medications with you to the doctor's office.

Finally, don't be afraid to discuss concerns with your doctor. Whatever you're afraid to mention could be a sign of a serious condition, or it may be the key to figuring out your problem. On the other hand, it might also be a concern that can be dismissed easily, ending your worries. Health-care practitioners are well equipped to deal with problems that you might find embarrassing. If you keep silent, you're only hurting yourself.

IMMUNIZATIONS

Preventing serious illnesses and disease is easier than having to fight them once they strike. For example, smallpox was not eradicated worldwide until the 1980s. Thankfully, the first steps toward defeating this dreaded disease began with early experimentation with immunization, the use of vaccines to prevent disease.

Vaccines have now been developed that prevent such diseases as influenza, mumps, chicken pox, measles, polio, and whooping cough. Prior to immunizations, diseases such as the mumps and the chicken pox were like rites of passage for every child—a part of growing up, and those such as polio and whooping cough claimed many lives.

Immunizations, however, are not unique to children. Some are intended for adolescents, young adults, and senior citizens.

What Is Immunization?

Immunity occurs through adaptation. When the immune system comes in contact with a foreign substance (called an antigen) it produces substances known as antibodies to destroy the invaders. If the antibodies cannot overcome the antigen, sickness occurs. However, once the illness has ended, the body "remembers" the antigen. If it reappears, the system can immediately produce antibodies and destroy it.

Immunization is the injection or implantation of a vaccine, microorganism, antibody, or antigen into the body in order to protect against, treat, or study a disease. A vaccine is a preparation introduced into the body to prevent a disease by stimulating the body's own natural antibodies against it and building the body's immunity to, or inability to contract, that disease.

Immunization can be passive or active. In passive immunization, antibodies from another person who has been infected with the disease are collected and made into a serum. The serum is then injected into the person who will be protected. Passive immunization provides immediate, but short-lived protection against specific diseases.

In active immunization, a killed or modified microorganism that does not cause disease is injected into the person who will be protected. Inside the body, the immune system produces antibodies against the modified microorganism, creating immunity. When the real organism invades the body, antibodies are easily produced to eradicate it. Active immunization provides long-lasting immunity.

How Is It Accomplished?

Vaccines are generally administered via injection, either intramuscularly (IM), intradermally (into the skin, or ID), or subcutaneously (under the skin, or SC). Some, such as the polio vaccine, can be received orally. Vaccines contain a very small amount of the disease—just enough for the body to recognize it and produce antibodies to defend against it. Once the antibodies are produced, the body is protected from the disease, even when exposed to it. Some immunizations, such as that for tetanus and diphtheria (Td), require repeated doses, or boosters, at scheduled intervals (for example, the Td booster is recommended every ten years) to ensure the body's continued defense against it.

Talk with your practitioner about immunization to be sure you are up to date on your vaccines. You can also call your local health department for information on when immunization is recommended and where it is available.

Why Is Immunization Important at Different Ages?

According to the U. S. Department of Health and Human Services, successful childhood immunization alone will not necessarily eliminate specific disease problems. Many of the remaining outbreaks of specific diseases now occur in older adolescents and adults. Persons who were never infected (and therefore do not have immunity) or were not immunized with vaccines against diphtheria, tetanus, measles, mumps, rubella, and poliomyelitis may be at risk of these diseases and their complications.

Risks of Vaccination

Most people suffer no ill effects from immunization. Some injections may cause pain or swelling at the site, fever, or fatigue. Some vaccines, such as measles, may result in a very mild form of the disease. However, for most people, the benefits of immunization outweigh any possibility of adverse effects.

Those with immune system disorders and those with cancer should not be immunized because of the effect the vaccine might have on the weakened immune system.

TRAVEL AND IMMUNIZATIONS

Immunization for specific diseases should be well thought out in advance, for some vaccines need to be in the body's system before exposure to the disease, some are given in a series of shots over a period of weeks, and some cannot be given along with others.

Basic vaccinations that you should already have include tetanus, diphtheria, polio, influenza, pneumococcal pneumonia, measles, mumps, and rubella (German measles). Vaccinations that are often required for international travel are yellow fever and cholera. And other vaccinations specific to a particular region or often recommended for international travel include malaria, hepatitis A and B, Japanese B encephalitis, typhoid, plague, rabies, and meningococcal meningitis. Because different countries require certain immunizations and sometimes alter them due to changing worldwide health trends, it is wise to contact the Centers for Disease Control and Prevention, a local or state health department, or a doctor in order to confirm exactly which immunizations you will need for your trip.

ON-LINE HEALTH RESOURCES

The advent of the Internet, the electronic medium made up of millions of networked computers worldwide, has revolutionized the way in which we can search for information, help, and support on health concerns. A worldwide library of health information is waiting for you on the Internet. In cyberspace, you can find anything from the symptoms of prostate cancer to statistics on hair loss products, read the latest research, learn about cutting-edge treatments, and even "talk" directly to experts.

The Internet can not only put a great deal of information into your hands, but also put you in touch with others who have a certain condition. On-line discussion groups can provide information on personal experiences, tips on how to cope with a condition, and often a surprising amount of support and encouragement.

Don't hesitate to bring the information you've found to your practitioner. Doctors don't know everything. The field of medicine is constantly changing, and it is easy for professionals to miss a new study or treatment posted on-line that may help you. A practitioner can also help steer you away from inaccurate health information. Keep in mind that some practitioners don't welcome outside information. If yours is one of them, encourage him or her to take a look at what you've found. (If you meet with a great deal of opposition, perhaps you should consider finding another practitioner.)

Getting On-Line

To gain access to the Internet, you need a computer, mouse, modem, phone line, and an Internet provider. The provider acts like a cable TV service, hooking you into the Internet for a base monthly fee or a per hour charge. Providers can be local or national. National providers include Prodigy, CompuServe, and America Online. While local services are often less expensive, national services provide a lot of extras you won't get with a local Internet connection—interactive discussions with celebrities, special interest sites, and some support forums. Be sure the provider you choose has a local phone number for access—otherwise, you'll be paying a long-distance phone bill in addition to your Internet fees.

If you don't have a computer or a modem, you may be able to gain access to the Internet at your local library or a nearby college. Some restaurants and cafes may even offer access.

Once you are on the Internet (or in cyberspace, as it is also called), there are several ways to get information. Your provider usually offers databases, information, and support groups as well as access to the Internet. You'll be assigned an e-mail, or electronic mail, address, and will be able to send and receive messages and files via computer. You also can sign up for mailing lists on various topics. Those on the list receive all messages sent to people on that list, allowing them to communicate and share information about a particular subject.

Internet newsgroups—electronic "places" where people with similar interests can communicate—are also available for more interactive communication. In these areas, you can send or receive messages on a particular subject. Thousands of newsgroups are available, many devoted to health and medical topics. You can also "talk" with other people, post opinions, or seek help through newsgroups, and sometimes you'll receive good leads on articles, helpful sites on the Internet, and other sources of information.

Finally, there's the World Wide Web. This is a network of information sites, called "home pages," set up by individuals or organizations. The pages (whose addresses usually begin "http://www.") can contain pictures, advertisements, and information and are updated regularly. Web pages are often cross-referenced and linked so that you can move between sites without typing in commands. Some sites give you the opportunity to be put on an electronic mailing list where updates, announcements, and news are sent to your e-mail address. While there is little interactive communication on the Web to date, it may become more versatile in the future.

Getting Around

An impressive array of men's health information exists on the Net, but searching out the information that you need on this electronic medium can be overwhelming since there's so much available.

Internet services provide users with a search engine, software that will search for a specific topic (such engines include Yahoo, Altavista, Infoseek, and Magellan). You can ask these search tools to check the Internet for a topic as broad as "men's health" or as specific as "impotence." Once you enter your topic, you'll get a listing of sites, including a brief description of each, that relate to your topic. Then it's up to you to decide if you want to "click" and enter the site.

When you're getting started, you may want to enlist the help of a computer-savvy friend to help you find your way around. Books are available on the subject that may be helpful. (See Suggested Reading, page 495.)

Avoiding the Pitfalls

Though there's a wealth of information available on the Internet, not all of it is credible. Some sites pitch "miracle cures" or offer inaccurate or potentially dangerous medical information. Frauds may present themselves as experts or physicians. The key is to sort through these "junk sites" to find the best information.

Anyone who has the tools can create and post a home page on the Internet, so it's important to find out the source of any Net information. An easy way to do that is to look for source words, such as the name of a university or college, national health organization, or well-known publication, when you review site lists brought up by a search engine. Since not all sites offer their credentials in their brief on-line descriptions, you may have to enter a home page before you find the source of the material.

If you're exchanging information with others in a newsgroup, you'll want to be leery about who's on the other end of the response—anyone can claim to be an expert or a doctor.

Suggested Sites

To help you get started locating men's health information on the Net or World Wide Web, check out these recommended sites. The addresses for the pages are listed within the parentheses.

Men's Health

1. *A Man's Life* (http://www.manslife.com). This on-line magazine includes health and fitness articles and news along with an interactive section that allows you to send questions to a medical doctor.

2. *Dear Doc* (http://deardoc.hlthnet.com). The men's health section is a question-and-answer format with posted answers that includes topics such as allergies, male breast cancer, balding, penile concerns, ulcers, and vasectomy. This site is interactive, and you may send your questions to a family doctor.

3. *Doctor's Hospital Health Source* (http://

www.doctors-10tv.com/alt/men/ men.htm). An Ohio-based physicians network runs this site. A men's health section includes topics such as baldness, testicular cancer, and prostate problems.

4. *Duke University Health Information On-Line* (http://h-devil-www. mc.duke.edu/h-devil). The section on men's health has four topics: premature ejaculation, testicular self-examination, erection problems, and urinary tract infection. The "Answer Page" provide answers to questions submitted through the site and includes hundreds of responses on subjects from jock itch to hangovers.

5. *The Hairloss Information Center* (http:// hairloss.com/index.htm). With a consumer focus, this site gives the scoop on baldness drugs, spray-on hair, and hair transplants. It includes an interactive feature where your questions can answered by e-mail.

6. *House Calls* (http://www.housecall.com). A search for men's health topics will pull up links to men's health forums/newsgroups and additional information on specific health concerns. Links to the National Health Council and the American Academy of Family Physicians home pages are included.

7. *New York Times Syndicate*—Your Daily Health (http://nytsyn.com). Here you will find the latest health and medicine news as well as a special section devoted to men's health.

8. *The Prostate Cancer Infolink* (http://

www.comed.com/prostate/). Part of CoMed Communications Internet Health Forum, this site offers the latest information on prostate cancer. Current clinical reviews and information on getting medical help are included. This site includes an interactive forum that allows you to ask questions and share experiences.

9. *The University of Texas-Houston Medical Information Center* (MEDIC) (http:// medic.med.uth.tmc.edu). The "Men's Health Issues" section includes these topics: exercise for a healthy heart; fat and cholesterol; prostatic cancer screening; and benign prostatic hyperplasia.

10. *USA Today* (http://www.usatoday.com). General health and specific men's health topics can be found under the Health Index in the Life section of this site. Topics under men's health include: baldness, birth control, infertility, prostate, and sexual health.

11. *Williams College Peer Health Homepage* (http://wso.williams.edu/peerh/men). The "Men's Health Issues" section is short but includes these topics: jock itch, prostatitis, male self-examination, and male problems with sexual functioning.

12. *World Wide Web Virtual Library* (http:// www.vix.com/pub/men/health/ health.html). The section of this site called "Men's Health Issues" is broken into physical and mental health segments. You'll find articles on topics such as health and gender, studies on cardiac problems, information on health legislation regard-

ing prostate cancer, a men's health products area, and tips for preparing healthy meals. There's also information on sexual addiction and suicide.

General Health

1. *CNN Food and Health Main Page* (http://www.cnn.com). This site presents news on health, fitness, and food topics through the "Food and Health" section.

2. *HealthLinks* (http://www.hslib.washington.edu). This University of Washington Health Sciences Center site offers vast health information, including health reference guides and articles from the center's *HealthBeat* publication. Links to other health sites on the Internet are offered.

3. *Healthwise* (http://www.columbia.edu/cu/healthwise). Columbia University's Health Education and Wellness program offers a team of professionals who will answer questions from this site. The site archives the answers and allows you to search them.

4. *Physician's GenRx Web Site* (http://www.icsi.net/GenRx/). Descriptions of drugs are provided in a database. A free registration is necessary before you can access the information.

INTERNET LINGO

- *BBS.* Bulletin Board Systems where you can send and receive messages. BBSs can originate from a single computer with a modem or from a complicated network such as those used by a commercial service.

- *Commercial service.* Term for large on-line services (with monthly access fees) that allow you to access the Internet and World Wide Web (America Online, CompuServe, Prodigy, etc.) and provide special forums and features.

- *FTP (File Transfer Protocol).* The standard used to transfer files between computers.

- *Gopher.* A menu-based guide, organized by subject, to directories on the Internet.

- *Home page.* A site on the World Wide Web or Internet that is created by an individual, group, or organization. Home page addresses begin "http://www."

- *Hypertext.* A way of retrieving information by choosing highlighted words (the hypertext) within the text on the screen.

- *Hypertext transfer protocol (http).* Command that precedes most typical Internet addresses.

- *Internet.* An electronic medium made up of millions of networked computers around the world. It is also known as cyberspace, the information highway, or the Net.

continues

- *Net.* A term used to refer to the entirety of cyberspace: the Internet, commercial services such as America Online, CompuServe, and BBSs.

- *Newsgroups.* Usenet areas, organized by subject, where you can send and receive messages or post opinions. See: Usenet.

- *Posting.* Sending a message to a newsgroup, bulletin board, or other public message area.

- *Search engine.* See: Web browser.

- *Server.* A software program on a computer that allows other computers to share its resources.

- *Usenet.* A collection of networks and computer systems that exchange messages and are organized by subject into newsgroups. See: Newsgroups.

- *Universal resource locator (URL).* The term for an on-line Internet address.

- *Web browser.* A software program that works with World Wide Web servers on the Internet to allow subscribers to easily search and view Web pages. Netscape is a popular Web browser.

- *Web page.* A document with hypertext, graphics, sounds, and links to other Internet resources.

- *World Wide Web.* A network of information sites, also known as the Web, that contains pictures, advertisements, and information. The sites are cross-referenced and linked with hypertext to allow readers to move between sites without typing commands.

MEN'S ROLES IN PREGNANCY

A few generations ago, pregnancy was considered "women's work." An expectant father's biggest role—after conception, of course—was that of a chauffeur, making sure his partner got to the hospital in time for her to be whisked away into the delivery room. The father-to-be was left behind to pace the hospital waiting room, awaiting news of the baby's arrival and the health of the mother and child.

But times have changed. Approximately 80 percent of American fathers now attend the births of their children. Fathers play a much greater role in child-care than ever before, and their participation begins long before a child is even born.

The Stages of Pregnancy

A pregnancy is divided into three parts, each called a trimester. The first trimester consists of weeks one through twelve; the second, weeks thirteen through twenty-six; and the third, weeks twenty-seven through forty.

Of course, it all begins with conception, which occurs when a woman's egg is fertilized by a man's sperm in her reproductive tract. The fertilized egg then implants in the lining of the uterus (or womb), and its cells begin to divide rapidly, developing into the fetus. Within four weeks, the heart, head, mouth, eyes, lungs, brain, spinal column, and genitals of the child are beginning to develop.

By the sixth or seventh week, the limbs and some internal organs, such as the stomach and the liver, are developing. By the eighth week, the fetus is about one inch long and weighs only a fraction of an ounce. At twelve weeks, the fetus is three inches long. The fingernails and toenails have developed, and the arms, hands, legs, toes, and feet are fully formed. By the end of the first trimester, the fetus contains most of its organs and tissues and has taken on a recognizable human form.

Pregnancy becomes noticeable during the second trimester. While at sixteen weeks the fetus weighs 4 ounces, by the end of twenty-six weeks, it has grown to 14 inches in length and weighs 2 pounds. The movements of the fetus can usually be felt by the twentieth week.

In the third trimester, the development of the heart, circulatory system, and respiratory system of the fetus is completed, and the fetus will reach a weight of about seven pounds, on average. The soft bones of the head remain flexible until after birth, to allow the baby to pass more easily through the birth canal.

The Importance of Support

A man's role in pregnancy is one of support. As a partner-in-reproduction, a man must offer encouragement and understanding to his partner, realizing that a woman's body undergoes drastic hormonal changes during pregnancy that might make her seem like a different person at times. Pregnant women often feel vulnerable due to frequent mood changes that leave them feeling as out-of-control emotionally as they do physically. An expectant father must be patient when dealing with these mood swings, realizing that they are as transient as a woman's physical changes during pregnancy.

At one time, fathers-to-be were expected by society to shield feelings of nervousness, anger, and sadness from their partners so as not to upset or worry them. However, psychological studies have shown that relationships between expectant parents are strengthened and closeness is increased when men share their concerns with their partners. So don't hesitate to share your feelings, including your fears, with your partner about becoming a father. And if you're feeling left out, let her know; it is probably unintentional on her part.

BECOMING A "PREGNANT" FATHER

Many men have contradictory feelings of joy, anxiety, and even fear about the impending birth of a child. The best way to relieve these feelings is to become an active, supportive participant in pregnancy. In other words, become a "pregnant" father:

1. Do not be a spectator. Get involved in the pregnancy. Attend as many obstetric appointments as you can—all if possible, and at least landmark visits, such as hearing the baby's heartbeat for the first time and seeing the baby on a sonogram monitor. Be active in planning for the baby's arrival. Add your input to parental decisions such as decorating the nursery and choosing clothes, a crib, stroller, and other items.

2. Help out. If you don't already, now is the time to start doing your share of household tasks such as laundry cooking, and cleaning. Also negotiate with your partner a division of labor for after the baby's arrival, leaving the details open to alterations, of course.

3. Take a "we're pregnant" attitude. Exercise with your partner, cut back on junk food, and quit smoking and drinking. This will help to encourage your partner's own program of good prenatal care and benefit your own health as well. Remember that secondhand smoke can be dangerous for the pregnant woman and the fetus, possibly contributing to birth defects.

4. Know what's coming. Educate yourself by reading about pregnancy and childbirth, attending childbirth classes with your partner, and talking with other fathers about their pregnancy, labor, and delivery experiences.

5. Get to know your baby. By the fifth month, you should be able to feel fetal movement by placing your hand or face on your partner's abdomen. By the end of the seventh month, the senses have developed, so let the baby become familiar with your voice by talking, reading, or singing to him or her.

6. Prepare for a change in lifestyle. Having a baby means going to fewer parties and movies-for-two, so be ready and willing to adjust your social life. Also anticipate a change in your relationship with your partner and promise each other that you'll make time to spend together.

Sex During Pregnancy

A big concern of many men is the topic of sexual intercourse during pregnancy. First of all, intercourse during pregnancy will not hurt the fetus or cause a miscarriage. Studies show that infants born to couples who had intercourse during pregnancy are no different from those of couples who abstained.

There are some times during pregnancy when you shouldn't have sex. In a high-risk pregnancy, a birth practitioner may put restrictions on intercourse. For example, a woman with a history of premature birth may be instructed to abstain because orgasm and nipple stimulation during pregnancy have been known to trigger contractions. Sexual intercourse should be avoided as well if there is any risk of transmitting a sexually transmitted disease to the woman—even if a condom is used for protection. The reason is that such diseases may be passed on to the child and may cause birth defects and other serious conditions. In addition, you should not have intercourse if the woman has vaginal bleeding or leakage of any fluid. Call a practitioner immediately if this occurs.

Almost every couple finds that their sexual relationship changes somewhat during pregnancy. Some women's sexual appetites diminish, while other women report having the best sex of their lives while pregnant. In most cases, surveys say, a woman's desire for intercourse decreases (often due to the nausea and other discomforts) during early pregnancy, while the man's desire remains the same. In middle stages of pregnancy, a woman's libido returns to normal or increases. In the last stages of pregnancy, both men and women report a decrease in desire.

For this reason, it is important to keep the lines of communication open regarding sexuality during pregnancy, and to remember that intimacy can be achieved in many different ways. If a partner is not comfortable with intercourse for whatever reason, try hand holding, reciprocal back massages, reading love poems, sharing a romantic candlelight dinner, or whatever else keeps the emphasis on love and away from lovemaking. In addition, hearing her partner's reassurance that her physical changes have not lessened his feelings for her can give a pregnant woman's fragile ego a much-needed boost.

Expectant couples may have to experiment with new positions in order to accommodate the woman's growing belly. Options to consider include the "spoon" and other positions where the man enters the woman from behind; a position in which a man sits on a chair, and the woman straddles him; or a position where the woman sits or lies on the edge of the bed, and the man enters her while standing between her legs.

Childbirth Methods and Options

Many decisions must be made regarding the birth of a child. For example, you'll need to discuss where it will take place, what childbirth method should be used, and whether pain-relieving drugs should be used during labor. Be active in these choices, discussing the options with your partner and her practitioner. Once a decision has been reached, you will need to follow through, learning your part in the birth method and acting as an advocate for your partner and child in the hospital to ensure that all goes as planned.

Common childbirth methods include the Dick-Read method, the Bradley method, the Lamaze method, and the LeBoyer method.

The Dick-Read method uses education and knowledge in combination with breathing control and relaxation techniques to eliminate fear, which creates tension and leads to pain. This method avoids medications and medical intervention, and was one of the first methods to encourage men to work with their partners in the delivery room. It is taught by the Read Natural Childbirth Foundation.

In the Bradley method, the man supports his partner with encouragement and coaching. The method uses darkness and solitude, a quiet environment, physical comfort, physical relaxation, controlled breathing, closed eyes, and the appearance of sleep to mimic the conditions found in the animal world. The Bradley method emphasizes good nutrition and is drug free, focusing on relaxation techniques, breathing techniques, and different birthing positions.

The Lamaze method teaches exercises to be used during childbirth, including different types of breathing techniques. It is based on the theory of conditioned reflexes; contractions are used as the stimulus to relax certain muscles through breathing techniques, which helps to block pain. Coaching by a partner is also important. While pain-relieving drugs are not usually used during labor with Lamaze, such medications may be used at times.

In the LeBoyer method, the focus is on reducing the trauma of birth. Labor and delivery take place in a darkened room, and the fetus is delivered with as little intervention as possible. Following birth, the baby is placed on the mother's abdomen and massaged. Then the partner washes the infant in warm water, and the baby is dried and wrapped.

In addition to these birth methods, a variety of birth positions may be used. The lithotomy position, where the woman lies on her back, is the standard position for childbirth, although many experts feel that it may make labor harder by forcing the woman to work against gravity. Other options include an upright position, such as sitting or kneeling, or lying on the side. Birthing under water is also an option. Special cushions, stools, and chairs have also been developed to help with childbirth. Keep in mind that midwives and birth centers, in general, are more likely to embrace an alternative birth position or method than a medical doctor or hospital.

Attending the Birth

Although it is almost a given in today's society that fathers will attend the birth of their children, their presence is certainly not mandatory. Despite going through all the preparations of childbirth, some men still do not want to attend the actual birth. If you feel this way, don't feel pressured to go through with it; your presence will most likely do more harm than good if your heart's not in it. And don't worry about losing out on early bonding: Studies have shown no correlation between fathers who don't attend births and their relationships with their children.

For more information:

American Society for Psychoprophylaxis in Obstetrics/Lamaze
1200 19th St., N.W., Suite 300
Washington, DC 20036-2422
800-368-4404
202-857-1128
http://www.lamaze-childbirth.com

Bradley Method Pregnancy Hotline
P.O. Box 5224
Sherman Oaks, CA 91413
800-423-2397
818-788-6662
http://www.bradleybirth.com

International Childbirth Education Association
P.O. Box 20048
Minneapolis, MN 55420
612-854-8660
http://www.icea.org

National Association of Parents and Professionals for Safe Alternatives in Childbirth
Rte. 1, Box 646
Marble Hill, MO 63764
573-238-2010

Read Natural Childbirth Foundation, Inc.
P.O. Box 150956
San Rafael, CA 94915
415-456-8462

RELAXATION THERAPIES

Relaxation is more than taking time away from the telephone, putting your feet up, and unwinding with a good book or movie. True, deep relaxation is a meditative state in which the mind is free of thoughts and worries—one that can relieve stress and provide a number of emotional and physical health benefits.

In today's stressful world, relaxation is necessary to counter the negative aspects of stress. (See Stress, page 101.) Whether you're dealing with a divorce, worrying about your job and financial future, or simply feeling tense because of a traffic jam, relaxation techniques can help restore your sense of balance and well-being and counteract the harmful toll stress takes on your body.

The Relaxation Response

Herbert Benson, M.D., is credited with introducing the concept of the relaxation response—the idea that practicing relaxation and meditation results in reduced tension, increased alpha (relaxed) brain waves, lower heart and breathing rates, slower metabolism, and decreased digestive acid secretion. This concept provides the basis for the use of relaxation techniques to improve health and reduce stress.

Benson's technique requires four basic elements:

1. A mental device, a constant stimulus of some sort—such as a word, a sound, or a phrase repeated either silently or aloud. This is called a mantra.

2. A passive attitude that disregards any distracting thoughts. Any distraction is blocked out by the repetition of the mental device.

3. Decreased muscle tension by taking a comfortable position that requires minimal muscle work.

4. A quiet environment with few environmental distractions.

To practice the relaxation response, think about the four basic elements. Sit in a comfortable position and repeat your chosen mantra over and over again to drive out all distractions until you're thinking about nothing at all. This will take practice; don't become discouraged if you find it difficult at first. If thoughts come into your mind, acknowledge them and let them fade away. Meditate this way for twenty minutes every morning and evening.

Relaxation Techniques

There is a wide variety of ways in which to achieve the relaxation response, ranging from deep breathing and meditation to hydrotherapy and aromatherapy. Some relaxation therapies such as biofeedback and hypnosis are used in conjunction with medical treatments and are also known as complementary therapies. (See Complementary Therapies, p. 436.) Additional resources for relaxation techniques are listed in Suggested Reading (p. 495).

Imagery

Imagery allows you to change your perception of a situation as a mental way to fight stress. It helps to promote deep relaxation, which causes a release of serotonin, a calming hormone that eases muscle tension and promotes healing. To practice imagery, stop what you are doing, close your eyes, and visualize a soothing scene—a beach with white sand and blue waters or the woods with birds singing and the scent of pine filling the air, for example. Spend five minutes or so examining and enjoying every detail of the picture. Hear the birds sing or feel the sting of the salt air. For a quick session of imagery, you might want to keep a pleasant picture or postcard in your wallet to look at in times of stress.

Progressive Muscle Relaxation

Muscle relaxation is a simple technique of contracting and relaxing of the muscles in order from the feet to the head. It is best used when lying down so that the muscle groups can be isolated, tensed, and released one by one. As you are tensing and releasing the muscles, compare how they feel when they are flexed with when they are relaxed. Note any areas that are already tense and make a conscious effort to relax them. Progressive relaxation breaks tense-mind/tense-muscle syndrome by teaching recognition of physical stress. Practice allows you to relax at will.

It is possible to practice a simpler version of progressive relaxation while sitting at a desk. Raise your shoulders to your ears as tightly as possible, then release them, making sure they are low at the finish. This will reduce the stress that builds in your shoulder, shoulder blades, and neck during the day.

Deep Breathing

This method focuses on slow, rhythmic breathing with deep inhalation and exhalation. To practice deep breathing, stand or sit straight and close your eyes for five minutes. Slowly take in a deep breath to the count of five. As you take in the air, let your abdomen and ribs expand up and out. Imagine the air entering every part of your body, into your head, your shoulders, your arms, your torso, and then your legs. When you exhale, imagine the air leaving through your toes. Deep breathing increases the volume of oxygen in the system and refreshes cells. It is often used in combination with other strategies.

Meditation

Meditation involves focusing on one object and ignoring external stimuli to promote relaxation. In fact, it was this ancient Eastern technique that was the inspiration for Benson's relaxation response. With meditation, oxygen consumption decreases; heartbeat, breathing, and metabolism slow; and blood pressure drops. To practice meditation, sit or lie comfortably with your eyes closed. Quietly repeat a chosen word, sound, or phrase (called a mantra) continuously, concentrating on it to prevent distraction. Breathe deeply, as described above. Practice ten to twenty minutes twice a day or whenever stressed. Classes on meditation may be available at a local YMCA or through the Yellow Pages.

Mindfulness

Mindfulness is simply focusing on the tangibles around you in order to relieve stressful thoughts. It serves to calm the mind and distract it from anxiety-producing thoughts about the past or the future. To practice mindfulness, focus on the objects, colors, and sensations around you. Look at the color of the walls or the texture of the carpet, for example, or concentrate on the sound of the traffic or the clock ticking. Mindfulness is often used to maximize relaxing effects of other strategies.

Aromatherapy

In aromatherapy, fragrant oils extracted from plants and flowers are used to promote relaxation. Fragrances can be imparted through scented candles, perfumes, skin lotions, or massage oils applied to the skin or added to warm bath water. Common scents used for relaxation include marjoram, lavender, geranium, chamomile, sandalwood, lily of the valley, roses, and apple spice. The smells prompt the signal portion of brain that controls emotions and memories, triggering a release of calming hormones and increasing relaxing brain waves. There are many books available on the details of aromatherapy, and courses or workshops may be available in your area. Check the Yellow Pages.

Hydrotherapy

Hydrotherapy uses water to change body temperature and promote relaxation. It includes swimming, bathing, or showering or use of a whirlpool or sauna. Warm water promotes the release of calming brain chemicals and stimulates healing throughout the body by increasing blood flow. Warm or hot water dilates blood vessels while cold constricts them. Both help improve circulation, enhancing relaxation. Buoyancy takes pressure off taut muscles. Hydrotherapy is also widely used as a means of physical therapy.

Warm water promotes sleep and hot water relieves muscle tension. Herbs and aromatherapy oils may also be added to the water (in what's called hydrochemical therapy) to aid relaxation.

Music Therapy

This therapy focuses on the power of music to relax and soothe. It can be used alone or in combination with other strategies. Soothing music can help block negative and stressful thoughts.

As a result, blood pressure drops, heart and breathing rates slow, and calming brain chemicals are released. Muscle tension decreases.

Listen to flowing or relaxing music—perhaps using headphones—with your eyes closed. New-Age music, jazz, classical music, and recordings of natural sounds such as birds or waterfalls are available and may be good choices for music. Music with one beat per second is preferable because it mimics the body's natural rhythms.

Self-Hypnosis

Self-hypnosis involves a set of specific mental commands a person gives to himself in order to enter a light hypnotic trance, a state of concentration similar to sleep in which the body can regenerate and energize itself more easily. Aside from relaxation, it can also be used in treating conditions such as nicotine addiction.

Self-hypnosis should never be attempted without the advice of a professional hypnotist. To practice, close your eyes and repeat the series of commands—for example, "My arms and legs are heavy"—until you believe that command has been achieved. With practice, self-hypnosis can be induced with only a few commands.

Biofeedback

Biofeedback is a method of consciously controlling involuntary body functions through concentration, taught using electronic monitoring of body's responses. Biofeedback can result in slowing of breathing and heart rate, a change in body temperature, and a release in muscle tension. Once the method is learned, an individual can control such responses whenever necessary. Biofeedback monitors are available commercially, and you can find training at specialist centers, which are found in most cities.

QUICK RELAXATION TIPS

1. *Head to the gym.* A workout helps to release excess energy and remove tension from muscles. The stimulus also triggers the production of endorphins and epinephrine, brain chemicals. Epinephrine, the hormone produced in times of stress helps to sustain the activity and keep heart and breathing rates up. It is offset by endorphins, tension-lowering chemicals that create a sense of well-being.

2. *Laugh.* Watch a funny movie or show to help reduce stress. Laughing can increase heart and breathing rates, and it gets the blood pumping. It also stimulates the immune system and raises levels of a brain chemical called catecholamine, which is associated with the production of endorphins.

3. *Stop and smell the roses.* If you're feeling the need to relax, take pleasure in the smaller things in life—a sunset, a compliment, a joke, for example. Such focus works to slow you down and help you gain perspective.

4. *Practice good posture.* Holding yourself correctly takes strain off of muscles and helps you breathe easier. Standing up straight also gives you the appearance of confidence, which in turn may lead to a better self-image.

5. *Get a hobby.* Find an activity that you like and let yourself become absorbed in it—you'll reach a state of relaxation and hardly notice the time passing. In addition, hobbies can stimulate the mind and broaden your horizons.

For more information:

American Society of Clinical Hypnosis
2200 East Devon Ave., Suite 291
Des Plaines, IL 60018
847-297-3317

Association for Applied Psychophysiology and Biofeedback
(formerly the Biofeedback Society of America)
10200 W. 44th Ave., Suite 304
Wheat Ridge, CO 80033
303-422-8436
http://www.aapb.org

PLASTIC SURGERY

Plastic surgery is the alteration of a part of the body. Reconstructive surgery is a form of plastic surgery done to repair an injury or disfigurement. These procedures can include everything from creating a skin graft after a bad burn or removing a birthmark. Cosmetic surgery is done for aesthetic reasons, for example, to improve appearance, minimize the effects of aging, or change a facial feature. According to a survey of the members of the American Society of Plastic and Reconstructive Surgery, 12 percent of all cosmetic procedures done in 1994 were performed on men.

As the statistics show, more men are considering cosmetic surgery today than ever before. Though traditionally women have been more sensitive about their looks as they age, reports show that men are more concerned than ever about wrinkles, sagging skin, excess fat, and complexion. It is thought that new emphasis on the ideal male body in media and advertising are fueling the trend, as well as a greater social acceptance of cosmetic surgery for men. While in the past men were discouraged from plastic surgery except for reconstructive reasons, today they are encouraged to have the procedures done, and there are many more procedures available than ever before.

While plastic surgery can improve self-esteem and boost confidence, it does not radically change appearance or make a person look drastically younger. Its effects may also be temporary; for example, a face-lift may sag within a few years. Before choosing cosmetic surgery, think about your motives for the operation and talk them over with your practitioner. Make sure your expectations for the surgery are realistic.

REASONS FOR RECON- STRUCTIVE SURGERY IN MEN

Skin cancer	29 %
Auto accident	24 %
Sports injuries	19 %
Head/neck cancer	17 %
Violent crime	5 %
Domestic violence	2 %

Source: American Academy of Facial Plastic and Reconstructive Surgery Survey, 1993.

Common Cosmetic Procedures for Men

The top cosmetic procedures for men are rhinoplasty (nose surgery), blepharoplasty (eyelid lift), liposuction (fat reduction), reduction mammoplasty (breast reduction), rhytidectomy (face-lift), otoplasty (ear surgery), and dermabrasion (skin sanding).

1. *Rhinoplasty.* This procedure changes the shape of the nose by altering the soft cartilage and bone. It is done through an incision within the nose. After the procedure, there will be bruising around the eyes and some difficulty breathing that may last several weeks. Swelling may linger for several months. Although rhinoplasty is the most common procedure for men, it is one of the most complex and requires a great deal of skill. If the procedure is not done correctly, the nose may appear misshapen or may not function correctly.

2. *Blepharoplasty.* Tightening the eyelids can make a man appear younger by eliminating puffy or baggy eyes. The procedure removes excess fat and skin above and below the eyes. Excess skin from the upper lid is removed through an incision in the natural crease above the eye. Fatty tissue from the lower lid is removed through an incision just below the lower eyelid. Bruising may last up to ten days after the procedure. Complications may include dry eyes, temporary blurred vision, excessive tear production, hematomas (swellings containing blood), and scarring around the line of the eyelashes.

3. *Liposuction.* In liposuction, fat is suctioned out of the body through a long, thin tube inserted into a small incision. Liposuction is not for those who are overweight, contrary to popular belief. The procedure works best on people who are close to their ideal weight, but still have pockets of fat that don't respond to diet and exercise. It is not effective against cellulite (the dimpled skin found on the thighs), and it does not work well on those with sagging or inelastic skin. The procedure should be performed by a physician who is experienced in liposuction. Complications may include blood clots (which in rare cases can cause embolism and death), fluid loss, and infection. A girdle must be worn after surgery until bruising and swelling disappear.

4. *Reduction mammoplasty.* Breast reduction is popular among overweight men and men who develop fatty deposits in the breast area. These deposits are common among former weight lifters and develop as the muscle is slowly replaced by fat. There may be some scarring or unevenness with the surgery.

5. *Rhytidectomy.* In a face-lift, an incision is made following the hairline. Excess skin and fat are removed, and sagging skin is pulled up toward the hairline and repositioned. Swelling and bruising last for several weeks after the surgery, and at times surgical drains are implanted to drain blood and fluid that may collect under the skin. Possible complications include scarring, hair loss around the incision, and damage to the nerves within the face.

NUMBER OF COSMETIC PROCEDURES FOR MEN

Procedure	Total Men	Percent of Procedures Done in Men
Rhinoplasty	10,419	29
Blepharoplasty	8,642	17
Liposuction	6,639	13
Breast reduction in men	4,416	100
Rhytidectomy	2,583	8
Otoplasty	2,248	48
Dermabrasion	2,222	22

Source: American Society of Plastic and Reconstructive Surgeons, 1994.

6. *Otoplasty.* Protruding ears can be altered surgically. In this procedure, an incision is made in the crease behind the ear, and cartilage and skin are removed. Possible complications include infection, scarring, and a recurrence of the protrusion.

7. *Dermabrasion.* Skin sanding is a procedure used to remove small wrinkles and scars by wearing down high spots on the face, using a rotating wheel. It is done with a local anesthetic when a small area is being done; a general anesthetic and hospitalization may be required for a large area. Dermabrasion is a painful procedure that leaves a thin, oozing crust over the worn away skin that heals in a few weeks. If too much skin is removed, scarring may occur. If the procedure is done unevenly, it can result in blotchy skin.

PHALLOPLASTY

Yes, phalloplasty is what you probably think it is—a procedure to enlarge the penis. Penile enlargement has become a new, hot procedure in cosmetic surgery, offering to increase the length and width of the penis substantially. Surgeons estimate that some 10,000 to 15,000 of the expensive procedures have been performed in the United States since the early 1990s.

Phalloplasty became available in the late 1980s. It can be done by injecting fat from another part of the body into the penis to widen it, or it can be done by cutting the ligament that attaches the penis to the pelvic bone. This allows the part of the penis that is within the abdomen—about 1 to $^1/_2$ inch—to drop down.

The hype surrounding the procedure includes glowing testimonials from satisfied customers and reassuring statements from supportive cosmetic surgeons. However, phalloplasty is an unregulated procedure: Because it doesn't include any new implant or drug, no scientific studies or research have been done to test its safety. However, the dangers of the procedure are coming to light: sexual dysfunction (including erection problems), deformity, and infection. The fat-injection procedure often has lumpy, disfiguring results. In addition, it's temporary, because the body gradually reabsorbs and redistributes the implanted fat.

Last year, a group of surgeons formed the American Academy of Phalloplasty Surgeons with hopes of standardizing the procedure and making it safer. In the meantime, however, the fat-injection procedure cannot be recommended, and the procedure that alters the ligament should only be used for men with exceptionally small penises. If you're overweight, however, you may be able to lengthen your penis simply by losing weight. It is estimated that an overweight man will lengthen his penis by an inch for every 35 pounds he loses until he reaches an average weight.

Choosing a Plastic Surgeon

Friends, family, or another practitioner can provide you with a referral to a cosmetic surgeon. You'll want to look for a surgeon who is board certified in plastic surgery; this means that he or she has undergone testing and training as designated by the American Board of Medical Specialties. Keep in mind that physicians can call themselves specialists in a particular field even if they have no specialized training or qualifications. You might also look for membership in a medical society, such as the American Society of Plastic and Reconstructive Surgeons.

These affiliations are a good sign that a practitioner is up to date on new procedures and teachings in a specialty; however, it is not a definitive stamp of excellence. After all, a talented surgeon may not be board certified, while an inferior doctor may manage to receive certification.

A board-certified plastic surgeon can be found by consulting *The Official ABMS Directory of Board Certified Medical Specialists*, published by Marquis Who's Who, which is available in most libraries. Board certification can be verified by calling the American Board of Medical Specialties at 800-776-CERT.

In addition to the qualifications of a plastic surgeon, you'll want to consider their manner. A plastic surgeon should answer all of your questions about the procedure and discuss with you your motivations and expectations. The surgeon should fully explain possible complications, alternatives to surgery, and potential outcomes. Avoid high-pressure surgeons who assure you that nothing will go wrong. Also, get a second opinion before undergoing a procedure.

Cosmetic surgery can be costly, and many practitioners ask that part of the fee be paid up front. Since most insurance plans do not cover cosmetic surgery (though they may cover reconstructive surgery), costs and payment methods should be explained.

QUESTIONS TO ASK

Questions to ask a potential surgeon include:

- What training do you have in the procedure I want? How many of these types of procedures do you perform in a year?

- Are you board certified in surgery?

- How safe is the operation? What are the possible side effects and complications?

- How long will the effects of the treatment last?

- What are the risks and benefits of the surgery?

- Where can the operation take place? In the office? In a hospital?

- What will happen to me before, during, and after the procedure? Are my expectations of the surgery realistic?

- What are your fees? In what ways can I pay?

- Will my insurance cover all or part of the costs of the procedure?

- Can I contact your former patients to learn more?

For more information

American Board of Plastic Surgery
7 Penn Center
1635 Market St.
Philadelphia, PA 19103-2204
215-587-9322

American Society of Plastic and Reconstructive
Surgeons
444 E. Algonquin Rd.
Arlington Heights, IL 60005
800-635-0635

Facial Plastic Surgery Information Service
1110 Vermont Ave., N.W., Suite 220
Washington, DC 20005
800-332-3223

LONG-TERM CARE

Without a doubt, long-term care has changed greatly in the past twenty years. Once, a person who needed care was usually limited to two options: moving in with a family member or entering a nursing home. Today, however, many more choices are available, ranging from home health care to assisted living and continuing care facilities.

This expansion in available care is primarily due to our aging population—there are simply more older people today than ever before. In 1965, when Medicare began, 18 million Americans were 65 or over. Today, 34 million have reached or passed their 65th birthday. The population needing care has grown older as well. In the 1950s, the average age of a person in a nursing home was about 70. Today, the average age is more than 80.

But age is not the only reason long-term care has changed. Nursing home scandals in past decades sparked reform, leading to an overhaul of the industry. Additionally, the recognition that

elderly individuals have different and varying needs also provoked the creation of other long-term-care options.

An estimated 7.2 million Americans age 65 or older currently need long-term care, as do 5.4 million children and working-age adults. The most common causes for needing long-term-care services by the elderly are arthritis and heart disease.

Determining Long-Term-Care Needs

Individuals need long-term care when a condition or illness limits their ability to carry out the activities necessary to maintain themselves or their households—or when they are at risk of harming themselves or others. These activities, called activities of daily living, or ADLs, are basic tasks such as eating, bathing, using the bathroom, and getting around the house. Other activities include traveling outside the home, handling money, cooking, doing housework, using the telephone, or taking medications. Because it may be difficult to determine the need for care based on a medical condition or illness, a person's need for care is often gauged by how well he or she can perform ADLs.

One person to talk with about the need for care is the individual's practitioner—he or she may be able to estimate the person's condition as well as how it may change in the future. You may also want to seek advice from a professional case manager. Case managers, who are usually nurses or social workers, are trained to assess an individual's needs, identify appropriate (and affordable) services, monitor the care provided, and follow up on an ongoing basis to reassess needs as appropriate. They can be hired through Medicaid (the largest government provider of long-term-care services) or an insurance company.

When determining the needs of an older loved one—or when thinking of your own future—you may want to contact your local Area Agency on Aging. Created as a result of the 1965 Older Americans Act, the Area Agency on Aging has more than seven hundred outlets in the fifty states. These agencies were established to set up a comprehensive and coordinated system to provide services to the elderly. You can find a listing for the agency closest to you in the Blue Pages of the phone book.

Home Health Care

Home health care delivers medical and personal services to partially or fully dependent people in their homes, helping people to stay in their homes longer and avoid costly hospitalization if possible. The goal of the care is to restore or stabilize health or to maximize independence while minimizing the effects of disability or disease.

Home health care may be intensive, intermediate, or maintenance. Intensive home care is similar to the care found in a hospital or nursing home and includes house calls, chemotherapy, intravenous feeding, blood tests, and x-rays. Intermediate home care does not require such hospital or nursing home care, but rather focuses on tasks such as providing physical or speech therapy, taking blood pressure or helping to administer medications. Maintenance care involves help with nonmedical tasks such as cooking, shopping, bathing, dressing, or eating.

Those who provide home health care include social workers, nurses, rehabilitation therapists, physical therapists, occupational therapists, speech therapists, respiratory therapists, home health aides, and homemakers.

Home health care is generally less expensive than nursing home care. In 1994, the federal General Accounting Office found that the Medicaid program in Washington State spent $419 per person per month for home care services and $2,023 for comparable care in a nursing facility. However, many aspects of home health care—for example, housekeeping, shopping, and prescription drugs—may not be covered by many forms of insurance, including Medicare.

More than 15,000 agencies nationwide provide home health care. These include the Visiting Nurse Association, private and public nonprofit agencies, the Veterans Administration, and for-profit organizations run by individuals or corporations.

If you are looking for individuals or agencies to provide home health-care services, start close to home. Tell your friends and family members what you think you need, based on the assessments you've made, and ask their advice. Some sources that may help you find the services you need include your practitioner; your hospital's discharge planner or social worker (if care is needed after hospitalization); the county health department; United Way and other community service organizations; your church or synagogue, retirement group or similar organizations; the local Area Agency on Aging; and the Visiting Nurse Association.

Community Services

The following community services are used as part of home health care to help otherwise independent seniors stay in their homes longer:

1. *Adult day care.* These programs provide health services, rehabilitation, and activities to seniors who may be temporarily or

permanently incapacitated. The arrangement provides services for the individual, as well as a break for full-time caregivers.

2. *Emergency response systems.* These commercial systems provide a small button transmitted that can be activated with light pressure if a fall or sudden illness requiring medical attention occurs.

3. *Homemakers.* These individuals offer a range of services, from providing transportation, meals, and personal care to paying bills, doing shopping, and doing light housekeeping. Some may be trained to perform simple health care tasks, such as taking blood pressure readings.

4. *Meals on Wheels.* Most Meals on Wheels programs deliver a midday meal five days a week, and possibly a ready-to-heat meal for the evening.

5. *Personal contact services.* This may involve a visiting volunteer or a prearranged phone call. The services are designed to check on the person's health and progress and provide some companionship.

6. *Transportation.* For those who can no longer drive, free and low-cost transportation services can provide rides to grocery stores, senior centers, social events, and medical offices.

Housing Options for Long-Term Care

Housing for Independent Living

For individuals who do not need regular health monitoring and can care for themselves with little or no assistance, housing options are available that provide independence, as well as some aid through the use of community services or home health care when necessary.

Five categories of housing are available to seniors in many communities:

1. Their own apartments or houses.

2. An apartment or small house on the property of a family or caregiver.

3. A retirement apartment or community of homes.

4. Congregate housing, an option in which each person has a private bedroom and bathroom, but all other rooms are shared.

5. Shared housing, in which several unrelated people live together and share expenses and responsibilities.

Costs vary, according to the type of housing, the location, and the number of services (if any) provided.

Continuing Care Communities

There are about 1,300 continuing care communities in the United States. This option is part housing complex, part activity center, and part health-care system. This facility serves as a lifelong home to residents (most sell their houses before entering), offering different levels of care as people's needs change as they grows older. For example, a continuing care community may have private homes and an on-site hospital or nursing home for those residents with health-care or medical needs.

When you enter a continuing care facility, you can expect to pay an entrance fee (usually $20,000 to $40,000). There are also monthly payments, which may increase annually (usually between

2 to 5 percent). Because continuing care is essentially a lifetime commitment, make sure there are no hidden fees or exclusions on health care before signing the contract and have a qualified attorney help you through the process.

To find a continuing care community, you can consult *The Consumer's Directory of Continuing Care Retirement Communities* or *The Directory of Retirement Facilities*, two sources available at most libraries.

Assisted Living Residences

Assisted living residences are a special combination of housing and personalized health care designed to respond to the individual needs of those who need help with the activities of daily living. They provide housing, meals, and various services to residents, including help with shopping, bathing, taking medications, and other needs. Housing may consist of a private, fully-equipped apartment in some of the larger, newer facilities, or simply a private or semiprivate room in other areas.

An estimated one million Americans currently live in assisted living residences. Most people who use assisted living residences have conditions such as arthritis or heart disease that hinder their ability to live on their own. However, they're usually alert and able to walk with little or no assistance. According to a 1994 survey by the Assisted Living Facilities Association of America, the average monthly room rate is between $2,000 and $3,500. However, there may also be monthly fees for meals, housekeeping, laundry, and transportation.

Contact local sources such as the Area Agency on Aging or the local department of housing for more information on such facilities in your area. You can also contact the Assisted Living Facilities Association of America, listed on page 138.

Nursing Facilities

With the increasing availability of alternatives such as home health care and assisted living, you or your loved ones may never need a nursing facility, also called a nursing home or convalescent home. A nursing facility may serve as a temporary placement for someone who is recovering from an injury or condition, or it may become a permanent home. In short, a nursing facility is a home for people who have difficulty caring for themselves while rehabilitation on all levels is undertaken.

The basic cost per day in a nursing facility is between $100 and $200, and a stay of a year can range between $40,000 and $70,000. There may be additional fees for supplies and services. To find a nursing facility, consult the usual local sources. *The Directory of Nursing Homes* may also be available at your local library.

WHAT TO LOOK FOR IN A NURSING FACILITY

When choosing a nursing facility, you need to look beyond the spotless reception area or well-groomed lawns and into a number of important health and safety issues.

- Ask about licensure and certification. Nursing facilities must be licensed in all states. A license means the home has been inspected and has met certain standards established by law. Nursing facilities may apply for Medicare and Medicaid certification, in which they agree to certain conditions and accept the rate paid by these programs. Medicare and Medicaid will not pay for care provided by a facility that is not certified. A nursing facility can voluntarily apply for accreditation from the Joint Commission on Accreditation of Healthcare Organizations. To become accredited, a facility must undergo an evaluation including a self-review, on-site visit by experts and a written report.

- Make sure the facility meets your needs. Find out the "typical profile" of a resident in that facility and be sure that it matches what you're looking for. A facility may specialize in a certain condition such as Alzheimer's disease or may offer only certain levels of care.

- Call the facility and arrange for a tour. While you're there, observe activities, talk with residents and visiting family members, talk with the nurses or nurses' aides (an excellent source of information about the place), and eat a meal. Try to get a feel for what everyday life is like for those who live there.

- Check out the physical layout. Also while at the facility, notice the state of the building and grounds. The area should be neat and well maintained, wheelchair ramps should be in place, and the facility should be located in a safe neighborhood, close to public transportation. There should also be areas outside where residents can sit or walk.

- Evaluate the facility for safety and comfort. For example, corridors should be well lit and uncluttered, a fire safety system should be in place, and grip bars should be in place in the showers and bathrooms. You should also notice the atmosphere of the facility. Are the people who work there pleasant? Are there enough windows to provide sunlight? Is there air-conditioning? Do residents have enough privacy?

- Ask about the availability of the staff. Check to see if there is always a physician on the premises or on call twenty-four hours a day, and ask if there is a registered nurse on duty all the time. Find out if residents have access to a pharmacist, as well.

- Find out about patient rights. Some facilities do not allow patients to select their own doctors or hospitals, for example. Ask if there are any limits or policies that may limit patient rights, and find out if the facility subscribes to the Patient's Bill of Rights from the American Hospital Association (see Medical Rights, p. 476).

continues

- Survey your community. Don't forget that friends, neighbors, coworkers, and members of the clergy may be able to give you some information about the facilities you are considering. Asking around can give you a good idea of a facility's reputation.

- Find out about all costs up front, and get them in writing. You should have a qualified attorney look over any contract before signing.

Paying for Long-Term Care

The Health Care Financing Administration's Office of the Actuary estimates that nearly $118 billion was spent on long-term care in 1994, and this does not include costs for specialized independent housing such as continuing care communities. Nearly 36 percent of these long-term-care costs were paid privately, primarily out of pocket by the elderly and their families.

Several federal and state programs help pay for long-term care, but in nearly all cases, coverage is limited, is based on eligibility, and may vary from state to state. Limited coverage is provided by Medicare, and only if certain conditions are met. Medicare is health insurance, and it does not cover housekeeping, transportation, chores, or other social services. It only covers serious illness or injury, not ongoing care of a chronic condition, so once a person's condition stabilizes, coverage ends. To be covered, services must be provided by a Medicare-certified agency or facility.

Medicaid is the largest government payer for long-term-care services. States administer the program on behalf of the federal government, and the eligibility criteria are decided by the government and the states. To be eligible for Medicaid in most cases, an individual must have a low income and few assets (though there are exceptions). As a result, many people become eligible for Medicaid only after they've spent all of their own assets on medical care—often after they're living in a long-term-care facility.

The Medicaid program generally pays for all levels of care in certified facilities for an indefinite period of time for eligible recipients. This institutional care can include care in an assisted living or nursing facility. Medicaid also requires that states provide home health services—including part-time nursing care, medical equipment, and speech therapy—to eligible recipients who would otherwise qualify for nursing facility care.

For information on Medicaid, contact your county department of social services, health, or welfare. The local Area Agency on Aging may also help.

A REMINDER TO VETERANS

Retired and honorably discharged veterans of the United States Armed Services may be eligible for medical care through the Veterans Administration (VA). While focus has tended to be on temporary hospital care, VA facilities are offering more home health and skilled nursing facility care. A few assisted living units have been built, and depending on bed availability, other VA facilities may provide long-term residential care. If you are a veteran and live near a VA medical facility, explore what services are available and your eligibility for them. For more information, contact the Veterans Affairs Department, 810 Vermont Ave., N.W., Washington, DC 20420; 800-827-1000; 800-829-4833 (TDD); or on-line at http://www.va.gov. (See Department of Veterans Affairs, p. 492.)

For more information:

American Association of Homes and Services for the Aging
901 E St., N.W., Suite 500
Washington, DC 20004-2037
202-783-2242
http://www.aahsa.org

American Health Care Association
1201 L St., N.W.
Washington, DC 20005
202-842-4444
http://www.webplus.net/ahca

Assisted Living Facilities Association of America
10300 Eaton Pl.
Farifax, VA 22030
703-691-8100

Health Care Financing Administration
200 Independence Ave., S.W., Room 423-H
Washington, DC 20201
202-619-0257

National Academy on Aging
1275 K St., N.W., Suite 350
Washington, DC 20005
202-408-3375
http://www.geron.org

National Association of Meals Program
1414 Prince St., Suite 202
Alexandria, VA 22314
703-548-5558

National Association of Area Agencies on Aging
1112 16th St., NW, Suite 100
Washington, DC 20036
202-296-8130

National Council on Aging
409 Third St., S.W., Suite 200
Washington, DC 20024
202-479-1200
http://www.ncoa.org

DEATH AND DYING

Many people undoubtedly owe their lives to advances in medical technology. However, high-tech medical care is also frequently used to prolong the last stages of life—a scenario unfortunately more common today due to the increase in the incidence of cancer and AIDS. Such advances have brought to light many issues surrounding death and dying—dying with dignity, the right-to-die, and even controversy about the definition of death—issues of the young and old, men and women alike. You may have to deal with such issues if you find yourself in the role of caring for an ailing loved one, or you may want to consider documenting your wishes surrounding your own death.

Grief

Grief is an emotional response to a loss or death, involving feelings such as anger, pain, frustration, sadness, guilt, anxiety, and disappointment. Even if a death or loss has been expected, you may feel overwhelmed by the feelings of loneliness, loss, anger, or disbelief. You may feel that you are moving in slow motion, or you may find that you experience swings in mood and energy. You may also experience physical symptoms related to stress such as diarrhea, shortness of breath, and an upset stomach.

Everyone experiences grief differently, but most people agree that it is important to express grief rather than suppress it. Men are less likely than women to share their feelings with others or to seek out support from those around them. But "bottling up" emotions can lead to depression, withdrawal from society, sudden outbursts, insomnia, and even physical illness.

Grief is typically marked by four stages: shock, denial, depression and withdrawal, and acceptance. However, these stages often overlap and may not be experienced in any particular order— many men often become stuck in the depression and withdrawal stage. However, the process of mourning and working through grief, though difficult, can provide relief.

During this time, it is important that you take care of yourself to help you deal with the stress:

- Take care of yourself. Keep warm (shock and emotional stress can cause body temperature to drop), rest, and eat well. Try to avoid alcohol and caffeine, as they will only add to your stress.

- Use a relaxation technique. Practice deep breathing. Those under stress tend to hold their breath or breathe shallowly, which can result in fatigue and anxiety. Close your eyes for a moment and breath deeply; inhale through your nose and exhale through your mouth. Think of inhaling new, cleansing air and exhaling old air. (See Relaxation Techniques, page 124.)

- Vent your feelings. Talk to family members, friends, support groups, or members of the clergy about your emotions. You may want to exercise or pick up a hobby to direct some of your energies.

- Take your time. There is no set time frame for grieving, a process that is often rushed by today's society. The grieving period is different for everyone and can span from several months to several years. However, if you experience intense feelings of anger and withdrawal for more than two weeks, you may want to talk with a counselor to sort out your emotions and begin the healing process.

- Think about the future. While leaving a loss behind may feel like a betrayal, it is important to think about how your life has changed and what you will be doing next.

- Accept help. Let others care for you. Let friends and family make a meal for you, take care of the house, or even just listen about your deceased loved one and your feelings. Such support can be healing for them as well as for you. Out of their love for you, friends and family need to give you the gift of their support.

The Definition of Death

Death was simple to define thirty years ago. If your heart stopped, if you stopped breathing, and if your eyes were dilated, you were dead. Today, the definition of death includes the irreversible loss of all brain functions, including the functions of the brain stem, which controls only the reflex functions such as breathing. Death is indicated by an unresponsiveness to stimuli, no movement or breathing, a lack of reflexes, and a flat electroencephalogram (EEG).

Changes in the definition of death have been brought about in large part by the technology available in intensive care units. Machines used in the intensive care unit—performing artificial ventilation and circulation, feeding by intravenous tubes, and elimination of waste—are capable of keeping a body alive, can sustain a body by performing its usual, basic functions, even if the brain has been irreversibly damaged. With these advancements, individuals who are incapable of living on their own can be kept alive indefinitely.

Under the modern definition of death, an individual may be considered alive even after he or she has suffered what is called cognitive death—in this situation, only the brain stem is still functioning, rendering the person able to breathe and sleep, but incapable of awareness or thought. This state, called persistent vegetative state (PVS) affects about ten thousand people in the United States.

As a result, there is a growing concern over the quality of life and the quality of the end of life. Right-to-die issues center around the legal right to reject mechanical life support and be allowed to die. You can protect your right to die with documents called advance directives, written statements that state how you want medical decisions made should you become incapacitated. The two most common forms of advance directives are a living will and durable power of attorney for health care.

Living Wills

When the patient's quality of life has greatly diminished and medical treatment only delays death, the question of how far medical treatment should go arises. A living will, also called a declaration to physicians, expresses your intentions for you. It is a document that states what kind of life-prolonging treatment you want or don't want. You may use a form, provided by state agencies or the organization Choice in Dying, or simply write a statement expressing your preference.

A living will should define the limits you want to put on medical treatment, including available technology and advance treatments that could sustain your life. You can decide whether or not to be put on a respirator or dialysis machine, be resuscitated, or be nourished intravenously. You can also make clear what treatments, for example, blood transfusions or artifical resuscitation, you want or do not want under any circumstances.

You may want to discuss these matters with your practitioner or lawyer. If you're interested in knowing more about the criteria used to determine death, ask your doctor about his or her standards or call the hospital and speak to the chief of staff or an administrator.

A living will should make your intent perfectly clear. Obviously, you cannot plan for every medical disaster that is possible, and you cannot possibly know what you would want done under every circumstance. Be sure to inform your physician, family, and attorney that you have a living will and inform them of its content. Also remember that you can revoke or change a living will at any time.

If you have specific questions concerning living wills in your state, you might wish to speak with your attorney and physician, as each state

FLORIDA LIVING WILL

INSTRUCTIONS

PRINT THE DATE

Declaration made this _____ day of _____, 19_____.

PRINT YOUR NAME

I, _____, willfully and voluntarily make known my desire that my dying not be artificially prolonged under the circumstances set forth below, and I do hereby declare:

If at any time I have a terminal condition and if my attending or treating physician and another consulting physician have determined that there is no medical probability of my recovery from such condition, I direct that life-prolonging procedures be withheld or withdrawn when the application of such procedures would serve only to prolong artificially the process of dying, and that I be permitted to die naturally with only the administration of medication or the performance of any medical procedure deemed necessary to provide me with comfort care or to alleviate pain.

It is my intention that this declaration be honored by my family and physician as the final expression of my legal right to refuse medical or surgical treatment and to accept the consequences for such refusal.

In the event that I have been determined to be unable to provide express and informed consent regarding the withholding, withdrawal, or continuation of life-prolonging procedures, I wish to designate, as my surrogate to carry out the provisions of this declaration:

PRINT THE NAME, HOME ADDRESS AND TELEPHONE NUMBER OF YOUR SURROGATE

Name: _____

Address: _____

_____ Zip Code: _____

Phone: _____

© 1995
CHOICE IN DYING, INC.

FLORIDA LIVING WILL — PAGE 2 OF 2

I wish to designate the following person as my alternate surrogate, to carry out the provisions of this declaration should my surrogate be unwilling or unable to act on my behalf:

PRINT NAME, HOME ADDRESS AND TELEPHONE NUMBER OF YOUR ALTERNATE SURROGATE

Name: _____

Address: _____

_____ Zip Code: _____

Phone: _____

ADD PERSONAL INSTRUCTIONS (IF ANY)

Additional instructions (optional):

I understand the full impo—— —is declaration, and I am emotionally and mentally competent to make t.. declaration.

SIGN THE DOCUMENT

Signed: _____

WITNESSING PROCEDURE

TWO WITNESSES MUST SIGN AND PRINT THEIR ADDRESSES

Witness 1:

    Signed: _____

    Address: _____

Witness 2:

    Signed: _____

    Address: _____

© 1995
CHOICE IN DYING, INC.

Courtesy of Choice In Dying   9/95
200 Varick Street, New York, NY 10014 1-800-989-WILL

has its own laws. On a federal level, however, there is a law called the Patient Self-Determination Act, which went into effect in late 1991. It requires workers of all federally funded institutions—hospitals, health maintenance organizations, hospices, skilled nursing facilities, and facilities accepting Medicare or Medicaid customers—to inform patients of their right to establish an advance directive. In most instances, the federally funded health-care institutions in your state will be able to fully explain your state's provision for advance directives. If an institution has moral or ethical codes that conflict with advance directives, they should inform you of their policies. In any case, do not hesitate to ask about their policies regarding advance directives.

While a living will expresses your wishes regarding health care, it still has it shortcomings. There is no guarantee that what you want will be carried out. The document can still leave room for legal, ethical, medical, and personal value uncertainties, and it is limited by the laws in each state. Nevertheless, it does make your wishes known to your family and friends, giving them guidance in making health-care decisions for you.

FREE INFORMATION ON ADVANCE DIRECTIVES

The following Congressional Research Service (CRS) reports are available from your U.S. Senators' offices at the U.S. Capitol, Washington, DC 20510 or from your Congressional Representative at the U.S. Capitol, Washington, DC 20515. Or call in your request to the capitol switchboard at 202-224-3121. Include the full title and the publication number, noted after the title, in your request.

- Treatment and Appointment Directives: Living Wills, Power of Attorney, and Other Advance Medical Care Documents (#91-87A)

- Life-Sustaining Technologies: Medical and Moral Issues (#91-45SPR)

- Advance Directives and Health-Care Facilities (#91-117EPW)

- Advance Medical Directives (#91-27A)

- Birth, Life and Death: Fundamental Life Decisions and the Right to Privacy (#90-180A)

- The Right to Die: Fundamental Life Decisions After Cruzan v. Director, Missouri Dept. of Health (#90-371A)

- A Survey of Statutory Definitions of Death (#91-635A)

FLORIDA DESIGNATION OF HEALTH CARE SURROGATE

INSTRUCTIONS

PRINT YOUR NAME

Name: _____

    (Last)   *(First)*   *(Middle Initial)*

In the event that I have been determined to be incapacitated to provide informed consent for medical treatment and surgical and diagnostic procedures, I wish to designate as my surrogate for health care decisions:

PRINT THE NAME, HOME ADDRESS AND TELEPHONE NUMBER OF YOUR SURROGATE

Name: _____

Address: _____

_____ Zip Code: _____

Phone: _____

If my surrogate is unwilling or unable to perform his duties, I wish to designate as my alternate surrogate:

PRINT THE NAME, HOME ADDRESS AND TELEPHONE NUMBER OF YOUR ALTERNATE SURROGATE

Name: _____

Address: _____

_____ Zip Code: _____

Phone: _____

I fully understand that this designation will permit my designee to make health care decisions and to provide, withhold, or withdraw consent on my behalf; to apply for public benefits to defray the cost of health care; and to authorize my admission to or transfer from a health care facility.

| FLORIDA DESIGNATION OF HEALTH CARE SURROGATE — PAGE 2 OF 2 |

ADD PERSONAL INSTRUCTIONS (IF ANY)

Additional instructions (optional):

I further affirm that this designation is not being made as a condition of treatment or admission to a health care facility. I will notify and send a copy of this document to the following persons other than my surrogate, so they may know who my surrogate is:

PRINT THE NAMES AND ADDRESSES OF THOSE WHO YOU WANT TO KEEP COPIES OF THIS DOCUMENT

Name: _____

Address: _____

Name: _____

Address: _____

SIGN AND DATE THE DOCUMENT

Signed: _____

Date: _____

WITNESSING PROCEDURE

TWO WITNESSES MUST SIGN AND PRINT THEIR ADDRESSES

Witness 1:

    Signed: _____

    Address: _____

Witness 2:

    Signed: _____

    Address: _____

Courtesy of Choice In Dying   9/95
200 Varick Street, New York, NY 10014 1-800-989-WILL

Durable Power of Attorney for Health Care

A durable power of attorney for health care (sometimes called a DPA) is a document that names an agent or surrogate who will carry out your wishes regarding medical treatment. While a living will is only about the final moments of life, the durable power of attorney can be drafted to give your agent the authority to make decisions about other areas of medical treatment—not just the termination of life support. The best strategy is to have both a living will and a durable power of attorney.

The individual you choose to represent you to your doctors is called an agent or proxy. According to your state's laws, your agent may not be legally bound to carry out your wishes as you have outlined them in your DPA. In any case, he or she will be legally able to speak for you, so it is very important to choose your agent carefully, considering someone who knows you as an individual and who will respect your wishes regarding treatment.

If a DPA has been outlined, the physician and your agent can make decisions about your medical care together: The doctor can provide your agent, just as he would a patient, with up-to-date information, medical facts, and options, and the agent can provide him with the reasons and circumstances behind your wishes. Without a DPA, there will be no one who can legally speak for you, and the decisions about your medical care will be left to a stranger who may have the best intentions but knows nothing about you, your history, personal circumstances, or your family.

As with any legal document, it is important to keep your DPA in safekeeping. Your family, physician, chosen agent, and attorney should be made aware of your wishes regarding medical treatment and should also hold a copy of the document.

Do Not Resuscitate Order

A do not resuscitate order, called a DNR order, is another document that can be used to help you to gain more control over the circumstances of your death. It means that cardiopulmonary resuscitative measures (CPR) will not be started, should respiration or heartbeat fail. These orders also mean that you will not be placed on long-term mechanical life support equipment.

It is important to talk to the attending physician about a DNR order before being admitted to a hospital, if possible. Discuss the matter with family members so they are aware of your wishes and document a DNR order in a living will. Also, convey this information to whomever holds your durable power of attorney. No matter how important a DNR order may seem under certain circumstances, it is revocable if you change your mind. And if you do, document your decision as well.

Assisted Suicide and the Death with Dignity Act

In the last two decades, right-to-die issues have given rise to the assisted suicide controversy. Assisted suicide, also called euthanasia or aid-in-dying, should not be confused with refusing treatment or being allowed to die. Assisted suicide is the actual assistance in causing death, providing the means to stop the heart from beating, the lungs from breathing, and the entire brain from having any activity, perhaps by administering drugs. Doctors are not legally able to assist in these "mercy killings," as they are considered criminal acts. The Hippocratic oath, under which doctors swear to protect life (and disallows them from intentionally causing death), ethically prevents them from taking part.

The Hemlock Society, an organization formed in 1980 to campaign for the right of terminally ill patient to choose voluntary euthanasia, is sponsoring a bill called the Death with Dignity Act that would let physicians and nurses legally provide aid-in-dying measures to terminally ill patients. Thirteen states also introduced aid-in-dying legislation that would allow legal options for those who are dying.

The bill is meant to keep the decision-making process with the patient and health-care provider and out of court. It is also designed to do the following:

1. Permit a competent terminally ill adult the right to request and receive physician aid-in-dying under carefully defined circumstances

2. Protect physicians from liability in carrying out a patient's request

3. Combine the concepts of Natural Death Acts and Durable Power of Attorney for Health Care laws and makes them more usable

4. Permit a patient to appoint an attorney-in-fact to be reviewed by a hospital ethics or other committee before the decision is acted upon by the physician

5. Require a competent adult person to sign a Death with Dignity directive in order to take advantage of the law

6. Require hospitals and other health-care facilities to keep records and report to the Department of Health Services after the death of the patient and then anonymously

7. Permit a treating physician to order a psychiatric consultation, with the patient's consent, if there is any question about the patient's competence to make the request for aid-in-dying

8. Forbid aid-in-dying to any patient solely because he or she is a burden to anyone, or because the patient is incompetent or terminal and has not made out an informed and proper Death with Dignity directive

9. Forbid aiding, abetting, and encouraging a suicide, which remains a crime under the Act

10. Forbid aid-in-dying to be administered by a loved one, family member, or stranger

11. Forbid aid-in-dying for children, incompetents, or anyone who has not voluntarily and intentionally completed and signed the properly witnessed Death and Dignity directive

12. Keep the decision-making process with the patient and health-care provider and out of court

13. Make special protective provisions for patients in skilled nursing facilities

14. Permit doctors, nurses, and privately owned hospitals the right to decline a dying patient's request for aid-in-dying if they are morally or ethically opposed to such action

Hospice Care

A hospice is a special facility designed solely to assist dying patients and their families. According to the National Hospice Organization, the hospice enables the patient to live as fully as possible, makes the entire family the unit of care, and centers the caring process in the home whenever appropriate.

Hospice care places emphasis on providing comfort and relief from symptoms, preparation for death, and support for survivors. Care can be provided in the home or in professional facilities with a homelike setting, but the idea is to allow death with dignity and keep the family close to the patient, away from the high-tech surrounds of a hospital. In fact, the active contributions and support of family members are welcomed.

Medicare now provides for hospice coverage both in and out of the home. Check with your local Social Security office or the Hospice Association of America for more information on Medicare.

Hospice Organizations

There are several hospice organizations throughout the country, some with their own specialties, such as terminally ill children. These groups can provide you with a wealth of information on care for the terminally ill, as well as put you in touch with support groups, help you with Medicare reimbursement problems, and refer you to homemaker-health aides.

For more information:

Children's Hospice International
2202 Mount Vernon Ave., Suite 3C
Alexandria, VA 22301
703-684-0330
http://www.chionline.org

Choice In Dying
200 Varick St., Suite 1001
New York, NY 10014

800-989-WILL
212-366-5540
http://www.choices.org

Hospice Association of America
228 7th St., S.E.
Washington, DC 20003
202-546-4759
http://www.nahc.org

Living/Dying Project
75 Digital Dr.
Novato, CA 94949
415-456-3915

Hospice Education Institute
190 Westbrook Rd.
Essex, CT 06426
860-767-1620

National Hemlock Society
P.O. Box 101810
Denver, CO 80250-1018
800-247-7421
http://www.hemlock.org/hemlock

National Hospice Organization
1901 N. Moore St., Suite 901
Arlington, VA 22209
703-243-5900
http://www.nho.org

National Institute for Jewish Hospice
8723 Alden Dr., Suite 652
Los Angeles, CA 90048
213-467-7423

RTS Bereavement Services
Lutheran Hospital-La Crosse
1910 South Avenue
La Crosse, WI 54601
608-791-4747

St. Francis Center
4880A MacArthur Blvd., N.W.
Washington, DC 20007
202-333-4880

Health Conditions

Despite the complexity and intricacies of the human body, most of us are able to live the majority of our lives without illness or health disorders. Yet when disease strikes, a man's life can be altered—sometimes permanently.

Understanding the conditions that beset you is an essential aspect of curing or coping with them. Individuals informed about their own conditions are in a better position to care for themselves than those who aren't sure what is happening—or what will happen. Informed people can also interact more easily with medical practitioners. Knowing about the diseases, ailments, and conditions that afflict you allows you to make better, more educated decisions about available treatments.

This section provides information on some of the most common and most important medical conditions affecting men today. Listed in alphabetical order, these discussions provide facts on specific conditions, their symptoms, their diagnosis, and their treatment. There are also, in many cases, tips on how to reduce your risk for a condition and on how to take care of yourself if you are facing that illness. Additional resources follow most topics.

By knowing more about what is happening to you, you will be better able to participate in your own health care.

ALCOHOL AND ALCOHOLISM

Many people enjoy alcoholic beverages from time to time—in moderation, alcohol may even have some health benefits. Yet it has addictive properties, and excessive use may lead to alcoholism, also called alcohol dependence. In 1992, according to the National Institute of Alcohol Abuse and Alcoholism, nearly 13.8 million Americans—of which 9.7 million were men— had problems with drinking. An estimated 8.1 million problem drinkers are alcoholics. A 1994 survey from the U.S. Department of Health and Human Services reports that men are more than four times as likely as women to report heavy alcohol use. Rates are highest among the unemployed.

According to the National Council on Alcoholism and Drug Dependence, alcoholism is a disease characterized by a periodic or continuous inability to control drinking, a preoccupation with alcohol, use of alcohol despite its consequences, and distortions in thinking, most notably denial.

Dependence on alcohol is psychological and physical. Emotional distress and cravings for alcohol are signs of psychological dependence—a person may need to drink to relax, for example. Physical dependence, when the body has adapted to the presence of alcohol and needs it to function, manifests itself in withdrawal symptoms that occur when alcohol is not available. These include sweating, diarrhea, vomiting, trembling, cramps, confusion, and, in extreme cases, seizures and coma, which may lead to death.

How Alcohol Works

Alcohol, also known as ethanol or ethyl alcohol, is a colorless liquid made by fermentation. Alcohol is a depressant, a drug that slows the central nervous system and acts as a mild anesthetic and tranquilizer. But it is probably most well known for boosting the body's levels of the brain chemicals dopamine, serotonin, and endorphins, which promote feelings of self-confidence, relaxation, and happiness.

Alcohol is absorbed into the bloodstream through the membranes of the mouth and the esophagus as well as the stomach and the intestines. The rate of absorption varies according to the type of beverage consumed (the higher the percentage of alcohol, the faster it is absorbed) and the amount of food in the digestive system at the time.

Once absorbed, about 10 percent of the alcohol is eliminated through perspiration and breathing, while the other 90 percent is metabolized by an enzyme in the liver. Some research indicates that men may have more of this enzyme than women and metabolize the same amount of alcohol faster, which is possibly why women tend to have higher blood-alcohol levels

than men have after the same number of drinks, even after taking into consideration body size. Women also tend to have a higher percentage of body fat and a lower percentage of water, which means the alcohol becomes more highly concentrated in a woman's system than in a man's.

Habitual drinkers acquire a tolerance to alcohol, meaning that more alcohol is needed to obtain the same feelings of relief and relaxation. As more alcohol is consumed on a regular basis, the liver breaks it down at a faster rate, meaning a greater intake is necessary to achieve the same blood-alcohol level. At the same time, nerve cells in the brain become less responsive to a given amount of alcohol. Tolerance is one of the warning signs of alcoholism.

Causes of Alcoholism

Alcoholism is not a result of a weak will or poor self-control. In fact, there is no single cause for alcoholism, but rather a number of contributing physical and environmental factors. According to studies, men have a 3 to 5 percent risk of alcoholism, while women have a 1 percent risk.

Studies show that a person whose parents or other relatives were alcoholics are at greater risk of alcoholism than people with nonalcoholic parents or relatives. The reasons behind this are not certain—the tendency may be genetic, environmental, or both.

It is also thought that some people may genetically be unable to properly metabolize alcohol, which could result in a tendency to alcoholism. Ethnicity plays a role as well. Native Americans and those of Irish background are at increased risk of alcoholism, and Jewish and Asian Americans are at decreased risk.

Alcohol dependence may also start with the use of alcohol to "self-medicate"—a person may

EFFECTS OF INCREASED BLOOD-ALCOHOL LEVEL BY PERCENTAGE

.02 (one drink)	Some drinkers may feel warmth and relaxation.
.04	Most people feel relaxed, talkative, and happy. Skin may flush.
.05	The first sizable changes begin to occur. Lightheartedness, giddiness, lowered inhibitions, and less control of thoughts may be experienced. Both restraint and judgement are lowered; coordination may be slightly altered.
.06	Judgement somewhat impaired; ability to make a rational decision about personal capabilities is affected, such as one's driving ability.
.08	Definite impairment of muscle coordination and a slower reaction time; driving ability suspect. Sensory feelings of numbness of the cheeks and lips. Hands, arms, and legs may tingle and then feel numb. Legally impaired in some states.
.10	Clumsy; speech may become fuzzy. Clear deterioration of reaction time and muscle control. Legally drunk in most states. It is illegal to operate a motor vehicle with this or greater blood-alcohol content (BAC) in most states.
.15	Definite impairment of balance and movement. The equivalent of a 1/2 pint of whisky is in the bloodstream.
.20	Motor and emotional control centers measurably affected; slurred speech, staggering, loss of balance, and double vision can all be present.
.30	Lack of understanding of what is seen or heard; individual is confused or stuporous. Consciousness may be lost at this level ("passes out").
.40	Usually unconscious; skin clammy.

Source: U.S. Department of Health and Human Services, Public Health Service, National Institute on Alcohol Abuse and Alcoholism, Rockville, Maryland.

drink because of stress, loneliness, or other factors in order to relax, forget any problems, and feel better emotionally and physically. Men, who traditionally act as the providers for their families, may drink because of financial problems or pressures in the workplace. As a person's tolerance to alcohol grows, consumption increases, setting the stage for alcoholism.

Other social factors, especially availability and acceptance of alcohol in a person's culture and social circle, also contribute to alcoholism. As a result, alcohol dependence is more prevalent in some countries and groups than in others. Men might be particularly susceptible to alcoholism since they're usually encouraged to drink socially.

Drinking patterns vary between men and women, with men having higher levels of heavy drinking and higher rates of alcohol disorders and drinking-related problems. Patterns also vary, according to ethnic background. African-American men are least likely to drink, white men are most likely to drink, and Hispanic men fall somewhere in between.

Symptoms

Development of alcohol dependence can be divided into four main phases, which most often overlap and merge:

1. In the first phase, tolerance to alcohol develops in a heavy social drinker.

2. In the second phase, a drinker experiences memory lapses relating to events occurring during drinking episodes.

3. In the third phase, there is a loss of control; the drinker can no longer stop drinking whenever he wants to.

4. In the final phase, there are prolonged binges of drunkenness, with the drinker suffering observable mental or physical complications.

Behavioral signs of alcohol dependence can include personality changes (such as irritability, jealousy, uncontrolled anger, and selfishness); irrational or inappropriate behavior; neglect of personal appearance; furtive behavior (hiding bottles, for example); and prolonged periods of intoxication.

Physical symptoms include nausea and vomiting, shakes, abdominal pain, numbness or tingling, weakness in the legs and hands, irregular pulse, unsteadiness, confusion and poor memory. Sudden withdrawal of alcohol may cause withdrawal symptoms, including delirium tremens, or D.T.'s.

The Dangers of Alcoholism

While the physical and psychological need for alcohol is the most apparent problem associated with alcoholism, a number of other, secondary disorders may affect people who consume large amounts of alcohol:

- Gastritis, pancreatitis, peptic ulcers, liver disease (including cirrhosis) and liver cancer, as well as oral cancers. Alcohol can have a direct toxic effect on the body's cells and tissue.

- Heart disease, high blood pressure, heart failure, and stroke. Alcohol can damage the heart muscle and increase blood pressure considerably.

- Kidney disease and failure. Heavy drinking taxes the kidneys by increasing urine output.

- Impaired sexual performance. Though alcohol can increase sexual confidence, it can hinder libido, erections, and orgasms. Heavy drinking decreases testosterone levels and has a feminizing effect over time. Breast tissue may enlarge, and pubic hair may disappear.

- AIDS/HIV and sexually transmitted diseases. Evidence shows there is a link

SIGNS OF PROBLEM DRINKING

The following questions developed by the National Institute on Alcohol Abuse and Alcoholism may be used to help determine if you or someone you know has a drinking problem or may be an alcoholic:

- Do you think and talk about drinking often?

- Do you drink more now than you used to?

- Do you sometimes gulp drinks?

- Do you often take a drink to help you relax?

- Do you drink when you are alone?

- Do you sometimes forget what happened when you were drinking?

- Do you keep a bottle hidden somewhere at home or at work for a quick "pick-me-up?"

- Do you need a drink to have fun?

- Do you ever start drinking without really thinking about it?

- Do you ever drink in the morning to relieve a hangover?

- Do you ever feel that you need a drink?

- Do you become irritable when drinking?

- Do you drink to get drunk?

- Has your drinking harmed your family or friends in any way?

- Does drinking change your personality, creating an entirely new you?

- Are you more impulsive when you are drinking?

"Yes" answers to any of these questions may be an indication of a drinking problem.

between alcohol use and behavior that increases the risk for contracting a sexually transmitted disease.

- Nutritional deficiencies. Alcoholics who satisfy their caloric requirements with alcohol may suffer from deficiencies, particularly the lack of vitamin B_1, or thiamine. The deficiency of thiamine, also known as beriberi, may lead to nervous system disorders and, in severe cases, heart failure.

HEALTH BENEFITS OF ALCOHOL

Moderate alcohol consumption—no more than two drinks a day—can benefit your health, according to some experts. (Keep in mind that a drink equals 12 ounces of beer, 5 ounces of wine or 1¹/₂ ounces of liquor.) The Framingham Study, a well-known study on heart disease, reported an association between moderate drinking and a reduced risk of coronary heart disease. Other studies have shown that moderate drinkers have a lower risk of stroke than those who don't drink. In addition, other research has established a link between moderate alcohol use and higher levels of high-density lipoprotein, the "good" cholesterol.

Despite these benefits of alcohol, anyone who is at high risk for alcohol-related problems should never drink—the dangers far outweigh any health benefits. Also, those who don't drink shouldn't start just because of the health benefits, which can be gained through eating well and exercising just as easily.

Treatment

According to a study from the National Alcohol Research Center, the number of men and women seeking treatment for alcoholism is steadily growing. However, men still outnumber women by far. Married men were found to seek treatment more often than single men, and younger men sought treatment more often than older men.

There are many places to turn for an alcoholic who wants to recover. By the time an alcoholic searches for help, he may have already become addicted to the substance and may require it in order to function. For this reason, physical and emotional assistance is needed.

Doctors, members of the clergy, or community health or social workers can help an alcoholic seek treatment. Most hospitals have inpatient or outpatient clinics to aid alcoholics. There are also divisions of public and private hospitals exclusively designed for the treatment of alcoholism. In addition, state alcohol abuse agencies provide programs for the prevention, detection, treatment, and rehabilitation of alcohol abusers. Check the blue pages in your phone book for contact information.

Alcoholics who are physically dependent require medical help, called detoxification, to get over withdrawal symptoms when they quit drinking. Detoxification is then followed by long-term treatment. Treatment involves three forms of therapy:

1. *Psychological treatments.* These therapies involve psychotherapy, a form of talk therapy that involves changing behavior and seeking the emotional roots of problems and that is usually performed in a group setting.

2. *Social treatments.* These forms focus on problems at work and at home and includes family members in the treatment process.

3. *Medical treatments.* This type therapy is needed by alcoholics who suffer serious withdrawal symptoms. The drug Antabuse (disulfiram), which causes nausea and vomiting when a person drinks, may be prescribed. In addition, a new drug called Revia (naltrexone hydrochloride) was approved in 1995. Revia works by reducing alcohol cravings and promoting

abstinence from alcohol. These medications are used as part of a comprehensive treatment program.

No single treatment is best for all alcoholics. Sometimes the forms may be combined.

Self-Help Groups

Alcoholics have also been shown to benefit from self-help organizations. For example, Alcoholics Anonymous (AA) is a fellowship of men and women who share their experiences, strengths, and hopes so they may solve their common problem and help others to recover from alcoholism. There's no membership fee, and the only requirement is a desire to stop drinking. AA is not affiliated with any sect, political party, institution, or other organization and has a strict policy of anonymity. During meetings alcoholics pass along their personal stories, describe the sobriety they have found in AA, and invite newcomers to join the informal fellowship. A 12-step program toward recovery forms the basis of AA's self-help treatment plan.

AA is made up of more than two million recovered alcoholics in the United States, Canada, and other countries, and about 65 percent of its membership is men. Families and friends of alcoholics can seek help from Al-Anon. Alateen is a group available for teenage children of alcoholics. These groups can help those close to alcoholics understand and deal with their problems.

Drinking and Driving

According to the National Council on Alcoholism and Drug Dependence, alcohol is a leading cause of traffic accidents in the United States. Almost half of all traffic fatalities are alcohol-related, and men are involved in the majority of fatal crashes. The U.S. Department of Transportation National Highway Traffic Safety Administration reports that 56,155 American drivers were involved in fatal crashes in 1995 while driving under the influence. Of those drivers, 41,216 (or 73 percent) were men.

You should never drive or operate machinery after drinking. The following table is a general guideline for how long to wait after drinking before attempting to drive. (Again, one drink equals $1^1/_2$ ounces of liquor, 12 ounces of beer, or 4 ounces of wine or champagne.)

Body Weight (lbs.)	1 drink	2 drinks	3 drinks	4 drinks	5 drinks	6 drinks
100–119	0 hrs	3 hrs	6 hrs	10 hrs	13 hrs	16 hrs
120–139	0 hrs	2 hrs	5 hrs	8 hrs	10 hrs	12 hrs
140–159	0 hrs	2 hrs	4 hrs	6 hrs	8 hrs	10 hrs
160–179	0 hrs	1 hrs	3 hrs	5 hrs	7 hrs	9 hrs
180–199	0 hrs	0 hrs	2 hrs	4 hrs	6 hrs	7 hrs
200–219	0 hrs	0 hrs	2 hrs	3 hrs	5 hrs	6 hrs
over 200	0 hrs	0 hrs	1 hr	3 hrs	4 hrs	6 hrs

For more information:

Alcoholics Anonymous Worldwide Services Office
475 Riverside Drive
New York, NY 10115
212-870-3400
http://www.alcoholics-anonymous.org

Al-Anon and Alateen Family Groups
Headquarters, Inc.
1600 Corporate Landing Pkwy.
Virginia Beach, VA 23454
800-356-9996
800-245-4656 (New York)
800-443-4525 (Canada)
757-563-1600

National Council on Alcoholism and Drug
Dependence
12 W. 21st St.
New York, NY 10010
800-NCA-CALL
212-206-6770
http://www.ncadd.org

National Clearinghouse for Alcohol and
Drug Information
Drug Abuse Information and Treatment
Referral Line
Box 2345
Rockville, MD 20847-2345
800-662-4357
800-662-9832 (Spanish)
800-228-0427 (hearing impaired)
301-468-6433
http://www.health.org

ALLERGIES

About fifty million Americans suffer from the sneezing, runny noses, itching, and rashes caused by allergies. These symptoms occur when the body's immune system, which protects against invading substances, becomes hypersensitive to usually harmless substances such as dust, molds, pollen, and certain foods. Any substance that stimulates the immune system to cause an allergic reaction is called an allergen.

If you've ever suffered poison ivy, had a mosquito bite, or sneezed after smelling a coworker's perfume, you're familiar with an allergic reaction. But you might not be familiar with exactly what occurred to create that response. When the immune system comes in contact with an allergen, it produces a type of blood protein called an antibody, a protein designed to eliminate the foreign substance from the body. Antibodies attach themselves to cells in the respiratory and gastrointestinal tracts, skin, and blood. These cells then release potent chemicals—histamines, prostaglandins and leukotrienes—that cause common allergic symptoms.

Symptoms

Allergy symptoms vary, according to the individual and the allergen. The most common allergic reaction is allergic rhinitis, with symptoms similar to a cold—clear and watery nasal discharge, nasal congestion, itchy nose and eyes, watery eyes, and sneezing. Allergic rhinitis may be an ongoing reaction, or it may occur seasonally. Seasonal allergic rhinitis is also known as hay fever (a misnomer since it has nothing to do with hay or fever). Because hay fever is often a reaction to molds, spores, or the pollens of grass, trees, and weeds, people with this type of allergy usually suffer the most during the spring and fall.

Rashes and skin irritation may result from allergic contact dermatitis, a reaction to contact with a particular substance. Such allergens include poison ivy, sun, dyes, cosmetics, metal compounds, and certain medications. Atopic dermatitis, or eczema, is usually a reaction to something eaten or inhaled. It is marked by a blistering and crusting rash that appears on the skin.

Food, drug, and insect sting allergies result from the consumption of various foods (milk, eggs, shellfish, nuts, soybeans, wheat products, chocolate), the ingestion or injection of certain drugs (most commonly penicillin and related antibiotics, sulfonamide drugs, barbiturates, insulin, anesthetics, and anticonvulsant drugs), or the sting venom of certain insects (such as wasps, bees, and ants). Symptoms of food allergies include hives, abdominal pain, vomiting and nausea, swelling, and diarrhea. Drug allergies can cause difficulty in breathing, wheezing, hives, itching, and skin rashes. Insect stings can cause hives, itching, and constricted sensations in the throat and chest.

With many types of allergies, symptoms can quickly escalate to a rare, potentially life-threatening reaction known as anaphylaxis or anaphylactic shock. With anaphylactic shock, blood pressure drops suddenly, air passages tighten, the throat becomes swollen, and hives may appear. Such a reaction usually happens only a few seconds or minutes after the person has come in contact with the allergen and can cause death if not treated immediately. While almost any allergen can cause such a reaction, it occurs more commonly after a bee sting or an injection of a new medication. Legumes and shellfish may also trigger a reaction. For those who have severe reactions to bee stings or foods, emergency kits, which usually contain an injection of epinephrine, are available.

LATEX ALLERGIES

One allergy that recently received special attention due to the increase in the protective use of condoms and rubber gloves is a reaction to latex. The proteins in latex cause allergic symptoms in about 1 percent of the general public and in 7 to 10 percent of health-care workers. A latex reaction most commonly produces a red, itchy skin rash on the areas touching the substance, but some people develop eye and respiratory problems and even anaphylactic shock.

Those who have suffered a serious allergic reaction should avoid latex. However, if you've had a mild, topical allergic reaction to latex condoms, there are a few things you might want to try before you give up on them. First, try another brand or one without lubrication, since you may only be allergic to a certain brand or you may be reacting to the condom's lubricant or spermicide rather than to the latex. As an extra preventive against rash, put a steroid cream (hydrocortisone) on your skin before putting on the condom. While latex condoms offer the best protection from the spread of HIV and other sexually transmitted infections, those who are severely allergic to latex should consider sheepskin condoms.

Diagnosis

The medical specialist who deals with allergies is known as an allergist, though a primary-care practitioner can also diagnose and treat allergies.

To diagnose specific allergies, a doctor may order a blood test to check for the presence of antibodies. There also are several skin tests available. In the scratch test (rarely used today), the doctor makes a series of short, superficial scratches on the skin—usually the forearm—and then rubs different extracts of suspected allergens into them. More common, the skin-prick test involves placing a drop of allergen extract on the arm or back. Then, a small needle pricks the skin under the drop. In the intradermal test, the allergen-containing solution is injected directly into the skin. A patch test, in which a small amount of an allergen is placed on the skin and covered by an adhesive patch, is used to diagnose contact dermatitis. In each of these tests the patient reacts positively to the substance if a red, itchy welt develops at the test area after fifteen to twenty minutes.

Pinpointing specific food allergies is a more complicated process. After skin and blood tests suggest certain foods are allergens, there are two choices to confirm a suspected food allergy. Avoidance is the simplest—the food is removed from the diet and the person is observed to see if allergic symptoms disappear. If they do, the food is reintroduced into the diet to see if symptoms recur. If they do, the food is then assumed to be a trigger.

The second, more scientific approach is blind testing, in which the person is given a dose of a suspected food allergen or a placebo, an inactive substance. This allows the doctor to determine whether the food really triggers a reaction.

Treatment

Once an allergy has been diagnosed, a doctor may prescribe an antihistamine, decongestants, or corticosteroids.

- *Antihistamines.* Antihistamines work best when taken before you come in contact with an allergen, since the antihistamine's job is to bind to tissue sites such as the cells lining the breathing tubes before histamines do so. Antihistamines are available over the counter and through a prescription.

  Proven to be useful for all types of allergies, antihistamines include Benadryl, Tavist, Chlor-Trimeton and Tacaryl. However, these types of antihistamines cause drowsiness. To counteract that sleepiness, some manufacturers combine the antihistamine with a decongestant that has an "upper" effect. Antihistamines sometimes also are combined with pain relievers to reduce headaches and pain associated with allergies. Newer antihistamines such as Claritin, Zytrec, Allegra, and Hismanal are nonsedating and have proven very effective in reducing allergy symptoms.

- *Decongestants.* By constricting blood vessels, decongestants shrink swollen mucous membranes to stop nasal congestion. And unlike antihistamines, decongestants are effective when an allergy attack is underway.

  Sold as pills, drops, or sprays, popular over-the-counter decongestants include Sudafed, Afrin, and Neosynephrine. Decongestants are stimulants and should be used with caution. Side effects include raised blood pressure, rapid heart rate, headaches, and jitteriness. Plus, nasal spray decongestants may become addictive and should be used for three to five days at most.

- *Corticosteroids.* Hormonelike anti-inflammatory drugs, corticosteroids are usually used to treat respiratory and skin allergies. Corticosteroids come as a spray or inhalant for respiratory tract problems, as injectables or topical formulas for allergic skin rashes, and in intramuscular, intravenous, and oral forms for systemic therapy. While nasal corticosteroids are safe to use for longer periods of time, the systemic forms should only be used in short-term allergy treatment.

When administered in low doses for short periods, corticosteroids have few side effects, although headaches, an upset stomach, and fluid retention are possible. Prolonged use of high doses may result in elevated blood pressure, gastric ulcers, weight gain, and psychological disorders.

When an allergy patient does not respond to medications alone, immunotherapy may be the answer. Immunotherapy helps to desensitize allergy suffers through a series of gradually potent injections of whatever the patient is allergic to—for example, ragweed, animal dander (the minute particles of skin that come from hair or feathers), and mold. With a 75 to 90 percent effectiveness rate, the shots should allow the patient to build a tolerance to the allergen and reduce or eliminate allergic symptoms. If successful, the course of treatment can continue for up to five years. However, a person may have a reaction to an injection, either a minor local reaction such as swelling at the site or a rare, more serious systemic reaction, involving difficulty breathing, hives, stomach pains, difficulty swallowing, and fainting. In addition, injections are not available to treat every type of allergy.

A new version of this treatment that is under study is nasal immunotherapy in which the allergen is absorbed into the body through a nasal spray. The advantage of the spray is that there are few side effects.

SELF-CARE FOR ALLERGIES

Probably the best way to control allergies is to minimize exposures to the allergens. Here are some ideas on how to do that:

- Keep windows and doors closed when the pollen count is high. Some radio and television stations (for example, all-weather stations) announce pollen levels. The pollen count usually increases daily from 4 P.M. to 10 A.M.

- Check the weather. On dry, sunny, and windy days in the spring, summer, and fall, there's probably pollen in the air, so it might be best to stay inside if you're allergic. Humid or rainy days are better for those with allergies to pollens: Offending plants don't pollinate on

continues

humid days, and rain keeps pollen out of the air. (However, rainy days may be worse for those with allergies to mold.)

- Use an air conditioner or air purifier, particularly in the bedroom. Be sure to clean the filter regularly.

- Use a dehumidifier to help reduce the growth of dust mites, molds, and fungi during summer humidity. Again, keep the machine clean to avoid molds.

- Avoid doing yardwork, mowing the lawn, or raking leaves if you're allergic to pollen or molds or wear a filter or mask to keep allergens out of your system.

- Clean your home as often as possible to remove pollen, dust, mold, and animal dander. Avoid dust-gathering knickknacks and draperies, bedspreads, and carpeting, especially in the sleeping area.

- Wash your bedding, synthetic pillows, and mattress pads often in hot water.

- Encase your mattress and pillows in plastic to reduce dust mite waste in the air.

- Avoid hanging clothes, sheets, and blankets outside to dry.

For more information:

Allergy Information Referral Line
American Academy of Allergy, Asthma and
Immunology
611 E. Wells St.
Milwaukee, WI 53202
800-822-2762

American College of Allergy, Asthma and
Immunology
1645 Oakton St.
Des Plains, IL 60018
800-842-7777

ALZHEIMER'S DISEASE AND DEMENTIA

Alzheimer's disease is much more than simple forgetfulness. It is a progressive, degenerative disease in which an individual's brain cells gradually deteriorate, causing thinking, behavior, and memory to become impaired. These problems result in an inability to function normally, which eventually causes death. Besides being considered the only cause of death in many of its victims, Alzheimer's disease, which has no cure, is also often considered a contributing cause of death when it couples with other conditions.

Ten percent of men in the United States over age 65 have Alzheimer's disease. In 1993, Alzheimer s disease caused 16,754 deaths, 98 percent of which were Americans age 65 and over. More women than men have Alzheimer's, which currently is the fourth leading cause of death in all developed countries, affecting twenty million estimated people worldwide. However, men have a higher death rate than women, though the mortality gap between genders decreased between 1979 and 1993, according to the National Center for Health Statistics. According to the Alzheimer's Disease Education and Referral Center, the disease may afflict more than twelve million Americans by the year 2040.

Risk Factors

The exact cause of Alzheimer's is unknown, though there are a number of theories as to its origins. These theories include genetic defects or predispositions to the disease, a deficiency of brain hormones, exposure to environmental toxins, and immune system dysfunction.

Current studies indicate that Alzheimer's kills two times more whites than African Americans. Although Alzheimer's usually sets in at age 65 or older, with incidence increasing with age, there are rare cases of people in their 30s to 50s getting the disease.

Symptoms

The development of Alzheimer's disease is usually divided into three stages. In the early stage, symptoms include short-term memory loss, difficulty concentrating or learning, social withdrawal, and difficulty calculating numbers or finding certain words. In the moderate stage, symptoms progress to include long-term memory loss, poor judgement, speech difficulties, disorientation (resulting in the person often getting lost), behavior, and personality changes, insomnia, fear, and depression. In the severe stage, symptoms include lack of recognition of friends and relatives, an inability to function independently, an inability to speak or understand speech, and delusions, hallucinations, and paranoia. Eventually, an Alzheimer's patient becomes unable to use his muscles and is mute, immobile, and incontinent.

Diagnosis

Pinpointing Alzheimer's disease can be very difficult—in most cases, a definitive diagnosis cannot be made until an autopsy is done after death. However, Alzheimer's disease is often confused with a number of treatable conditions, so tests must be done to rule out other possibilities. Diagnosis begins with a physical examination and a medical history. Then, neurological tests—noninvasive tests that evaluate brain function—are done. These tests may be nothing more than a series of questions or exercises, as basic as examining a person s reflexes or testing his ability to walk and balance. Other tests can include mental status checks, which are usually a series of questions testing memory. If these simple tests prove to be inconclusive, a doctor may decide to order laboratory tests, including standard blood and urine screenings, to rule out other conditions. Thorough neurological and physical exams are recommended to determine if Alzheimer's is present.

If these tests are inconclusive, other techniques may be used to help diagnosis. An electroencephalogram (EEG) uses electrodes attached to the scalp to measure the brain's electrical activity. Computerized tomography (CT) uses x-ray technology to create a three-dimensional image of the brain. Magnetic resonance imaging (MRI) involves the use of magnetic waves to create cross-sections of the brain. In addition, positron emission tomography (PET) and single photon emission computer tomography (SPECT) show how the body's systems are functioning. These tests can reveal injuries, tumors, or areas of dead tissue in the brain and can show how well the brain is functioning. Again, these tests are used to diagnose Alzheimer's through process of elimination. Definitive diagnosis cannot be done until after death.

Treatment

A limited number of treatment options are available for those with Alzheimer s disease. Pharmaceutically, doctors consider a drug called tacrine (Cognex) to be the best option. Although other drugs are still being tested for their treatment value, tacrine increases the levels of a chemical called acetylcholine in the brain. This substance helps relay messages through nerve cells; although it decreases the symptoms of Alzheimer's, it does not cure the disease. A serious side effect of this drug is liver damage. Other effects include vomiting, nausea, and diarrhea. Other substances are being tested now that may be used to treat Alzheimer's in the future, including cholinergic drugs, which aim to stimulate the body's production of substances that promote brain neuron functioning.

In early 1997, a new drug called Aricept (donepezil hydrochloride) was approved for marketing by the Food and Drug Administration. The drug is similar to tacrine in that it helps relay messages through the nervous system, but does not treat the disease itself. Possible side effects include nausea, diarrhea, and vomiting. Unlike tacrine, it does not carry a risk of liver disease. It also needs to be taken less frequently than tacrine. It is best used in the early stages of the disease because it may not be helpful as Alzheimer's progresses.

Other drugs are used to treat the symptoms of Alzheimer's disease. For example, antianxiety drugs may help treat restlessness and behavioral problems. Depression, insomnia, and delusions may also be treated with specific drugs.

Options for Care

A variety of caregiving options are available to those with Alzheimer's and their families. The first step is to determine, with the help of a practitioner, the needs of the individual, and then the resources of the individual and the family should be considered. With these needs and limits in mind, a decision can be made as to appropriate care. Options include home health care by the family (supplemented with care by a part-time health care worker or an adult day care program) and various levels of long-term, nursing-home care. (See Long-Term Care, p. 132.)

Home Health Care

Despite a variety of care options, over 70 percent of those with Alzheimer s are cared for at home, according to the American Association of Retired Persons. Although most Alzheimer's caregivers are, in fact, women, a significant number of men care for their ailing wives or partners. According to a long-term care survey, 28 percent of caregivers are men, a number that is expected to grow. Home health care involves providing a safe environment for the patient and helping him or her through daily activities such as dressing, eating, and grooming. Activities and exercises can be done to keep the person active and interested, and certain techniques can help to combat memory loss. Home care may also involve dealing with difficult situations such as sudden outbursts, hallucinations, wandering, and sleep disturbances.

Home health care can take its toll on the caregiver, who must watch the personality and intellect of a loved one slip away. Those who must care for a loved one with Alzheimer's and do

CARING FOR SOMEONE WITH ALZHEIMER'S

While caregivers are tending to Alzheimer s patients at home, certain procedures can be followed to make this task more effective, more successful, and easier for both the caregiver and for the patient:

- Make the home as safe as possible.

- Remove sharp, heavy, or breakable objects that could cause harm.

- Install locks on doors to prevent wandering.

- Insulate items, such as heaters, that could cause burns.

- Arrange furniture to ease the walking path.

- Install nightlights and light all areas that could be hazardous, such as stairs.

- Improve communication techniques. Be sure to speak slowly, carefully, and emphatically. Body language, such as hand gestures and eye contact, can also help. Do not speak for the person, but rather offer encouragement and give your loved one adequate time to respond. Eliminate any distractions and focus solely on what the patient is trying to tell you.

- Follow a routine. This can lend a sense of stability to the individual's confusing environment and help eliminate sleep problems.

- Do not take things personally. Angry reactions or outbursts are not intentional on the part of a person with Alzheimer's—personality and behavioral changes are a symptom of the disease. If outbursts occur, remain calm, speak in a soothing tone, and try to distract the person from the focus of attention. Trying to reason with an Alzheimer's patient is rarely effective and may make the situation worse.

- Be patient. The calmer you remain, the better your chances of successful communication.

so in their own home have higher levels of depression and lower levels of positive health habits (such as eating right, exercising, and taking care of their own health) when compared with others who are not caregivers. This could be attributed to the fact that caregivers often ignore their own way of life to improve their patient's. For example, while encouraging a patient to eat right and maintain exercise habits, the caregiver becomes preoccupied with the patient and doesn't eat correctly or exercise regularly. Caregivers also often feel short on time and energy.

There are available services to help care for an ailing loved one. As the disease progresses, home care may become impossible as the person with Alzheimer's will require constant supervision and advanced medical care.

Other Forms of Dementia

Alzheimer's disease is a form of dementia, which is defined as a loss of intellectual function. Dementia is severe enough to interfere with a person's daily functioning and gradually grows worse. Although Alzheimer's accounts for some 75 percent of all cases of dementia, there are more than seventy other conditions that can cause dementia, a loss of brain function. Some forms of dementia—such as those brought on by drug use, depression, brain injuries, and curable diseases such as syphilis and tuberculosis—are reversible. However, the following conditions are among those that are not reversible:

1. *Parkinson's disease.* This disorder of the central nervous system causes a deficiency of the brain chemical dopamine, which plays a role in transmitting messages in the brain. It results in tremors, stiffness in the joints and limbs, speech impediments, and difficulty moving. In the late stages, memory loss may develop. It affects more than one million Americans each year, and more men than women. Drug treatment can alleviate symptoms but cannot reverse the damage or stop the progression of the disease. (See Parkinson's Disease, p. 330.)

2. *AIDS.* Dementia is a secondary effect of AIDS that occurs when the virus attacks the brain. One-third of those with AIDS experience dementia. Again, drugs can be used to slow the development of symptoms, but cannot cure the condition. (See AIDS/HIV, p. 391.)

3. *Multiple sclerosis.* In this condition, the protective covering of the nerve fibers in the brain and spinal cord is destroyed, affecting bodily functions. Symptoms include poor coordination, pain, double vision, lack of energy, and problems with mental functioning. It occurs in people between the ages of 20 and 40 and may progress and regress in cycles. The ratio of women to men sufferers is three to two. Treatment involves treating the muscular problems; there is no treatment for dementia that results.

4. *Huntington's disease.* This disease usually begins between the ages of 35 and 50. It is a degenerative brain disease that results in involuntary movement of the muscles, intellectual decline, memory loss, slurred speech, and psychiatric problems. It is a genetic disorder, and there is no treatment available to stop its progression, although drugs can be used to treat symptoms.

5. *Wilson's disease.* In this genetic disorder, copper accumulates in the liver and is released into the rest of the body. If the metal accumulates in the brain, it can destroy brain tissue, resulting in tremors, rigid muscles, speech problems, and dementia. It is a rare disease that usually occurs in adolescence. Drugs can be used to remove the copper from the system and halt the progression of the disease.

6. *Vascular dementia.* This occurs when blood flow to the brain is blocked, resulting in brain damage. Stroke and embolism, for example, can cause vascular dementia. Reducing the risk of stroke and treating high blood pressure can stop the progression of vascular dementia, but cannot reverse the symptoms.

7. *Pick's disease.* This condition is similar to and often mistaken for Alzheimer's. It results in

personality changes, behavioral changes, disorientation, memory loss, and deterioration of language abilities. It is marked by the presence of Pick bodies—round, densely packed protein deposits—in the brain. Treatment can control symptoms, but not halt the progress of the disease.

8. *Lewy body dementia.* Also very similar to Alzheimer's, Lewy body dementia is marked by protein deposits known as Lewy bodies that form in the brain.

9. *Creutzfeldt-Jakob disease.* A rare disease, Creutzfeldt-Jakob occurs quickly— memory loss, behavior changes, and mental deterioration occur in the early stages, and death can occur within a year of the onset of symptoms. It is thought to be caused by a virus, and no treatment is available.

For more information:

Alzheimer's Association
919 N. Michigan Ave., Suite 1000
Chicago, IL 60611-1676
800-272-3900
312-335-8700
http://www.alz.org

Alzheimer's Disease Education and Referral Center
P.O. Box 8250
Silver Spring, MD 20907-8250
800-438-4380
301-495-3311
http://www.alzheimers.org/adear

American Health Assistance Foundation
15825 Shady Grove Rd., Suite 140
Rockville, MD 20850
800-437-2423
301-948-3244
http://www.ahaf.org

American Heart Association
7272 Greenville Ave.
Dallas, TX 75231
800-AHA-USA1
214-373-6300
http://www.amhrt.org

American Parkinson's Disease Association
1250 Hylan Blvd., Suite 4B
Staten Island, NY 10305
800-223-2732
http://www.apdaparkinson.org

Huntington's Disease Society of America
140 W. 22nd St., 6th floor
New York, NY 10011
800-345-4372
212-242-1968
curehd@hdfa.ttisms.com

Multiple Sclerosis Association of America
706 Haddenfield Road
Cherry Hill, NJ 08002
800-833-4672
http://www.msaa.com

National Family Caregivers Association
9621 E. Bexhill Dr.
Kensington, MD 20895-3104
800-896-3650
301-942-6430

National Multiple Sclerosis Society
733 Third Ave.
New York, NY 10017-3288
800-344-4867
212-986-3240 (New York)
http://www.nmss.org

National Parkinson's Foundation
1501 N.W. Ninth Ave.
Miami, FL 33136
800-327-4545
http://www.parkinson.org

Parkinson's Disease Foundation
William Black Memorial Research Building
Columbia-Presbyterian Medical Center
650-710 W. 168th St.
New York, NY 10032
800-457-6676
212-923-4700
http://www.parkinsons-foundation

ARTHRITIS

More than one hundred different diseases can be called arthritis, and they all have two things in common—they affect the joints and cause pain. Arthritic disorders are among the most common ailments; some fourteen million American men suffer from one form or another. Arthritis is also our number one disabler: two million men find their daily activities severely limited by it, according to the Arthritis Foundation.

Ankylosing spondylitis, gout, osteoarthritis, and rheumatoid arthritis (each described below) are among the forms of arthritis that affect men. While the typical arthritis sufferer is a woman over age 45, gout and ankylosing spondylitis are found almost exclusively in men. The most

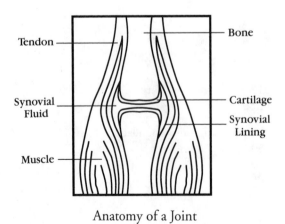

Anatomy of a Joint

common form of arthritis, osteoarthritis, appears to affect both genders equally. In fact, it is more common in men than in women before the age of 45; after that it is more common in women than in men. Women are three times more likely than men to develop rheumatoid arthritis, another common form of the disease that most often occurs between the ages of 35 and 50.

The Anatomy of a Joint

A joint is any place within the body where two or more bones meet. Joints allow movement and flexibility, and there are hundreds of joints in the body. The wrists, elbows, knees, and ankles are some obvious examples of joints; however, there are also joints in the skull (the sutures between the plates of the skull that harden once the brain has reached full size), the middle ear (which allow the tiny bones to vibrate), and even where the roots of your teeth are embedded in the jaw.

Joints are held together by muscles. Tendons connect the muscles to the bone. Ligaments are strong, fibrous bands that attach bone to bone, wrapping around the entire joint to keep it stable. In a healthy joint, the ends of the bone are covered with cartilage, a smooth tissue that allows the bones to glide across each other easily. In addition, each joint is encased in a fluid-filled joint capsule. The cells inside the capsule form the synovial membrane, or synovium. This membrane secretes synovial fluid, which lubricates the joint.

Ankylosing Spondylitis

Ankylosing spondylitis (AS) is a form of inflammatory arthritis that primarily attacks the spine.

Though it is relatively rare (about 300,000 Americans are believed to suffer from it, according to the Arthritis Foundation), AS is most commonly found in a group that has few specific health problems—young men between the ages of 16 and 35. Ankylosing spondylitis tends to run in families; the genetic marker HLA-B27 is found more often in people with this condition than in the rest of the population.

AS starts as inflammation in the joints and ligaments that support the lower back. This inflammation causes pain and stiffness in the lower back and hips and can be distinguished from other lower-back ailments because the pain is usually worsened by rest or inactivity and relieved by movement and exercise.

The progression of AS varies in individuals—some men never experience more than moderate stiffness and pain; others eventually suffer a great loss of mobility. AS can result in the spine and chest bones fusing and becoming rigid, possibly causing difficulty breathing. Early diagnosis and proper treatment can help to prevent or slow this process.

Diagnosis

The cause of AS is unknown, but it has a large genetic component. The gene present in over 90 percent of the people with AS has been identified, but simply carrying that gene does not mean a person will develop AS. However, a blood test that shows the presence of the gene, coupled with the symptoms and x-rays that reveal bony growths in the lower spine and hip joints, confirms the diagnosis. Because not everyone who carries the gene or has a parent with AS develops it, it is suspected that bacteria may trigger the inflammatory process, but that has not been proven.

Treatment

The aim of AS treatment is to relieve pain and stiffness, preserve mobility, and prevent deformities. The most common medications for AS are nonsteroidal anti-inflammatory drugs (NSAIDs) such as ibuprofen and naproxen. These relieve pain and stiffness, which allows the person with AS to exercise, maintain good posture, and live as normally as possible.

It is equally important that a man with AS maintain good posture at all times, even when sleeping. This helps keep joints from fusing at undesirable angles. Keep you spine straight, your shoulders back, and your head up while sitting, standing, and walking. At night, sleep flat, not curled up, on a hard mattress; the Arthritis Foundation suggests trying to sleep on your stomach without a pillow.

Regular exercise, tailored to your needs by a physical therapist, is also necessary. Exercises that strengthen your neck and back will help maintain your posture, and aerobic exercise and deep breathing will keep your chest and rib cage flexible. Many men with AS find that swimming is the best exercise for them, since it promotes both flexibility and deep breathing. Most men with AS can continue to work as long as their jobs do not require a lot of bending, lifting, or working in a crouched position. The ideal situation is one in which you can alternate sitting (with a cushion if necessary) and standing with rest intervals throughout the day.

Gout

Despite its image as a disease of rich old men, gout can strike anyone at any age. Men in their forties are actually the group most likely to suffer their first bout of gout. Gout usually afflicts only one joint (most often the big toe), causing intense pain and swelling around the joint. Proper diagnosis and treatment of gout are important, because, left untreated, gout will recur more frequently and do lasting damage to the joint; occasionally, it may spread to other joints as well.

Gout flares up when an excess of uric acid in the blood (called hyperuricemia) causes tiny, needle-shaped crystals to form in a joint. The crystals cause the joint lining to become inflamed. Persistent, untreated gout results in the buildup of crystal deposits called tophi under the skin. These lumps accumulate near the afflicted joint, or on the toes, fingers, and elbows, even in the outer edge of the ear. If tophi are not treated, they can damage joints.

Hyperuricemia occurs when the body makes too much uric acid or when the kidneys can't eliminate it fast enough. There are several causes of each condition, some preventable and some not. For example, diuretic drugs (which promote urination) can reduce the kidneys' ability to clear uric acid, as can an inherited kidney disease. Obesity, excessive amounts of alcohol, and heavy consumption of foods high in purines, such as organ meats and gravies, can also contribute to gout.

Not everyone who has hyperuricemia will develop gout (though such people have an increased risk of kidney stones). But when there is excess uric acid, a joint injury, a severe illness, chemotherapy, or an eating and drinking binge can trigger an attack.

Diagnosis

To diagnose gout, apart from observing the characteristic pain and swelling of gout, your doctor will take a blood sample to measure your levels of uric acid. To eliminate the possibility that what

you are suffering is pseudogout, or infectious arthritis, the doctor will most likely also take a sample of synovial fluid and examine it under a microscope for uric acid crystals.

Treatment

Once diagnosed, the treatment for gout must be tailored to the individual and may need to be modified over time. The immediate goal is to alleviate the symptoms of the acute attack, usually with the drug colchicine, NSAIDs such as ibuprofen or naproxen, or corticosteroids such as prednisone. Then your doctor will determine

---

SELF-CARE FOR GOUT

Once you've been diagnosed with gout, there are a number of ways you can help to prevent recurrent attacks. Try the following tips:

- Be sure to drink plenty of liquids—at least ten to twelve 8-ounce glasses of water, juice, and other nonalcoholic fluids every day. This helps your kidneys eliminate excess uric acid.

- Maintain a healthy weight. Obesity has been linked to high blood levels of uric acid.

- Avoid drinking alcohol.

- Completely avoid foods rich in substances called purines, which boost uric acid production. These include organ meats (including liver and sweetbreads), sardines and anchovies, mushrooms, and all meat broths and gravies.

the best way to prevent future attacks by lowering the levels of uric acid in your blood and urine, and reducing your body's production of it. He or she will most likely prescribe allopurinol, a drug that slows the body's rate of uric acid production, and/or probenecid or sulfinpyrazone, drugs that prevent uric acid deposits in joints and dissolve the ones already there. The latter two drugs are also used to prevent and/or dissolve tophi. There is no cure for gout, so you may need to take these drugs for the rest of your life to prevent symptoms.

Osteoarthritis

Osteoarthritis is the "wear and tear" form of arthritis. It is caused by the breakdown of the cartilage that covers the end of each bone. Healthy cartilage is smooth, which allows joints to move freely, and tough, to act as a shock absorber between bones. But in osteoarthritis, the cartilage breaks down in slow stages. First, it becomes soft, frayed, and less elastic. In time, large sections wear away completely, letting the ends of the bone rub together. The bone ends thicken, and the joint may even change shape, grow spurs (bony growths), and develop fluid-filled cysts. All of this makes joint movement painful.

No one is sure what causes osteoarthritis, or even if it is actually age-related; but heredity, obesity, injury, and overuse all appear to play roles in osteoarthritis. For example, a long-term study from the Johns Hopkins School of Medicine found that men who are 20 pounds overweight in early adulthood are three-and-a-half times more likely than those who are not overweight to develop osteoarthritis of the knee and hip by age 65.

Osteoarthritis can affect virtually any joint in the body, but the most likely sites are the hips, knees, spine, fingers, and big toes. (Men are especially likely to suffer from osteoarthritis of the hip.) The pain is usually not symmetrical in the early stages. It usually begins as an ache or stiffness after unusual exercise or periods of inactivity. The pain can become severe, but it often differs from joint to joint; osteoarthritis in a knee may cause catching or grating, whereas spinal arthritis may cause numbness in the legs. Often, osteoarthritis in the fingers will cause the formation of large nodes in the knuckles.

Diagnosis

Generally, osteoarthritis is diagnosed by your medical history and a physical examination of the painful joints. An x-ray may be done to determine the amount of damage within a joint. In addition, fluid may be drawn out of a joint, using a needle to rule out other causes of arthritis. The fluid is tested for the presence of infection or tiny crystals of uric acid, which signal gout. Blood tests may also be done to rule out the possibility of rheumatoid arthritis.

Treatment

There is no cure for osteoarthritis, but its symptoms can be treated. Acetaminophen (Tylenol) is often recommended because it relieves pain with the fewest side effects. NSAIDs such as aspirin and ibuprofen reduce inflammation as well as pain and may be helpful. However, these may irritate the stomach—using coated aspirin or taking medication with meals can prevent irritation. Severe pain may require prescriptions of NSAIDs and, rarely, corticosteroid shots directly into the joint. Topical therapy, with creams that contain aspirin compounds or capsaicin (the hot element in chili peppers), relieves pain for many people.

PREVENTING OSTEOARTHRITIS

Statistics showing the prevalence of osteoarthritis suggest that it is an inevitable part of getting older. But doctors are not convinced that this is true, and indeed, it might be possible to prevent osteoarthritis by taking certain precautions in your younger years:

1. Be smart about exercise. Exercise can be the best prevention against osteoarthritis because it strengthens muscles, helps maintain a healthy weight, and works to keep joints flexible. However, don't overdo high-impact exercises such as running. If your knees start to suffer overuse, don't hesitate to change your regimen.

2. Protect your knees against injury during sports in your teens, twenties, and thirties. Wear protective gear such as knee and elbow pads when playing contact sports.

3. Practice good posture. Standing and sitting up straight can help reduce pressure on the joints, especially those of the spine.

4. Learn to perform your job without stressing your joints. If your job requires repetitive movements or movements that stress the joints, be sure to vary your activities and working position as much as possible. (Farmers and carpet layers, for example, have high rates of arthritis because of wear and tear on the hips and the knees.)

5. Wear a seat belt to prevent injury to your knees (and other body parts) in a car accident.

Drug therapy is often coupled with exercise and physical therapy, along with a number of other nonmedical, alternative treatments. (See Alternative Arthritis Treatments, p. 172.)

Sometimes severely damaged joints require surgery. One procedure, called osteotomy, corrects bone deformity by cutting the bone and repositioning it. It is most commonly done on the knee, as is arthroscopic debridement. In arthroscopic debridement, the doctor inserts a small probe and removes floating bits of cartilage and bone that interfere with movement and cause pain. Total joint arthroplasty involves resurfacing, or relining, the ends of bones so they can move more freely against each other; it is also the term used for total joint replacement, in which the joint is removed and a metal, ceramic, or plastic device is inserted in its place.

Self-care is also a valuable part of arthritis treatment. Learning to pace yourself during the day and making sure to get adequate rest at night are two of the most important ways to cope with osteoarthritis. Accept that you may not be able to do some things as quickly or as easily as before, but focus on what you can do, rather than what you can't. There are many devices available for use around the house such as automatic can openers that make everyday chores easier; two other items that will add to your comfort and well-being are a firm mattress, and comfortable, well-fitting shoes.

Rheumatoid Arthritis

Rheumatoid arthritis (RA) causes inflammation in the joints and other parts of the body, including the connective tissue that surrounds organs such as the heart and lungs. In this debilitating form of arthritis, the synovial membrane becomes inflamed. The membrane thickens and becomes tough and fibrous, causing pain when the joint is moved. The symptoms may come (in what's called a flare-up) and go (in a remission). If left untreated, the affected joints may become deformed.

RA differs from osteoarthritis in that it occurs in younger individuals, usually people between 20 to 40 years of age. It also tends to be more painful than osteoarthritis and occurs in symmetrical joints. Rheumatoid arthritis can also cause fatigue, weight loss, fever, and general malaise, while osteoarthritis symptoms are limited to joint pain.

No one knows what causes RA, though many think that it is an autoimmune disease—a disease in which the body's immune system malfunctions and destroys its own tissues. Rheumatoid arthritis also has a genetic factor—if a parent or sibling has the disease, you are three to five times more likely than the rest of the population to have it. If you suspect RA, seek treatment as soon as possible; studies show that the sooner treatment is received, the better the chances of recovery.

Diagnosis

Initially, a medical history and physical examination are done to help diagnose RA. However, diagnosis often involves blood tests, including a complete blood count (which measures the amounts of red and white blood cells and platelets in the blood), a sedimentation rate test (which shows how fast the blood cells cling together), and a test for rheumatoid factor (a protein that signals the presence of inflammation). Using the results of these tests, practitioners can usually make a definitive diagnosis. In difficult cases, imaging techniques such as magnetic resonance imaging (MRI) may be used for diagnosis.

Treatment

As with osteoarthritis, treatment focuses on relieving symptoms rather than curing the disease. Aspirin and other NSAIDs are often prescribed to relieve pain because of their anti-inflammatory properties. Steroid drugs such as prednisone and cortisone are used occasionally in the treatment of RA to relieve pain by reducing inflammation; however, they are not effective against osteoarthritis, which usually doesn't involve much inflammation. Steroid drugs are used only for short periods in small doses because potential side effects include weight gain, nervousness, insomnia, increased body hair, muscle wasting, lowered resistance to infection, and mood swings.

A number of drugs, known as remittive agents, are thought to slow the progression of RA. These include gold salts (taken orally or as injection), Plaquenil (a malaria drug), penicillamine, and methotrexate. These drugs work slowly, over a few weeks or more, to bring about a remission or partial remission. However, there is little scientific evidence that they are effective, despite the fact that they sometimes work.

As with osteoarthritis, surgery may be used as a last resort. Procedures include synovectomy, removal of the lining of the joint, which in RA becomes inflamed and grows wildly. Synovectomy is done with the aid of arthroscopy, in which a flexible fiberoptic scope is inserted into the joint to view the structures. An affected joint might also be fused or altered (for example, the angle or length of the bones changed), or the entire joint might be replaced. Joint replacement is a last resort used only when medical treatments have failed and the painful joint is beyond repair.

For more information:

Ankylosing Spondylitis Association
P.O. Box 5872
Sherman Oaks, CA 91413
800-777-8189
310-652-0609 (California)
http://www.spondyl.org

Arthritis Consulting Services
4620 N. State Rd. 7, Suite 206
Fort Lauderdale, FL 33319
800-327-3027

Arthritis Foundation
30 W. Peachtree St.
Atlanta, GA 30309
800-283-7800
404-872-7100
http://www.arthritis.org

National Institute of Arthritis and Musculoskeletal and Skin Diseases
NIH Information Clearinghouse
Box AMS
9000 Rockville Pike
Bethesda, MD 20892
301-495-4484

ALTERNATIVE ARTHRITIS TREATMENTS

Drug therapy is only a small part of the treatment recommended for osteoarthritis and rheumatoid arthritis. The following therapies have also been shown to help some people relieve symptoms of the diseases:

1. *Exercise.* Low-impact aerobic exercise such as walking, swimming, stationary cycling, and water exercises—as well as specific stretching exercises—can loosen joints, increase range of motion, strengthen muscles, and relieve arthritis pain. In addition, exercise helps to maintain a healthy weight, especially important since obesity is often considered the cause of some types of arthritis. Talk with your practitioner or a physical therapist about recommended exercises.

2. *Physical therapy.* Physical therapy restores or preserves the range of motion in joints and strengthens the muscles surrounding them. You may need to consult a physical therapist only long enough to learn some simple exercises you can do at home, or you may need regular therapy, which can also include supervised exercise, massage, and weight training. A physical therapist can help you learn how to use supportive devices such as splints, canes, braces, cervical collars, or crutches, as well as how to do everyday tasks with as little pain as possible.

continues

3. *Heat and cold treatments.* Applying heat to joints increases blood flow and loosens joints, and cold treatments can help to relieve pain.

4. *Hydrotherapy.* Soaking in a whirlpool or hot tub may be helpful for your arthritis, loosening tight joints while providing buoyancy to reduce some of the pressure on affected joints.

5. *Diet therapy.* Though there is no definitive evidence, some experts believe certain foods are linked to arthritis symptoms. In some studies, milk and cheese were found to cause symptoms. Other research shows foods in the nightshade family (potatoes, bell peppers, tomatoes, eggplant, and chili peppers) trigger arthritis flare-ups.

   In addition, studies show that those with arthritis should avoid foods that contain omega-6 fatty acids (vegetable oils such as safflower, sunflower, sesame, and soy), which produce inflammatory chemicals in the body. At the same time, they should eat foods that contain omega-3 fatty acids (mackerel, sardines, and salmon), which have an anti-inflammatory effect.

6. *Vitamin and mineral therapy.* Experts recommend that those with arthritis get their recommended dietary allowance of all the vitamins and minerals. While there are no specific vitamins and minerals thought to help arthritis, the disease can deplete the body's stores of a number of nutrients, including vitamins A, B_6, C, and E, selenium, pantothenic acid, and copper.

7. *Acupuncture.* This complementary therapy, which involves the insertion of small, thin needles under the skin, may help relieve arthritis symptoms temporarily in some individuals.

8. *Herbal therapy.* Herbs that may be helpful include arnica, meadowsweet, cayenne pepper, devil's claw, and feverfew.

BACK PAIN

Eight out of ten adults will suffer from lower-back pain at some time in their lives, and most will have more than one episode. According to the National Center for Health Statistics, back pain is the number two reason, behind cold symptoms, that people cite for seeing a doctor. Men tend to suffer more back pain than women, most likely because men tend to hold jobs that carry a high risk for back pain—construction, trucking, and sedentary office jobs, for example.

Back pain rarely indicates serious damage to your back. Most lower-back problems are not serious and disappear within a few days to several weeks.

The Anatomy of the Back

The back is a complex integration of bone, nerves, and muscle. The spine, or backbone, consists of thirty-three cylindrical vertebrae stacked on top of each other to form a column. The top seven vertebrae are known as the cervical vertebrae. The twelve in the midback are known as thoracic vertebrae, and the five in the lower back are called lumbar vertebrae. The nine vertebrae at the very base of the spine usually grow together by adulthood to form the sacrum and the coccyx, or tailbone.

Cushions known as discs separate the vertebrae from each other. These round, flat discs—made of collagen and filled with water—act as shock absorbers. The facet joints—paired connective joints that act as hinges between the vertebrae—hold the spine together, along with nerves, muscles, ligaments, tendons, and cartilage. The spinal cord runs through a long, hollow canal formed by openings in the vertebrae.

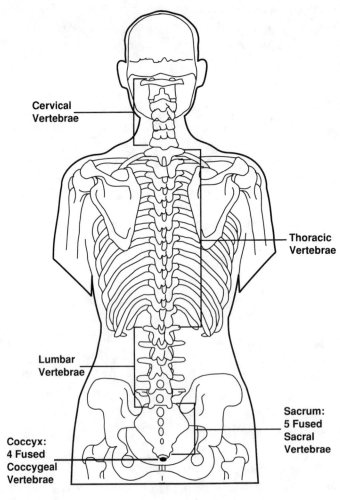

Cervical
Vertebrae

Thoracic
Vertebrae

Lumbar
Vertebrae

Sacrum:
5 Fused
Sacral
Vertebrae

Coccyx:
4 Fused
Coccygeal
Vertebrae

Anatomy of the Back

Types of Back Pain

Back pain can occur anywhere in the spine; however, it is most common in the lumbar spine, or lower back, which must endure more stress and strain than any other part of the back. Acute problems, which occur suddenly and heal quickly, last less than three months—usually a few days to several weeks.

Pain in the back is most often due to three factors: strained or sprained muscles, a problem with a spinal disc, or a problem with a facet joint. These factors may occur alone or in combination, often making it difficult to pinpoint the cause of the pain. In fact, the overwhelming majority of back pain is idiopathic; in other words, no one knows what causes it.

Most often, pain is attributed to muscle strains, sprains, and spasms. The terms *strain* and *sprain* are similar in that both are used to describe an overworked muscle, ligament, or tendon. A strain consists of an overstretching or minor tearing of a muscle or ligament in the back, and a sprain is a significant tear in the muscle. Strains and sprains can be caused by sudden, unaccustomed exercise or a violent motion (on the job, during sports, or in an accident); however, just twisting your body the wrong way can cause a ligament to tear. A muscle spasm occurs when muscles painfully contract. Many spasms are defensive reactions by the muscles to protect an injured area.

Back pain can also be caused by a herniated, or "slipped," disc, a condition that occurs when the protective cushion bulges beyond its normal placement in the spine and presses on the spinal nerves. It can cause shooting pain in the buttocks and legs (called sciatica), numbness, tingling, weakness, and in its most severe state, loss of urinary control.

Finally, facet joints can become worn, or the synovial membrane, the delicate membrane that lines the facet joint, can become inflamed—perhaps by arthritis (inflammation of one or more joints) or even gradual wear and tear caused by normal movement over the years. A facet joint can also be damaged if the adjoining disc becomes herniated because, without that protective cushion, the vertebrae become compressed and rub together.

Less commonly, back problems can be caused by other conditions, including osteoporosis (in which vertebrae become brittle and easily damaged), scoliosis (in which a curve develops in the spine), infections (such as meningitis, an infection of the spinal cord), and ankylosing spondylitis (a rare condition in which the spine gradually fuses).

Risk Factors

Many factors may put you at risk for lower-back pain. Obesity is a major factor because it puts added stress on the spine. For example, the large stomach of an obese man shifts his center of gravity forward, making the erector spinae (the muscles that keep the spine erect) work extra hard to maintain upright posture. This exertion puts more pressure on the spine at the facet joints and the discs, causing lower-back pain.

A sedentary lifestyle is also a risk factor. Long periods of standing and sitting cause the vertebrae to become compressed during the course of the day. In addition, inactivity tends to lead to weight gain and poor muscle tone (especially of the abdominal muscles), other risk factors for back pain. Weak and inflexible back muscles, typical in those who are not physically fit, may become strained trying to support the spine.

Many risks are linked to occupations. Frequent bending and twisting, lifting, forceful movements, and repetitive work (such as on assembly lines) are also risk factors. Vibrations, usually either from factory work or from traveling for long periods in a car or truck, can also aggravate the spinal column and cause back pain. In addition, emotional stress may exacerbate back problems; studies show people who don't like their jobs are at higher risk for back pain than those who enjoy what they do.

Diagnosis

Back problems can be diagnosed and treated by your primary-care physician, orthopedist or orthopedic surgeon (who specializes in bone and muscle disorders), neurologist or neurosurgeon (who specializes in nerve and brain disorders), osteopath (a physician whose training emphasizes the musculoskeletal system) or chiropractor (who must complete four years at a chiropractic college, where he or she receives extensive training specifically in the musculoskeletal system).

WHEN TO SEEK PROFESSIONAL CARE

If your back pain could be characterized in any of the following ways or is being accompanied by any of the following symptoms, you should seek professional care:

- Your back pain is constant and severe and hasn't improved after three days of bed rest.

- Your back pain is moderate but has persisted for more than a month despite efforts to relieve it.

- Your back pain disappears only to reappear on a regular basis.

- Your back pain is accompanied by a noticeable change in your bowel habits.

- In addition to your back pain, you're experiencing weakness in one or both of your legs.

- In addition to your back pain, you're having trouble raising the toes on one or both of your feet.

- Your back pain is accompanied by unexplainable weight loss.

- Your back pain is accompanied by a fever that is not associated with a cold or flu.

- Your back pain is accompanied by swelling in joints such as your fingers, wrists, elbows, ankles, or knees.

- Your back pain has been waking you up at night.

The practitioner will discuss symptoms, take a medical history, and do a physical examination. If the back pain has lasted longer than a month, diagnostic tests may be done to gather information. These include blood tests; x-rays; a magnetic resonance imaging (MRI) scan, which uses magnetic forces to create an image of the back; and a computerized tomography (CT) scan, which creates a three-dimensional picture of the back. Electromyography (EMG), a technique that measures the electrical impulses within the muscles, may be done to test for nerve damage.

Because the back is so complex, it may be difficult for a practitioner to tell the exact cause of the back pain. However, only about one person in two hundred will have a serious medical condition, according to the Agency for Health Care Policy and Research.

Self-Care Treatment

If your back pain does not require an immediate trip to the doctor, you can try treating yourself using self-care techniques. A *short* period of bed rest is usually recommended after the onset of severe back pain, but lying down for more than two or three days weakens muscles and bones and may extend the length of recovery needed. If you do opt for bed rest, be sure to get up and walk around every few hours, even if your back hurts.

Also, during the first forty-eight hours after your back symptoms begin, apply a cold pack or a bag of ice to the area for five to ten minutes at a time every few hours to numb the area and reduce inflammation. After forty-eight hours, a heating pad or hot shower or bath should be used two to three times daily to increase blood flow to the area, promoting healing. Over-the-counter medications such as acetaminophen, aspirin, and

ibuprofen may also provide some relief. Because aspirin and ibuprofen may irritate the stomach, take only as many as you need to relieve the pain and do not exceed the maximum dosage of six tablets in a twenty-four-hour period.

Until your back feels better, you should avoid heavy lifting and sitting for extended periods of time. Exercise stimulates the production and release of endorphins, the body's natural painkillers, and it improves the flow of blood and oxygen throughout the body. You should continue to exercise even after your back has healed because one of the best ways to prevent more back problems is to keep fit. Low-impact aerobic exercises such as walking, bicycling (mobile or stationary), and swimming (except the butterfly stroke) are considered the best and fastest way to get rid of back pain, but avoid jogging, which can jar the spine, and tennis and golf, which require vigorous twisting movements.

Medical Treatment

While at one time practitioners widely prescribed strong painkillers and muscle relaxants for back pain, they now often recommend nothing but over-the-counter pain relievers such as aspirin, ibuprofen, and acetaminophen, which studies show help just as much and with fewer side effects. Prescription-strength versions of these drugs are also available. Corticosteroids, drugs such as cortisone and prednisone, may be prescribed for short periods to reduce inflammation and pain, but they have side effects that include weight gain, nervousness, insomnia, increased body hair, muscle wasting, lowered resistance to infection, and mood swings. Corticosteroids may be taken orally or injected.

Both osteopaths and chiropractors use spinal manipulation—the use of hands to apply pressure to the spine in different directions and

BACK PAIN PREVENTION

Try these tips to protect your back:

1. Take advantage of ergonomics. Use a chair, possibly one that reclines slightly, with good lower-back support. This is especially important if you sit for long periods. If you stand all day, try resting one foot on a small stool to take pressure off your back.

2. Call a time-out. When driving long distances, stop every hour to walk around your car to stretch your legs and back. (While on the move, place a pillow or rolled-up towel behind your lower back to support your spine and minimize vibrations.) If you're working at a desk, take time now and then to stand, stretch, and walk around the office.

3. Practice good posture. Slouching as you sit puts twice as much pressure on the spine than sitting up straight does.

4. Exercise right. Obesity, poor muscle tone, and poor flexibility are all risk factors for back pain—and all factors that exercise can help remedy. Experts recommend a combination of aerobic exercise and strength training. But remember to warm up before each workout to avoid pulling muscles.

5. Quit smoking. Smoking can put you at higher risk for disc injuries. It is thought to affect muscle health by hindering the removal of waste products from the muscles.

6. Adopt a proper sleeping position. Most experts recommend sleeping on your back with a pillow under your knees or on your side with a pillow between your bent knees—but don't sleep on your stomach. A firm mattress will also do your back good.

locations in order to "adjust" the spine. Not long ago, the practice of spinal manipulation was deemed quackery by the American Medical Association (AMA). But in 1987, after a lengthy lawsuit in which chiropractors accused the AMA of conspiring to monopolize medicine, the AMA changed its stance. A recent study by the Agency for Health Care Policy and Research found spinal manipulation to be a viable treatment for some patients. It should only be done by a trained professional.

Complementary therapies are often used to treat back pain with varying degrees of success.

These include use of TENS (transcutaneous electrical nerve stimulation), massage, biofeedback, acupuncture, and hydrotherapy. (See Complementary Therapies, p. 436.) In addition, back braces, traction, or ultrasound (a procedure that uses the vibrations of sound waves to treat injured tissue and reduce inflammation) are sometimes prescribed, though their benefits are not proven.

One more treatment is available specifically for a herniated disc—a procedure known as chemonucleolysis. In the procedure, an enzyme called chymopapain is injected into the disc to

HOW TO LIFT HEAVY OBJECTS

1. Take your time. Think about what you're going to do before you do it.

2. Place your feet shoulder-width apart to create a solid base of support.

3. Bend at the knees, *not* at the waist. Let your spine curve naturally.

4. Tighten your stomach muscles.

5. Position the person or object directly in front of, and close to, your body.

6. Lift with your legs, not your back.

7. Do not twist your body. Point your toes in the direction you want to move and pivot in that direction.

8. Don't try to be a superhero. If an object is too heavy or has an awkward shape, get help.

Decompression surgeries include discectomy, removal of all or part of a disc that's pressing on a nerve. In laminectomy with discectomy, the lamina (the bony plate on the back of the vertebrae) is removed along with the disc to relieve pressure. In microdiscectomy, the disc is removed through a tiny opening with the help of a microscope. This procedure is less invasive than the others and has a shorter recovery time. Percutaneous discectomy involves removing the disc with suction. Spinal fusion surgeries involve the use of bone grafts, metal implants, rods, and pins to immobilize and strengthen the vertebrae.

Many experts maintain that much of the back surgery done in the United States is unnecessary. Seek a second opinion and get all the information on the risks and benefits of a recommended procedure before consenting to it. In most cases, putting off surgery for several weeks will not make back problems worse.

For more information:

Agency for Health Care Policy and Research
Publications Clearinghouse
P.O. Box 8547
Silver Spring, MD 20907
800-358-9295
http://www.ahcpr.gov

American Academy of Orthopaedic Surgeons
(AAOS)
6300 N. River Rd.
Rosemont, IL 60018-4262
800-346-2267
http://www.aaos.org

American Physical Therapy Association
1111 N. Fairfax St.
Alexandria, VA 22314
703-684-APTA
http://www.apta.org

shrink it and relieve the pressure on the adjacent nerves. It is successful 75 percent of the time, but it may cause temporary severe back spasms and a painful recovery. This procedure is usually done by a surgeon in a hospital.

Surgery

There are two general categories of back surgery: decompression (done to relieve pressure on a nerve or other spinal structure) and fusion (done to fuse a spinal structure together to prevent painful or damaging movement). People with nerve problems, fractures, or dislocations are the most common candidates for surgery.

Back Pain Association of America
P.O. Box 135
Pasadena, MD 21122
410-255-3633

International Chiropractors Association
1110 N. Glebe Rd., Suite 1000
Arlington, VA 22201
703-528-5000

National Institute of Arthritis and Musculoskeletal
and Skin Diseases
NIH Information Clearinghouse
Box AMS
9000 Rockville Pike
Bethesda, MD 20892
301-495-4484

BIRTH DEFECTS AND GENETIC DISORDERS

Birth defects, also called congenital defects, are abnormalities that are present in a child at birth. Birth defects range in severity from cosmetic abnormalities to genetic disorders and structural problems that could mean serious mental retardation or death. A genetic disorder is any condition that is caused by a fault within a gene, the genetic materials within a person's cells that determines growth and development.

It is important to note that genetic disorders and birth defects are not always the same thing. Birth defects may be caused by a genetic disorder, but they are not always triggered by a fault within a gene—they can also be caused by problems during a child's development in the womb (for example, talipes), or they can be caused by exposure to medications, toxins, drugs and alcohol, diseases such as rubella, or damage during delivery. On the other hand, genetic disorders may not be apparent at birth (for example, hemophilia and sickle-cell anemia).

The Role of Genetics

A genetic disorder can be passed from parent to child in three different ways: through dominant genes, recessive genes, or x-linked recessive genes.

A child has a 50 percent chance of inheriting the condition if one parent has a dominant gene. Diseases caused by dominant genes are called autosomal dominant disorders. If both parents are carriers of recessive genes that carry an illness, there is a 25 percent chance that each child will inherit the condition, a 50 percent chance that each child will be a carrier who does not have the disorder, and a 25 percent chance that each child will be unaffected. Diseases caused by recessive genes, called autosomal recessive disorders, are often severe and can lead to early death.

The X and Y chromosomes determine if a child is male or female. If the mother is a carrier of an X-linked recessive disorder, there is a 50 percent chance each son will receive the abnormal X chromosome and be affected and a 50 percent chance each daughter will be a carrier.

Screening for Birth Defects

Genetic counseling involves a series of questions, and possibly some genetic tests, to determine if you or your partner has any genetic anomalies or family history of disease that may be passed on to a child. These tests help anticipate any possible problems with the pregnancy. Certain ethnic groups are screened for genetic disorders that are more prevalent within their groups than in the general population: for example, thalassemia (also called Cooley's anemia) screening in people of Mediterranean descent; Tay-Sachs screening in people of Jewish descent (specifically Eastern European, or Ashkenazi);

FINDING A GENETIC COUNSELOR

To find a genetic counselor or genetic services program or to get more information about genetic counseling, start by contacting any or all of the following groups:

American Board of Medical Genetics
9650 Rockville Pike
Bethesda, MD 20814
301-571-1825

This group certifies genetics professionals and publishes a roster of board-certified members.

National Center for Education in Maternal and Child Health
2000 15th St., N., Suite 701
Arlington, VA 22201
703-524-7802

This center operates a clearinghouse for publications on genetics. It also publishes a directory of clinical genetic services centers throughout the United States.

March of Dimes Birth Defects Foundation
1275 Mamaroneck Ave.
White Plains, NY 10605
914-428-7100

Genetic counselors may also be found at university medical centers, private hospital settings, state or federal departments of health, private practices, or through health maintenance organizations or managed care plans.

and sickle-cell disease screening in the African-American population.

Look to a genetic counselor to answer these questions:

- Do I, my child, or another relative have a genetic disease?

- What does being a carrier mean?

- Is any member of my family a carrier of a genetic disease?

- What are the chances that my future children or other members of my family will have a particular genetic problem?

- What can be expected for me or for a family member with a genetic disorder?

- Where can good treatment and care for this disorder be obtained?

Keep in mind that genetic counseling offers no guarantees and offers no solutions—it merely provides information. A risk of a particular disease does not guarantee that a child will have the condition, and family history free of genetic defects does not guarantee a healthy infant.

Common Genetic Disorders and Familial Diseases

Achondroplasia. This form of dwarfism is caused by a dominant gene. A child with achondroplasia has a relatively normal torso and short arms and legs. Problems can arise due to the common symptoms of this disorder that include swayback, crowded teeth, spinal cord compression, bowlegs, and ear infections. Psychological problems may also arise.

Cleft lip and palate. This is an incomplete fusion in lip or palate (roof of mouth) caused by hereditary and/or environmental factors. These conditions can be corrected with reconstructive surgery. Heredity factors are identifiable in 25 percent of cases. Nongenetic factors may be identified and include maternal diabetes, alcohol abuse, anticancer drugs, and seizure medications.

Cystic fibrosis (CF). Caused by a recessive, defective gene, this is the most common fatal genetic disease among Caucasians. It causes a malfunction in the workings of the lungs and the pancreas. In those with the condition, thick mucus builds up in the lungs, making breathing difficult and encouraging the growth of bacteria, which leads to pneumonia and other bronchial diseases. While ultimately fatal, people with CF can live well into adulthood with the help of treatments that introduce healthy genes and enzymes into the systems. Prenatal testing reveals the disease in many cases.

Diabetes mellitus. This is a disorder of insulin production by the pancreas or interference with the effect of insulin on cells, which results in high levels of sugar in the blood. Up to 25 percent of the U.S. population may carry a predisposition toward diabetes.

Down syndrome. The number twenty-one chromosome pair does not divide normally at conception. Risk for this condition increases with maternal age. People with Down syndrome are short in stature and generally have slanting eyelids; broad, flat noses; small ears; and short, stubby fingers. There may be moderate to severe mental retardation, and congenital heart defects are common. Down syndrome can be prenatally detected by screening programs and testing, most notably amniocentesis (in which a needle is used to sample amniotic fluid for testing).

Duchenne-type muscular dystrophy. This is an x-linked disorder that appears in boys between ages 6 and 9. Muscles weaken over time, forcing the child into a wheelchair by the teen years. It affects all muscles, including the heart and those used in breathing. Although orthopedic devices are available for those with the disease, there is no cure.

Gaucher disease. This condition affects the liver, spleen, and bone marrow and appears anytime from childhood on through adulthood. It is seen most commonly in Ashkenazi Jews.

Glaucoma. This is characterized by higher than normal pressure inside the eye that, if untreated, can lead to blindness. It is hereditary in 10 to 15 percent of cases. The genetic trigger is not well understood, but people of African ancestry suffer from it more than those of European background. Greater pigmentation in very dark eyes may be a factor.

Hemophilia. The defective gene is located on the X, or female, chromosome and is recessive. In hemophilia, which affects men almost exclusively, blood does not clot normally and can lead to uncontrolled, even fatal bleeding. In December 1995, the Centers for Disease Control and Prevention (CDC) showed 16,866 men—and 3,851 women—affected by the disease. One man in every 7,500 is born with the disorder. Screening is available for women who may carry the disease.

Symptoms of hemophilia include many large or deep bruises; internal bleeding into the joints, causing pains and swelling; blood in the urine or stool; and prolonged bleeding from cuts or injuries after surgery or tooth extraction. Minor cuts and scrapes are not usually cause for major problems for people with hemophilia. Rather, it is the internal bleeding that is of concern. The large joints and limb muscles— for example the knees, ankles, and elbows— are common sites for internal bleeding.

There is no cure for hemophilia. Treatment is geared toward preventing and controlling bleeding episodes, using medication and clotting factors. In addition to medication, called factor replacement therapy, physical therapy can help damaged joints function better.

High cholesterol. Familial high cholesterol is an autosomal dominant trait. There is a flaw in the gene that controls production of low-density lipoprotein (LDL) receptors. One person in five hundred is affected. If left untreated, the person receiving gene from one parent may have a first heart attack in his or her thirties or forties.

Huntington's disease. A dominant gene results in lethal disease not apparent at birth. Early symptoms, including clumsiness or tics, appear between the ages of 35 and 45. Symptoms worsen to include twisted facial expressions, uncontrollable writhing of the body, and severe emotional problems that resemble manic depression or schizophrenia. Deterioration can continue ten to twenty years until death. Genetic testing can be used to detect carriers of the disease.

Hypertension. Hypertension, or high blood pressure, may be triggered in some cases by an autosomal dominant gene, but the exact genetic functioning unknown. Some researchers claim the problem lies in how sodium is carried across cell membranes. Others argue that inherited problems in eliminating sodium from the body are the culprits. Others cite excessive sensitivity to stress.

Marfan syndrome. This disease of connective tissue is caused by a dominant gene. Symptoms may be mild or severe, may be present at birth or not until adulthood. Affected individuals are often tall, slender, and loose-jointed. A pattern of abnormalities can affect the heart, blood vessels, lungs, eyes, bones, and ligaments. It can sometimes cause sudden death in adults unaware they had the disorder.

Neurofibromatoses. These are inherited disorders of the nervous system caused by abnormal genes and gene mutations. The severity of symptoms can vary greatly. A common sign can be six or more large tan spots on the skin, often present at birth. Benign tumors may appear under the skin, often during adolescence. Tumors can also develop on the auditory (hearing) nerves, the brain, and spinal chord. Most cases are mild, but some children can have learning disabilities, speech problems, seizures, and problems with hyperactivity.

Phenylketonuria (PKU). This inherited enzyme deficiency prevents proper breakdown of the amino acid phenylalanine. It can lead to severe mental retardation and physical problems; however, a special diet low in this amino acid can avert these problems. It is routinely screened for at birth.

Sickle-cell anemia. In this condition there is crescent-shaped, rather than round, hemoglobin (pigment) in red blood cells. Abnormal cells are more likely to get caught in the spleen and die, leaving person with a shortage of red-blood cells, and thus a shortage of oxygen. Sickle cells stuck in arteries can result in injury to the brain, lungs, and kidneys. Symptoms may not appear until six months of age. It is common in people of African descent and can cause death. Blood tests are available to diagnose carriers of the trait.

Spina bifida and anencephaly. Together these neural tube defects (NTDs) are among the most common birth defects in the United States. Anencephaly (missing brain) is always fatal. Spina bifida, which results in a gap in the bone that surrounds the spinal cord, can be slight or severe. Severe cases include paralysis, lack of bladder and bowel control, and hydrocephalus (water on the brain.) Neural tube defects can be caused by a combination of hereditary and environmental factors. Over 95 percent of the cases of NTDs can be detected by screening early in pregnancy.

Tay-Sachs disease. A recessive, defective gene results in body's inability to produce an enzyme that normally breaks down fatty deposits in the brain and nerve cells. The disease is common among Ashkenazi Jews. Symptoms, which include behavior changes, paralysis, and blindness, may not appear until six months of age. There is no treatment available, and death usually occurs before age four.

Thalassemia. This is a blood disease triggered by recessive gene commonly found among those of Italian or Greek descent, but the disorder can affect those of Middle Eastern, southern Asian, or African descents. Thalassemia refers to various types of anemia. The most harmful is Cooley's anemia. Children appear normal at birth but become pale and weak within the first year or two of life. Without treatment, major organs become enlarged with heart failure and infection, which may lead to death.

Wilson's disease. In this condition, copper accumulates in the liver and is released into the rest of the body. If metal accumulates in the brain, it can destroy brain tissue, resulting in dementia. It usually manifests itself during adolescence.

Nongenetic Birth Defects

There are also a number of birth defects with no genetic cause. These include the following:

Cerebral palsy (CP). This refers to movement and posture problems resulting from brain injury, possibly because of oxygen deficiency in the womb. It is considered a birth defect if injury occurs before or during birth. CP is often expressed by abnormal muscle control, loss of sensation, and some degree of hearing impairment. Physical and speech therapy are available for those with the condition, which may slowly progress over time.

Fetal alcohol syndrome (FAS) and drug-addicted infants. Severe birth defects can be brought on by the use of alcohol and drugs during pregnancy. Intoxicants pass through the placenta to developing baby. FAS infants are undersized at birth, have small heads, mild to moderate retardation, short attention spans, and behavioral problems. There may be joint abnormalities and congenital heart disease. Narrow eyes and short, upturned noses are characteristic of FAS children. Infants born to heroin addicts are often born addicted themselves and may suffer withdrawal symptoms severe enough to cause brain damage or death. Cocaine and marijuana users give birth to infants smaller than normal.

Rh disease. Problems can arise for unborn baby if the mother lacks the Rh factor in her blood (Rh-negative) and the father has the factor (Rh-positive). If the fetus is Rh-positive and is a second or later pregnancy, the mother's antibodies will attempt to destroy baby's blood cells. A maternal vaccine is now available to prevent antibodies from forming in the mother's blood.

Rubella. Severe birth defects can result if the mother is exposed to rubella (German measles) in early pregnancy. Defects include blindness, deafness, microcephaly (small-sized head), mental retardation, cerebral palsy, and congenital heart defects. The woman is immune to rubella if she already has had the disease or if she is vaccinated prior to becoming pregnant.

Talipes (clubfoot). This is the second most common birth defect in the United States. Scientists are not sure why boys are twice as likely as girls to develop clubfoot. In the worst cases of clubfoot, the entire foot is twisted inward and downward. It is thought to occur when the fetus holds a fixed position in the uterus for a long time, possibly when fetal movement is limited by insufficient amniotic fluid.

For more information:

Alliance of Genetics Support Groups
35 Wisconsin Circle, Suite 440
Chevy Chase, MD 20815
301-652-5553

American Association on Mental Retardation
444 N. Capital St., N.W., Suite 846
Washington, DC 20001-1512
800-424-3688
202-387-1968 (District of Columbia)

American Cleft Palate Educational Foundation
1829 E. Franklin St., Suite 1022
Chapel Hill, NC 27514
919-933-9044

Children's Wish Foundation
P.O. Box 28785
Atlanta, CA 30358
800-323-9474
404-393-9474 (Georgia)

Cooley's Anemia Foundation
129-09 26th Ave., Room 203
Flushing, NY 11354
800-522-7222
http://www.thalassemia.org

Cystic Fibrosis Foundation
6931 Arlington Rd.
Bethesda, MD 20814
800-344-4823
301-951-4422
http://www.cff.org

Huntington's Disease Society of America
140 W. 22nd St., 6th Floor
New York, NY 10011-2420
800-345-4372
212-242-1968
curehd@hdfa.ttisms.com

March of Dimes Birth Defects Foundation
1275 Mamaroneck Ave.
White Plains, NY 10605
914-428-7100

National Down Syndrome Congress
1605 Chantilly Dr., Suite 250
Atlanta, GA 30324
800-232-6372
ndsc@charitiesusa.com

National Down Syndrome Society
666 Broadway
New York, NY 10012
212-460-9330
http://www. ndss.org

National Hemophilia Foundation
110 Greene St., Suite 303
New York, NY 10012
800-42-HANDI
212-219-8180
http://www.hemophilia.org

National Multiple Sclerosis Society
733 Third Ave.
New York, NY 10017-3288
212-986-3240 (New York)
http://www.nmss.org
800-344-4867

Sickle Cell Disease Association of America, Inc.
200 Corporate Pointe, Suite 495
Culver City, CA 90230-7633
800-421-8453

Spina Bifida Association of America
4590 MacArthur Blvd., N.W., Suite 250
Washington, DC 20007-4226
800-621-3141
410-825-0213 (Maryland)
http://www.infohiway.com/spinabifida

United Cerebral Palsy Association
1660 L St., N.W., Suite 700
Washington, DC 20036
800-USA-5UCP
202-776-0406
http://www.ucpa.org

CANCER

According to the American Cancer Society, more than 760,000 American men were diagnosed with cancer in 1996, accounting for 56 percent of the total number of cancer cases diagnosed that year. Today, one in every five deaths among all Americans is cancer-related.

This general discussion of cancer, useful terminology, and common treatments and their side effects is followed by entries on types of cancer, specifically breast cancer, colorectal cancer, lung cancer, lymphoma, oral cancer, prostate cancer, penile cancer, skin cancer, and testicular cancer.

What Is Cancer?

Cancer occurs when cells divide and multiply without order. To stay healthy, the body naturally makes new cells to replace old ones. But when the cells begin to reproduce, even though new cells are not needed, without control or order, normal cells may malfunction or be crowded out and starved of nutrients by the new cells. As a result, the body can no longer function as it should.

The rapidly multiplying cells may form a mass of tissue, called a growth or tumor. There are three different types of tumors: benign tumors, malignant tumors, and precancerous lesions.

A benign tumor is not cancerous and can usually be safely removed. This type of tumor does not spread to other parts of the body and is rarely life-threatening. A malignant tumor is cancerous. Its cells can invade other organs throughout the body and affect their proper function. It can spread by invading neighboring tissues or by entering the bloodstream through the lymph nodes (the nearby glands that are part of the immune system) and traveling to various parts of the body. The spread of cancer is called metastasis.

A precancerous lesion is any limited area of the body that shows abnormal, though not necessarily cancerous, changes—for example, a lesion may consist of rapidly growing normal cells. Lesions can be the result of an injury or disease. If left untreated, lesions have the potential of becoming malignant.

Symptoms

The American Cancer Society lists seven basic warning signals of cancer. If you have any of these symptoms, talk with a practitioner as soon as possible. Early detection and treatment greatly increase the chances of being cured, so listen to the body's warning signals. Do not wait until there is pain. Pain is not an early indication of cancer; on the contrary, it is usually a late

CANCERS AMONG MEN—CASES AND DEATHS REPORTED IN 1996

Cancer	Cases	Deaths
Prostate	317,100	41,400
Lung	98,900	94,400
Colorectal	67,600	27,400
Lymphoma	33,900	13,250
Melanoma of the Skin	21,800	4,600
Oral	20,100	5,380
Testicular	7,400	370
Penile	1,000 (estimated)	250

symptom. It's important to remember that these symptoms can also be related to other conditions that are not cancerous—a trip to the doctor can put your worries to rest.

The seven warning signs include

1. A change in bowel or bladder habits

2. A sore that does not heal

3. Unusual bleeding or discharge

4. Thickening or a lump in any part of the body (for example, in the testicles)

5. Indigestion or difficulty swallowing

6. An obvious change in a wart or mole

7. Nagging cough or hoarseness

Risk Factors

According to the National Cancer Institute, our current understanding of what causes cancer is not complete, but it is clear that cancer is not caused by an injury such as a bump or bruise. And although being infected with certain viruses may increase the risk of contracting certain types of cancer (for example, the HIV virus may increase the risk for lymphoma), cancer is not contagious.

Doctors know that there are specific factors that can increase the risk of contracting cancer— these are known as risk factors. While some factors are inherited and cannot be avoided, others—scientists say roughly 80 percent—are environmental or lifestyle factors that can be avoided. In either case, just because you have a particular risk factor does not mean you will get cancer. In fact, according to the National Cancer Institute, most people at risk do not. But you can lower your risk by avoiding those factors whenever you can—and by getting regular checkups. That way, if cancer develops, it is likely to be detected and treated while it's still in an early stage, greatly increasing the chance for a cure.

Some of the factors that are known to increase the risk of cancer include tobacco use, diet, sunlight, alcohol, radiation, chemicals and other substances in the home or workplace, and a familial history of cancer.

Tobacco use. The National Cancer Institute reports that tobacco causes cancer. In fact, one-third of all cancer deaths in the United States each year are attributed to smoking tobacco, using "smokeless" tobacco, and being regularly exposed to environmental tobacco smoke without actually smoking. In addition, cigarette smoking is a major cause of heart disease, stroke, chronic bronchitis, and emphysema.

For those who smoke one pack a day, the chance of getting lung cancer is about ten times greater than for nonsmokers. Smokers are also more likely than nonsmokers to develop several other types of cancer besides lung cancer, such as oral cancer (cancer of the mouth and throat) and cancer of the larynx, esophagus, pancreas, bladder, and kidney. The use of smokeless tobacco also causes oral cancer. Exposure to environmental tobacco smoke, or secondhand smoke, increases the risk of lung cancer for nonsmokers: The risk of contracting lung cancer increases 30 percent or more for a nonsmoking spouse of a smoker.

Diet. What you eat can increase—or decrease—the risk of contracting cancer. Doctors believe there is a link between a high-fat diet and certain cancers such as cancer of the breast, colon, and prostate. Obesity (weighing 20 percent more than your ideal weight) also appears to be linked to increased rates of cancer of the prostate, pancreas, and colon. Nevertheless, there are foods that some believe can help protect against some forms of cancer: foods high in fiber, vitamins, and minerals (such as fruits and vegetables); whole grain breads; legumes; and rice.

Sun. According to the American Cancer Society, about 90 percent of the estimated 800,000 skin cancers reported in 1996 could have been prevented by protection from the sun's rays. Ultraviolet radiation from the sun damages the skin and can cause skin cancer. The damage is permanent and cumulative. Sun lamps or tanning booths that emit ultraviolet radiation are also unsafe.

Alcohol. Drinking large amounts of alcohol increases the risk of cancer of the mouth, throat, esophagus, and larynx. Alcohol can also damage the liver and lead to liver cancer.

Radiation, chemicals, and other substances. Although x-rays taken for medical purposes lead to very little exposure and far outweigh the risks, repeated exposure to radiation can be harmful. Talk with a doctor or dentist about the use of shields to protect areas of the body not pictured in the x-ray. The risk of cancer can increase with exposure to various substances that are commonly found in the workplace. According to the National Cancer Institute, asbestos, nickel, cadmium, uranium, radon, vinyl chloride, benzidine, and benzene are well-known examples of carcinogens (substances or agents known to cause cancer) in the workplace. It is important to follow work and safety rules to avoid contact with dangerous materials.

Hereditary factors. A small number of cancers, including melanoma and cancers of the breast and colon tend to occur more often in some families than in the rest of the population. The National Cancer Institute reports that it is not always clear whether this familial pattern is connected to heredity, factors in the family's environment and lifestyle, or chance. Recently, researchers have been able to pinpoint the genetic markers that signal an increased risk of cancer, making genetic testing a possibility for some cancers in the future. If a close relation has had cancer, talk to a doctor and follow recommendations for cancer prevention and early detection.

Diagnosis

Many cases of cancer are first discovered during a routine physical, an important reason to see your practitioner regularly. If cancer is suspected, diagnostic tests, which may include imaging, endoscopy, and laboratory tests, are available. If these diagnostic tests show a tumor or other abnormality, a biopsy (removal of a sample of tissue for analysis) will be done to determine if it is cancerous or benign.

Imaging

Imaging is a process that produces pictures of the inside of the body to determine if a tumor is present. There are several ways of producing an image, including x-rays, radionuclide scanning (in which the patient swallows radioactive substance, and a scanner measures the radioactivity in certain organs to provide a picture of any abnormal areas on paper or film), and ultrasound (use of sound waves to create an image of internal structures). Magnetic resonance imaging (MRI) uses magnets and computers to create a picture that can show the size, shape, and location of a tumor and whether the cancer has spread to other parts of the body. Computerized tomography (CT) scans use a beam that rotates around the body to create a three-dimensional x-ray. The computer then creates a complete picture of the selected area. CT scans can show the relationship of a tumor to other structures, show the size of the tumor, and show whether it has spread to other organs.

PREVENTING CANCER

The following general recommendations are thought to help reduce your risk of cancer:

- Don't smoke. Smoking is the most preventable risk factor for cancer.

- Drink alcohol in moderation—no more than one to two drinks per day.

- Shun the sun. Avoid the sun between 11 A.M. and 3 P.M., when the sun is high overhead and its ultraviolet rays are strongest. Use protective clothing or sunscreen rated SPF 15 to 30 to block most of the sun's harmful rays.

- Eat a high-fiber, low-fat diet. Be sure to get at least five servings of fruits and vegetables a day.

- Watch out for health risks in the environment. If you work around any harmful substances, follow safety rules to keep any risk of cancer to a minimum.

- Get regular examinations by your practitioner. Remember that checkups and preventive screenings go a long way toward catching cancer early, when it is most easily cured. Screening is especially important if you are at high risk for cancer—for example, if it runs in your family. (See Physicals and Preventive Screening, p. 109, for information on recommendations for cancer screening.)

- Practice self-examination regularly. Learn how to do testicular self-examination. (see p. 227 for instructions.) To spot skin cancer, examine your skin regularly.

Endoscopy

The doctor can examine many areas inside the body by using a thin, lighted tube called an endoscope, during a procedure known as an endoscopy. For example, the tube can be inserted through the mouth for a look at the lungs or the stomach, through the anus for a view of the rectum or colon, and through a small incision to examine internal organs such as the gallbladder. Many of these procedures can be done in a practitioner's office.

The newer flexible scopes owe their success in large part to the development and application of fiberoptics technology. Fiberoptic devices are thin, flexible tubes containing bundles of glass filaments that can transmit light around bends and curves to illuminate the inside of the body. In some cases forceps, scissors, or other tiny instruments can be threaded through channels in the scope to facilitate surgical procedures. In addition, the pictures taken by the lens of the scope can be fed to a television monitor for better viewing by practitioners. During the exam, the doctor can also collect tissue or cells, a procedure called a biopsy, to examine them for cancer. (See Medical Testing, p. 462.)

Laboratory Tests

Laboratory tests such as blood and urine tests are also commonly performed and may show if cancer has affected the body in any particular way. There is no single laboratory test that can detect cancer, but tests may show any changes the body may be undergoing. An example of a laboratory test is the prostate-specific antigen (PSA) test for prostate cancer, a blood test that indicates levels of PSA in the blood. Elevated levels may indicate a problem with the prostate.

Biopsy

A biopsy is the collection of a sample of tissue from the suspicious area or growth for microscopic examination. In most cases, a biopsy is the only sure way to determine if a problem may be cancer.

There are several types of biopsies:

1. *Needle aspiration biopsy.* A small amount of tissue is collected via suction through a thin, hollow needle inserted into the suspicious tissue. Needle aspiration biopsy is inexpensive and less invasive than other types of biopsy. It can be done in a practitioner's office. It is also known as aspiration biopsy, fine needle biopsy, or suction biopsy.

2. *Core needle biopsy.* This method uses a slightly larger needle than needle aspiration biopsy. A tiny cutting instrument is inserted through the needle to cut away tissue for collection. It is slightly more invasive than needle aspiration biopsy, but is considered more accurate because more tissue is collected for examination.

3. *Excisional biopsy.* This involves the surgical removal of the tumor for examination. It can also serve as a treatment for the cancer when the entire tumor or suspicious area is removed.

4. *Incisional biopsy.* In this method, part of a tumor or suspicious area is surgically removed for examination.

The tissue removed is examined by a specialist in the examination of human tissue, known as a pathologist. The pathologist will determine whether or not cancer is present, and if it is, what type it is and what stage it is at. A positive biopsy indicates the presence of cancer, and a negative biopsy means that no cancer has been found. Biopsies are not always accurate: They can be categorized as false negative (meaning no cancer has been found when it actually is present) or false positive (meaning the biopsy indicates cancer when there is, in fact, none). The accuracy varies, according to the type of cancer and the type of biopsy.

It may take several days or weeks for the results of a biopsy to be returned. However, analysis can be done almost immediately if necessary. For example, if a biopsy is taken during an invasive surgical procedure, it may be analyzed while the person is undergoing the operation. If the biopsy turns out to be positive, suspicious areas can be removed during the same procedure.

Stages of Cancer

When cancer is diagnosed, the doctor needs to know how much the cancer has grown. As a result, cancer is classified according to stages that indicate how large a tumor is or how far the cancer has spread from its original site. The stages of a cancer vary slightly, according to its type, but generally range from stage 0 (the earliest stage, known as *in-situ* cancer) to stage 5 (cancer that has spread, or metastasized, throughout the body). Another stage, recurrent cancer, indicates cancer that has reappeared even though there was no evidence of it after previous treatment was completed.

The stages of cancer are used to determine what treatment should be followed. The earlier a cancer is diagnosed, the easier it is to cure.

Treatment

There are several basic methods of treating cancer, used individually or combined. The type of cancer, its stage, and the age and overall health of the patient determine the method used.

Surgery is a local treatment of cancer; that is, it involves only the area of the body that is affected by cancer. It is used to remove the cancerous tissue and, if the cancer has spread, the surrounding tissue and the nearby lymph nodes. For most forms of cancer, surgery is the primary treatment, though other treatments may be used along with—or instead of—surgery.

Radiation therapy, also called radiotherapy, involves the use of high-energy rays to destroy the reproductive material of cancerous cells and prevent them from multiplying. It is generally used after surgery as an adjuvant, or supplemental, therapy to destroy any cancer cells that may remain.

Radiation therapy affects only the cells in the treated area. It can be administered externally (radiation is administered by a machine) or internally (an implant of radioactive material is placed directly into or near the tumor). Common side effects include tiredness; red, sunburned skin in the treated area; nausea and vomiting; hair loss; and loss of appetite. Radiation therapy also may cause a decrease in the body's white blood cells, those that help the body fight infections. Radiation administered in the area of the pelvis may also cause a reduction in sperm count and fertility. The specialist who administers radiation therapy is known as a radiation oncologist.

Chemotherapy is a treatment that uses anticancer drugs to kill cancer cells. Unlike surgery or radiation therapy, chemotherapy is systemic rather than local, meaning its effects are not limited to the area of the body that is affected by cancer. Instead, the drugs (administered orally or through a vein) travel through the bloodstream and throughout the body. While the prescribed dose is chosen to try to limit damage only to cancer cells, chemotherapy affects normal cells as well.

Chemotherapy is given in cycles of a treatment period that is followed by a recovery period, then another treatment period, and so on. The type of drugs used to kill the cancer cells and the number of treatments depend on the type of cancer and its stage.

The side effects experienced also depend on the type of drug used and the dose. Generally, anticancer drugs affect cells that divide rapidly such as blood cells and those cells that line the digestive tract. As a result, those who have chemotherapy are vulnerable to infections, bruise easily, and feel tired. They also experience loss of appetite, nausea and vomiting, as well as hair loss and mouth sores. Infertility may be another side effect of chemotherapy. Whether or not this loss in fertility is permanent depends on the type of drugs used and the patient's age.

Hormone therapy can be used on the certain types of cancer that depend on hormones to grow—prostate cancer and breast cancer among them. Doctors may recommend therapy designed to prevent cancer cells from getting the hormones they need. This can be done through surgically removing the hormone-producing organs (such as the testicles) or by using drugs that stop hormone production or change how the hormones work. This type of treatment is systemic, like chemotherapy, affecting cells throughout the body.

Patients can experience a number of side effects, including nausea and vomiting, swelling, and weight gain, and, in some cases, hot flashes. Men may experience impotence, loss of sexual desire, and loss of fertility. How long these symptoms last or if they are permanent depends on whether or not a surgical procedure is done, the type of drugs used, and the stage of the cancer.

Biological Therapy, also called immunotherapy, is the injection of a substance into the body—for example, the protein interferon—to enhance the body's natural defenses against cancer. It is a relatively new form of treatment, and it is still considered experimental. It can also be used to help protect the body from some of the side effects of treatment such as infections that may occur during chemotherapy. Biological therapy has its own side effects, including flulike symptoms such as chills, fever, muscle aches, weakness, loss of appetite, nausea, vomiting, and diarrhea. Some patients get a rash and some bleed or bruise easily. The side effects a patient experiences depends on the type of biological therapy used. They are usually short-term and gradually go away after the treatment stops.

Bone Marrow Transplantation may be used for some particularly aggressive or recurrent forms of cancer (such as lymphoma, lung cancer, leukemia, and brain cancer), a bone marrow transplant may be done. Bone marrow, the tissue that produces new cells and helps to maintain the immune system, can be damaged by the high doses of chemotherapy and radiation that may be needed to treat some forms of cancer. In a bone marrow transplant, the bone marrow is removed and stored, then replaced after the

SIDE EFFECTS AND SEXUALITY

Cancer treatments such as radiation therapy and chemotherapy by nature affect some of the healthy tissues of the body—there is no way to limit their cell-killing capacity to only the dangerous, cancerous cells. As a result, there may be some temporary or permanent effect on sexuality and fertility.

In men, the treatment may affect sperm production, lowering sperm counts and affecting fertility. Treatment, in some cases, may also lead to impotence—the inability to have an erection. However, cancer treatments have been refined and improved to reduce the risk of impotency. Younger men are more likely than older men to regain fertility after treatment.

One option for a man concerned about fertility is a donation to a sperm bank before treatment. If the man become infertile due to treatment, but wants to have a biological child, the sample of sperm can be used in an assisted fertility technique. (See Infertility, p. 412.)

Sexuality is usually affected during treatment. Radiation and chemotherapy, which have side effects such as fatigue and nausea, often lower the sex drive, or libido—and the stress of having cancer can affect libido as well. Changes in appearance such as hair loss can also leave a person feeling unattractive. However, healthy sexuality will most likely return after treatment ends.

The American Cancer Society offers two publications, *Sexuality and Cancer* and *For the Man Who Has Cancer and His Partner*, which deal with these issues. They are available free by calling 800-ACS-2345.

high-dose treatment is completed. (If an individual's marrow is removed and replaced, the transplant is known as an autologous transplant. But in some cases, bone marrow may also be donated by a genetically compatible donor.) In this way, the cell-producing bone marrow is preserved rather than destroyed by the cancer treatment.

Bone marrow transplants are new and very expensive procedures, usually costing more than $100,000, and often they are not covered by insurance, even though they are no longer considered experimental. Because they are so complex, such transplants should only be performed at reputable hospitals or health centers with a great deal of expertise.

For more information:

(Note: Resources for information about specific cancers are listed at the end of those topics.)

American Cancer Society
1599 Clifton Rd., N.E.
Atlanta, GA 30329-4251
800-ACS-2345
404-320-3333
http://www.cancer.org

American Institute for Cancer Research
Nutrition Hotline
1759 R St., N.W.
Washington, DC 20009
800-843-8114 (nutrition hotline)
202-328-7744 (Washington, DC)
http://www.aicr.org

Biological Therapy Institute Foundation
P.O. Box 681700
Franklin, TN 37068-1700
615-790-7535

Cancer Care Inc.
1180 Avenue of the Americas
New York, NY 10036
800-813-HOPE
212-302-2400
http://www.cancercare.org

CHEMOcare
2 North Rd., W.
Chester, NJ 07930
800-55-CHEMO
908-879-4039 (New Jersey)

International Cancer Alliance
4853 Cordell Ave., Suite 11
Bethedsa, MD 20814
800-ICARE-61
http://www.icare.org/icare

National Cancer Institute
Cancer Information Service
9000 Rockville Pike
Bethesda, MD 20892
800-4-CANCER
800-638-1234 (Alaska)
800-524-1234 (Hawaii)
301-496-5583
http://cancernet.nci.nih.gov

For information on alternative cancer treatments:

Cancer Control Society
2043 N. Berendo St.
Los Angeles, CA 90027
213-663-7801

Committee for Freedom of Choice in
Cancer Therapy
1180 Walnut Ave.
Chula Vista, CA 91911
619-429-8200

International Association of Cancer Victors
and Friends
7740 W. Manchester Ave., Suite 203
Playa del Ray, CA 90293
310-822-5032

People Against Cancer
604 East St.
P.O. Box 10
Otho, IA 50569-0010
515-972-4444
http://www.dodgenet.com/nocancer

CANCER TREATMENTS: QUESTIONS TO ASK

New and improved technology has greatly increased the number of treatments available for cancer. Because of the number of options available, choosing a particular treatment may be difficult, and there are many questions to be asked. According to the National Institutes of Health, here are some questions you may want to ask your doctor:

- What is my diagnosis?

- What is the stage of the disease?

- What are my treatment choices? Which do you recommend for me? Why?

- What are the chances that the treatment will be successful?

- Would a clinical trial be appropriate for me?

- What are the risks and possible side effects of each treatment?

- How long will treatment last?

- Will I have to change my normal activities?

- What is the treatment likely to cost?

Breast Cancer

Breast cancer, the growth of abnormal cells in the breast tissue, is rare for men, accounting for only 1 percent of all breast cancer cases. The American Cancer Society estimated that there were 1,400 new cases of male breast cancer in the United States in 1996 (compared with 184,300 female cases). According to the American Cancer Society, one man will develop breast cancer for every one hundred women—1:100 roughly the ratio of the amount of breast tissue in men to that in women.

Little is heard about breast cancer in men in the United States, despite the tremendous educational push about breast cancer for women, and most men probably don't know they are able to get the disease. In addition, physicians often aren't alert to its symptoms, so breast cancer in men is typically found at a later stage. According to one study, men diagnosed with breast cancer before it spread to the lymph nodes (nearby glands that are part of the immune system) had an 84 percent chance of surviving ten or more years. In those whose cancer was caught after it had spread to the lymph nodes, the ten-year survival rate was only 14 percent. About 240 men die from breast cancer each year.

Risk Factors

The risk of breast cancer increases with age—most men with breast cancer are over the age of 60. Recent studies have also shown that men who come from families with a history of breast cancer in men or women are at higher risk than

WOMEN WITH BREAST CANCER

The closest most men come to being touched by breast cancer is when the disease affects a woman in their lives such as a wife or partner. With a breast cancer diagnosis come changes in priorities, relationships, traditional roles, and emotions. To cope with these changes and help a woman in your life with breast cancer, consider the following suggestions from Y-ME National Breast Cancer Organization:

- *Keep talking.* Communication through a fight with breast cancer—from diagnosis to coming home after treatment—is extremely important. Tell your partner what you're feeling and listen to how she feels, making sure you understand her message.

- *Participate in her care.* While breast cancer can make you and your partner feel helpless, learning more about the disease and its effects can give you an idea of your choices and put you both more in control. Accompany your partner to doctor visits and take notes and ask questions while you are there. Be at the hospital as much as possible. Act as a patient advocate during treatment or even provide some care for her yourself.

- *Expect imbalance.* The normal roles in relationships often change with breast cancer—everyday priorities change and the normal balance of give and take is altered. Strive to remain flexible and make a commitment to get through any rough times together.

- *Adjust to physical changes.* Breast surgery, especially mastectomy, and other treatments can leave a woman feeling frightened, uncomfortable, and unhappy with her appearance—as well as physically ill. You may also have feelings of fear and loss. Talk about your feelings and work together to adjust to physical and sexual changes—for example, look at scars together or change the position of intercourse to whatever is most comfortable for her. One-fourth to one-third of all couples have sexual difficulties after surgery, so communication is especially important in this area.

- *Support yourself.* Women with breast cancer need a lot of support, but those who stand behind them do as well. Talk with family and friends about your feelings and needs. You can also talk with another man who shares your concerns by calling the Y-ME Men's Hotline at 800-221-2141. You will be matched with a volunteer who will return your call at the time and place you choose. Women diagnosed with breast cancer can also call this hotline number to speak with a survivor of breast cancer.

(Source: "When the Woman You Love Has Breast Cancer," Y-ME National Breast Cancer Organization, 212 W. Van Buren St., 5th Floor, Chicago, IL 60607-3908; 800-221-2141.)

those who don't—although that risk is less than that of a woman in the same family.

Abnormal hormonal activity is thought to be a risk factor for breast cancer in men. Such hormonal problems include hyperestrogenism, a condition characterized by abnormal secretion of the female hormone estrogen; gynecomastia, enlargement of the male breasts (see the box below); and Klinefelter's syndrome, a chromosomal disorder marked by decreased or absent sperm production, underdeveloped testicles, lack of secondary sex characteristics (such as voice change or beard growth) and gynecomastia. A man with Klinefelter's syndrome is said to be twenty times more likely to develop breast cancer than a man with no risk factors.

Diet also may play a role. While the American Cancer Society notes that the role of dietary factors in breast cancer has not been firmly established, breast cancer incidence rates for countries throughout the world correlate with variations in diets, especially fat intake—high fat intake generally means a higher cancer rate.

Other factors that may be associated with increased breast cancer risk and that are currently under study include alcohol consumption, physical inactivity, and exposure to carcinogens (such as pesticides or radiation).

Symptoms

A lump or thickening in the breast—especially one that does not go away—is the most common sign of breast cancer. Usually the lump occurs beneath the areola, the colored area around the nipple, because that is where the breast tissue is most concentrated in men. Because men have less breast tissue than women, lumps are typically easier to spot. Noncancerous, or benign, lumps are generally firm, well-defined masses. Cancerous, or malignant, lumps tend to be hard, irregular, and painless.

Other signs and symptoms of breast cancer are swelling, dimpling, skin irritation, scaliness, pain, tenderness of the nipple, and nipple discharge. Sometimes the nipple is drawn into the chest, changes shape, or becomes crusty.

GYNECOMASTIA

Female hormones, heavy consumption of alcohol, liver disease, and certain prescription drugs can all contribute to the development of breast tissue in men, a condition known as gynecomastia. This condition occurs in some 30 to 40 percent of men during their lifetimes. While it is noncancerous, it is a risk factor for breast cancer, so men with a history of gynecomastia may want to perform breast self-examinations on a regular basis as a precaution.

This swelling of the breasts is most often attributed to high levels of estrogen, a female hormone that is produced by the male body as well. Gynecomastia most often occurs during the hormonal surge of puberty and after age 50. Alcohol consumption contributes by lowering the body's levels of testosterone, the off-setting male hormone. In addition, if there is a problem with the liver (the organ that removes estrogen from the body) levels of the female hormone will also rise. Medications can also cause gynecomastia.

Breast tissue may also swell in men who are overweight. This condition is known as pseudogynecomastia and has no connection with risk of breast cancer.

IF YOU HAVE BREAST CANCER

It is hard to be diagnosed with any sort of cancer, but breast cancer can be especially difficult for a man to deal with. Breast cancer is a rare disease in men, and as a result not much is known about it. It may be difficult to find a physician or center that has had experience treating this type of breast cancer. In addition, few studies have been done on the disease—and it's unlikely that more will be done—because it is difficult to find enough men with the condition to do reliable research.

Also, because breast cancer is typically thought of as a woman's disease, and is often linked to "feminizing" hormonal disorders, a man may feel his masculinity is being threatened. Treatment may involve removal of the testicles and doses of female hormones. Radiation and surgery may leave a man with a loss of arm strength, which can interfere with work or sports.

If you're involved in a battle with breast cancer, it's important to remember that there are organizations and support groups available. Contact the American Cancer Society, the National Cancer Institute and other organizations listed below for referrals to groups that may be able to help you deal with breast cancer. A number of on-line sites also bring men with the condition together for support and discussion.

While most breast lumps are not cancerous, the only way to find out for sure is through a physician's exam and testing. If you have any of the symptoms of breast cancer, talk with your practitioner as soon as possible—many men ignore symptoms or are embarrassed to mention them to their doctors, possibly delaying diagnosis and treatment.

Diagnosis

If breast cancer is suspected, the doctor will take a personal and family medical history and perform a physical exam of both breasts and the lymph nodes in the neck and armpit.

A mammogram, an x-ray of the breast done by compressing it between two plates, can be used to confirm the location of suspicious tumors and spot many of those that are too small to feel. Ultrasound, a procedure that creates an image of tissue by using sound waves, now is being used in conjunction with mammograms to more accurately diagnose breast lumps or irregularities. Thermography, a test that detects lumps by measuring the heat emitted from the breast, is also sometimes used; however, it is not as accurate as mammography or ultrasound.

Once the abnormalities are pinpointed, your doctor may do a biopsy, a procedure in which cells are removed for microscopic analysis. Cells and tissue may be drawn out by using a thin, hollow needle, called a needle aspiration biopsy, or through a larger needle by using a tiny cutting tool, called a core needle biopsy. (Core needle biopsies are widely considered to be more accurate than needle aspiration, as they collect more tissue for diagnosis.) Tissue may also be removed surgically for examination in what is called an excisional biopsy.

After the cells are collected, testing will determine what type of breast cancer cells—

HOW TO PERFORM A BREAST SELF-EXAMINATION

If you're at risk for breast cancer, this self-examination may help you to catch any cancer at an early stage:

1. Place your right arm behind your head.

2. Using the finger pads of the middle three fingers on your left hand, feel for lumps or thickening in your right breast area.

3. Move around the breast in a circular way, being sure to go over the entire breast area.

4. Examine your left breast by using the right hand's finger pads.

5. Remember what your breasts feel like most of the time so you'll recognize a change in the future.

6. See your doctor right away if you find any lumps, thickening, or other symptoms of breast cancer.

if any—are involved. Certain types of breast cancers spread faster than others. Additional tests like x-rays, blood work, and bone and liver scans may be done to determine the stage of the cancer and whether it has spread. The results of these tests dictate the type of treatment you receive.

If Klinefelter's syndrome is suspected, karyotyping—a test that looks at the patterns of the chromosomes—can be done to confirm that diagnosis.

Treatment

Treatment of breast cancer depends on the individual and the stage at which the cancer is diagnosed. In breast cancer in men that is discovered in its early stages, surgery is most often used. Surgical treatment may involve lumpectomy (removal of only the tumor and surrounding tissue) or mastectomy (surgical removal of the breast and possibly the lymph nodes). While women with breast cancer usually choose lumpectomy to save as much breast tissue as possible, men are usually treated with mastectomy and the removal of lymph nodes since the cosmetic results are not as important.

Radiation therapy may be done after surgery to destroy any remaining cancer cells—or it may be used instead of surgery for people who are not strong enough to have surgery. Surgery or radiation may result in stiffness in the treated area, decreased shoulder function, or fluid retention in the arm. Chemotherapy is used rarely.

In more advanced cancer cases, hormone therapy is commonly used. The breast cancers in men tend to be affected by the levels of hormones in the body—one reason that abnormal hormonal activity is a risk factor. As a result, when hormone levels drop, the cancers often shrink. Tests may be done to determine how receptive the breast cancer will be to hormone therapy.

Hormonal treatment options include orchiectomy, removal of the testicles, to stop hormone production. The adrenal glands may be removed as well in a procedure known as an adrenalectomy, or the pituitary gland can be removed in a procedure called a hypophysectomy. Orchiectomy is usually used first; it shrinks tumors in two-thirds of all cases. Recently, drugs known as antiestrogens (for example, tamoxifen) have begun to be used to treat breast cancer in men. To date, these drugs have been effective in 50 percent of cases.

Anyone who has had breast cancer should have regular follow-up exams throughout his life since it's possible for cancer to return many years after the initial treatment. Though men with breast cancer are not likely to develop breast cancer in the other breast (a tendency that is common in women), they are likely to develop another type of cancer elsewhere in the body.

For more information:

American Cancer Society
1599 Clifton Rd., N.E.
Atlanta, GA 30329-4251
800-ACS-2345
404-320-3333
http://www.cancer.org

Breast Cancer Information Clearinghouse
http://nysernet.org/bcic/

National Alliance of Breast Cancer Organizations (NABCO)
9 E. 37th St., 10th Floor
New York, NY 10016
212-889-0606
http://www.nabco.org

National Breast Cancer Coalition
1707 L St., N.W., Suite 1060
Washington, DC 20036
202-296-7477

http://www.natlbcc.org

National Cancer Institute
Cancer Information Service
9000 Rockville Pike
Bethesda, MD 20892
800-4-CANCER
800-638-1234 (Alaska)
800-524-1234 (Hawaii)
310-496-5583
http://cancernet.nci.nih.gov

Male Breast Cancer Homepage
http://interact.withus.com/interact/mbc

Y-ME National Breast Cancer Organization
212 W. Van Buren St., 5th Floor
Chicago, IL 60607-3908
800-221-2141
312-986-8228
708-799-8228
http://www.y-me.org/

Colorectal Cancer

Colorectal cancer is the growth of abnormal cells in the large intestine (the colon is the main section of the large intestine, and the rectum is the last 8 to 10 inches of the colon). This form of cancer is the second most common cancer in the United States, and the third leading cause of death from cancer in men. According to the American Cancer Society, a total of 67,600 new cases of colorectal cancer (also called colon and rectal cancer) occurred in men in 1996—and an estimated 27,400 men died of the disease the same year.

That's the bad news. The good news is that colorectal cancer is highly treatable if it's caught early. But you need to be on the lookout for it. Colorectal cancer is hard to detect in some cases because symptoms may not appear until the cancer is advanced—often not until growths in the

PREVENTION OF COLORECTAL CANCER

You can take steps to prevent colorectal cancer simply by avoiding the factors that put you at risk. While there may be nothing you can do about a family history of the disease or the development of polyps in the colon, you can do the following:

- Eat a low-fat, high-fiber diet to aid digestion. High-fiber foods include whole-grain cereals, breads, pasta, vegetables, and fruit. Also, reduce your total fat intake to 30 percent or less of your total calorie intake.

- Get enough exercise. Experts recommend at least twenty minutes of moderate activity most—if not all—days of the week.

- Maintain a healthy weight. Eating right and getting enough exercise are half the battle if you're looking to lower your weight.

- Avoid smoking and drinking.

It's also important to get regular checkups, especially if you have a family history of the disease. The American Cancer Society recommends an annual digital rectal examination (DRE) beginning at age 40, as well as a fecal occult blood test (FOBT) every year after age 50 (some studies recommend the FOBT annually after age 40). Once every three to five years, a sigmoidoscopy, a diagnostic test in which a flexible scope is inserted into the rectum and colon, should be done. If you have polyps, have your practitioner monitor their growth. If you are have several risk factors for colorectal cancer, noncancerous polyps can be removed to reduce risk.

colon have become large enough to obstruct the digestive tract. By that time, the cancer may have already spread to the liver, lymph nodes, or other parts of the body, making it much harder to treat.

The statistics reflect this tendency. According to the American Cancer Society, some 91 percent of those diagnosed at an early stage survive for more than five years. However, if the cancer has spread to nearby organs or lymph nodes, the five-year survival rate drops to 63 percent. For those whose cancer has spread throughout the body, the survival rate is only 7 percent.

Risk Factors

Factors that increase your risk of colorectal cancer include:

- *A personal or family history of colorectal cancer.*

- *Polyps.* Polyps develop in the mucosa that lines the colon. The mucosa is a pinkish tissue made up of millions of tiny, tubular passages that absorbs the remaining water and minerals from the digested material as it travels through the colon. New mucosal cells take over for old cells that slough off every four to five days. When new cells emerge faster than old ones can be discarded, cells accumulate and create a polyp, a small bump on the lining of the colon. Polyps are not cancerous, but they may develop into colon cancer and should be monitored by a physician.

- *Inflammatory bowel disease.* This disease includes Crohn's disease, an inflammation of the intestines, and/or ulcerative colitis, a condition in which sores occur in the colon.

- *A high-fat, low-fiber diet.* Dietary fat is thought to increase the amount of bile acids in the colon, acids that may damage the lining of the organ. A low-fiber diet contributes to slow digestion, possibly allowing these damaging substances to linger in the colon.

- *A sedentary lifestyle.* Exercise helps speed digestion and quickly move along any possibly harmful chemicals in the digestive tract.

- *Obesity.* Extra pounds increase the risk of colon cancer.

- *Drinking alcohol.* People who consume three or more alcoholic beverages a day may have a significantly higher risk of developing rectal cancer than those who abstain.

Symptoms

Early colorectal cancer and polyps usually have no symptoms. But if they do occur, symptoms include rectal bleeding; bloody or black stools; pain in the lower abdomen; cramping and gas pains; bloating or a full feeling even after a bowel movement; loss of appetite; loss of weight; and fatigue. Diarrhea, constipation, or unusually narrow stools lasting for more than ten days are also symptoms.

While these symptoms may be a sign of other problems, you should visit your practitioner if they persist for more than ten days.

Diagnosis

To detect colon or rectum cancer, a doctor will utilize a series of tests. In the digital rectal examination (DRE), the practitioner inserts a lubricated, gloved finger into the lowest four inches of the rectum to check for abnormalities. An occult stool blood test, a laboratory test to detect blood in the stools, may be done.

Other diagnostic procedures include a lower gastrointestinal (GI) series, in which the colon is examined by x-ray after a contrast dye, known as barium, is administered. The barium allows the internal structures to be visible on x-ray. Computerized tomography (CT) uses x-ray technology to create a three-dimensional image, and magnetic resonance imaging (MRI) involves the use of magnetic waves to create cross sections of the area.

Finally, a sigmoidoscopy or colonoscopy may be done. In a sigmoidoscopy, a flexible, fiberoptic tube is inserted into the rectum to inspect the lower portion of the colon. A colonoscopy inspects the upper portion of the colon. During either of these procedures, photographs may be taken, or a tissue sample may be collected (in a procedure called a biopsy) for microscopic analysis.

Treatment

The most effective method of treating colorectal cancer is surgery to remove the tumor and nearby lymph nodes. If the cancer is limited to a polyp, the polyp can be removed in a procedure called

THE FOOD CONNECTION

Recent medical studies suggest that what you eat and drink may affect your chance of getting colorectal cancer. Here are some of the findings:

- A high-fat, low-fiber diet may double your risk of colon cancer.

- Men who eat an abundance of foods containing calcium and vitamin D such as fortified milk and salmon (which helps the body absorb calcium) may reduce their risk of colorectal cancer by a third.

- A study of people who had noncancerous colorectal polyps removed showed that vitamins C and E may reduce the recurrence of polyps, which may develop into cancer.

- Eating cruciferous vegetables such as broccoli, cauliflower, and cabbage on a regular basis may reduce the risk of cancer in the gastrointestinal tract.

a polypectomy, done during a colonoscopy by inserting instruments through the fiberoptic scope. Polyps can also be removed through an opening in the abdomen. If the cancer is more extensive, a section of the colon containing the tumor and surrounding tissue can be surgically removed in a procedure called a wedge resection. If the lymph nodes are removed as well, the procedure is known as a bowel resection. Surgery is most often accompanied by radiation therapy or chemotherapy to destroy any remaining cancer cells.

In most cases where a section of the colon is removed, the remaining segments are reattached. When necessary, a colostomy is done—this involves the creation of a hole in the abdominal wall through which waste passes into a bag the outside of the body. A colostomy is permanent in about 15 percent of cases when the cancer is extensive and part of the colon must be completely removed. Otherwise, the temporary colostomy bag is removed after the colon heals from the operation. Ostomy surgery does not affect fertility or the ability to have an erection.

For more information:

American Cancer Society
1599 Clifton Road, N.E.
Atlanta, GA 30329-4251
800-ACS-2345
404-320-3333
http://www.cancer.org

National Cancer Institute
Cancer Information Service
9000 Rockville Pike
Bethesda, MD 20892
800-4-CANCER
800-638-1234 (Alaska)
800-524-1234 (Hawaii)
310-496-5583
http://cancernet.nci.nih.gov

United Ostomy Association, Inc.
19772 MacArthur Blvd., Suite 200
Irvine, CA 92612-2405
800-826-0826
714-660-8624
http://www.uoa.org

Lung Cancer

Lung cancer, the uncontrolled growth of abnormal cells in the lung, is the leading cause of death from cancer among men. Approximately 95,000 men die of lung cancer every year, according to the American Cancer Society.

Lung cancer has a high mortality rate because it is usually discovered after the cancer has spread, or metastasized, from the lungs to other parts of the body. In 85 percent of those diagnosed, the cancer has already metastasized. According to the American Cancer Society, 46 percent of patients with localized lung cancer (that has not spread to other parts of the body) live for five or more years after diagnosis. Yet only 13 percent of patients with lung cancer that has spread live five or more years after diagnosis.

Types of Lung Cancer

There are two main types of lung cancer: small cell carcinoma (or oat cell carcinoma) and nonsmall cell carcinoma.

Small cell carcinoma accounts for 20 percent of all lung cancer cases. It is the most aggressive type and is more likely to have spread by the time of diagnosis. It is also called oat cell carcinoma because the cells are shaped like grains of oats.

Nonsmall cell carcinoma has three subtypes. The first, squamous or epidermoid cancer, accounts for 30 percent of all lung cancers and grows from the flat, scaly cells that line that air passages. Adenocarcinoma, the second type, accounts for 30 percent of all lung cancers, and is more common among women. This tumor begins in the mucous membrane of both the smaller and larger respiratory tubes of the lungs. While it can be caused by cigarette smoke, adenocarcinoma is the form that is more likely to be caused by other sources such as industrial substances and chemicals. Finally, large cell carcinoma is responsible for about 10 percent of all lung cancers. It develops in the lungs as large, round cells. The remaining 10 percent of lung cancers are uncommon forms.

Smoking and Lung Cancer

Most lung cancer deaths are related to cigarette smoking—90 percent of lung cancers among men are caused by smoking. The lesson is a simple one: The longer a person smokes, the more likely he is to die of lung cancer. (See Smoking, p. 95.) According to the American Cancer Society, a two-pack-a-day smoker who has smoked more than forty years has a lung cancer mortality rate that is twenty-two times higher than a nonsmoker. But those who quit smoking can lower their risk of lung cancer by half. Ten years after kicking the habit, the bronchial lining returns to normal. In fact, 87 percent of lung cancers would eventually disappear if no one smoked cigarettes, says the American Cancer Society. While smoking a pipe or cigars also can lead to lung cancer, they are more likely to lead to oral cancers, cancers of the mouth, throat, larynx, and esophagus. (Smokeless tobacco also causes oral cancers.)

The risk of lung cancer is also higher for those around smokers. Secondhand smoke breathed by nonsmokers contributes to about three thousand lung cancer deaths annually in the United States, according to the American Cancer Society. One study found that nonsmokers married to heavy smokers have two to three times the risk of lung cancer compared with those married to nonsmokers.

Other Causes of Lung Cancer

Industrial substances and chemicals may also contribute to lung cancer. These include radon (see box), arsenic, nickel, chromates, coal gas, mustard gas, vinyl chloride, and asbestos. Smoking can compound your risk of lung cancer from exposure to these substances. For example, asbestos workers who smoke increase their risk of developing lung cancer by sixty times.

Air pollution and heavy doses of radiation may also contribute to lung cancer, although no scientific proof exists today to definitely link these concerns to the disease.

Symptoms

Because the lungs are large, cancer can be present for many years without being detected. In 85 percent of cases, lung cancer is not diagnosed until it has spread from the lungs. Early symptoms of lung cancer—coughing, wheezing, and shortness of breath—are often mistaken for a cold or bronchitis or ignored. Other symptoms include coughing up blood, ongoing chest aches and pains, fever, weakness, weight loss, and repeated bouts of pneumonia. Advanced symptoms of the disease include hoarseness, shortness of breath, swollen lymph nodes in the neck, difficulty swallowing, shoulder, back, or arm pain and drooping of the upper eyelids.

There may also be headaches, blurred vision, dizziness, and bone pain.

If any of these symptoms are present, visit your practitioner. Symptoms such as a chronic cough and shortness of breath are not normal and need medical attention.

Diagnosis

To identify lung cancer and the type and extent of the disease, doctors will first start with a medical history to determine if the patient smokes and if so how frequently. Then a physical examination will check how well the heart and lungs are functioning.

A number of techniques can be used to locate suspicious areas. Chest x-rays can locate larger tumors in the lungs. Tomograms, x-rays that show a thin layer of lung at a time, can reveal small cancer growths not visible on a standard x-ray. In addition, magnetic resonance

THE RADON CONNECTION

Radon, a radioactive gas, is the second leading cause of lung cancer (after smoking) in the United States today. According to the Environmental Protection Agency (EPA), there are about 14,000 deaths each year in the United States that result from breathing radon.

Where does radon come from? Radon is a naturally occurring decay product that is created when uranium in rock and soil gradually breaks down. You can't see, taste, or smell radon. It seeps up from the ground and gets into the air through cracks in solid floors, construction joints, cracks in walls, gaps in suspended floors, gaps around service pipes, cavities inside walls, and the water supply. When windows and doors are shut, radon levels can build up in your home. The problem can be corrected by sealing cracks in the home and installing insulation and vents.

The EPA says nearly one out of every 15 homes in the United States may have elevated radon levels. Radon problems are more common in some areas of the country than others, but the only way to know if your home, school, or workplace has a radon problem is to test for it. You can get low-cost do-it-yourself tests through the mail or at a hardware store, or you can hire a professional contractors to do the testing for you. Be sure to hire an EPA-qualified or state-certified radon tester. The National Safety Council offers a radon hotline at 800-SOS-RADON.

PREVENTING LUNG CANCER

- Don't smoke. Ask your doctor about ways to stop smoking, or contact the American Lung Association or National Cancer Institute for information and referrals to support groups in your area. (See "Smoking" for tips on how to quit.)

- If you don't smoke, avoid secondhand smoke and encourage a smoke-free environment at home and at work.

- Stay away from pollution. For example, just walking or jogging along a busy street can increase your risk of lung cancer. Exercise in the early morning or evening after the sun has set, when pollution levels are lowest, or cover your face with a mask to filter out pollution. Experts say pollution levels are at their worst in the late afternoon. Also, stay indoors on days when pollution levels are reported to be high.

- Avoid industrial chemicals on the job. If you work around chemicals or fumes, protect yourself with a face mask or other protective equipment. You may even want to talk with your employer about ways to make the workplace a safer place in which to breathe.

- Have your home checked for radon if you live in an area known for such problems.

- Get your vitamins and minerals. Studies show vitamins C and E may help protect against lung cancer. Vitamin C can be found in citrus fruits, red bell peppers, broccoli, and papaya, and vitamin E can be found in eggs, wheat germ, whole-grain cereals, and sunflower and almond oils.

- Eat watercress. Studies show the vegetable contains phenethyl isothiocyanate (PEITC), a compound that is thought by some to prevent lung cancer. The National Cancer Institute is currently conducting trials to test its effects. And even if it doesn't turn out to prevent lung cancer, you can't go wrong. Watercress is still high in calcium, vitamin C, and beta carotene.

imaging (MRI) may be done. This technique uses magnetic waves and computers to create a picture that can show the size, shape, and location of a tumor and whether the cancer has spread to other part of the body. Computerized tomography (CT) uses a beam that rotates around the body to create a three-dimensional x-ray. The computer then creates a complete picture of the selected area. For example, CT scans can show the relationship of a lung tumor to other chest structures and show the size of the tumor and whether it has moved into other organs.

If an abnormal area is located, a biopsy— a procedure in which tissue collected for microscopic examination—is done. A biopsy is the only test that can confirm the presence of cancer, and there are many different types of biopsy.

A biopsy may be done through sputum cytology, the microscopic examination of cells coughed up from the lungs or the bronchial tubes (the air passages from the windpipe to the lungs). While it can't show a tumor's location, sputum cytology can determine if the cells are cancerous and, if so, the type of lung cancer present.

Bronchoscopy is a procedure where a tube with lighting and a magnifying device is inserted through the nostril or mouth into the bronchial tubes. While viewing abnormal areas through bronchoscopy, samples of tissue are taken and tumors are viewed for location and size.

Needle biopsy involves the insertion of a long, thin needle into the tumor to draw out a tissue sample for lab testing. A fluoroscope, an x-ray machine that projects images on a fluorescent screen, is used to guide the needle. Lymph node biopsy involves the surgical removal of lymph nodes in the neck if they are enlarged or abnormal, to check for the spread of cancer. Radionuclide scans show if cancer has spread to other areas of the body. A small amount of radioactive material that can be absorbed only by cancer cells is injected into the patient to highlight any abnormal areas. A scan can then provide an image of those areas.

Thoracotomy is exploratory surgery usually done if other tests are negative but there is still concern that cancer is present.

Treatment

As with many cancers, surgery, radiation, and chemotherapy are used to treat lung cancer. Depending on the size and location of the tumor, part or all of the lung will be removed during surgery. Tissue from around the tumor will be removed and examined for cancer cells. For the first few days after surgery, patients usually need a machine to aid breathing. Physical activity may be limited after surgery, depending on the amount of lung removed and overall health. Many patients undergo rehabilitation following surgery. In addition, support groups are available for survivors of lung cancer. Contact the American Lung Association or the American Cancer Society for more information.

Following surgery, radiation therapy can be used to attack any remaining cancer cells. Radiation therapy also may be used instead of surgery, when it is not a viable option, to destroy cells and relieve pain and other symptoms. The side effects of radiation include exhaustion (which subsides about a week after that last treatment), dry or sore throat, and scarring of the lungs.

Chemotherapy, the injection of cancer-killing drugs into the system, can also be used. According to the American Cancer Society, chemotherapy has increased survival rates for about 70 percent of patients with small cell lung cancer. For other types of lung cancer, chemotherapy is used when the cancer cannot be controlled by surgery or radiation. Side effects of chemotherapy include hair loss, nausea and vomiting, changes in blood count, and a feeling of tiredness.

For more information:

American Cancer Society
1599 Clifton Rd., N.E.
Atlanta, GA 30329-4251
800-ACS-2345
404-320-3333
http://www.cancer.org

American Lung Association
1740 Broadway, 14th Floor
New York, NY 10019-4374
800-LUNG-USA
212-315-8700
http://www.lungusa.org

National Cancer Institute
Cancer Information Service
9000 Rockville Pike
Bethesda, MD 20892
800-4-CANCER
800-638-1234 (Alaska)
800-524-1234 (Hawaii)
310-496-5583
http:/cancernet.nci.nih.gov

Office on Smoking and Health Hotline
Centers for Disease Control and Prevention
4770 Buford Hwy., N.E., Mailstop K-50
Atlanta, GA 30341-3724
800-CDC-1311 (recorded message)
770-488-5705
http://www.cdc.gov/tobacco

Smokenders
4455 E. Camelback Rd., Suite D150
Phoenix, AZ 85018
602-840-7414
smokenders@aol.com

Lymphoma

Lymphoma is a cancer that develops in the lymphatic system. According to the American Cancer Society, lymphoma is the fifth most common cancer in men, with 33,900 new cases in men reported in 1996.

Lymphoma occurs when cells in the lymphatic system, part of the body's immune system, grow abnormally and without control. (See Lymphatic System, p. 16.) There are two main types of lymphomas: non-Hodgkin's lymphoma and Hodgkin's disease. Though they have many of the same characteristics, these are two different conditions that are treated differently. The main developmental difference between Hodgkin's disease and non-Hodgkin's lymphoma is a distinct type of cell, called the Reed-Sternberg cell, which appears only in Hodgkin's lymphoma.

Hodgkin's disease is more likely to develop and spread predictably than non-Hodgkin's lymphoma, making it easier to cure. Non-Hodgkin's lymphoma more often develops outside the lymph nodes in organs such as the bones and the liver and may grow rapidly.

Non-Hodgkin's Lymphoma

According to the American Cancer Society, an estimated 52,700 new cases of non-Hodgkin's lymphoma were reported in the United States in 1996; of those, 29,900 were in men. In addition, since the 1970s, the incidence rates have increased approximately 75 percent. The rise can be attributed to an increase in cases of HIV, which is associated with non-Hodgkin's lymphoma, and increases in levels of chemicals and pollution.

There are at least ten types of non-Hodgkin's lymphomas. They are usually grouped according to how fast they grow: low grade (slow growing), intermediate grade, and high grade (rapidly growing). Survival rates reported for lymphomas vary widely, according to the stage of the lymphoma and the type of cancer cells present. The American Cancer Society reports that the overall five-year survival rate for non-Hodgkin's lymphoma is 51 percent.

Hodgkin's Disease

Hodgkin's disease is relatively rare. It accounts for less than 1 percent of all cancer cases in the United States, according to the National Cancer Institute. It most often affects young people between the ages of 15 and 34 and people over the age of 55. The American Cancer Society reports there were an estimated 7,500 new cases of Hodgkin's disease in the United States in 1996; 4,000 of those were men. Unlike non-Hodgkin's lymphoma, the incidence rates for the disease have declined since the 1970s, especially among the elderly. The survival rates for this disease, as with non-Hodgkin's lymphoma, vary widely. The American Cancer Society reports that the overall five-year survival rate for Hodgkin's disease is 80 percent.

Risk Factors

The risk factors for non-Hodgkin's lymphoma and Hodgkin's disease are similar. In fact, no one is sure what causes lymphoma. Men are slightly more likely than women to get lymphoma, which rarely occurs in people under the age of 44. It is known that the condition, in part, involves reduced immune functions and exposure to certain infectious agents. It's suspected that occupational exposure to herbicides and other chemicals increases the risk of contracting lymphoma.

Persons who undergo organ transplants are at higher risk due to an altered immune function. In addition, those who are infected with human immunodeficiency virus (HIV) and HTLV-1 (human T-cell leukemia/lymphoma virus-1) are at higher risk of contracting lymphoma. This happens because HIV attacks and destroys the immune system, leaving the individual with AIDS vulnerable to infections and certain cancers. Most AIDS-related lymphomas are non-Hodgkin's lymphoma, but according to the American Cancer Society, Hodgkin's disease cases have also been reported.

Symptoms

Again, the symptoms of non-Hodgkin's lymphoma and Hodgkin's disease are similar. A painless swelling in the lymph nodes located in the neck, groin, or underarm is the most common symptom of lymphoma. Other signs of the disease include fever, fatigue, weight loss, night sweats, itching, and reddened patches on the skin. There may be nausea, vomiting, or abdominal pain. If the condition has progressed, there will be evidence of a weakened immune system—the body will no longer be able to fight off infections.

It's important to note that these symptoms are also commonly caused by the flu or other infections. However, if these symptoms last longer than two weeks, see a doctor. Early detection of lymphoma increases the chance for a cure.

Diagnosis

A blood test and x-rays of the chest will generally be the first step in diagnosing lymphoma. Lymphangiography, in which a contrast dye is injected into the lymph vessels to highlight the lymphatic system, may also be done. If cancer is suspected, it can be definitively diagnosed through a lymph node biopsy. During this procedure, tissue from an enlarged lymph node is surgically removed and examined. A pathologist, an expert in the diagnosis of tissues, examines the specimen to tell if the cells are cancerous. The pathologist will also check for the presence of the Reed-Sternberg cell, which would indicate Hodgkin's disease rather than non-Hodgkin's lymphoma.

If cancer is diagnosed, an examination is done to find evidence of how far it has spread in order to determine its proper treatment. A doctor will again conduct a physical exam, order blood tests, x-rays (including a chest x-ray), and possibly, another biopsy. A computerized tomography (CT), a three-dimensional x-ray, may be done to see if the disease has spread to the chest, pelvic, or abdominal regions. Lymphangiography can also help determine the extent of a cancer.

A gallium scan, a form of radionuclide scanning, can also be prescribed. During this procedure, the patient drinks a liquid containing traces of radioactive gallium, a metal that is absorbed by the body after several days. Using a special "gamma camera" that emits minute bursts of light (photons), doctors can essentially view a map of the body, seeing how well each organ absorbed the gallium and whether there are tumors present.

A cancer specialist may also order a bone scan, in which a machine generates a picture of the bones so doctors can determine if they are affected by cancer. A bone marrow biopsy is another test used to determine how far the cancer has spread. During this test, a long, strong needle punctures the bone and extracts marrow samples for analysis. A pathologist then determines whether cancer cells are present.

Treatment

The type of treatment used depends on the type of cells present, the cancer's location in the body and its stage and the age and overall health of the patient. The methods of treating lymphomas can be complex. Hodgkin's disease, though rare, is more predictable in its growth and is therefore treated differently from non-Hodgkin's lymphoma, which develops less predictably.

For both types of cancer, the main components of treatment are radiation therapy and chemotherapy. Rarely, surgery is used to remove tissue, a gland, or an organ affected by the cancerous cells. If surgery is performed, it will usually be followed by radiation or chemotherapy to kill any remaining cells.

More recently, bone marrow transplantation has begun to be used in those with recurrent or especially aggressive lymphoma. This procedure, which is no longer considered experimental, allows a person to withstand unusually high doses of chemotherapy or radiation by removing and storing bone marrow—the tissue that creates new blood cells—and replacing it after the treatment is completed. In this way, the bone marrow that would otherwise be destroyed by chemotherapy or radiation is preserved to create new cells to bolster the immune system. Bone marrow transplantation is a complex, expensive treatment, however, and should only be done by a hospital or center with experience in the procedure. Be aware, also, that many health insurers do not cover the cost (usually more than $100,000) of bone marrow transplants.

For more information:

American Cancer Society
1599 Clifton Rd., N.E.
Atlanta, GA 30329-4251
800-ACS-2345
404-320-3333
http://www.cancer.org

Leukemia Society of America
600 Third Ave.
New York, NY 10016
800-955-4LSA
212-573-8484
http://www.leukemia.org

Lymphoma Research Foundation of America, Inc.
8800 Venice Blvd., Suite 207
Los Angeles, CA 90034
310-204-7040

National Cancer Institute
Cancer Information Service
9000 Rockville Pike
Bethesda, MD 20892
800-4-CANCER
800-638-1234 (Alaska)
800-524-1234 (Hawaii)
310-496-5583
http://cancernet.nci.nih.gov

Oral Cancer

Cancer can appear in any part of the oral cavity, the area that includes the lip, tongue, mouth, and throat. It is more than twice as common in men as in women, and it occurs most often after age 40, though it can develop at any age. The most frequent cause of oral cancer is tobacco use—smoking, chewing tobacco, and dipping snuff (keeping fine, powdered tobacco tucked under the lip or tongue).

The American Cancer Society estimates that there were 29,490 new cases of oral cancer in 1996—with 20,100 of them in men. Some 8,260 men died from the disease in the same year. Of those who are diagnosed with oral cancer, 81 percent will live for more than one year after diagnosis. The five-year survival rate is 52 percent, and the ten-year rate is 41 percent.

Risk Factors

According to the National Cancer Institute, tobacco use accounts for 80 to 90 percent of oral cancers. Smokers are four to fifteen times more likely to develop oral cancer than nonsmokers. Studies have indicated that smokeless tobacco users are at particular risk, which increases significantly for long-time dippers or chewers. People who stop using tobacco, even long-time

---

PREVENTING ORAL CANCER

When most people think of the health risks of smoking and drinking, they think of lung cancer or a liver disease such as cirrhosis. But oral cancer can be just as serious—sometimes resulting in the loss of areas of the mouth or teeth, or even death. To help prevent oral cancer:

- Stop smoking and using tobacco products. You may think you're avoiding the risks of lung cancer by chewing tobacco or dipping snuff, but you're still at high risk of oral cancer. But even smoking a pipe can increase the risk for lip cancer. While quitting tobacco can be difficult, people who quit can greatly reduce their risk—even if they have been long-time users. Check your phone book for local organizations to help you quit using tobacco or contact the American Cancer Society or the National Cancer Institute for a referral to a group in your area. (See "Smoking" for tips on how to quit.)

- Drink moderately. Heavy drinking can increase the risk of oral cancer and greatly multiply the risk of someone who smokes.

- Protect your lips. The sun's ultraviolet rays can cause lip cancer, so keep your lips covered with a lip balm that contains sunscreen with a skin protection factor (SPF) of at least 15. You may also want to wear a hat with a brim to shade your face.

- Have regular checkups. A doctor or dentist should examine the mouth for changes in the color of the lips, gums, tongue, or inner cheeks, and for scabs, cracks, sores, white patches, swelling, or bleeding. Oral exams are especially important for people over age 50 and for those who use alcohol or tobacco products.

users, can greatly reduce their risk of developing oral cancer.

Another cause of oral cancer is excessive consumption of alcohol. In fact, those who drink heavily but don't smoke may have a higher risk than people who do smoke. In addition, the risk for developing oral cancer is multiplied for people who use both alcohol and tobacco, because scientists believe the two substances increase each other's harmful effects. One source estimates the risk to be more than thirty-five times that of someone who neither drinks nor smokes.

Lip cancer may be caused by exposure to the sun's ultraviolet rays, and certain nutritional deficiencies—a lack of vitamins B and A, for example—have also been linked to oral cancer. Another possible cause is poorly fitting dentures and bridges, as well as sharp or broken teeth, that chronically irritate or infect the gums.

Studies show that oral cancer sometimes develops in people who have a history of leukoplakia, the presence of whitish patches inside the mouth, or erythroplakia, red velvety patches inside the mouth. Because cancer may develop in these otherwise harmless patches, monitoring is necessary if they occur.

Symptoms

Once a month, examine your mouth (cheeks, gums, tongue, lips, and mouth lining) by looking in a mirror. Check for any of the following changes or symptoms:

- A sore that bleeds easily and doesn't heal

- A lump or thickening

- A red or white patch that persists

- Soreness or a feeling that something is caught in the throat

- Difficulty chewing or swallowing

- Difficulty moving the tongue or jaws

- Numbness of the tongue or other area of the mouth

- Swelling of the jaw that causes dentures to fit poorly or uncomfortably

Although these symptoms may be caused by less serious problems, it is important to see a dentist or doctor if any persist more than two weeks.

Diagnosis

Diagnosis usually begins with an examination of the mouth by a doctor or a dentist, and x-rays may be done. If an abnormal area is found, tissue is collected for microscopic examination in a procedure called a biopsy to determine if it is cancer—a biopsy is the only definitive test for oral cancer. A doctor, often an oral surgeon that specializes in surgery of the mouth, removes part or all of the abnormal area, and a pathologist, a specialist in the examination of tissue, looks for cancer cells in the tissue. If cancer is present, further tests may be done to find out whether the cancer has spread to other parts of the body.

Treatment

Treatment for oral cancer depends on several factors, including the location, size, type, and extent of the tumor; the stage of the disease; and the patient's age and overall health.

The principal method of treatment for oral cancer is surgical removal of the affected area, followed by radiation therapy to destroy any remaining cells. Chemotherapy and hyperthermia, which uses a special machine to heat the body for a certain period of time to kill heat-sensitive cancer cells, are now being tested as additional alternative treatments for oral cancer patients. Patients are usually advised to have any needed dental work done before treatment for oral cancer begins, since treatment can make the mouth more sensitive and susceptible to infection.

As with other cancers, treatment for oral cancer can cause unpleasant side effects. These depend on the type and extent of the treatment, the specific area being treated and each individual's reaction to the treatment. Some side effects are temporary, and some are permanent. Surgery to remove a large tumor inside the mouth may require partial removal of the palate, tongue, or jaw, alterations which could change the person's ability to chew, swallow, or talk, and which might change appearance. Radiation therapy often makes the mouth sore and dry, making it hard to chew and swallow. Weight loss can be a serious problem for people undergoing oral cancer treatment, because eating is often difficult. Many patients will not be able to wear dentures during radiation therapy and up to a year after treatment. Be sure to talk with your practitioner before treatment about any possible effects.

Rehabilitation options for patients who have been treated for oral cancer include dietary counseling, surgery, a dental prosthesis, speech therapy, and other services. Some patients need reconstructive and plastic surgery to rebuild the bones or tissues of the mouth. Patients fitted with a prosthesis may need special training to use the device.

For more information:

American Association of Oral and Maxillofacial Surgeons
9700 Bryn Mawr Ave.
Rosemont, IL 60018
800-467-5268

American Cancer Society
1599 Clifton Rd., N.E.
Atlanta, GA 30329-4251
800-ACS-2345
404-320-3333
http://www.cancer.org

National Cancer Institute
Cancer Information Service
9000 Rockville Pike
Bethesda, MD 20892
800-4-CANCER
800-638-1234 (Alaska)
800-524-1234 (Hawaii)
301-496-5583
http://cancernet.nic.nih.gov

National Institute of Dental Research
31 Center Dr., MSC2190
Building 31, Room 5B49
9000 Rockville Pike
Bethesda, MD 20892-2190
http://www.nidr.nih.gov

Support for People With Oral and Head and Neck Cancer, Inc.
P.O. Box 53
Locust Valley, NY 11560-0053
516-759-5333
http:www.spohnc.org

Penile Cancer

Penile cancer is the growth of cancerous cells on the skin and tissues of the penis. Penile cancer is rare in the United States, but some 25 percent of the men who get this disease die from it. Approximately one thousand cases are reported each year in the United States, which accounts for less than .02 percent of all male cancers in the country.

Most penile cancer affects the glans (the tip of the penis) or the foreskin (the fold of skin that covers the glans). Because such cancers tend to be slow growing, the penis can be preserved in most cases where the cancer is diagnosed early.

Risk Factors

Penile cancer is most common in elderly men and African Americans, and the rate of incidence increases steadily after age 55.

Some believe that lack of circumcision, removal of the foreskin, is a risk factor for penile cancer possibly because of hygienic factors. The belief is that if the penis is not kept clean, smegma, a buildup of mucus and other secretions, can collect under the foreskin and cause irritation and inflammation of the glans and contribute to the development cancer. Almost all cases of penile cancer occur in men who are not circumcised at birth, and areas of the world where circumcision is uncommon have higher rates than countries where boys are regularly circumcised. However, studies have shown that cleanliness is a factor in penile cancer because in Sweden, where circumcision is rare but cleanliness is high, there are few cases of penile cancer. (See Circumcision, p. 419.)

The risk of penile cancer is higher for smokers than for nonsmokers, with the risk increasing sharply even if only ten cigarettes a day are smoked. Some experts theorize that carcinogens from the smoke may be present in smegma, triggering the growth of abnormal cells.

Studies suggest that the human papilloma virus (HPV) may be responsible for a small percentage of penile cancer cases. HPV, a sexually transmitted virus, can cause penile cellular changes that, left untreated, may lead to cancer. HPV can cause genital warts, though it has no symptoms in many cases.

Symptoms

Symptoms include a red spot, crust, wartlike growth, or sore on the penis, unusual liquid coming from the penis (abnormal discharge), pain, a lump in the groin, or bleeding during erection or intercourse. These may also be symptoms of a sexually transmitted disease. If any of these signs are present, visit a practitioner for an examination.

Diagnosis

Because the penis is easily accessible, diagnosis is usually straightforward, beginning with an examination of the penis. To definitively diagnose cancer, a small sample of tissue from the affected area of the penis is taken in a procedure called a biopsy, and the cells are examined under a microscope. If cancer of the penis is found, more tests will be done to see if the cancer has spread to other parts of the body. One such test is a needle aspiration, in which a needle is used to draw fluid out of a lymph node (a gland that is part of the immune system) in the groin area. The fluid is then examined to see if the cancer has infected the lymph nodes. In another test, lymphangiography, a special dye is injected that is absorbed into the lymphatic system. A scan is then done that creates images of the areas affected by the dye.

Treatment

The most common treatment for all stages of penile cancer is surgery. The cancer is removed surgically using one of several methods.

1. *Wide local excision.* The cancer and some normal tissue on either side of the abnormal area are surgically removed.

2. *Microsurgery.* The cancerous area, but little normal tissue, is removed. To do this, the doctor removes the cells while looking through a microscope.

3. *Laser surgery.* The cancerous area is destroyed using a narrow, concentrated beam of light.

4. *Penectomy.* The penis is partially or totally amputated. While it is the most drastic, amputation is the most common and most effective treatment for penile cancer. Lymph nodes may be taken during this procedure, too. In partial penectomy, part of the penis is removed. Some patients remain capable of erection, orgasm, and ejaculation. In total penectomy, the entire penis is taken. This leaves patients significantly impaired sexually, but stimulation of the remaining genital tissue, including the mons pubis, the perineum, and the scrotum, can produce orgasm for some.

Other treatments include radiation therapy and chemotherapy. Radiation therapy may be used to kill cancer cells and shrink tumors with x-rays or other high-energy rays. Radiation may be used alone or after surgery to kill any remaining cells. Chemotherapy uses drugs to kill cancer cells. For very small surface cancers, fluorouracil cream—a chemotherapy drug—is put on the skin of the penis. Other chemotherapy treatments are given by pill or by injection and travel through the body to kill cancer cells outside the penis. Again, it may be used alone or after surgery.

Biological therapy may also be used to treat penile cancer. It involves the injection of a substance into the body—for example, the protein interferon—to enhance the body's natural defenses against cancer. It is a relatively new form of treatment, and it is still experimental.

For more information:

American Cancer Society
1599 Clifton Rd., N.E.
Atlanta, GA 30329-4251
800-ACS-2345
404-320-3333
http://www.cancer.org

Biological Therapy Institute Foundation
P.O. Box 681700
Franklin, TN 37068-1700
615-790-7535

National Cancer Institute
Cancer Information Service
9000 Rockville Pike
Bethesda, MD 20892
800-4-CANCER
800-638-1234 (Alaska)
800-524-1234 (Hawaii)
301-496-5583
http://cancernet.nic.nih.gov

Prostate Cancer

Prostate cancer, the rapid growth of abnormal cells in the prostate gland, is the second leading cancer killer of men after lung cancer. Approximately 317,000 men are diagnosed with the disease annually in the United States, and 41,400 men die each year. The number of newly diagnosed cases rises each year, possibly because heightened awareness of the disease and better diagnostic methods are better able to identify men with the condition.

The prostate gland is part of the male reproductive system. It is about the size of a walnut and is located near the rectum just below the bladder. The gland surrounds the urethra, the tube that allows urine and semen to pass out of

PREVENTING PROSTATE CANCER

To help prevent prostate cancer:

- Eat vegetables. Studies show that people who consume more vegetables are also less likely to develop prostate cancer. Beta-carotene, which is found in green leafy vegetables such as spinach and broccoli, has been noted as a possible factor in lowering cancer risk.

- Fill up on tomatoes. Recent research shows the risk of prostate cancer is dramatically reduced in men who eat ten or more servings of tomato products a week. Experts believe that lycopene, the substance that gives tomatoes their red color, has a positive effect on the prevention of prostate cancer. Tomato sauce, tomatoes, and pizza were at the top of the list. Strawberries and guava also contain lycopene.

- Maintain a healthy weight. Men who are overweight have a higher risk of prostate cancer.

- Eat less fat. Studies have linked a high intake of saturated fat with an increased risk of prostate cancer. And cutting back on fat can also help you stay in a healthy weight range, which further reduces risk. Another bonus: Researchers say a lower fat intake may help to prevent the spread of cancer in those who already have the disease.

- Get enough vitamin E. Researchers say that vitamin E can reduce risk by 34 percent. It can be found in eggs, whole-grain cereals, wheat germ, sunflower oil, and almond oil. The recommended dietary allowance is 15 I.U. (international units) for men.

the body. The major function of the prostate is the production of prostatic fluid, which becomes part of semen.

Though in some cases prostate cancer may develop quickly, it usually grows very slowly, making it easy to treat and cure. (In fact, in some men it may grow so slowly that no treatment may be required.) Fifty-seven percent of all prostate cancers are discovered in their earliest stages, a time when the five-year survival rate is 98 percent. The survival rate for all stages of prostate cancer combined is 85 percent, a rate that decreases beyond five years after diagnosis. Some 61 percent of men diagnosed survive ten years, while 49 percent survive fifteen years.

Risk Factors

African-American men are more likely to get prostate cancer than other men; the American Cancer Society reports incidence rates are 37 percent higher for African Americans than for white men. Studies have also shown that men living in Europe and North America have higher rates of prostate cancer than men in other parts of the world. The incidence of cancer also increases with age, meaning risk increases as you grow older. Around 80 percent of those diagnosed with prostate cancer are over 65.

Another group at risk are those with a family history of the disease. Recently, research has incorporated genetics into the picture as scientists look for a possible gene or genetic link that might trigger the onset of cancer.

Diet and nutrition might also play a role in the development of prostate cancer. Specifically, studies have linked fat consumption to higher incidences of prostate cancer. This may account for the higher overall rates found in North America in relation to other parts of the world where fatty acid consumption accounts for a smaller portion of a person's diet.

Symptoms

In the early stages there are no outward symptoms. As the disease progresses, the major symptoms include problems with urination such as difficulty in starting and stopping the flow, frequent nighttime visits to the bathroom, a weak urine flow, or blood in the urine. These symptoms are similar to those of a condition called benign prostatic enlargement (BPH), or enlarged prostate. (See Prostate Disease, p. 333.) However, while in BPH these symptoms develop gradually, the onset is usually rapid if the cause is cancer. Additional symptoms of prostate cancer include painful ejaculation and lower back, pelvis, and thigh pain. If any of these symptoms occur, it's necessary to see a family physician for further testing to determine the trouble.

Diagnosis

Because of the initially slow progression of the disease, prostate cancer often goes undetected for a long time before it is found and diagnosed. Many times it is discovered by accident while screening for another condition. The two most common tests used to screen for prostate cancer are the digital rectal examination (DRE) and the prostate-specific antigen (PSA) test.

In a digital rectal examination (DRE), a doctor inserts a gloved, lubricated finger into the rectum to examine the prostate for lumps or other abnormalities. A DRE does not diagnose cancer per se; it is used only to locate abnormalities that may be cancerous. While the DRE is the standard test for prostate cancer, studies show that the DRE may not be effective in catching cancer before it spreads. Often, tumors in their early stages are too small to be felt or are located in the back of the gland where the physician cannot feel them. Nonetheless, the American Cancer Society recommends that all men over the age of 40 have a DRE as part of their yearly physical.

The prostate-specific antigen (PSA) test is a simple blood test that works by measuring levels of a protein called prostate-specific antigen, generated by the prostate gland. This enzyme is produced by both the normal cells and any cancerous cells. However, cancerous cells produce higher amounts of PSA than the normal cells; therefore, higher PSA levels may indicate cancer. Similarly, an enlarged prostate gland also produces more PSA.

Like DRE, the PSA test does not definitively diagnose cancer, it only indicates that it may be present. Only a biopsy—a procedure that collects tissue for examination—can confirm or rule out cancer. The PSA test is also used to monitor the growth of prostate cancer after diagnosis.

The test measures PSA levels in nanograms per milliliter. Currently, a level below 4 ng/ml is considered normal, while a level between 4 and 10 ng/ml is considered an elevated level. A level higher than 10 ng/ml is a strong indication of cancer. However, because acceptable PSA levels increase with age, some experts believe the standard should be adjusted according to the age of the patient. Evidence also shows that African-American men tend to have higher PSA levels. One study in the *New England Journal of*

Medicine that takes into account these factors suggests a level of 2.0 for men in their 40s; 4.0 for men in their 50s; 4.5 for men in their 60s; and 5.5 for men in their 70s.

Another test, the transrectal ultrasound, is also done to screen for cancer. This test, which uses sound waves to create an image of the prostate gland, is not considered to be extremely reliable, too often producing high numbers of positive results when there is no cancer present.

If a screening test alludes to a problem, other tests are done to confirm the diagnosis. These include blood work, x-rays, and imaging tests such as a computerized tomography (CT) scan, which creates a three-dimensional x-ray of the region, or an magnetic resonance imaging (MRI) scan, which uses magnetic waves to create an image of tissue. To confirm the presence of cancer, a biopsy, a procedure in which a tissue sample is removed for analysis, must be done.

A biopsy can be done without anesthesia. One method uses a spring-loaded device (a "gun") that is inserted through the rectum and guided by ultrasound. The device uses a fine needle to collect a tissue sample; the "gun" works so quickly that it can barely be felt. A fine, thin needle can also inserted through the rectum to aspirate, or suction, cells out of the prostate for examination. Biopsies are safe, though they carry a small risk of infection. Once the biopsy is done, the collected cells are examined to determine if cancer is present, and if it is, how far it has progressed.

Treatment

The type of treatment received depends upon the severity of the cancer as well as other factors such as age, risk of the treatments, quality of life issues, and present health. Nontreatment is also an important option to consider.

Surgery. The radical prostatectomy, done when the cancer is confined to the prostate gland, is a surgical procedure that entails removing the prostate gland and seminal vesicles (two structures located underneath the bladder that contribute to the production of semen) to eradicate the cancer. The surgery is considered very successful in treating cancer and has a ten-year survival rate of 77 percent for larger tumors and 94 percent for smaller tumors. However, in some cases additional surgery or treatment may be needed after surgery especially if the cancer has spread beyond the prostate at the time of treatment.

Prostatectomy is a serious surgery that carries a risk of infection, injury to the bladder (which may result in urinary incontinence), and erection problems, though refinements in surgical methods that spare crucial nerves have limited the chance of complications. The risk of impotence is estimated to be 30 percent, though some estimates go as high as 50 percent. In addition, several studies have found that about 40 percent of men who have had prostatectomy have urinary incontinence, though this figure varies as well.

Radical prostatectomy is usually not recommended for men over age 70 because it is not proven to add any years to life and because there may be serious side effects. Prostatectomy is usually not used once the cancer has spread beyond the prostate gland.

Radiation Therapy. Radiation therapy is another method for attacking prostate cancer. It may be used by itself to treat small cancers or cancers that have spread beyond the gland. It may also be used to supplement radical prostatectomy, killing any cells that may have been left behind after the procedure. Types of radiation treatment include external beam radiotherapy and brachytherapy. External beam radiotherapy is administered by a machine that directs the

THE CONTROVERSY OVER PSA TESTING

There are many questions about the accuracy—and the value—of the PSA test. Experts agree that the PSA test is more accurate than the DRE, mainly because it can detect cancers before they can be felt. However, the PSA test is very sensitive and often gives false-positive or false-negative results. Also, some believe it may push people toward treatment they don't really need.

A false-positive result is when the test indicates cancer, when in fact there is no disease. Research shows that only one-third of those with high PSA levels will eventually be diagnosed as having prostate cancer. In other words, the false-positive rate can be as high as 66 percent. With a false-negative result, the test reports there is no sign of cancer when cancer is actually present. Studies show that 20 to 40 percent of men with prostate cancer have normal PSA levels.

Many factors other than cancer are thought to affect PSA levels—so many, in fact, that the test loses much of its reliability. These include the presence of other conditions such as BPH and prostatitis, the timing of rectal exams, and the sites of biopsies. Other factors such as prostate stones, prostate trauma, hormone levels, and urinary infections also alter PSA readings. Different types of cancer cells may trigger different levels of PSA. Even a patient's age has been linked to changes in PSA levels: As a man grows older, the amount of PSA produced appears to rise. Certain medications may also affect the PSA test. For example, evidence shows that finasteride (Proscar), a drug used to treat BPH, tends to artificially lower PSA amounts.

Experts also question the value of the PSA test, even when it's correct. Because prostate cancer is so often slow-growing, it often does not require treatment, which in itself may carry health risks. Some fear that such early detection of the cancer will lead men to choose unnecessary treatment when it may do more harm than good. In addition, there's no evidence that treatment saves lives: Some studies show that men who receive aggressive treatment for prostate cancer live just as long as those who do not.

Because of the controversy surrounding PSA, recommendations on when and how often to have the test vary. The American Cancer Society and the American Urological Association recommend that all men over the age of 50 have a PSA test each year and that men at risk of the disease should have the test annually after age 40. The U.S. Preventive Services Task Force, the American Academy of Family Practitioners, and the American College of Physicians recommend against routine testing and suggest that men talk with their doctors about the risks and benefits of the test. The National Cancer Institute has no recommendation—it's holding out until more evidence is available.

What this means is that the choice is yours. For example, if you fall into one of the groups at high risk of prostate cancer, screening may be to your advantage. Be sure your test is accompanied by a DRE to help avoid a false-negative diagnosis (but have the blood drawn first, as the DRE might interfere with PSA levels). You'll also want to abstain from ejaculating for twenty-four to forty-eight hours before a PSA test, since this may affect the results. And if you have high PSA levels, remember that they do not necessarily mean cancer—seek a second opinion before going ahead with any treatment or invasive diagnostic procedure.

x-rays to the area of treatment. Brachytherapy is done by implanting radioactive "seeds" or pellets inside a patient where they emit radiation for approximately one year. There is no evidence that use of seeds is any safer or more effective than traditional external beam radiotherapy.

Some of the side effects from these treatments include rectal problems and urinary troubles. In addition, there is also a risk of impotence—some experts believe the risk is similar to that of surgery; others believe radiation therapy is safer. Chemotherapy has not proven useful in treating prostate cancer.

Hormonal Therapy. In certain instances, hormonal therapy may be used to prohibit the production of testosterone, the hormone that feeds the cancer. This can be done by injecting medications or hormones into the system or by removing the testicles. In many cases, the tumor growth slows or even shrinks in size; however, in others, the treatment has little effect and the cancer begins to spread again. This method is used in men with advanced cancers who can't have surgery or radiation. Side effects resulting from the hormonal changes include erection problems, tender breasts, and hot flashes.

PROSTATE CANCER TREATMENT: CHOOSING WHAT'S RIGHT FOR YOU

There are a variety of treatments for prostate cancer—including nontreatment—and there are numerous serious, often permanent side effects that go along with some of them. Weighing the pros and cons of a particular option can be difficult. It may be a choice between putting off treatment and letting the cancer grow and undergoing major surgery that carries a risk of impotence and incontinence. To help find out what the right choice is for you:

- Get the facts. Once you've been diagnosed with prostate cancer, talk at length with your physician and do some research of your own into your condition. The more you know about the condition, the more you can participate in your care and make the best choices.

- Find out the statistics. Ask your doctor for specifics about the risk of side effects such as erection problems and incontinence. If you're undergoing a procedure or diagnostic test, you're entitled to know all of its drawbacks as well as its benefits—this disclosure is known as informed consent. If you don't feel you know enough, don't go through with the procedure until you're satisfied.

- Evaluate yourself. Consider what's important to you and how you will react to the treatment option and any side effects. For example, one man may be more willing to risk side effects to become cancer free, whereas another may not want to risk his quality of life to treat a condition that may never advance.

- Don't rush into it. Take the time you need to research your condition, evaluate therapies and get second or even third opinions from other doctors.

Other Options

There are a few other treatments sometimes used for prostate cancer. Cryosurgery (cryoablation) is a relatively new form of treatment—still considered experimental by most doctors—that involves using liquid nitrogen to freeze the cancer cells. It is used when cancer is contained exclusively within the prostate. An experimental drug, suramin, appears to be able to shrink prostate tumors; however, it does have powerful side effects. Biological therapies, which bolster the body's own defenses against cancer, are also sometimes used.

In addition, nontreatment, or watchful waiting—taking no action to treat the cancer—should be considered as an option. Because prostate cancer tend to grow slowly and because treatment often has serious side effects such as impotence, it may be worth holding off on treatment and simply monitoring the progress of the disease. Although 30 to 40 percent of men over the age of 50 have prostate cancer, evidence suggests that only 4 to 8 percent have cancer that is significant or requires treatment.

In addition, cancer cells appear to multiply at a slower rate in older men, and most men with prostate cancer die with the disease rather than because of it. Studies show that a man over 70 with early-stage prostate cancer usually has a good prognosis even if he receives no treatment, and the National Cancer Institute advises no treatment for men over age 70.

Be sure to talk with your practitioner about the possibility of nontreatment and get a second opinion before undergoing any treatment or procedure.

For more information:

American Cancer Society
1599 Clifton Road, N.E.
Atlanta, GA 30329-4251
800-ACS-2345
404-320-3333
http://www.cancer.org

American Foundation for Urologic Disease
1128 N. Charles St.
Baltimore, MD 21201
800-242-2383
410-468-1800
http://www.acess.digex.net.-afud.org

Mathews Foundation for Prostate Cancer Research
817 Commons Dr.
Sacramento, CA 95825
800-234-6284
916-567-1400
mathews@sna.com

National Cancer Institute
Cancer Information Service
9000 Rockville Pike
Bethesda, MD 20892
800-4-CANCER
800-638-1234 (Alaska)
800-524-1234 (Hawaii)
301-496-5583
http://cancernet.nic.nih.gov

US TOO International, Inc.
930 N. York Rd., Suite 50
Hinsdale, IL 60521-2993
800-808-7866
630-323-1002
http://www.ustoo.com

Skin Cancer

As the largest organ of the body, skin protects the inner organs and tissues from bacteria and injury and regulates the body's temperature. The skin also plays an important role in the sense of touch. Cancer of the skin is the most common of all cancers, even though it can be prevented in most cases.

In 1996, according to the American Cancer Society, 21,800 men (and 16,500 women) were diagnosed with malignant melanoma, the most serious form of skin cancer. That same year, 4,600 men died of the same condition. In addition, there are more than 800,000 cases a year of basal cell and squamous cell skin cancers, two highly curable forms of skin cancer. While most skin cancers are easily cured, they can destroy skin and tissue and spread if untreated.

Types of Skin Cancer

Basal cell cancer accounts for about 75 percent of skin cancers. It typically develops on the face and ears in the layer of cells that forms the base of the skin, taking the form of a white or gray, raised, pearly nodule (a small, irregular mass) that may become an open sore. This type of skin cancer is slow growing and usually does not spread. But untreated, basal cell cancer can spread to nearby areas and invade the bone and other tissues beneath the skin.

Basal cell cancer, which grows within the deepest layers of the skin, can recur in the same place or develop anew elsewhere on the body. Within five years, 35 percent of patients diagnosed with one basal cell cancer will develop a second basal cell carcinoma.

Basal cell cancer was once considered a disease of the older generation, but it is being diagnosed more and more in younger people, possibly because tanning, outdoor activities, and styles of clothing that expose more skin have become more popular.

Squamous cell cancer accounts for about 20 percent of all skin cancers. These cancers arise from the epidermis—the topmost layer of the skin—and usually appear on sun-exposed areas like the face, ear, neck, and hand. They generally begin as small, round, painless lumps, or as flat, crusty, red areas, which may grow to resemble warts. They can also develop in lesions such as scars or open sores.

Squamous cell cancers usually are more aggressive than basal cell cancers. They likely will invade structures beneath the skin and are more likely to spread to other parts of the body, such as lymph nodes, bone, and tissues underneath the skin.

Malignant Melanoma is the most serious and most deadly skin cancer. While melanoma was once rare in this country, the incidence rate has increased about 4 percent per year since 1973 and doubles every decade. Incidence rates are more than forty times higher among whites than African Americans.

Melanoma starts in melanocytes cells, specialized skin cells that produce the pigment melanin. Normally, melanin—when exposed to sunlight—turns darker to produce a tan that helps protect the skin from burning.

Melanoma usually occurs where there is a mole, though it can appear anywhere on the body. The tumors most frequently appear on the chest, back, and abdomen, and are common in white men. While melanoma is rare in African Americans, it can occur on the palms, skin under the nails, and the soles of their feet. Melanoma may take the form of an eye tumor in older adults, affecting the choroid layer of the eye. Eye tumors usually have no symptoms and eventually result in detachment of the retina and deterioration of vision. Treatment involves destroying the tumor with laser surgery if it is small or removing the eye to prevent the cancer from spreading to the brain.

Melanoma is almost 100 percent curable if detected early. But while melanoma accounts for only 5 percent of skin cancers, it is responsible for 75 percent of the deaths. That's because melanoma is more likely than other forms of skin cancer to spread to other body parts such as bone or lymph nodes, making it difficult to cure. If the melanoma is diagnosed in an early stage, the five-year survival rate is 94 percent. However, once the cancer has spread to the surrounding regions, the rate drops to 60 percent. In cases where the cancer spreads to distant parts of the body, the survival rate is only 16 percent.

Risk Factors

Overexposure to the sun is the main cause of skin cancer. Fair-skinned people, especially those with red or blond hair, are most likely to get skin cancer because their cells have less melanin, meaning they sunburn more easily. Risk is very low among African Americans because of the amount of melanin present in the skin. Asian and Hispanic men are also less likely to get skin cancer than the general population.

Those who freckle and burn rather than tan are also at higher risk, as are people who live or vacation regularly in sunny places, especially those near the equator. Other risk factors include exposure to ultraviolet radiation through tanning beds and sun lamps; frequent exposure to ioniz-ing radiation from x-rays; occupational exposure to coal tar, pitch, creosote, arsenic compounds, or radium. Some forms of skin cancer are com-mon in members of the same family.

Men are slightly more likely than women to develop skin cancers, possibly because outdoor jobs with sun exposure, as well as industrial jobs with exposure to certain chemicals, are held by men more than by women. Participation in out-door sports such as golf and swimming may also increase the risk of skin cancer.

Symptoms

Any unusual skin changes, especially a change in the size or color of a mole or other darkly pigmented growth or spot, may be a sign of skin cancer and should be checked by a physician.

Symptoms of skin cancer include scaliness, oozing, bleeding, or change of the appearance of a bump or nodule, the spread of pigmenta-tion beyond its border, a change in sensation, itchiness, tenderness, or pain. Look for a pale, waxlike, pearly nodule, or a red, scaly, sharply outlined patch—these may be basal cell or squa-mous cell cancers.

Small, molelike growths that increase in size, change color, become open sores, and bleed eas-ily from a slight injury may be melanomas. The American Cancer Society suggests the "ABCD Rule" for identifying melanoma:

- A is for asymmetry. One-half of the mole does not match the other half.

- B is for border irregularity. The edges are ragged, notched, or blurred.

- C is for color. The pigmentation is not uniform.

- D is for diameter greater than 6 millimeters.

The American Cancer Society recommends monthly self-examinations for skin cancer. This involves checking the entire body, using a mirror, for any skin changes or symptoms. A dermatologist, a specialist who deals with the skin, may also be helpful in checking for cancer. Children should also be examined monthly.

Diagnosis

Diagnosis begins with an examination by a practitioner. If there is a suspicion of cancer, a biopsy (removal of a small sample of tissue) of the irregular area will be done, usually right in the practitioner's office. The sample is then sent to a laboratory and viewed under a microscope by a pathologist (an expert in the examination of tissues) for cancer cells. If abnormal cells are present, the pathologist will determine what type of cancer cells they are and how far the cancer has progressed.

Treatment

Treatment for skin cancer includes surgery in 90 percent of cases. Small lumps or abnormal areas may be removed in a practitioner's office. In the early stages of cancer, abnormal cells may also be removed through electrodessication (tissue destruction by heat), cryosurgery (tissue destruction by freezing), or laser therapy (tissue destruction using a concentrated light beam).

TIPS FOR PREVENTING SKIN CANCER

- Try to avoid the sun when its rays are strongest—between 10 A.M. and 3 P.M. Avoiding solar radiation between 11 A.M. and 1 P.M. can reduce your exposure by half. The National Cancer Institute's "shadow method" states that if your shadow is shorter than you are, stay indoors since this indicates the UV rays are at their strongest. Also remember that ultraviolet rays are still present on cloudy days.

- If you must be in the sun, wear clothing to cover as much of the skin as possible. Use a hat to protect the head and face. Wear sunglasses with UV protection.

- The American Academy of Dermatology and the Skin Cancer Foundation recommend that a sunscreen with a sun protection factor (SPF) of at least 15 be used on all bare areas when you are outside. SPF 15 screens out 93 percent of the sun's burning rays, plus using it correctly for the first eighteen years of life can lower a person's skin cancer risk by 80 percent. The higher the SPF number, the longer it will take you to burn. For example, a SPF 2 provides only 50 percent protection, while an SPF 34 offers 97 percent protection.

- Do not use sun lamps or go to tanning salons, because they intensify UV rays.

- Avoid sun when using medications containing Retin-A, tetracycline, sulfa drugs, thiazide diuretics, or indomethacin. These make your skin more sensitive to sunlight and more apt to burn.

- Conduct a monthly skin examination, using a mirror, to be aware of any changes in your skin. See your doctor immediately if you find a suspicious mole, growth, or lump on your skin, or if there has been a change in size, shape, or color of an existing mole.

Radiation therapy is often the first treatment for hard-to-reach cancers such as those around the eyes and nose. For basal cell or squamous cell cancer, radiation therapy may follow surgery to reduce the chance of spreading.

Another option is microscopically controlled surgery, where a thin slice of the cancer is removed and the bottom layer is examined for cancer cells. The process is repeated until a cancer-free layer is found.

For malignant melanoma, the growth and usually nearby lymph nodes are surgically removed. Chemotherapy may be used for additional treatment of melanoma, though it's not usually effective. Biological therapy, an experimental therapy that uses substances to boost the body's immune system, is also an option. Though biological therapy has not been widely used in the past, several studies have recently shown biological therapy with substances such as interferon and interleukin-2 to improve survival rates for those with high-risk melanoma. Biological therapy is most often used as an adjuvant, or supplemental, therapy.

Surgery for skin cancer may be followed by reconstructive surgery if necessary. Techniques to reconstruct skin include skin grafts, skin and muscle flaps, and tissue expansion. In a skin graft, skin is transplanted from another part of the body to the damaged area, where it grows to provide cover. A skin and muscle flap transplants a section of skin and tissue from one part of the body to another and preserves the blood supply. Flaps are used when there has been loss of deep tissue. Tissue expansion involves stretching the existing skin to cover a damaged area. These methods may be used along with implants or bone grafts to recreate underlying structures.

For more information:

American Cancer Society
1599 Clifton Rd., N.E.
Atlanta, GA 30329-4251
800-ACS-2345
404-320-3333
http://www.cancer.org

National Cancer Institute
Cancer Information Service
9000 Rockville Pike
Bethesda, MD 20892
800-4-CANCER
800-638-1234 (Alaska)
800-524-1234 (Hawaii)
301-496-5583
http://cancernet.nic.nih.gov

Skin Cancer Foundation
P.O. Box 561
New York, NY 10016
800-SKIN-490
212-725-5176
info@skincancer.org

Testicular Cancer

Testicular cancer is a growth of abnormal cells within a testicle. The testicles, also known as the testes, are the male sex glands. They are encased in the scrotum, a pouch of skin located behind the penis. The primary functions of the testicles are to produce and store sperm and to produce male sex hormones that control the development of the reproductive organs and other male characteristics such as body and facial hair and a deep voice.

Although it accounts for only 1 percent of all cancers in American men, testicular cancer is the most common cancer in men between the ages of 15 and 34. The American Cancer Society estimated that 7,400 new cases of testicular cancer occurred in the United States in 1996.

An estimated 370 men died of the disease in 1996, significantly fewer than the estimated 41,400 who died of prostate cancer. Testicular cancer is about four times more common in white men than in African-American men.

The two most common types of testicular cancer are seminomas and nonseminomas. Seminomas, which make up about 40 percent of all testicular cancer, are comprised of immature germ cells. They are slow-growing and are usually found before they spread beyond the testicle. Nonseminomas, which make up about 55 percent, grow more rapidly and may spread before they are discovered. According to the American Cancer Society, 60 to 70 percent of men with nonseminomas have cancer that has spread to nearby lymph nodes.

Testicular cancer is almost always curable if it is diagnosed and treated early. The key to early detection is regular testicular self-examination (TSE). Although no scientific studies have been done to determine the effectiveness of TSE in preventing deaths from testicular cancer, it is clear that TSEs do increase a man's chances of detecting what could be a malignant tumor in his testicles. The American Cancer Society recommends that a man have a testicular examination done by a practitioner every three years after age 20 and every year after age 40, in addition to frequent self-examination.

Risk

Experts do not know the exact cause of testicular cancer. The risk of testicular cancer is three to seventeen times higher than average for boys born with undescended testicles (a congenital condition known as cryptorchidism). The risk increases if the condition is not surgically corrected in early childhood.

Other, less common, conditions to which testicular cancer has been linked are Klinefelter's syndrome (a chromosomal disorder characterized by men with small testicles, enlarged breasts, and a lack of secondary sex characteristics such as beard growth and voice change); gonadal aplasia (failure of testicular development); and hermaphroditism (development of both male and female sex characteristics). Low birth weight may be another minor risk factor, as well as a mother's history of unusual bleeding or spotting during pregnancy or a mother's use of alcohol or sedatives or exposure to x-rays while pregnant. Some men with testicular cancer also have a history of injury to the scrotum; however, many doctors believe such an injury does not cause cancer but simply calls attention to an already-present tumor.

Symptoms

Most cases are discovered by the patients themselves, either unintentionally or by self-examination. Symptoms of testicular cancer include the following:

- A lump in either testicle
- Enlargement of a testicle
- A feeling of heaviness in the scrotum
- A dull ache in the lower abdomen or the groin area (where the thigh joins the abdomen)
- A sudden collection of fluid in the scrotum
- Pain or discomfort in a testicle or in the scrotum
- Enlargement or tenderness of the breasts

Men who notice any of these symptoms should see a doctor immediately.

Diagnosis

In addition to reporting his personal and family medical history and getting a complete physical checkup, including careful examination of the scrotum, a patient will most likely have a chest x-ray and blood and urine tests done. If the physical exam and lab tests do not show an infection or another disorder, a practitioner will probably suspect that cancer is present.

Most tumors in the testicles are malignant, or cancerous, but the only way to know for sure is to examine a sample of tissue under a microscope, a procedure called a biopsy. However, the tissue sample can be obtained only by removing the entire affected testicle through the groin, a surgical procedure called radical inguinal orchiectomy. Surgeons do not cut through the scrotum or remove just a part of the testicle because if cancer is present, cutting through the outer layer of the testicle might cause the cancer to spread to surrounding tissues and lymph nodes. Testicle removal also can halt further growth if a malignant tumor is present. Removal of one testicle does not interfere with fertility or the ability to have an erection.

Treatment

Treatment of testicular cancer depends on the stage and cell type (seminoma or nonseminoma) of the disease, as well as the patient's age and overall health.

Because they grow slowly, seminomas are usually diagnosed before they have spread and are extremely sensitive and responsive to radiation treatment. Radiation therapy directed to the lymph nodes can usually remove cancer cells there, making surgical removal of the lymph nodes unnecessary.

Chemotherapy is another treatment option. The chemotherapy drug Platinol (cisplatin) is considered by many experts to be the drug of choice for treating testicular cancer, and it is often used after surgery or radiation in combination with other chemotherapy drugs. Other drugs used include Ilex (ifosamide), Vepesid (etoposide), Velban (vinblastine sulfate), and Blenoxane (bleomycin sulfate).

Nonseminomas grow rapidly are not usually caught before they spread; however, the cure rate is still quite high. Surgical removal of the lymph nodes is often necessary after the cancer has spread beyond the testicle because nonseminomas do not respond as well to radiation therapy. Treatment of nonseminoma patients also can include chemotherapy with various drug combinations.

Each method of treatment has side effects that vary from person to person and even from one treatment to the next. Contrary to the worries of many men, the loss of one testicle will not affect a man's ability to engage in sexual intercourse and will not make him sterile. A man with one healthy testicle can have a normal erection and produce sperm. A man can also have an artificial testicle, a prosthesis, implanted into the scrotum for cosmetic purposes.

Regular follow-up examinations are important in order to be sure the cancer is completely gone. Testicular cancer seldom recurs after a patient has been cancer-free for three years. Men who have been treated for cancer in one testicle have about a 1 percent chance of developing cancer in the remaining one. If cancer does appear in the second testicle, it is almost always a new disease rather than a result of cells that have spread from the first tumor. As before,

TESTICULAR SELF-EXAMINATION

Most cases of testicular cancer can be caught in the early stages, when it is most curable, with routine testicular self-examination. All men—not just those at high risk—should perform a TSE at least once a month.

The best time for a TSE is immediately after a warm bath or shower because the skin of the scrotum is relaxed from the heat, making it easier for you to find anything unusual. TSE is a simple procedure that takes only a few minutes:

1. While standing in front of a mirror, look for any swelling on the surface of the scrotum.

2. Using both hands, examine each testicle by placing your index and middle fingers underneath the testicle and your thumbs on the top. Gently roll the testicle between the thumbs and fingers. It is normal for one testicle to be larger than the other.

3. Feel for any abnormal lumps, approximately the size of a pea, on the front or sides of the testicle. The lumps are usually painless. Do not confuse the epididymis (a cordlike structure on the top and back of the testicle that stores and transports the sperm) with an abnormal lump.

4. If you do find a lump, make an appointment with your doctor immediately. The lump may be an infection that requires treatment or may be cancer—only a doctor can make the diagnosis. Be sure to see your doctor regularly in addition to practicing routine TSE. Your doctor should examine your testicles during a checkup. He or she can also check the way you do TSE.

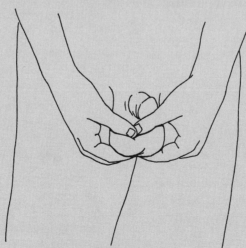

Testicular Self-Examination

Source: National Cancer Institute

patients should continue to do a testicular self-examination every month.

For more information:

American Cancer Society (ACS)
1599 Clifton Road, N.E.
Atlanta, GA 30329-4251
800-ACS-2345
404-320-3333
http://www.cancer.org

The National Cancer Institute
Office of Cancer Communications
Bethesda, MD 20892
800-4-CANCER
800-638-1234 (Alaska)
800-524-1234 (Hawaii)
310-496-5583
http://cancernet.nic.nih.gov

CHRONIC FATIGUE SYNDROME

Chronic fatigue syndrome (CFS) is a condition characterized by long-term, constant exhaustion and muscle pain. By definition, a syndrome is a collection of a number of symptoms rather than a specific disease. Because of the varying symptoms associated with CFS, this debilitating condition is often confused with a number of other conditions and is difficult to diagnose. It generally occurs suddenly, coming on over a few hours or a few days. An estimated 200 per 100,000 people are said to have the condition, which usually affects young adults, and women twice as often as men. It is also known as chronic fatigue immune dysfunction syndrome (CFIDS), and has also been called "yuppie flu," because of the myth that it occurs more often in young, upwardly mobile professionals.

Symptoms

Chronic fatigue syndrome is much more than a simple case of tiredness or lethargy. According to the Centers for Disease Control and Prevention, in order to be considered chronic fatigue syndrome, a condition must involve an unexplained, persistent, or recurring fatigue that has lasted for longer than six months. The fatigue interferes with daily activities, does not result from exertion, and does not improve with rest. In addition, four of the following symptoms must be present: impaired memory or concentration; recurrent sore throat; tender lymph nodes; muscle or joint pain; exceptional fatigue after usually tolerable exercise, which persists for more than twenty-four hours; severe headache; and unrefreshing sleep.

Minor symptoms include fever and chills, sudden mood changes, loss of appetite, cravings for strange foods, and visual problems.

Diagnosis

No tests can confirm the presence of chronic fatigue syndrome, and, in fact, many experts believe the problem to be psychological. For this reason, if you suspect you have CFS, you should find a practitioner who takes the condition seriously. You may want to get in touch with an organization or support group that deals with CFS; such a group may be able to provide a referral to a physician in your area.

To diagnose CFS, a practitioner must first rule out a number of other disorders, including HIV/AIDS, cancer, infections, fungal or parasitic disease, neuromuscular disease, mononucleosis, depression, and psychiatric problems. A person may also undergo tests such as a complete blood count (CBC), adrenal and thyroid function tests (which monitor the functions of hormone-producing glands), chest x-rays, or a urinalysis.

SELF-CARE FOR CHRONIC FATIGUE

Several lifestyle changes can be made to help reduce the debilitation caused by CFS. A person with CFS should do the following:

- Get plenty of bed rest, offset by a scheduled program of regular exercise. Activity helps alleviate the problems associated with fatigue.

- Eat a well-balanced diet. While specialized diets and vitamin regimens have not been proven effective in treating the syndrome, maintaining proper nutrition is important to keep energy levels up and to stay healthy. CFS sufferers may suffer loss of appetite or feel strong cravings for strange foods and often do not eat properly.

- Try complementary therapies. While there is no cure for CFS, acupuncture, Chinese medicine, homeopathy, and herbal therapies may provide relief from symptoms by raising energy levels, reducing stress, and alleviating headaches and muscle pain.

Blood may also be analyzed for the amounts of different substances such as alpha-interferon and lymphocytes that may indicate CFS.

CFS is difficult to diagnose mainly because its cause is unknown. At one time, CFS was thought to be associated with the Epstein-Barr virus, the herpes virus that causes infectious mononucleosis, and was known as chronic Epstein-Barr virus syndrome. Some believe CFS to be an autoimmune disease (a disease in which the body produces an immune response to attack its own tissues); others link it to fibromyalgia, an unexplained condition of muscle pain and disease. It has also been linked to Lyme disease, a tick-borne illness.

Treatment

Presently, no definitive drugs can cure or even alleviate the symptoms of CFS. Individual complaints, however, may be treated. For example, antidepressants may be prescribed for depression and analgesics for headaches. Some experimental drugs, such as the drug ampligen, are being developed for use against CFS.

While the condition cannot be cured, it does not get worse over time and often improves over the course of several years. Individuals affected by CFS live with the condition and often rearrange their lives around the limitations of CFS.

For more information:

Chronic Fatigue Immune Dysfunction Syndrome (CFIDS) Association
P.O. Box 220398
Charlotte, NC 28222-0398
800-442-3437

National Chronic Fatigue Syndrome and Fibromyalgia Association
P.O. Box 18426
Kansas City, MO 64133
816-931-4777

CIRRHOSIS

Cirrhosis is a disease of the liver caused by chronic damage to its cells that results in bands of fibrous scar tissue within the organ. These bands of damaged tissue result in impairment of the liver to perform its normal activities. When enough cells are damaged and the vital functions of the liver are significantly limited, death can result.

In the United States, according to the U.S. National Center for Health Statistics, approximately 16,500 men died in 1992 from causes directly related to chronic liver disease and cirrhosis. Men are twice as likely to die from cirrhosis than women.

Causes of Cirrhosis

Heavy alcohol consumption is the most common cause of cirrhosis in the Western world: Almost half of cirrhosis-caused deaths are associated with alcohol. The disease is linked to the amount rather than the type of alcohol consumed; people who drink at least eight to sixteen ounces of hard liquor—which is equivalent to 32 to 64 ounces of wine or 64 to 128 ounces of beer—daily for fifteen or more years will develop cirrhosis 30 percent of the time. The risk increases as the number of years of consumption goes up.

Viral liver disease is also a common cause of cirrhosis. Hepatitis B, an inflammation of the liver, which is mainly transmitted through sexual contact or sharing of IV needles, is the most common viral disease associated with cirrhosis.

Less common causes of cirrhosis include the following:

- *Inherited disorders or diseases of the bile ducts* (the network of ducts that carry bile—a liquid that transports waste products and helps to break up fats—from the liver to the gallbladder and on to the small intestine)

- *Hemochromatosis* (the abnormal accumulation of iron)

- *Wilson's disease* (accumulation of copper in the liver)

- *Cystic fibrosis,* in which the bile ducts become blocked

- *Heart failure that has led to long-term congestion of blood in the liver,* (cardiac cirrhosis)

- *Parasitic infection of the liver* (schistosomiasis), a condition particularly common in North Africa

Symptoms

Although many people with cirrhosis experience few symptoms, signs of the disease may include jaundice (yellowing of the skin and whites of the eyes), edema (fluid collection in the tissues), as well as symptoms such as fatigue, weakness, and loss of appetite. In men, cirrhosis may cause a sex hormone imbalance that leads to the enlargement of breast tissue and the loss of body hair.

Complications of cirrhosis include

- *Ascites* (a collection of fluid in the abdominal cavity). This condition is a result of low protein levels in the blood and high blood pressure in the veins leading to the liver.

- *Esophageal varices* (enlarged veins in the walls of the esophagus). These swollen throat veins are also caused by increased blood pressure in the veins leading to the liver. If the esophageal veins rupture, vomiting of blood can result.

- *Confusion and coma.* Impaired mental function can result as the liver becomes unable to detoxify materials poisonous to the brain.

- *Hepatoma* (a cancerous tumor originating in the liver).

Diagnosis

A physical examination and blood tests may suggest a diagnosis of cirrhosis. Confirmation of the diagnosis may be made by a biopsy of the liver, in which a needle is inserted through the skin to obtain a piece of the organ for examination under a microscope.

Treatment

Once the liver is scarred, the damage is irreversible. The treatment of cirrhosis is limited to preventing further damage and preventing or treating complications.

Swelling of the abdominal cavity (ascites) may be controlled by taking diuretics (drugs that increase the production of urine). Bleeding esophageal varices can be treated by injections of a solution via a flexible tube placed through the mouth into the esophagus. The injected agent works by scarring and blocking the veins. Mental confusion can be improved by reducing dietary protein intake, which helps to reduce the level of toxic waste products circulating in the blood.

Abstinence from alcohol, combined with the intake of a nutritious diet and a daily multivitamin supplement, can help prevent further liver damage.

When appropriate, the treatment of underlying diseases or disorders is prescribed. For instance, if a virus (as in hepatitis B) is found to be responsible for the liver damage, your physician may prescribe an antiviral drug. If cirrhosis is caused by the overload of certain metals (as in Wilson's disease and hemochromatosis), diuretics may prove to be helpful. In severe cases of cirrhosis, a liver transplant might be considered.

PREVENTING CIRRHOSIS

To prevent cirrhosis, drink moderately. Your risk of cirrhosis is slight if you limit yourself to two drinks a day—with a drink defined as a 12-ounce beer, a 5-ounce glass of wine or $1^1/_2$ ounces of liquor. Remember, also, that the quality of the alcohol you drink has no bearing on your risk of cirrhosis—the finest brandy has the same effect on the liver as the cheapest beer.

You should also watch out for hepatitis. Hepatitis C, spread through infected blood or sharing of IV needles, leads to cirrhosis in one-third of those infected. Hepatitis B, which is spread through infected blood and other bodily fluids (meaning that kissing, ear piercing, and sexual contact can lead to transmission), leads to cirrhosis in 5 to 8 percent of patients. A vaccine is available for hepatitis B, but not for C. (Hepatitis A, which is spread through contaminated food or drinking water, does not contribute to cirrhosis unless it becomes chronic.)

For more information:

Alcoholics Anonymous Worldwide Services Office
475 Riverside Drive
New York, NY 10115
212-870-3400
http://www.alcoholics-anonymous.org

American Liver Foundation
1425 Pompton Ave.
Cedar Grove, NJ 07009
800-223-0179
201-857-2626 (New Jersey)
http://www.liverfoundation.org

COLDS AND FLU

Influenza, commonly called the flu, and the common cold are viral infections that affect the respiratory tract. A cold involves the nose, throat, and surrounding air passages and, in general, has milder symptoms and a shorter recovery period than the flu. In contrast, the flu usually comes on suddenly with more severe symptoms, including a fever and the chills.

Causes of Colds and Flu

There are more than twenty identified families of viruses. About half of all cold viruses come from the rhinovirus family (the prefix *rhino* comes from the Greek for nose). The flu, on the other hand, comes from three families described as the type A, B, and C strains. The type A strain is responsible for most flu epidemics because it can alter its genetic makeup, making it difficult for a person to develop an immunity to it.

Colds and flu are spread when an infected person coughs or sneezes infected droplets, which cling to the hands or other surfaces. The infected person might pass the virus by touching or shaking the hand of another person or touching an object. The person who was touched or who touched an infected object then touches his or her mouth, eyes, or nose, introducing the virus into the body. Influenza is spread most readily in places where people gather such as schools, workplaces, and nursing homes.

Symptoms

Cold and flu symptoms include headache, aching muscles and joints, sore throat, cough, nasal congestion, and fatigue. The flu may also include chills and a fever that may reach 104°F.

Nausea, vomiting, and diarrhea are usually symptoms of a gastrointestinal problem rather than the flu, although many people misdiagnose themselves. Gastroenteritis, for example, is caused by germs from the rotavirus family. These short-lived infections can be treated with bismuth subsalicylate (Pepto-Bismol). (See Digestive System Disorders, p. 243.)

The first signs of a cold or the flu may appear about one to four days after the virus has been introduced in the body. While a cold passes in a few days, the flu usually lasts about a week and can be followed by fatigue and depression. Some people may become seriously ill and may need to be hospitalized for the flu. Twice as many men than women die from the flu and complications such as pneumonia.

Diagnosis

It is difficult to diagnose influenza because its symptoms are similar to those of many other illnesses. To determine if the influenza virus is present, a doctor might take a sample of throat cells with a cotton swab and have a culture prepared in a laboratory. Blood tests are another way to diagnose influenza; doctors look for the presence of antibodies that fight the virus.

Treatment

Antibiotics are ineffective against viruses, so colds and flu must be left to run their course. While there are over-the-counter (OTC) medications available to treat symptoms, many experts recommend against them. This is because the symptoms are signs of your body's attempts to rid itself of the virus. For example, a cough is an attempt to get rid of mucus in the respiratory tract; a fever creates a heated environment that makes killing viruses easier; and nasal congestion helps escort viruses out of the body. By suppressing these symptoms, you may actually be making it harder for your body's immune system to fight the virus, prolonging your illness. You might want to try letting the cold or flu run its course for a few days rather than taking medications.

If symptoms are extreme and you choose to self-medicate, helpful OTC medications include aspirin, ibuprofen, and acetaminophen (to ease muscles aches, join pain, fever, and headaches); decongestants (to relieve nasal stuffiness and improve breathing); cough medicines (to suppress a dry cough that interferes with sleep); and throat lozenges (to provide relief from a sore throat). Don't, however, take antihistamines for a cold or the flu. These have little effect on congestion.

There are caveats, of course, that go with each of these remedies. Aspirin should not be given to those under the age of 19 because of the risk of Reye's syndrome, a potentially fatal reaction. Decongestants can raise blood pressure, and nasal inhalants shouldn't be used for more than three days in a row because they can actually cause inflammation of the nasal passages. Cough medicine should be used sparingly, since it

SELF-CARE FOR COLDS AND FLU

Try these strategies and remedies to help get through your next cold or bout of flu:

- Blow your nose often. This can help get rid of mucus and congestion. But blow gently or you may drive infected mucus back into the ear passages, causing an earache.

- Squirt saline spray to clear your nostrils. You can buy saline spray or create your own by mixing $\frac{1}{4}$ teaspoon salt, $\frac{1}{4}$ teaspoon baking soda, and 8 ounces of warm water. Squirt the solution into one nostril while gently holding the other closed. Let the nostril drain, then repeat two or three times. Then do the same with the other nostril.

- Drink plenty of fluids. Hot fluids are best because they help relieve congestion. Stay away from alcohol, however, and use caffeine only in moderation.

- Eat chicken soup. Studies show that this age-old remedy contains an amino acid that helps break up congestion and clear clogged nasal passages.

- Steam yourself. Taking a hot shower, using a humidifier, or inhaling steam from a pot of boiling water helps drain nasal passages and relieve congestion.

- Use a salve or rub. Vicks VapoRub and other mentholated products applied under the nose and on the chest can help you breathe better by opening nasal passages wider. They can also help soothe raw or irritated skin.

- Help your immune system. Eating right and staying warm can help give your body the resources it needs to fight off the illness. Get plenty of proteins and vitamin C.

suppresses the mechanism the body needs to rid the respiratory tract of mucus.

For those individuals who suffer from a chronic illness or who have experienced complications associated with the flu, a doctor's treatment is necessary. In addition, if you have had a fever of 101° F or above, especially one that lasts for more than three days and is accompanied by a sudden, nonproductive cough, seek medical care immediately. This could be a sign of pneumonia, which can be fatal if left untreated.

Prevention

Because there are no known cures for the cold or the flu, the best strategy is to avoid getting them in the first place. Try the following tactics to reduce your risk and reduce the risk of transmitting an illness to another:

- Wash your hands. This is probably one of the most effective ways to cut your risk of colds and flu. Most people infect themselves with a cold or flu after touching their eyes, mouth, or nose after they've touched an infected person or object. To get rid of any germs that may be on your hands, wash them frequently with soap and hot water and avoid touching your face. Keep in mind that germs don't need to be spread personally—viruses can linger on surfaces such as phones, pens, and computer keyboards.

- Don't cover your mouth when you sneeze or cough. This causes the viruses to collect on your hands, where they will be easily transmitted to others. Instead, simply turn your head. Most experts believe that viruses must be passed by direct contact

and can't be transmitted by airborne droplets.

- Stay moist. Moisture helps your mucous membranes do their job: trapping foreign particles and germs that enter the respiratory tract. To keep the membranes in shape, drink plenty of water, use a humidifier or saline nasal spray or dab some petroleum jelly in each nostril.

- Get your vitamins and minerals. Be sure you're getting your recommended dietary allowance of these natural substances to help keep your immune system in condition. In particular, vitamin C and zinc have been shown to be especially helpful in staving off colds and flu. Herbs such as echinacea also help boost the immune system.

- Keep to yourself. When colds and flu are in the air, you may want to avoid any large gatherings to protect yourself from unwanted germs. Visiting sick friends may also be risky—those with an illness generally "shed" viruses that can be easily acquired. If you do visit, be sure to wash your hands.

- Boost your immune system. Be sure to eat right, avoid caffeine and alcohol and get enough exercise in order to give your body the greatest advantage in its fight against colds and flu. In addition, if you smoke, stop.

Immunizations for the Flu

There are several types of the influenza virus, called types A, B, and C. Type A is the most serious of the three and is responsible for most flu epidemics. It produces new strains regularly. The Centers for Disease Control and Prevention (CDC) predicts which strain of type A will affect the population during the flu season and develops the appropriate flu shot. The immunization does not eliminate the threat of contracting influenza (it immunizes about 60 to 70 percent of the people who receive the shot), but for individuals in high-risk groups, the vaccination is an important measure in preventing serious illness, complications, and even death.

It is a common misconception that the vaccine can actually cause influenza. All the viruses in the vaccine are already dead, so it is impossible to get influenza from the vaccine.

It usually takes about two weeks for the vaccine to build up enough protection against influenza, so it is important to be vaccinated in the fall, before "flu season" begins. In the United States, influenza is most common from December to April. People 9 years and older need one shot each influenza season, and children less than 9 years old may need a second shot after one month. It is important to be vaccinated every year since the strain of influenza changes and the vaccine is adjusted accordingly.

The CDC recommends the vaccine to people over 65, people who live or work in long-term-care or health facilities, people with compromised immune systems (such as those with HIV or cancer), children and pregnant women, as well as to anyone who wants to reduce his or her chance of catching influenza.

The Risks of Being Vaccinated

There are very small risks associated with the flu shot. Some people develop reactions to the vaccine, ranging from mild soreness to serious allergic reactions. The benefits of the vaccine, however, far outweigh the risks. For these individuals, the complications caused by influenza are far more serious.

If mild or moderate problems occur, they usually start soon after the vaccination is given and usually last up to two days. These include soreness, redness or swelling where the shot was given, fever and aches. If there is a reaction more serious than this, contact your doctor immediately.

The CDC recommends that before being vaccinated, tell the doctor or nurse if you have a serious allergy to eggs; have ever had a serious reaction to the influenza vaccine; were ever paralyzed by Guillain-Barre syndrome; or now have a moderate or serious illness.

For more information:

American Lung Association
1740 Broadway 14th floor
New York, NY 10019-4374
800-LUNG-USA
http://www.lungusa.org

DEPRESSION

Depression—the energy-draining, joy-blocking, motivation-sapping illness that turns life to black and gray—is so widespread in our society that it's called the "common cold of mental illness." It affects 11.5 percent of all men and 25 percent of all women. But depression isn't as innocuous as a cold, especially for men.

Even though statistics show that women are more than twice as likely to be depressed as men are, males are nearly five times more likely to commit suicide if they suffer from depression. In 1990, over 15,000 men killed themselves because of depression, compared with around 3,400 women. (See Suicide, p. 364.) Some experts believe that may be due to the fact that depression is underdiagnosed in men, who are culturally conditioned to repress negative feelings and emotions. Men are also less likely than women to seek medical help for any reason and are consequently less likely to seek treatment that may shorten the duration and intensity of a depressive bout—and reduce the risk of suicide.

In fact, a 1991 study showed that North American men seek help through counseling services only about half as often as women. Characteristics that are desirable in those being counseled—acknowledgment of personal problems, willingness to disclose one's feelings, tolerance of feeling vulnerable, and emotional awareness and expression—are often the opposite of the traditionally socialized male role. The reluctance to seek counseling also raises the possibility that many deaths that appear accidental (for example, car crashes, drug overdoses, and risky thrill-seeking accidents) are actually suicides committed by men with undiagnosed depression.

Depression consists of feeling sad, hopelessness, a general disinterest in life, and a sense of reduced emotional well-being. Unlike the occasional "blues" that most people experience, depression deepens and is persistent. It becomes a true depressive illness when it affects a person's behavior and physical state, often leading to insomnia, digestive problems, sore muscles, or head and backaches.

Causes of Depression

Depression can be caused by biological or physical changes or a combination of these factors. Whether the result of biological or psychological stressors, depression is indicative of an imbalance in brain neurotransmitters, which can be diagnosed and treated.

Biological depression is triggered by physical illnesses such as heart disease, diabetes, acquired immune deficiency syndrome (AIDS), cancer, and hormonal disorders such as thyroid imbalances. In addition, some people may have a genetic predisposition to depression. According to the American Psychiatric Association, major depression occurs one-and-a-half to three times as often among those with a parent, grandparent, or sibling with the disorder as among the general population. Another possible biological cause of depression in men is their naturally lower levels of the brain chemical serotonin, which is an important mood-regulator.

Psychological depression can be related to painful events or social circumstances such as the loss of job or difficult upbringing. Such depression is called reactive depression. If the depression lasts longer than two weeks and remains or increases in intensity, it may cause physical problems and calls for treatment.

Diagnosing Depression

The first hurdle a man (and often his physician), has to overcome is recognizing and accurately diagnosing his depression. For one thing, many men are likely to dismiss the physical complaints that often signal depression or blame them on stress. If a man does go to his general practitioner, it's likely the doctor will miss the signs of clinical depression. (On the other hand, many mental health specialists are likely to ascribe mental illness causes to purely physical ills.) One way to avoid misdiagnosis is for both doctor and patient to be aware of the symptoms that, taken together, almost definitely diagnose depression.

The American Psychiatric Association uses the following criteria to diagnose depression. To be clinically depressed, a person must have at least five of the symptoms listed (including the first two) for the same two-week period. The symptoms cannot be normal reaction to the death of a loved one.

1. Depressed mood (sometimes irritability in children and adolescents) most of the day, nearly every day

2. Markedly diminished interest or pleasure in all, or almost all, activities most of the day, nearly every day

3. Significant weight loss when not dieting (more than 5 percent of body weight in a month) or decrease/increase in appetite nearly every day

4. Insomnia or hypersomnia (excessive sleep) nearly every day

5. Psychomotor agitation or psychomotor retardation, an abnormal speeding up or slowing down of one's physical activities or mental processes, nearly every day, as observed by others

6. Fatigue or loss of energy nearly every day

7. Feelings of worthlessness or excessive or inappropriate guilt (which may be delusional) nearly every day (not merely self-reproach or guilt about being sick)

8. Diminished ability to think or concentrate, or indecisiveness, nearly every day

9. Recurrent thoughts of death (not just fear of dying) or of suicide without a specific plan, a suicide attempt or a specific plan for committing suicide

Depression may also manifest itself as a violent outburst or self-medication, in which a man uses alcohol or drugs to cope with difficulties. Withdrawal from family and friends is also a sign of depression.

The Spectrum of Depression

There are several types of depression, and—because treatment varies—it is important to have the type correctly diagnosed.

The most common type of depression is major depressive disorder, also called unipolar disorder, which is characterized by a combination of at least five of the conditions listed above. Types of major depressive disorders include melancholic depression, in which the individual appears to have permanently lost interest or pleasure in everything, and psychotic depression, marked by delusions, hallucinations, and a permanent sad mood. About 15 percent of those with major depressive disorders develop psychotic depression, which has a high risk of suicide.

About two million Americans suffer from manic-depressive disorder, or bipolar disorder, each year. This condition includes symptoms of alternating depression and mania. Mania is characterized by heightened mood, exaggerated optimism and self-confidence, increased physical and mental activity, impulsiveness, poor judgment, and reckless behavior. Generally, the mania phase lasts one to three months, and the depressive phase lasts six to nine months.

Dysthymia is "low-grade" chronic depression, characterized by low mood of at least two years' duration. Sufferers usually invest what little energy or enthusiasm they can muster for work, leaving nothing for family or social life. One expert calls this "dutiful self-denial." Dysthymia usually develops into more severe depression.

Another type of depression is seasonal affective disorder (SAD), which affects women more often than men and especially affects those living in the upper reaches of the Northern Hemisphere. With SAD, depression regularly begins in late fall or winter and persists until spring. Believed to be triggered by lack of exposure to sunlight, people with SAD tend to sleep, eat too many carbohydrates during the winter months, and become socially withdrawn. They also exhibit symptoms of classic depression.

Treatment

The worst mistake a depressed man can make is to think he can handle it on his own. Unfortunately, that mistake is made far too often: Only about one-third of people with depression seek help. It is essential to get help for depressive illness. Those with untreated severe depression have a suicide rate as high as 15 percent. In fact, suicide is the fifth highest killer of men ages 25 through 44 and has increased 26 percent in men over the past twenty years. With proper treatment, however, about 80 percent of those with major depression experience significant improvement and are able to lead productive lives.

There are many proven therapies—drug and nondrug—that relieve depression, but all of them require the services of a professional. Though some depressions lift on their own after six months to a year, many cases will never resolve on their own.

Therapists. Professional help can be sought from a psychiatrist, a psychologist, a primary-care physician, a social worker, a family therapist or a psychiatric nurse specialist. Therapists employ a range of approaches, depending on their background, education, and philosophies; in many cases, they combine drug treatment with talk and/or behavioral therapy. Choosing a therapist who is not a physician does not preclude

the use of drugs in treatment; psychologists who take this approach refer their clients to a personal physician for antidepressant prescriptions.

A psychiatrist is a licensed medical doctor who has completed four years of medical school and a residency. Psychiatry emphasizes physical causes behind mental illness. Psychiatrists are experienced in the use of antidepressants and other medications to treat depression.

A psychologist has completed four years in graduate school in psychology and usually holds a Ph.D. (doctor of philosophy) or a Psy.D. (doctor of psychology). Psychologists often have a subspecialty in clinical or counseling psychology and are licensed to practice psychology. Most psychologists cannot prescribe medications, though they often work with medical doctors who can.

Primary-care physicians such as family physicians, internists, and specialists in adolescent medicine are medical doctors who may be qualified to diagnose and treat patients with depression. However, primary-care physicians often refer cases to psychiatrists.

Clinical social workers usually complete a two-year graduate program to obtain a master's in social work (M.S.W.). Family therapists are usually licensed (though they aren't always) in marital and family therapy and have a degree in that type of counseling. A psychiatric nurse specialist, a registered nurse who has specialized training in treating mental or psychiatric disorders, may also treat a person with depression.

Psychotherapies. Common therapies employed by these therapists include cognitive and behavioral therapy and psychodynamic therapies. Cognitive and behavioral therapies work to help correct the self-defeating actions and thought processes that lead to depression in the first place.

Cognitive therapy focuses on positive thinking and optimism; behavioral therapy concentrates on encouraging positive behavior.

There are more than two hundred varieties of psychodynamic therapies, including psychotherapy and interpersonal therapies. These "talk therapies" focus on treating the root of the depression, often thought to be a childhood or past experience. Many are designed to lead patients to personal insight that shows them the origins of their depression and the behavioral patterns that trigger and sustain it. This approach involves expressing emotions and thoughts to a practitioner. Treatment with talk therapy can last anywhere from two to five sessions to years.

Antidepressants. Antidepressants are the class of medications most often used in the treatment of depression. These drugs work by stimulating or blocking certain brain chemicals, acting on receptors or impulses. Types of antidepressants include the following:

1. *Tricyclics* (Elavil, Norpramin, and Pamelor). These drugs affect the neurotransmitters, chemicals in the brain that influence the transmission of the signals that shape behaviors and feelings. Side effects include dry mouth, weight gain, constipation and difficulty urinating, drowsiness, and dizziness.

2. *Monamine oxidase inhibitors, or MAOIs* (Parnate and Nardil). MAOIs, as their name indicates, inhibit the production of the enzyme monamine oxidase that breaks down neurotransmitters. As a result, levels of neurotransmitters increase. Side effects include those of tricyclics, as well as rapid heartbeat and a decreased sexual drive. Certain foods such as figs, aged cheese, certain wines, and monosodium glutamate may react negatively with MAOIs, causing headache, nausea, seizure, stroke, and possibly coma. For this reason, MAOIs are usually prescribed for those who don't respond to tricyclic antidepressants.

3. *Selective serotonin reuptake inhibitors, or SSRIs* (Prozac, Zoloft, and Paxil). These drugs have become the preferred medications for treating depression. These work by slowing the rate at which the neurotransmitter serotonin is absorbed, thereby increasing neurotransmitter levels in the brain. There are fewer side effects with SSRIs than with other antidepressants. Side effects that might occur include nausea, diarrhea, anxiety, headache, and rash. Temporary side effects may include lowered sex drive, difficulty achieving orgasm, and erectile problems.

4. *Selective serotonin noradrenergic reuptake inhibitors, or SSNRIs* (Effexor). These are some of the newest drugs available for depression. SSNRIs function as SSRIs, but have a different chemical composition.

5. *Lithium.* This mood-stabilizing antidepressant is used in the treatment of manic-depressive disorder. Possible side effects include nausea, vomiting, muscle weakness, and increased thirst and urination. Careful monitoring is needed for those using lithium, which carries a risk of kidney and liver damage.

In addition to antidepressants, other medications may be used. To ease the anxiety and insomnia that often accompany affective disorders, sedatives (benzodiazepines) may be included in treatment. In addition, hallucinations and extremely disorganized thought patterns may be treated with neuroleptics (Risperdal and Mellaril).

Drug treatment can take several weeks to kick in and must be monitored. For some people, treatment may be stopped after a period of time. In severe cases, drug treatment can last many years to a lifetime.

Other Treatments

Aside from medications and therapy, light therapy and electroconvulsive therapy may be used in specific cases of depression. Light therapy is limited to people with seasonal affective disorder. It involves exposure to light (10,000 lux intensity) from a light box placed near the person for several hours daily. Usually effective after three or four weeks of treatment, light therapy may need to be supplemented with drug therapy and a timed light that goes on while the person is still sleeping.

In addition, electroconvulsive therapy may be used in rare cases. This "shock" therapy that fell into disrepute in the 1950s and 1960s is now given under anesthesia. It is generally reserved for people who have not responded to several months of drug therapy, or people with severe melancholic or psychotic depression.

For more information:

American Psychological Association
Office of Public Affairs
750 First St., N.E.
Washington, DC 20002
202-336-5700
http://www.apa.org

Depressives Anonymous: Recovery From
Depression
329 E. 62nd St.
New York, NY 10021
212-689-2600

National Foundation for Depressive Illness
P.O. Box 2257
New York, NY 10116
800-248-4344

National Institute of Mental Health
Inquiries Branch
5600 Fishers Ln.
Rockville, MD 20857
Depression/Awareness, Recognition and Treatment
(D/ART)
800-421-4211

National Depressive and Manic Depressive
Association
730 N. Franklin St., Suite 501
Chicago, IL 60610
800-826-3632
http://www.ndmda.org

National Mental Health Association
1021 Prince St.
Alexandria, VA 22314-2971
800-969-6642
703-684-7722
http://www.nmha.org

DIABETES

About 6 percent of the U.S. population is estimated to have diabetes—more than sixteen million Americans. About 45 percent of those with diabetes are men. However, only about half of those with diabetes know that they have it. Diabetes is the fourth leading cause of death by disease in the United States, killing more than 160,000 people each year.

Diabetes is a chronic disease that affects the body's metabolism—the way it turns food into energy. A healthy body changes carbohydrates such as sugars and starches—for example, fruit, bread, and vegetables—into a form of sugar called glucose. Glucose is carried to cells through the bloodstream, and insulin (a hormone made in the pancreas) helps it enter the cells. In those with diabetes, the pancreas does not make enough insulin or the body can't use the insulin correctly.

What makes this malfunction serious is that glucose then builds up in the bloodstream and damages other body parts. Diabetes hastens wear and tear on many crucial functions: Untreated, diabetes can cause damage to the kidneys, heart, eyes, feet, legs, nerves, and blood vessels. Major health problems caused by diabetes include blindness, kidney disease, amputations, heart disease, strokes, and birth defects. Women who have both diabetes and heart disease are more likely to die than men with the same conditions.

Type-I Diabetes

In type-I diabetes, also known as insulin-dependent diabetes, the body's own immune system attacks the cells of the pancreas that produce insulin. This results in disruptive swings in blood sugar levels, causing hyperglycemia (too much blood sugar) or hypoglycemia (too little blood sugar). Those with type-I diabetes are also at risk of ketoacidosis, which is a poisoning of the system with ketones (toxic acids that result from the breakdown of fats for fuel). Some ketones are excreted through the urine, which is why those with type-I diabetes test their urine. In extreme cases, ketoacidosis can cause unconsciousness, diabetic coma, or death.

Experts have not determined the cause of type-I diabetes, though there is a genetic link. Type-I diabetes cannot be prevented. It is usually diagnosed in those under 30 and was once known as juvenile diabetes.

Type-II Diabetes

Type-II diabetes, also called noninsulin dependent diabetes or adult onset diabetes, accounts for 85 to 90 percent of all cases of diabetes. People with type-II diabetes are most often diagnosed after age 30, are obese, and usually do not have ketones in their urine. In this condition, insulin is still produced by the body, but it does not function properly. It is believed that excess weight and a high carbohydrate intake causes the body's cells to become resistant to insulin. At the same time, the cells that produce insulin work overtime and eventually become exhausted, resulting in inadequate insulin production.

Type-II diabetes also has a genetic link, though it is generally believed it must be triggered by age or excess weight. Four out of five people with this condition are overweight.

Risk Factors

While most practitioners do not do routine tests for diabetes, you may want to be tested if you are in a high-risk category for the condition. Those most at risk to get diabetes are those who are overweight; people with a family history of diabetes; those who are 40 and older; African Americans; Hispanics; and Native Americans.

Some 2.6 million African Americans (9.6 percent) have diabetes. Hispanics are two to four times as likely as the general population to have diabetes—some 9.6 of Mexican-Americans, 9.1 percent of Cuban-Americans, and 10.9 percent of Puerto Ricans have the disease. In addition, some 12.2 percent of Native Americans have diabetes (compared with 5.2 percent of the general population.) Studies show that diabetes is reaching epidemic proportions and is a major cause of death for Native Americans.

Symptoms

Symptoms of diabetes include sudden weight loss; frequent urination; frequent hunger and/ or thirst; vision problems; weakness and fatigue; irritability; slow healing of cuts (especially on the feet); frequent infections; circulation problems, including tingling or numbness in legs, feet, or fingers; frequent skin infections; and itchy skin.

Diagnosis

To check for diabetes, your doctor will start with a routine blood test. In normal adults, blood-sugar levels range between 60 and 100 milligrams per deciliter—designated as mg/dl—of blood plasma when a person is fasting—that is, has not eaten in three or more hours. If fasting blood sugar is between 115 and 140 mg/dl, doctors may be concerned and may continue to monitor your blood glucose. If your fasting blood sugar is over 140 mg/dl, a doctor may use two other tests to confirm diabetes.

The fasting plasma glucose test is performed after a person hasn't eaten for eight to twelve hours. Several of these tests are given on different days, and diabetes is diagnosed if glucose levels are higher than 140 mg/dl on two successive tests.

The oral glucose-tolerance test is a fasting blood sample taken after a person eats a high-carbohydrate diet for three days. After that sample is taken, the patient drinks a glucose solution and blood samples are taken every thirty minutes for two hours, with another sample taken an hour later. The blood samples show how the body handles glucose. Normally, blood levels rise after the glucose is consumed and then return to normal. In those with diabetes, blood-

ERECTION PROBLEMS AND DIABETES

A special concern for men is that diabetes can affect sexual activity. According to the American Diabetes Association, erection problems occur among 50 to 60 percent of all men over age 50 who are diabetic. Blood vessel disease or nerve disease are the most common causes of problems in men with diabetes. Blood vessel disease will block the flow of blood to the penis. If the nerves to the penis are damaged, they may not be able to send signals and may limit blood flow, which can prevent an erection.

A man with diabetes should practice good blood glucose control in order to prevent nerve and circulatory damage and prevent any problems. If a man with diabetes is experiencing erection problems, he should see his doctor to determine the exact cause and receive treatment. Physical problems often account for erection problems in men, but the stress of the disease sometimes will create psychological reasons for the sexual malfunction.

sugar levels don't fall that quickly. Blood-sugar levels higher than 200 mg/dl one to two hours after a meal confirm diabetes. And if the blood sugar registers more than 200 mg/dl after the fasting segment of this test, there's no doubt that the person has diabetes.

Treatment

Although there is no cure for diabetes, the disease is treatable, and many of those with diabetes live normal lifespans and have active lifestyles. Each type of diabetes has a different treatment regimen. By injecting prescription insulin, those with type-I diabetes are able to regulate their sugar metabolism.

Although some people with type-II diabetes eventually become insulin dependent, most can control their sugar levels, and some can even reverse the disease process so insulin is produced and functions normally. What that takes is a disciplined routine of medication, weight loss, diet, and exercise.

Recently, there's been good news for those with type-II diabetes. The drug Glucophage (metformin hydrochloride), approved for sale in the United States, is effective in lowering blood sugar in those with type-II diabetes who do not respond to the traditional medications. Plus, researchers may be on the path to other treatments. They recently discovered a protein called PC-1 that is found in excessive quantities in those with type-II diabetes and appears to make cells "resistant" to insulin.

Prevention

Type-I diabetes cannot be prevented at present, but researchers are looking for ways to identify the predisposing genetic factors and the viral or environmental triggers of the disease. But you can reduce your risk of getting type-II diabetes if you

- Maintain a healthy weight.

- Eat low-fat foods.

- Get regular exercise. Exercise can help you lose weight that could trigger diabetes. In addition, evidence shows that building muscle mass through exercise triggers your muscle's use of insulin and may help prevent diabetes.

For more information:

American Diabetes Association
1660 Duke St.
Alexandria, VA 22314
800-232-3472
http://www.diabetes.org

National Diabetes Information Clearinghouse
Box NDIC
9000 Rockville Pike
Bethesda, MD 20892-3560
301-654-3327

American Dietetic Association
216 W. Jackson Blvd., Suite 800
Chicago, IL 60606-6695
800-366-1655
312-899-0040

American Association of Diabetes Educators
444 N. Michigan Ave., Suite 1240
Chicago, IL 60611
312-644-2233

DIGESTIVE SYSTEM DISORDERS

Many of the major digestive system disorders— gallbladder disease, ulcers, heartburn, hernias, and hemorrhoids—are addressed in their own, individual topics. However, some additional problems that deserve attention are addressed here briefly. Here you will find information on appendicitis; constipation; diarrhea; diverticulosis and diverticulitis; gastroenteritis; gastritis; inflammatory bowel disease (colitis and Crohn's disease); irritable bowel syndrome; lactose intolerance; polyps; and tumors of the small intestine and the stomach.

SYMPTOMS OF DIGESTIVE DISEASE

Though symptoms vary, according to the condition, the following are warning signs that a digestive problem may be present:

Long-lasting stomach pains accompanied by chills and shaking

Blood in the stools or black stool

Yellowing of the skin and whites of the eyes (jaundice)

Difficulty swallowing

Unexplained weight loss

A sudden change in bowel habits, for example, diarrhea or constipation, that lasts for more than a few days

Vomiting

Appendicitis

Appendicitis is inflammation of the appendix, a short, narrow organ that dangles from the first section of the large intestine. The function of the appendix and the cause of appendicitis are unknown.

Symptoms include pain in the abdomen, particularly the lower, right side; nausea and vomiting; lack of appetite; and the urge to pass stool or gas. It can be diagnosed through feeling the abdomen for tenderness and a rectal examination. Treatment involves surgery to remove the infected organ. If the organ is not removed, it may rupture and cause contamination of the abdominal cavity, called peritonitis, which is a potentially fatal condition.

Constipation

Constipation is the inability to move the bowels and pass stool or the infrequent passage of stool. Causes of constipation include obstruction, medications, or a change in how much water is removed from the waste in the intestine. A leading cause of constipation is a lack of sufficient fiber in the diet as a result of eating overrefined foods. Some people may think they're constipated just because they don't have a certain number of bowel movements per day or week. However, everyone is different. Regularity, and not frequency, is the key to good bowel health.

PREVENTING CONSTIPATION

While laxatives may be used to prevent or resolve constipation, they can also contribute to the problem if they're used incorrectly. To help keep things moving regularly, the following self-care tips may be more helpful than a laxative.

- Drink eight glasses of water each day.

- Eat a high-fiber diet.

- Exercise regularly.

- Don't put off going to the bathroom. Delays can dry out stool and contribute to constipation.

- Avoid enemas. While enemas may precede certain medical procedures, they're not meant for everyday use. Enemas can actually contribute to constipation by irritating the colon.

Treatment includes dietary changes and other self-care measures. Constipation may also be treated with glycerine suppositories, laxatives, and purgatives, although their use should be limited and then only under the supervision of a doctor. Persistent constipation should be a sign that further professional medical attention is needed.

Diarrhea

Diarrhea is characterized by frequent bowel movements. While not a disease, diarrhea could signal some underlying condition that may warrant further professional attention. However, most diarrhea can be self-treated and should resolve in about two to three days.

The probable cause of diarrhea is food or water that contains an organism (generally bacteria) that upsets the delicate balance of the large intestine. When this occurs, the normal process of passing food through the intestines is disrupted and the food passes too quickly through the system.

Most cases of diarrhea may be treated with over-the-counter medications; however, if symptoms do not resolve within two to three days, then professional assistance is needed because of the risk of dehydration. Diarrhea in at-risk people, for example, infants and the elderly, is quite serious, and professional medical attention should be sought at the first sign of it.

Diverticulosis and Diverticulitis

Diverticulosis and diverticulitis are conditions affecting the large intestine (colon) and are characterized by the formation of small pouches called diverticula at weak spots on the intestine wall. The condition is known as diverticulosis when the diverticula are merely present, and as diverticulitis when the diverticula become inflamed or infected. If not diagnosed and treated, diverticulitis may result in bowel blockages and abscesses. These conditions generally affect people over the age of 60; however, they have been diagnosed in people as young as 40.

Symptoms of diverticulosis are limited to tenderness or muscle spasms in the lower abdomen. Symptoms of diverticulitis include abdominal pain, fever, and increased white blood cell count. Diagnosis is done through a barium enema, in which a contrast material that makes the intestines visible on x-ray is given via enema. Treatment involves bed rest, stool softeners, and a liquid diet. If infection has occurred, antibiotics are prescribed. In severe cases, a section of bowel may be removed and the remaining portion temporarily attached to a hole in the abdomen to allow for the passage of waste. At a later date, the remaining bowel is reattached. This procedure is known as a temporary colostomy.

Gastritis

Inflammation of the stomach lining, known as gastritis, can be triggered by a number of situations. Smoking and drinking alcohol can cause gastritis, as can a problem with acid production in the stomach even if there is no ulcer present. Gastritis can also be caused by a number of medications or by a vitamin B_{12} deficiency. In most cases, gastritis is harmless and passes quickly. In rare circumstances, there may be internal bleeding.

Symptoms include pain or discomfort in the abdomen, nausea and vomiting, and diarrhea. Diagnosis is done according to symptoms, though a barium x-ray (in which a contrast material is swallowed to highlight the digestive system on x-ray) or gastroscopy (in which a fiberoptic tube is inserted via the mouth to view the stomach) may also be done. Treatment involves over-the-counter medications such as antacids or acid-reducers (Pepcid, Zantac). Vitamin B_{12} injections may be prescribed if a deficiency is diagnosed.

Gastroenteritis

Gastroenteritis, or infection and inflammation of the gastrointestinal tract, is extremely common. The Centers for Disease Control and Prevention estimate that over 25 million cases of gastroenteritis occur each year. Of these, about half can be attributed to viruses. Other causes include bacteria and parasites. Symptoms of the condition may include watery diarrhea, abdominal cramps, nausea and vomiting, fever, and headache. Gastroenteritis usually does not last longer than thirty-six hours. Some forms of gastroenteritis are often confused with the flu.

Types of viral infections include the rotavirus, Norwalk virus, and cytomegalovirus. While these conditions are generally not dangerous for those in good health, they may cause death in children, older adults, and in people whose immune systems are compromised, so treatment should be sought immediately if symptoms are present in such people. In healthy adults, the symptoms usually disappear on their own after a few days. Antibiotics are ineffective against viral infections, and antidiarrheal drugs only prolong the condition.

Types of bacterial infections include salmonella, Escherichia coli (E. coli), and shigella. The infections are generally transmitted through contaminated food and water. Again, these conditions usually resolve on their own. However, antibiotics may be prescribed.

Inflammatory Bowel Disease

Inflammatory bowel disease, or IBD, is an umbrella term that covers Crohn's disease and colitis. IBD should not be confused with irritable bowel syndrome, or IBS, which is characterized by involuntary muscle movement in the large intestine.

Colitis

Colitis is a form of inflammatory bowel disease that affects the colon. The chronic, progressive condition causes inflammation, small ulcers, and abscesses in the inner lining of the colon, which may lead to obstruction or perforation of the colon. There is no known cause of colitis, which occurs most often in people between the ages of 15 and 30, but there may be hereditary links. Colitis carries with it an increased risk of colon cancer.

In many people with colitis, there may be no symptoms. If they do occur, symptoms include bloody diarrhea, abdominal pain, frequent bowel movements, joint pain, fever, and weight loss. It is diagnosed by using proctosigmoidoscopy, in which a fiberoptic scope is inserted into the rectum to view the inside of the colon. A barium x-ray or a colonoscopy, insertion of a fiberoptic scope into the rectum to view the colon, may be done also. Treatment involves anti-inflammatory drugs such as sulfasalazine and corticosteroids. In cases that involve severe diarrhea, treatment may focus on preventing dehydration or malnutrition.

Some 25 percent of those with colitis require surgery at some time. Usually, ileo-anal anastomosis is performed, in which the colon is removed and the small intestine is attached directly to the anus to allow the normal passage of waste.

FOOD POISONING

Common types of food poisoning include gastroenteritis, in which unwashed or contaminated food or water is ingested, and botulism, which results from the ingestion of a toxin often found in improperly canned foods. Gastroenteritis usually occurs within six hours of eating the contaminated food. It usually is not serious and passes in about twelve hours. Botulism, which occurs twelve to thirty-six hours after eating, is very serious and requires medical attention immediately. It can be fatal. You should seek medical attention if you suffer sudden severe vomiting and diarrhea. Also, any sign of food poisoning in children, the elderly, or people with weakened immune systems should be treated immediately.

To help prevent food poisoning:

- Cook meat thoroughly. Beef is often contaminated with E. coli bacteria, which is destroyed by heat. While most strains are harmless, others can cause infections that lead to kidney failure and death. Young children, older people, and those with weakened immune systems (perhaps from cancer treatments or AIDS) are especially vulnerable to the dangers of E. coli.

- Watch the time. Food can be safely kept without refrigeration for up to two hours—one hour if the temperature is 85°F or higher. After that, the stage is set for bacterial growth. If you're in doubt about whether something has been out of the fridge too long, throw it away.

- Handle meat carefully. Wash your hands after working with meat, poultry, seafood, and eggs and don't let their juices touch other surfaces or foods. Wet, warm surfaces promote the growth of bacteria, and hands spread them around.

- Marinate your meat in the refrigerator and be sure you don't baste cooked meat with an uncooked marinade. Also, don't use the same utensils you used on the uncooked meat on the finished product.

- Avoid the half shell. Mollusks such as oysters, clams, and mussels filter water through their systems to feed and are often contaminated by bacteria and viruses in polluted water. Don't eat them raw—instead, cook them thoroughly to kill all bacteria. Discard any unopened mollusks.

For more information on food safety, contact the U.S. Department of Agriculture Meat and Poultry Hotline at 800-535-4555 or the Food and Drug Administration Seafood Hotline at 800-FDA-4010. These hotlines can answer questions and provide information about food safety.

Crohn's Disease

Crohn's disease, or ileitis, is a rare, chronic inflammation that can affect any part of the digestive system, though it most often affects the small intestine. It is a form of progressive inflammatory bowel disease that usually occurs in those between the ages of 15 and 35, and it may have genetic or environmental links. While some people with Crohn's disease may have few symptoms, in others it causes chronic diarrhea, abdominal pain, and complications such as bowel obstruction. Stress is known to exacerbate Crohn's disease and should be avoided.

Symptoms may include diarrhea, fever, weight loss, fatigue, cramps, and joint pain. It can be diagnosed through barium x-rays and colonoscopy. Treatment involves a change in diet, anti-inflammatory medications, and, rarely, corticosteroids to reduce inflammation. Vitamins and minerals may be prescribed if the disease is causing malabsorption problems. If the intestine becomes blocked, surgery is necessary to remove the obstruction—about 70 percent of those with Crohn's disease have at least one procedure. However, obstructions may recur after surgery. In severe cases that affect the large intestine, the section of intestine may be removed, and the small intestine will be brought through a hole in the abdominal wall to allow waste to pass out of the body. This procedure is called an ileostomy. If the small intestine is affected, the diseased portion will be removed and the remaining healthy portions will be stitched together.

Irritable Bowel Syndrome

Irritable bowel syndrome (called IBS) affects twenty-five to fifty-five million people in the United States and results in 2.5 million yearly visits to the physician. It is estimated that 5 to 19 percent of all men are affected by IBS. It is the most common disorder of the large intestine.

IBS, also called spastic colon and irritable colon syndrome, is an involuntary muscle movement in the large intestine. It is called a functional disorder because there are no signs of abnormality in the colon, such as a growth or intestinal bleeding. IBS is often mistaken for more complicated and serious digestive diseases such as inflammatory bowel disease.

Symptoms include gas, abdominal pain, diarrhea or constipation (or alternating bouts of each), nausea, feeling full after eating only a small meal, sensation of urinary urgency, incomplete emptying after urinating, fatigue, and pain during intercourse. Stress can often trigger IBS, though not everyone who has stress-related bowel problems has the disorder.

IBS is diagnosed through a process of elimination, making sure the symptoms are those of a more serious disease such as colitis or inflammatory bowel disease. Diagnosis involves a complete medical history and examination. A stool sample may be taken to test for blood in the stool. Also recommended is a proctosigmoidoscopy and a barium x-ray.

Many individuals find that a change in diet significantly reduces the effects of IBS. Fat (both animal and vegetable) is often a culprit because it stimulates contractions of the colon. Lactose (the natural sugar found in milk) and gas-producing vegetables such as broccoli and cabbage can also cause IBS symptoms to flare up. Doctors have also found that dietary fiber may lessen IBS symptoms in many cases. High-fiber diets keep the colon mildly distended, which helps to prevent spasms from developing, and reduce constipation.

A doctor may prescribe fiber supplements or an occasional laxative to relieve constipation.

Antispasmodic drugs may be prescribed to help reduce abdominal pain and the sensation of the urgency for a bowel movement. Antacids/antigas medications (such as Tums and Mylanta) and antidiarrhea medications (such as Imodium AD) are also used in treating the abdominal pain, cramping, and diarrhea. Antidepressant drugs are also used in treating IBS; studies have shown that these drugs help relieve the symptoms of IBS, independently of their antidepressant qualities. Smooth muscle relaxants (such as peppermint oil) help relax the smooth muscles of the gut and relieve cramping.

At times, mental health counseling and relaxation training can help relieve IBS symptoms. Emotional stress also stimulates colonic spasms in people with IBS, possibly because the colon is controlled partly by the nervous system, which is directly affected by the stressors in our lives. Biofeedback, a relaxation therapy that trains you to control usually involuntary bodily functions, may be especially helpful in treating IBS. (See Complementary Therapies, p. 124, and Relaxation Therapies, p. 436.)

Lactose Intolerance

Lactose intolerance is caused by a deficiency of the enzyme lactase in the digestive system. The enzyme is needed to digest lactose, the sugar in cow's milk. Symptoms of lactose intolerance may include cramps, bloating, diarrhea, and gas when milk or dairy products are consumed. It is estimated that more than thirty million Americans suffer from lactose intolerance, which occurs more often in people of Asian, African, or Mediterranean origin than in Northern and Western European whites. Some 75 percent of African Americans, Jewish, Mexican-American, and American Indian adults and 90 percent of Asian

American adults have lactose intolerance, according to the National Digestive Diseases Information Clearinghouse.

Treatment includes decreasing consumption of dairy products or use of an over-the-counter digestion aid. These aids are taken before eating or mixed with milk to help convert lactose into simple sugar.

Polyps

A polyp is a tumor, usually noncancerous, that grows from the lining of the large intestine. These common tumors affect two out of every three Americans over the age of 60. Symptoms, if they do occur, include blood in the stool, mucus discharge from the anus, or a change in bowel movements. They are usually diagnosed during a screening for colon cancer. While most polyps are not cancerous when they develop, some types may become cancerous—in fact, most colon cancers develop from polyps. For this reason, regular screening via colonoscopy is recommended for those with polyps. In some cases, surgical removal of the polyps may be recommended to prevent cancer. Polyps can be removed during colonoscopy, or an entire section of the colon may be removed by way of treatment.

Tumors of the Small Intestine

Tumors, or abnormal growths, may occur rarely in the small intestine. Most intestinal tumors are noncancerous, though a small percentage are cancerous.

Symptoms of a benign tumor include pain, bleeding, and nausea and vomiting. Symptoms of cancerous tumors include weight loss, nausea and vomiting, bleeding, and pain. Diagnosis is done with a barium x-ray, and surgery is usually recommended to remove all tumors, noncancerous and cancerous. The removed tissue is then analyzed for cancerous cells in a procedure called a biopsy. If cancer is found, chemotherapy and radiation may be used in addition to surgery.

Noncancerous tumors are not life-threatening. However, cancerous tumors may spread and should be treated promptly.

Tumors of the Stomach

Stomach tumors, growths within the stomach, affect twice as many men as women. Most stomach tumors are cancerous—the American Cancer Society reports fourteen thousand new cases of stomach cancer in men each year. The causes of stomach cancer are unknown, although there are thought to be dietary and hereditary links.

Symptoms, which resemble those of a peptic ulcer, include discomfort in the abdomen not helped by medications, blood in the stool, vomiting of blood or vomiting after meals, a bloated feeling, and weight loss. Diagnosis is done through a barium x-ray and an endoscopy, in which a fiberoptic tube is inserted through the mouth into the esophagus, stomach, and duodenum for a direct view of the digestive tract. Tissue may be collected during endoscopy for analysis in a procedure called a biopsy. Biopsy is the only definitive diagnosis for cancer.

Treatment involves surgery to remove the tumor and may be followed by radiation or chemotherapy. Treatment is generally successful when the cancer is caught early.

For more information:

Crohn's and Colitis Foundation of America, Inc.
444 Park Ave., S., 11th Floor
New York, NY 10016-7374
800-932-2423
212-685-3440
http://www.ccfa.org

Digestive Disease National Coalition
507 Capitol Ct., N.E., Suite 200
Washington, DC 20002
202-544-7497

National Digestive Diseases Information Clearinghouse
2 Information Way
Bethesda, MD 20892-3570
301-654-3810
http://www.niddk.nih.gov

DRUG ABUSE

Drug abuse is any deliberate misuse of a drug, a chemical entity that creates a specific biological response. All drugs—whether they be illicit street drugs, prescription medications, or legalized drugs such as nicotine or alcohol—are dangerous and have the potential of being misused. Drug abuse destroys lives, takes away all semblance of self-control through addiction, and can lead to dangerous, life-threatening health complications, including lung disease, heart disease, and AIDS.

The dark attraction of drugs lies in their abilities to alter mood and perception, relieve pain, gratify physical desires, and even enhance abilities. They can give a user a way to escape from reality, stressful problems, or an unpleasant environment. Yet addiction, a chronic, uncontrollable and compulsive behavior that is the hallmark of drug abuse, results after continued exposure to drugs. Some drugs are more addictive than others; narcotics and cocaine, for example, have highly addictive properties. Also, some users are more prone to addiction than others.

In general, abusers take drugs at regular, short intervals and exercise little or no self-control over their drug usage, pursuing the euphoric sense, or "high," in order to relieve feelings of inadequacy or depression or to escape from reality. Eventually, drugs are needed to maintain and cope with everyday life.

According to a 1995 survey from the Substance Abuse and Mental Health Services Administration, 7.9 million men in the United States had used an illicit drug within the past month, and 13.1 million had used within the past year. The highest rate of illicit drug use was among men between 18 and 25 years old.

Addiction

Drug abuse is normally characterized by certain drug-dependent states (addictions) in which the abuser finds himself psychologically dependent, physically dependent, and functionally dependent.

Psychological dependence, or habituation, is a type of compulsive neurotic behavior in which there is an emotional need and craving for and reliance upon drugs to maintain a sense of well-being.

Physical dependence, or true addiction, is a state in which the body physically needs the drug in such a way that, if the drug dosage were drastically reduced or stopped, withdrawal symptoms appear. Another manifestation of physical dependence is the tolerance the drug user gains in continued, repeated use of a drug. The user is tolerant of a drug when increasingly higher doses of the drug are needed to maintain the same drug effect.

Functional dependence describes the dependence of the body's functions on a certain drug to maintain a sense of well-being (a person may become functionally dependent even on laxatives or nasal sprays). One or all of these drug dependencies are characteristically present in patterns of excessive and/or regular drug abuse.

Types of Drugs

Drugs, specifically psychoactive drugs (those drugs which influence the mind), can be inhaled, ingested or injected. These different routes of administration allow drugs to be carried through the bloodstream, eventually to the central nervous system. Those drugs that are intravenously injected or inhaled affect the drug user at a faster rate than ingested ones. Drugs are classified into general categories.

1. *Depressants.* Drugs that slow down and relax signals passing through the central nervous system and are able to produce a physical dependency: for example, alcohol, barbiturates, sedatives, and tranquilizers.

2. *Narcotics or narcotic analgesics.* Painkillers that are addicting and produce an intense high: for example, opium, codeine, heroin, and morphine.

3. *Stimulants.* Addicting drugs that speed up signals to the central nervous system and produce alert, energetic behavior: for example, cocaine, amphetamines, caffeine, and nicotine.

4. *Hallucinogens.* "Psychedelic" drugs that produce hallucinations or changes in sensory perceptions: for example, LSD, ecstasy, mescaline, PCP, psilocybin, and cannabis (marijuana, hashish).

Signs of Drug Abuse

The signs and symptoms of drug abuse vary from person to person, but general signs of addiction and abuse can be recognized. These include the following:

SEX AND DRUGS

Rumor has it that many illicit drugs—especially marijuana and cocaine—increase sexual desire and performance, but the truth is quite the opposite. While some drug users report initial increases in enjoyment of sex, long-term use inevitably leads to some sort of sexual dysfunction, whether it be erection problems, loss of libido (sex drive), infertility, or an inability to experience orgasm.

Prolonged use of marijuana, for example, reduces testosterone levels, decreases libido, and lowers sperm counts. In one study, men who smoked pot four days a week for six months had lower testosterone levels. Some 35 percent had lower sperm counts, and 10 percent were impotent. Marijuana use also seems to encourage abnormal formation of sperm cells. It takes about two months without marijuana use for sperm to return to normal.

Chronic cocaine and crack (highly purified cocaine) use results in loss of desire, erection problems, loss of satisfaction, lower testosterone levels, lower sperm counts, and abnormal sperm development. In fact, in a New York University School of Medicine study of crack users found that twenty-four of thirty-eight men said they couldn't get an erection while using crack, and most reported that they could hardly feel the orgasm if they did have one. Cocaine also boosts blood pressure and heart rate, which, when added to the exertion of sex, could cause heart attack in some. Cocaine use also contaminates sperm cells, which could affect the fetus if pregnancy were to occur. Sexual dysfunction due to cocaine use usually disappears after two to three weeks away from the drug.

- Changes in personality or behavior: violent mood swings of euphoria, apathy, depression, changing friendships, secretiveness, lying, denial of problems, and demanding or stealing money.

- Decline in job performance or academic performance: poor work effort or poor grades, inattentiveness or distraction at job or at school.

- Changes in physical habits or appearance: weight loss, loss of appetite, change in sleeping habits, appearance of unusual skin lesions, puncture wounds, appearance of symptoms indicating the onset of severe health problems or diseases, persistent

cough, nasal congestion, red, bloodshot eyes, physical exhaustion, different clothes, and indifference to personal grooming.

- Withdrawal from parents, family and friends: solitary drug use, little or no communication with those around the user.

- Presence of drugs or drug paraphernalia: hypodermic needles, tubes, plastic bags, or other suspicious articles found on or around the user.

- Frequent intoxication of user: consistent intoxication or abnormal or hazardous behavior.

Symptoms

Drug addiction may also be suspected if a reduced dosage or complete cessation of the drug produces pronounced *withdrawal symptoms.* General withdrawal symptoms include aches and pains, anxiety, chills, cramps, convulsions, dehydration, diarrhea, dizziness, fever, hot flashes, insomnia, nausea, perspiration, psychotic behavior, tremors, vomiting, and weakness.

These symptoms occur because the body becomes dependent on its continuous presence in the body's system. When the drug is eliminated or reduced, the body experiences mental and physical symptoms. Some of the drugs that can produce marked withdrawal symptoms include alcohol, narcotics, nicotine and caffeine, tranquilizers, amphetamines, marijuana, and cocaine.

Treatment

The treatment of drug dependence and abuse consists of various treatment programs, most of them employing gradual detoxification and continued psychotherapy treatment. Treatment can be drug-free or maintenance, residential (halfway houses and therapeutic communities) or ambulatory (outpatient treatment facility), voluntary or involuntary (complete hospitalization), or a combination of several of these methods. Drug-free programs are aimed at abstinence, total withdrawal from the drug. Maintenance treatment involves detoxification by the administration of other drugs that relieve and prevent unpleasant withdrawal symptoms: for example, Antabuse (an antagonist drug for alcohol); methadone or naltrexone (an antagonist drug of heroin).

With any drug abuse treatment program, psychological and emotional support for the user is essential for the recovery of his mental stability.

Local or community support groups (for example, Narcotics Anonymous) and family members can provide invaluable support and encouragement for the rehabilitation of the drug user. Also, other support groups exist to help family members cope with another members' addictions. Local agencies, abuse centers, clinics and abuse hotlines can give information about drugs and drug abuse.

For more information:

Al-Anon and Alateen Family Groups
Headquarters, Inc.
1600 Corporate Landing Pkwy.
Virginia Beach, VA 23454
800-356-9996
800-245-4656 (New York)
800-443-4525 (Canada)
757-563-1600

American Council for Drug Education
164 W. 74th St.
New York, NY 10023
800-488-3784
http://www.acde.org

National Clearinghouse for Alcohol and
Drug Information
Drug Abuse Information and Treatment
Referral Line
P.O. Box 2345
Rockville, MD 20847-2345
800-662-4357
800-662-9832 (Spanish)
800-228-0427 (hearing impaired)
301-468-6433
http://www.health.org

National Council on Alcoholism and
Drug Dependence
12 W. 21st St.
New York, NY 10010
800-NCA-CALL
212-206-6770
http://www.ncadd.org

EYE DISORDERS

Most people take their eyes for granted. They think little about how they work, what can go wrong with them, and what they really mean to their overall lives. But without sight, the world shrinks. This topic looks at some of the most common eye problems.

Refractive Errors

The most common eye disorders are refractive errors in which the shape of the eye doesn't permit it to refract, or bend, light rays properly. As a result, vision becomes blurred. According to the National Eye Institute, part of the National Institutes of Health, about 120 million people in the United States have refractive errors. Myopia (nearsightedness), hyperopia (farsightedness), presbyopia (aging eyes), and astigmatism (distorted vision) are different types of refractive errors.

Myopia

People who are myopic see well up close but have trouble with distant objects. The reason is the "length"—the front-to-back distance—of the eye. The normal eye focuses images on the retina. The myopic eye is elongated, so images of distant objects focus in front of the retina, not on it. Myopia is often diagnosed in children when they are between 8 and 12 years old. It tends to get worse during the teenage years when the body grows rapidly and to stabilize between the ages of 20 and 40. Then, at 40, focusing on close objects typically becomes a problem.

Genetics may play a significant role in myopia. According to studies, if one or both of your parents are myopic, then you have a greater chance of becoming myopic by age 18 than someone whose parents were not myopic. Another risk factor is close-vision activity—primarily reading. While one in four Americans is myopic, the condition is extremely rare in

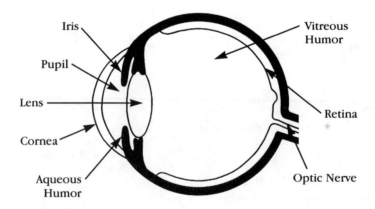

Schematic section of the human eye

Source: American Optometric Association

illiterate societies, presumably because of the close-vision factor.

Hyperopia

Farsightedness is a condition in which the eye is "shorter" front to back than normal. Hence, the images of close objects such as the words on this page aren't in focus when they reach the retina.

Presbyopia

This is a reduced elasticity of the lens of the eye that is responsible for difficulty focusing. Starting as early as age 20, the lens slowly loses its elasticity. By about age 40, the lens is significantly rigid and cannot change shape enough to bring close objects into focus. This condition gradually worsens with age.

Astigmatism

Astigmatism is caused by a defect in the cornea rather than a problem with the lens of the eye. Whereas a normal cornea is smooth and round, someone with an astigmatism has a comparatively oval cornea that curves more in one direction than the other. As a result, the eye cannot focus clearly on either near or distant objects.

Diagnosis

If you're experiencing blurry vision and headaches, then it's time to visit an eye specialist. The American Academy of Ophthalmology recommends that eye examinations should be conducted on an as needed basis for people under 40. Between the ages of 40 and 65, people need to be examined every two years due to the risk of age-related conditions. After age 65, exams should occur annually.

If you experience problems with your vision, don't hesitate to see an eye-care professional.

Some vision-related symptoms are sometimes signs of serious problems such as diabetes, high blood pressure, blood clots, and arteriosclerosis.

Treatment

Eyeglasses and contact lenses are the most common methods of correcting refractive errors such as hyperopia, astigmatism, myopia, and presbyopia. They work by compensating the shape of your eye and refocusing light rays on the retina. While there is no surgical solution for hyperopia or presbyopia, several surgical options exist for myopia and astigmatism.

Ophthalmic lenses, or glasses, are commonly used to correct vision. They are also sometimes used as protective devices in sports or industrial settings.

Contact lenses are thin sheets of plastic that are made to fit the cornea, the front surface of the eye. The lenses correct vision as glasses do, while providing good peripheral vision and reducing distortion. Because they do not fog up or fall off, contacts are well-suited for those with an active lifestyle and those who do not wish to wear glasses for cosmetic reasons. The amount of daily care and cleaning varies with the type of lens.

Surgery can be used to change the eye's focus by changing the contours of the cornea. One procedure is radial keratotomy (RK), which may help those with nearsightedness and some with astigmatism. In this procedure, an ophthalmologist makes several deep incisions, or keratotomies, around the edge of the cornea in a radial, or spokelike, pattern. This flattens out the cornea and shortens the eye. It is estimated that approximately 90 percent of people who undergo RK will have their vision improved to at least 20/40.

CHOOSING AN EYE SPECIALIST

There are three main types of professionals who specialize in eye care.

1. *Ophthalmologist.* An ophthalmologist is the only medical doctor with special training and skill to diagnose and treat all diseases of the eye. Typically, an ophthalmologist has completed medical school, an internship, and at least three years of specialized training, called a residency. Board-certified ophthalmologists have also passed an examination from the American Board of Ophthalmology.

2. *Optometrist.* This is a doctor of optometry (but not a physician) whose main duty is to determine the need for corrective lenses. Optometrists have completed college and four years of optometry school. They are licensed in all states to use pharmaceuticals to diagnose eye diseases, and in most states they may prescribe drugs. They cannot perform surgery and generally refer those with serious conditions to ophthalmologists.

3. *Optician.* An optician is trained to follow the eyeglass prescription written by an ophthalmologist or optometrist, grind lenses, and help fit them to the wearer. Opticians in some states can fit and dispense contact lenses. However, opticians cannot examine eyes or prescribe corrections.

Complications of RK may include infection, difficulty fitting contact lenses, glare or starbursts around the eyes, temporarily fluctuating vision and the need for additional surgery or corrective lenses. RK is not effective for people with severe myopia, and there is concern that it may weaken the cornea, making it more vulnerable to rupture if it were to receive a direct hit. In addition, some people who have the surgery experience overcorrection of their vision and need reading glasses for farsightedness. RK is an outpatient procedure.

The newest procedure is photorefractive keratectomy (PRK), which was approved by the Food and Drug Administration (FDA) in 1995 for mild to moderate cases of nearsightedness. In this procedure, a laser is used to scrape a few thousandths of an inch of tissue off the surface of the cornea with high-energy, ultraviolet radiation. The outpatient procedure takes about fifteen minutes, with eyedrops used to anesthetize the cornea. PRK is said to improve vision to 20/40 (about the level needed to drive a car) in some 90 percent of patients. The price of PRK is estimated at $1,500 to $2,500 per eye.

Studies indicate that it may take several months to bring one's vision up to par after PRK, while RK works within days. After PRK, the eye may be painful and teary for several days until the corneal epithelium grows back. While there is some initial improvement in vision, it takes three to six months until healing is complete. More than 70 percent of patients report some halo glare after PRK, especially at night, in the first few months after the surgery.

In addition, 3 to 7 percent of patients in the trials experienced complications. Shaving away the cornea holds a risk of scarring and hazy vision. In 1 to 3 percent of patients, vision becomes worse. According to the FDA, some 4 percent of patients have hazy vision for up to a year after PRK. The FDA also cautions patients that the procedure cannot be reversed.

If you're considering RK or PRK, talk with a practitioner about the pros and cons of the procedure. Ask about side effects and risks and find out if your expectations for the surgery are realistic. Also, be sure to get a second opinion: because the expensive procedures take such little time, there's a risk that they'll be pressed on consumers by overeager doctors.

Floaters and Flashes

A floater is a tiny clump of gel or cellular debris within the clear jellylike fluid, called the vitreous humor, that fills the eye. The small clumps cast shadows on the retina, creating small, fuzzy black spots that appear to be floating in front of the eye. They occur as the vitreous humor degenerates, usually during middle age. However, they are also common in those who are nearsighted and in people who have had cataract or laser eye surgery.

Floaters are not serious, only annoying. Eventually, the brain learns to compensate for the floaters, and they become less noticeable. There is no treatment for floaters. You can move floaters temporarily out of your field of vision by rapidly moving your eyes back and forth. This pushes the floaters out of the center of the vitreous humor, out of your line of vision.

Flashes occur when the vitreous humor rubs or pulls on the retina. These, too, are no cause for concern if there are no other symptoms

and occur more frequently with age. However, if flashes are persistent and are accompanied by a number of new floaters, this could indicate a torn retina, a serious condition that requires immediate treatment.

Torn and Detached Retinas

A retinal detachment is a separation within the retina. It occurs when a hole or tear in the retina allows vitreous fluid to leak inside. The fluid may cause the retina to detach from the back of the eye, something like wallpaper peeling off a wall. It's estimated that between eighteen and thirty thousand Americans develop detached retinas each year. Those at risk for detach retinas include those with glaucoma, diabetes, acquired immune deficiency syndrome (AIDS), a family history of the condition, and those who have had eye surgery or eye trauma.

Symptoms include flashes of light or sparks followed by numerous small floaters or spots. It can be diagnosed by an eye-care professional during an eye examination. Because a tear can lead to a loss of vision, prompt surgery is usually recommended to correct the problem. This surgery can be done by using a laser or by using cryotherapy (or freezing) to seal the retina back into place. Alternatively, a gas bubble may be injected into the vitreous space inside the eye to force the retina back into place. As a rule, these procedures are successful.

Color Blindness

Color blindness, an inherited genetic condition, is the result of mutations in the photopigment gene. Color blindness occurs when the pigment in certain cones (the retinal cells responsible for central and color vision) of the eye is missing, the pigment is abnormal, or those cones that have pigment do not work as well as others. Color blindness is far more common in men than in women, with about one in twelve men (but only one in two hundred women) in North America and Europe being born with some form of color blindness.

The variation of pigment accounts for different types of color blindness, but in most cases only one cone is affected and leads to a problem distinguishing between red and green. Those with red-green color blindness are known as protanopes. Deuteranopes make mistakes with blue-greens and purples. Tritanopes confuse yellow with violet. Tetartanopes confuse yellow with blue. Some color blind people have trouble distinguishing light tints and dark shades.

There are color vision defects that develop as the result of lesion of the macula, optic nerve, or visual cortex. Also, eye changes from cataracts or the toxic effect of chemicals can alter color perception.

Diagnosis and Treatment

Most people with color blindness realize their condition without a doctor's diagnosis. However, color blindness can be diagnosed with simple tests that involve picking out a shape from a different color background. Those with color blindness will not be able to see the shape.

There is no treatment for color blindness, but people who have grown up with the condition usually adjust and perceive colors from other clues such as the position of traffic lights.

Age-Related Macular Degeneration (AMD)

The leading cause of blindness in people over 60 and a normal part of the aging process, AMD is damage or a breakdown of the macula, the tiny area in the center of the retina that's responsible for central vision. This disease affects distance and close central vision, making activities such as reading difficult or impossible.

About 90 to 95 percent of AMD is "dry," or characterized by the slow breakdown and death of the layer of light-sensing (photoreceptor) cells in the macula. The remaining cases are from "wet" AMD, in which abnormal new blood vessels grow and leak beneath the macula. Although "wet" AMD accounts for a small percentage of cases, it is responsible for 90 percent of all blindness from AMD.

Risk Factors

According to the National Advisory Eye Council and the National Eye Institute, approximately 1.7 million people over the age of 65 in the United States in 1995 had some visual impairment as a result of AMD, with about a hundred thousand of those having rapid loss of vision. Men have a lower risk of developing AMD than women, but smoking and genetic factors may play a role in the development of AMD. Some studies also found an association between AMD and hypertension, cardiovascular disease, atherosclerosis, hyperopia, light skin and eye color, and cataracts.

Symptoms

While AMD is painless, the most common symptom is blurred vision, particularly in dim light. With "wet" AMD, straight lines appear crooked because fluid from the leaking blood vessels gathers and lifts the macula. In both cases, a small blind spot may form permanently in the middle of the field of vision.

Diagnosis

There are several tests an eye-care professional can administer to detect AMD:

- Your macula can be examined for damage through an ophthalmoscope, an instrument used in eye examinations to give a clear view of the retina and macula.

- You can be shown an Amsler grid, which is similar to graph paper but has a dot in the center. You'll be asked if you see wavy lines or blind spots in your central vision.

- A fluorescein angiogram will detect abnormal blood vessels under the retina. In this procedure, a fluorescent dye is injected into your arm, and the retina is photographed as the dye passes through the blood vessels in the back of the eye.

Treatment

There's no treatment for "dry" AMD, which takes many years to impair vision seriously. "Wet" AMD, which is far more destructive, may be stopped with laser surgery if caught in the first few weeks after onset. This treatment, photocoagulation, involves aiming a laser light onto the back of the eye, sealing leaking membranes, and destroying new blood vessels through concentrated heat. The procedure is fairly effective, leaving a scar that creates a blind spot but stops the creation of new blood vessels in some people. In others, it only delays the disease's progress for a year or two because recurrent blood vessels form on the edge of the scar. According to the National Eye Institute, only 25 percent of "wet" AMD patients benefit from photocoagulation since those who are leaking blood through the fovea, or center of the macula, cannot be treated by lasers.

PREVENTING AMD

AMD may be somewhat preventable by avoiding smoking and harsh sunlight. Always wear sunglasses that block ultraviolet rays. And recent studies have found that there's a significantly lower risk of "wet" AMD among people who eat a diet rich in dark green, leafy vegetables and yellow or red vegetables—foods high in the antioxidant vitamins A, C, and E. Lowering your intake of saturated fats and cholesterol-rich foods also may lower your risk of AMD.

Diabetic Retinopathy

The most common diabetic eye disease, retinopathy is a condition in which the blood vessels in the retina are diseased and may swell and leak fluid. In others, new blood vessels grow on the surface of the retina. Either way, these changes result in vision loss or blindness.

Diabetic retinopathy is the most common cause of vision loss in Americans age 20 to 74. According to the National Eye Institute, 8,000 Americans become blind each year as a result of diabetic eye disorders. Most people with diabetes develop some degree of retinopathy during their lifetimes.

Diabetic retinopathy begins as nonproliferative, or background, retinopathy, which is the mild form of the disease that doesn't usually affect vision. The small blood vessels in the central retina gradually narrow and weaken, and small bulges, or microaneurysms, develop on the vessels. Eventually, theses bulges tear or break and then bleed. The greatest threat at this stage is that the fluid from the vessels may leak into the macula and cause it to swell, putting pressure on other areas of the eye. This leads to blurred vision.

If the retinopathy progresses to proliferative retinopathy, the new blood vessels branch out in and around the retina. Eventually the vessels tear and leak blood into the vitreous humor. As the eye tries to repair the damage, scar tissue forms, damaging the retina and resulting in partial loss of sight. In advanced cases, the vitreous humor may pull the retina away from the back of the eye, resulting in total vision loss.

Diabetic retinopathy can often be prevented with the control of blood-sugar levels and high blood pressure, a healthy diet, good eye care, and by not smoking.

Diagnosis

If you have diabetes and experience blurred vision, light flashes, changes in color vision or contrast sensitivity—the ability to discern an object from its background—see an eye-care professional for an examination. Early detection is important in the treatment of diabetic retinopathy, so a yearly eye examination is recommended for anyone with diabetes.

Treatment

In the early stages of diabetic retinopathy, photocoagulation, the laser procedure used for age-related macular degeneration, is used. In advanced stages, photocoagulation may be used along with a high-risk operation known as vitrectomy. In this procedure, an ophthalmologist removes blood and membranes that may be blocking vision from the vitreous humor and cuts the scar tissue that can cause the retina to detach. The extracted vitreous body and blood are then replaced with saline or air or other gases or occasionally with silicone oil.

Cataracts

A cataract is a clouding in the transparent lens of the eye that blocks or distorts light, causing loss of vision. The lens consists mostly of water and protein. Eventually, some of the protein may clump together and start to cloud a small area of the lens, creating an area called an opacity. Over time the opacities increase in number, clouding more of the lens, until the amount of light entering the eye and striking the retina is markedly reduced.

Cataracts are a normal part of aging and rarely occur in the young. The process may begin in a person's forties or fifties, but usually it isn't until the sixties that vision is affected. According to the U.S. Department of Health and Human Services, about half of Americans ages 65 to 74, and about 70 percent of those age 75 and older, have cataracts.

Opacities initially form in different parts of the lens, so there are different types of cataracts. Nuclear sclerosis, the most common type of opacity, is a condition in which the nucleus gradually becomes more dense and opaque. A cortical cataract makes the outer shell of the lens become more opaque. And when most clouding is centered on the back surface of the lens, it's a posterior subcapsular cataract.

Risk Factors

People with diabetes under the age of 70 have a 30 to 40 percent greater chance of having a cataract than a person without diabetes. Malnutrition and certain medical problems can lead to cataracts. There is some risk involved with treating conditions such as asthma and arthritis with steroids, since steroid use may result in cataracts in some people. A cataract can result from an injury to the eye or ongoing exposure to intense heat or electric shock. Plus, the use of alcohol, smoking, and exposure to ultraviolet light, x-rays, and radiation have been linked to cataract formation. In fact, recent studies show that people who spend a lot of time in the sun develop cataracts earlier than others. A high dietary intake of vitamin A may reduce the risk of cataracts.

Symptoms

The most common symptom of cataracts is cloudy or blurred vision—almost as though you're looking through water (*cataract* means "waterfall" in Latin). Other changes start slowly and become more noticeable over time—colors look faded or yellow and there may be glare from sunlight, the light from a lamp or an oncoming car's headlights at night.

Diagnosis

A routine eye exam will diagnose cataracts. The Snellen chart test (the familiar test with rows of different-size letters) gives a measure of your visual acuity. In the slit-lamp exam, the eye-care professional focuses a vertical slit of light onto your cataract to see how dense the cataract is and to determine whether your cornea is healthy enough to withstand surgery if recommended.

Treatment

Currently, there are no nonsurgical treatments that can restore the natural lens to its clear state. About 1.35 million Americans have cataract surgery each year, according to the National Eye Institute. Improvements in surgical techniques now allow for removal of cataracts at any stage, although minimum standards are agreed upon in the medical profession. Vision must be reduced to 20/40 before surgery will be considered.

There are three main types of cataract surgery:

1. *Intracapsular.* The lens is removed entirely. This procedure is obsolete and primarily used in developing countries these days.

2. *Extracapsular.* Through a small incision, the cataract is removed in parts with a scalpel, and the nucleus is removed in one piece.

3. *Photoemulsification* (PE). In this most advanced, and most common, procedure, the nucleus is broken up and liquefied by the vibrations of a handheld ultrasound probe. Then it's aspired through a needle. The incision is very small and sometimes there are no stitches needed.

Every cataract extraction is followed with the implantation of a plastic lens, usually in the space between the iris and the vitreous humor, to correct blurry vision. It's held in place by two spring-like fibers. To picture it, imagine a contact lens with a question mark extending from the top and bottom.

After surgery, vision usually is restored in a matter of weeks. Cataract surgery improves vision in 90 to 95 percent of all cases, although vision is not restored to 20/20. In fact, most people who undergo cataract surgery can expect to wear eyeglasses or contact lenses for the rest of their lives. Cataracts cannot grow back.

Glaucoma

Glaucoma is a disease of the optic nerve, the bundle of nerves that carries images from the retina to the brain. In most cases of glaucoma, the normal fluid pressure inside the eyes, known as the intraocular pressure (IOP) slowly rises and puts direct pressure on optic nerve fibers. Untreated, the disease may lead to vision loss, as the fibers die, or even to blindness.

The space between the iris and cornea is filled with a clear solution called the aqueous humor that is produced by ciliary tissues around the lens. Normally, this fluid flows out of the inner part of the eye through the pupil and then is absorbed into the bloodstream through the trabecular meshwork—the system of tiny drainage canals all around the outer end of the iris. This continual production, flow, and drainage help bathe and nourish the lens, iris, and cornea. (This is not the same as tears.)

According to the National Eye Institute, about two million people in the United States have glaucoma, and 80,000 are blind from open-angle glaucoma. Glaucoma is the third leading cause of blindness in the United States, behind macular degeneration and cataracts. Men have a higher rate of glaucoma but a lower rate of eye pressure than women. And while high IOP has come to be equated with glaucoma, there are cases where people with high IOP never develop glaucoma.

Glaucoma can affect anyone, but it's most common in people over age 60. It is also five times more prevalent among African Americans than whites. A family history of the disease, high blood pressure, and smoking may be risk factors for glaucoma.

Open-Angle Glaucoma

Open-angle glaucoma is where the fluid drains too slowly out of the eye. In this condition, the angle where the iris meets the cornea is as wide and open as it should be, and the entrances to the drainage canals are clear. The problem is that the drainage canals are clogged inside. About 90 percent of people with glaucoma have this type.

Open-angle glaucoma is a chronic condition that progresses slowly as the eye's drainage canals become more and more clogged and the pressure within the eye gradually increases. Usually this buildup happens without pain or discomfort. It may takes years before there is any visual change. Age seems to bring on this disorder, but no one knows why it develops.

Closed-Angle Glaucoma

Closed-angle glaucoma is a rare structural problem that occurs when the drainage canals may be blocked altogether. The angle between the iris and cornea is not as wide and open as it should be. Therefore, when the pupil enlarges too much or too quickly, the outer edge of the iris impinges on the drainage canals. An acute condition, closed-angle glaucoma can suddenly change for the worse. Symptoms and damage are usually very noticeable: blurred vision, severe headaches or eye pain, nausea and vomiting, and rainbow halos around lights at night.

Diagnosis

The primary test for glaucoma is tonometry, which measures the IOP. This may be done with an air tonometer, which directs a puff of air against the eye and measures the time it takes to flatten the cornea. However, this has been largely superseded by newer types of tonometers. After numbing the eye with anesthetic drops, the practitioner presses the instrument lightly against the cornea. The pressure causes a slight indentation, and the tonometer registers the eye's resistance.

Since pressure isn't always a sign of glaucoma, the other standard test is ophthalmoscopy, which allows the practitioner to see whether the optic nerve has been damaged. The eye-care professional may also use a slit-lamp microscope to inspect the drainage system and optic nerve for signs of damage.

If pressures are high or the optic nerve looks unusual, most doctors will do one or two special glaucoma tests. Perimetry is a test that produces a map of the complete field of vision. A computer flashes points of light around a bowl-shaped area while the individual touches a switch as soon as he thinks he sees the light, however dim. Perimetry is useful because it detects very small changes in peripheral vision, where glaucoma makes its first inroads.

Gonioscopy is done by numbing the cornea and placing a handheld contact lens on the eye. This allows the doctor to look sideways into the eye to check whether the angle where the iris meets the cornea is open or closed.

Treatment

Treatment is started if the pressure in both eyes is more than 30 mm/Hg and the optic nerve is cupped, or the visual field map shows some abnormal patterns that are typical of glaucoma damage. Some eye-care practitioners withhold treatment from those with mildly or moderately elevated IOP until there's evidence of glaucomatous damage. They do this because only a small portion of patients actually develop damage, and the cost and side effects of treatment are considerable.

The main objective of treatment is to lower IOP, either by decreasing the amount of aqueous humor that's produced or by increasing its outflow. For open-angle glaucoma, that's typically done with both eyedrops and pills that fall into the categories of beta blockers, epinephrine-related drugs, miotics or carbonic anhydrase inhibitors. Treatment for glaucoma is for a lifetime, so the effectiveness of the drugs will decrease over time, and new ones will have to be prescribed. And glaucoma medications may cause side effects such as breathing problems, mental and physical lethargy, irregular heartbeat, high blood pressure, and headaches. While the degree of side effects will vary from person to person, most should become less noticeable after a week or two of using the medication.

Recent research has established that laser therapy may be a more effective treatment since it's relatively noninvasive. The procedure known as trabeculoplasty burns 100 tiny holes in the trabecular meshwork, allowing the aqueous humor to drain faster from the eye. Laser treatment may only be performed once for glaucoma and is not a cure, so medication and possibly microsurgery become necessary.

During microsurgery, a tiny piece of the iris is removed in a preventive iridectomy. Then, in a procedure called a trabeculectomy or sclerostomy, the surgeon makes a tiny opening in the sclera, the white part of the eye. This new opening allows the aqueous humor to bypass the clogged drainage canals.

Certain behaviors can help to control glaucoma, including regular aerobic exercise to lower IOP, not smoking, and maintaining normal blood pressure. And researchers are investigating the possibility that open-angle glaucoma may be controlled or prevented by consuming antioxidant nutrients found in dark green leafy and yellow or red vegetables such as broccoli, spinach, and carrots.

For more information:

American Academy of Ophthalmology
P.O. Box 7424
San Francisco, CA 94120-7424
415-561-8500

American Foundation for the Blind
11 Penn Plaza, Suite 300
New York, NY 10001
800-232-5463

American Optometric Association
243 N. Lindbergh Blvd.
St. Louis, MO 63141
314-991-4101

Association for Macular Diseases
210 E. 64th St.
New York, NY 10021
212-605-3719

Glaucoma Research Foundation
490 Post St., Suite 830
San Francisco, CA 94102
800-826-6693
415-986-3162

Lighthouse National Center for Vision and Aging
111 E. 59th St.
New York, NY 10022
800-334-5497
http://www.lighthouse.org

National Eye Health Education Program
National Eye Institute
National Institutes of Health
Box 20/20
Bethesda, MD 20892
301-496-4001

FOOT CONDITIONS

The fifty-two bones in your two feet—twenty-six in each—account for one quarter of the bones in your body. According to the American Podiatric Medical Association, the average person takes eight thousand to ten thousand steps each day. Over a lifetime, these steps add up to about 115,000 miles—more than four times around the earth's circumference. Given these figures, it's no wonder that 75 percent of Americans will suffer from foot health problems at least once in their lives.

Podiatric physicians, also known as a podiatrists, are licensed health-care professionals who specialize in the care of feet. These practitioners are not medical doctors; instead, they have undergone a four-year course of study for the degree of doctor of podiatric medicine (D.P.M.) They provide 39 percent of all foot care. (Orthopedic physicians provide 13 percent, physical therapists and others provide 11 percent, and all other physicians provide 37 percent.) Podiatrists are trained to care for all of the following foot disorders.

Athlete's Foot

Athlete's foot, or *tinea pedis*, is a common fungal infection of the feet. It occurs most frequently among teenage and adult males. Symptoms of athlete's foot include peeling, cracking, and itching skin, especially between the toes.

A pair of feet contains approximately 250,000 sweat glands and excretes up to a half-pint of moisture each day. For this reason, feet are a great home for the athlete's foot-causing fungus, which thrives in moist, damp places. Not drying feet well after swimming or bathing and wearing tight shoes and socks can contribute to the development of athlete's foot, as can sweaty feet and a warm climate. Athlete's foot does not usually affect people who regularly walk barefoot because their feet stay well ventilated. Athlete's foot is commonly thought to be very contagious, easily contracted just from walking barefoot in the locker room (hence, its name). However, experimental, unsuccessful attempts to infect healthy skin with athlete's foot have proved otherwise. For unknown reasons, some people are very susceptible to athlete's foot whereas others can have the fungus on their skin and never develop an infection.

Most of the time, athlete's foot will not disappear by itself but instead will cause the skin to blister or crack, leaving it susceptible to bacterial infection. In recent years, several former prescription treatments have become available over-the-counter to relieve the cracking, burning, and itching of athlete's foot. These antifungal creams and powders should be applied for the entire length of time directed even if the symptoms subside.

Athlete's foot can be prevented by following these easy instructions:

- Wash your feet at least once a day.

- Keep your feet thoroughly dry. After showering, you may want to apply cornstarch or powder to the toes to absorb moisture.

- Avoid tight shoes, especially in warm weather. Sandals are the best summer footwear.

- Wear cotton socks, rather than those made of synthetic materials. White socks are better than colored socks, which can add to heat buildup inside shoes. Change socks at least once a day.

- Expose your feet to light and air as much as you can. Go barefoot at home if possible. However, if you are prone to athlete's foot, don't go barefoot in locker rooms or around swimming pools where you could come into contact with the fungus.

- Sprinkle an antifungal powder into your shoes during warm months.

Calluses

A callus is a buildup of dead, thickened, yellowish-red skin that cushions the foot from excess pressure (often a result of being overweight) and friction (caused by ill-fitting shoes). Calluses usually form on the ball of the foot, the heel, or the underside of the big toe. Provided they do not hurt or become infected, calluses are no cause for worry.

Some calluses, however, have a deep-seated "core," or *nucleation*, which can make them very painful when they are under pressure. Painful calluses may be caused by a poorly aligned bone or crooked toe. A dropped metatarsal (when one of the small, round bones behind the toes is much lower than the ones on either side of it), bunions, hammertoes, and other biomechanical problems can also cause more serious calluses.

Most calluses can be corrected simply by wearing comfortable shoes. Losing weight may also help reduce pressure. A nonmedicated callus pad or a moleskin—a soft cloth with one velvety side and one sticky side—can be used to cover the callus and alleviate discomfort. To soften a callus, soak the foot daily in warm water and use an abrasive brush or pumice stone (a rough-edged stone that can be purchased in a drugstore) to flake away dead skin. Apply a moisturizing cream to the area a few times daily.

Podiatrist Suzanne M. Levine of the New York College of Podiatric Medicine suggests the following solution for getting rid of unwanted calluses. Mix five or six crushed aspirin tablets with one tablespoon of lemon juice and apply the paste to the callus. Put the entire foot into a plastic bag and cover it with a warm towel for at least ten minutes. Unwrap the foot and use a pumice stone to scrub the callus and flake away the dead skin.

In extreme cases, calluses can be cut away by a podiatrist. However, if the pressure or friction that caused the callus continues, the callus will recur.

Corns

A corn is a hard, thickened, round, yellow area of the skin's surface layer. Corns usually form on or between the toes. As corns thicken, the tissues underneath may become very irritated. Like some calluses, corns may have a deep core where the corn is thickest and most painful. A corn that is swollen, reddish, or painful has become inflamed.

Corns are the result of friction and pressure on the feet. This pressure can be caused by tight-fitting shoes or socks, deformed and crooked toes, a seam or stitch inside the shoe that rubs against a toe, a too-loose shoe in which the foot slides forward with each step or prolonged walking on a declining slope.

If a corn constantly rubs against the side of a shoe, it will grow and become painful. Pain may also stem from friction between a corn and a bone where a bursa lies. Bursa are fluid-filled sacs that overlay and protect joints in the body. If such friction occurs, the bursa will become swollen and painful.

Despite the claims of television commercials, over-the-counter corn removal remedies do not work. Most of them contain salicylic acid, a caustic substance that can cause blisters and infection, in addition to the primary corn problem.

To treat a corn at home, soak the foot in warm water and Epsom salts. Then apply moisturizing cream and wrap the area in plastic for at least fifteen minutes. After removing the plastic, rub the corn with a pumice stone in a side-to-side motion to remove the hard skin. Nonmedicated pads applied around the corn may relieve pain-causing pressure.

The pain relief provided by treatment of corns will be temporary if pressure and friction continue. The only lasting solution to alleviate the pain of corns and prevent the development of more corns is to buy shoes that do not cramp the feet. When corns are caused by an imbalance in the feet, a podiatrist might recommend custom-made orthotic inserts. In severe cases, a podiatrist might also recommend that crooked or deformed toes or bony prominences be surgically straightened.

Warts

A wart is a hard, circular, benign tumor that is skin-colored and rough to the touch. There are several different kinds of warts. Those that develop on the feet—usually on the soles—are called plantar warts. They tend to grow in clusters, but they also can appear alone. Blood vessels that feed the wart often are visible as black dots. When pressure is applied at its sides, a wart is more painful than a corn or callus.

Blisters

A blister is actually a protective device that defends against friction between a shoe and the skin of a foot. Once a blister has formed, it is best to leave it alone and allow it to heal on its own. According to the American Podiatric Medical Association, blisters should not be popped. Apply moleskin or an adhesive bandage to the blister and leave it on until it falls off on its own, most likely in a bath or shower. Keep feet dry and always wear socks to provide a cushion between your feet and shoes. If a blister breaks, clean the area with alcohol or an iodine solution, apply an antibiotic cream, and cover it with a sterile bandage. To avoid blisters, steer clear of shoes that are too short or too narrow.

Bunions

A bunion is a bony bump on the edge of the big toe that causes the joint to become inflamed. It often causes the big toe to drift toward the smaller toes, even resting under or over the second toe. Symptoms of a bunion include redness, swelling, and pain along the inside of the foot, just behind the big toe.

Bunions are one of the most common deformities of the forefoot. A common cause of bunions is an abnormality in foot function, for example, a turned-out joint at the base of the big toe. People with a family history of bunions are thought to be genetically predisposed to developing them. Rheumatoid and psoriatic arthritis are other possible contributing factors. Tight-fitting shoes can also accelerate the formation of a bunion. Bunions are more common in women than in men, possibly due to differences in foot shape and hormone levels and the use of high-heeled shoes.

A painful bunion is caused by friction and inflammation of the toe's bursal sac, which can lead to bursitis. To relieve pressure on bunions, wear wide sandals or shoes with a wide and deep toe box or with a hole cut out of them. Orthotic inserts, special insoles, or arch supports may also be helpful.

The best way to treat painful, red, swollen bunions is to apply an ice pack three to four times a day for fifteen to twenty minutes each time. Another way to reduce inflammation is to soak the feet (bunions often appear on both feet) in warm water and vinegar (1 cup per gallon of water). Use nonmedicated commercial bunion pads (available at drugstores) if you wish to protect bunions from shoe pressure.

Besides applying special pads and dressings, a podiatrist may inject steroid and local anesthetic around a bunion to reduce swelling. He or she may also use splints or digital orthotics to realign the big toe joint. Other possible podiatric treatments include ultrasound, electrogalvanic stimulation, paraffin baths, and whirlpool massages. Bunion surgery—which usually is done in the podiatrist's office—is the only way to correct the deformity, thus completely eliminating the bunion.

Hammertoe

A hammertoe is a deformity of one of the middle toes—most often the second—in which the joint becomes bent and twisted into a claw like

CARING FOR YOUR FEET

Here a few easy things you can do to keep your feet healthy, clean, and odor-free:

- Wash your feet daily and be sure to dry them thoroughly.

- Examine your feet regularly for calluses, corns, and other disorders.

- Trim your toenails straight across with clippers designed for toenails. Leave nails slightly longer than the ends of your toes.

- Always wear comfortable shoes. Afternoon is the best time to shop for shoes because feet swell during the day. Be sure to try on both shoes; one foot may be larger than the other, and you should fit the larger one.

- Change your shoes daily to allow each pair to air out. Change your socks at least once a day, more often if your feet sweat a lot.

- To eliminate foot odor, try soaking your feet in a vinegar and water solution. Foot powders and antiperspirants might also do the trick.

- Massage your feet frequently.

- Take up walking. It's excellent exercise for your feet as well as for your entire body.

- To prevent injury, wear protective footwear (such as steel-toed boots) when using power machines such as lawnmowers and chainsaws and when moving heavy objects.

position. Hammertoe usually stems from muscle imbalance. The two types of hammertoe are flexible (the joint can be straightened with the fingers) and rigid. The most common cause of hammertoe is heredity—congenital foot shapes such as a high arch or a sagging arch. The condition may also result from injury.

To relieve the pain of hammertoe, which is caused by an aggravated bursal sac, cover the area with padding such as a corn pad, lamb's wool, or a bandage. Minor surgery may be necessary to correct hammertoe. Soft tissue or tendon surgery is performed on flexible hammertoe. Rigid hammertoe may require the removal of a small piece of bone. Both surgeries are in-office procedures that require the wearing of a splint or surgical shoe for one to four weeks afterward.

Ingrown Toenails

Ingrown toenails occur when toenails cut into the skin along the margin of the nails. Signs of infection include redness, swelling, increased warmth, and pain. The most common cause of ingrown toenails is improper trimming. Toenails should always be cut straight across—never on a curve—and they should not be cut too short. Tight-fitting shoes or socks are another cause.

An ingrown toenail will usually heal if pressure is kept off of it, so wear sandals or shoes with a hole cut in them. Discomfort might be somewhat relieved by soaking the area in a basin of warm water two to three times daily. If the nail becomes infected, try soaking it in a water and iodine solution, cut or trim the nail if necessary, clean the nail groove and apply an antibiotic cream. If pain persists, see a physician or podiatrist. Minor surgery may be necessary to drain infection, surgically correct a chronic ingrown toenail, or remove a deformed toenail so that it will not grow back.

Aching Arches and Plantar Fascitis

A common cause of aching arches and deep pain on the bottom surface of the heel is plantar fascitis, or inflammation of the plantar fascia. The plantar fascia is a wide band of tissue that extends along the sole of the foot from the heel to the toes. It helps to secure the arch. Heel spurs—calcium deposits at the point where the plantar fascia meets the heels bone—are commonly associated with plantar fascitis, which can be exacerbated by obesity.

The arches of walking feet should dip only slightly when the feet roll from the heel toward the toes. If the arches touch the ground, pain will most likely result. Besides plantar fascitis, aching arches can be caused by ligaments, arthritis, flat-footedness, a change of routine, and tendinitis (inflammation of tendons in the feet). Rest and ice are the best treatments for aching arches and heel pain. An elastic bandage wrapped around the arch may help support it, as will shoes with extra arch supports and insoles. If pain persists, see a physician or podiatrist.

For more information:

American Academy of Orthopedic Surgeons
6300 N. River Road
Rosemont, IL 60018-4262
847-823-7186

American Academy of Podiatric Sports Medicine
1729 Glastonberry Rd.
Potomac, MD 20854
800-438-3355

American Podiatric Medical Association
9312 Old Georgetown Rd.
Bethesda, MD 20814
800-FOOTCARE
301-571-9200
http://www.apma.org

GALLBLADDER DISEASE

The gallbladder is a small organ located underneath the liver on the right side of the body. The major function of the pear-shaped sac is to store a digestive-aiding substance called bile and secrete it into the small intestines and other organs when it is needed to help break down food.

Bile is produced by the liver and contains various substances such as fats, cholesterol, and salts. It travels to the gallbladder through the common bile duct (which also leads to the small intestines) and the cystic duct, a small duct that branches off the common bile duct. Three cups of bile can be made by the liver each day, and the gallbladder can store about one cup of concentrated bile.

During digestion, the muscular gallbladder contracts and releases stored bile back through the cystic duct into the common bile duct, where it travels to the intestines to aid digestion. The bile is absorbed in the intestine and returns to the liver through the bloodstream.

Gallstones

The most common form of gallbladder disease is gallstones. These hard, solid lumps form when materials in the bile such as cholesterol and pigments turn hard and crystallize. Gallstones can form as a result of various factors, including a buildup of bile in the gallbladder, an overload of cholesterol in the bile, or the existence of proteins in the bile and liver that promote crystallization. Contrary to possible belief, too much calcium in the diet does not cause gallstones.

Types of stones include cholesterol stones and pigment stones. Cholesterol stones account for 80 percent of the total number of gallstones.

They are white or yellow and composed mostly of cholesterol. These are formed when the bile is too high in cholesterol and there are not enough salts present to keep the concentration liquid. Pigment stones are made mostly from calcium salts and account for roughly 20 percent of all gallstones. Pigment stones can cause conditions such as the formation of fibrous liver tissue, which results in the loss of functional liver cells (cirrhosis), digestive tract infections, and heredity blood cell disorders. A person with mixed stones has both pigment stones and cholesterol stones.

Gallstones can be produced in a vast array of sizes, some extremely small and others as large as a golf ball. The number of stones may vary from one stone to up to several thousand in some cases.

Risk Factors

Yearly, over one million United States residents will discover that they have gallstones. It is estimated that 10 percent of the American population—about twenty million people—have gallstones. However, women are two to three times more likely to have gallstones than men, especially during ages 20 to 69 because pregnancy, oral contraceptives, and estrogen replacement therapy increase the risk for gallstones. However, once men reach the age of 65, their chances of having a gallstone greatly increase.

Also at risk are people who suffer from obesity because they tend to have more cholesterol in their bile. They also tend to release bile more slowly. This, in turn, leads to the formation of stones. Extensive fasting, rapid weight loss, and an extremely low-calorie diet also tends to bring

---

PREVENTING GALLSTONES

- Maintain a healthy weight. Those who are overweight are six times more likely to get gallstones than those at a healthy weight.

- Lose weight slowly. Rapid weight loss boosts the levels of cholesterol in the blood, meaning more cholesterol will end up in the bile, promoting gallstone formation. Weight lost a few pounds at a time is also more likely to stay off.

- Don't fast or use crash diets. If you don't eat, bile is not released to help aid digestion and builds up in the gallbladder.

- Eat small meals several times a day. This results in a regular release of bile from the gallbladder. However, do not use this advice as an excuse to eat several regular meals. Instead, spread your regular calorie intake out over the course of the day.

- Watch your cholesterol. Again, high levels of blood cholesterol mean that the bile may become saturated with cholesterol, leading to gallstones.

- Get plenty of fiber. Studies show that men who eat fiber release bile from their gallbladders more often and have fewer gallstones. Good sources of fiber include whole-grain products, fruits, and vegetables.

about gallstones. It is believed that foods high in starch, fiber, and cholesterol lead to gallbladder stones when eaten in excess. Native Americans have the greatest amount of risk for developing stones. In fact, most Native American men have gallstones by the time they reach age 60. Mexican men and women of all ages also tend to be at greatest risk.

Symptoms

Most gallstone patients have "silent stones," gallstones without symptoms. However, pain in the right, upper abdomen can occur when a gallstone comes out of the gallbladder and becomes lodged in a duct. This pain usually lasts less than an hour—though it can last several hours—until the stone drops back into the gallbladder. Gallstone pain can spread from the abdominal area to the shoulders, back, and chest on the right side of the body. For this reason, gallstone pain is often mistaken for a heart attack.

Other symptoms that may occur with gallstones include the following:

- Vomiting during attacks.

- Intermittent attacks. Gall attacks can occur weeks, months, or years apart.

- Cholecystitis. When gallstones become stuck in the cystic duct (the small duct between the gallbladder and the common bile duct), the flow of bile is blocked. This results in a condition called cholecystitis, also called inflammation of the gallbladder. This is a common problem caused by gallstones. However, a more uncommon problem occurs when gallstones get stuck in the ducts between the liver and the intestine, thus preventing bile flow from the gallbladder and liver. This results in pain and jaundice (skin turning a yellowish color) or an inflammation of the pancreas. Persistent pain, jaundice, and fever are warning signs of blockage. If these blockages remain for an extensive amount of time, irreversible damage may occur to the gallbladder, liver, and pancreas. These can be fatal.

- Intolerance of fatty foods, indigestion, frequent stomach pain and constipation should not be attributed to gallstones. A true gallstone attack occurs no more than one to three times a year.

Diagnosis

Stones can be spotted during an abdominal x-ray or ultrasound and are often first diagnosed after an x-ray is taken because of another complaint. However, when a doctor is looking specifically for gallstones, an ultrasound is the most-used tool. This entails sending sound waves through the abdomen to create an image of the gallbladder. When stones have formed, the sound waves bounce off of them and reveal their location. Ultrasounds are painless and do not involve radiation.

Treatment

The most-used treatment of gallstones is a surgical procedure called cholecystectomy. Every year, over 500,000 Americans undergo gallbladder surgery. Two types of cholecystectomy exist: the standard cholecystectomy or a procedure called a laparoscopic cholecystectomy.

A cholecystectomy entails removing the stones or the entire gallbladder if necessary, through a 5- to 8-inch incision. Hospital stay for this procedure is about a week, with additional time for recovery at home. A person can function normally without a gallbladder, and there are no known long-term ill effects from gallbladder removal.

The laparoscopic technique is used in approximately 85 percent of the current 600,000 gallbladder surgeries performed each year. It involves inserting a small surgical camera through a small incision into the abdomen, giving the surgeon a close-up picture of the patient's insides. The gallbladder is identified, and the cyst formation is removed, not the entire gallbladder. This procedure is less painful, has fewer complications, and heals more quickly than the standard procedure. There are potential side effects to both of these procedures, including infections that become potentially dangerous.

Alternatives to surgery do exist, including oral medicines such as Actigall and Chenix. These are made from natural acids located in bile and are used to help people who cannot tolerate surgery. Treatment from these medications may be required for months to years before gallstones

are dissolved, and these medications do have side effects, such as diarrhea.

Another option is a procedure called lithotripsy. In lithotripsy, the stones are broken apart into fine pieces by shock waves. The waves can be administered by using a machine called a lithotripor, which is placed against the abdomen, or while the person is seated in a tub of water, which serves to conduct the shock waves. The tiny pieces then pass out of the system with the bile. At times, medications are prescribed to help dissolve the remnants of the stones. Lithotripsy requires general or local anesthesia, but no incision.

Other Conditions

The gallbladder can also be affected by cancer. Gallbladder cancer usually affects those with gallstones, though it occurs rarely—only in three people per 100,000 each year. Symptoms include jaundice and pain in the upper right side of the

CONTROVERSIAL SURGERY

There is some controversy over which surgical gallbladder stone treatment—the cholecystectomy or the laparoscopic cholecystectomy—is more effective and necessary. Recent studies at the University of Pennsylvania found that the newest laparoscopic method is responsible for the "alarming rise" in gallbladder surgeries and that since its introduction in 1989, removals rose 22 percent.

Statistics also show that the laparoscopic technique now accounts for over 85 percent of gallstone operations each year. However, there may not be any advantage to laparoscopy over the traditional technique. An April 1996 study from the journal *Lancet* found that laparoscopic cholecystectomy offered no benefit over traditional cholecystectomy in terms of recovery time, postoperative pain, length of hospital stay, or time back to full activity. However, others studies have shown laparoscopic surgery to be more effective in reducing recovery times.

With the increasing rate of gallbladder surgery, it is wise to remember that only those suffering from severe and reoccurring gallstone attacks should undergo surgery. Talk with your practitioner about the pros and cons of each type of surgery, and be sure to get a second opinion if surgery is recommended.

abdomen, but is usually painless. As a result, it often is not diagnosed until after it has spread, making it hard to treat. Diagnosis is done by using an ultrasound, and surgery to remove the tumor is the main form of treatment.

In other rare instances, the gallbladder may be empty when it becomes blocked by a gallstone. As a result, the organ fills with mucus secreted by the gallbladder walls, creating a distended gallbladder known as a mucocele.

Congenital or genetic defects may also affect the gallbladder. For instance, a person may be born without a gallbladder, with an oversized gallbladder or with two gallbladders. These abnormalities rarely cause any physical problems.

For more information:

Digestive Disease National Coalition
507 Capital Ct., N.E., Suite 200
Washington, DC 20002
202-544-7497

National Digestive Diseases
Information Clearinghouse
2 Information Way
Bethesda, MD 20892-3570
301-654-3810
http://www.niddk.nih.gov

National Institute of Diabetes and Digestive and
Kidney Diseases
Building 31, Room 9A-04
31 Center Dr.
Bethesda, MD 20892-2560
301-496-3583
http://www.niddk.nih.gov

HAIR LOSS

If your self-esteem is following your hair down the drain, take comfort in the fact that you're not alone. For most men, hair loss is a fact of life, one that cannot be changed with medica-tions, surgery, special vitamins, or shampoos. Over two-thirds of all men will experience some degree of hair loss, or *alopecia*, in their lifetimes. Those who become bald usually have significant loss by age 35.

Male-Pattern Baldness

In most cases, hair loss can be attributed to what is known medically as *androgenetic alopecia*, commonly known as male-pattern baldness. Men with male-pattern baldness have an inherited sensitivity to androgens (male hormones). At a genetically predetermined time, the follicles in the scalp begin to convert testosterone to a hormone called dihydrotestosterone, which causes the follicles to shrink. As a result, hair grows in thinner until all that remains is vellus—fine, colorless hair that most people call "peach fuzz." (Consequently, eunuchs—castrated men whose bodies do not produce testosterone—never suffer from hair loss.)

The genetic tendency of male-pattern baldness is usually inherited from the mother's side of the family, meaning that if your mother's father was bald, you may be bald yourself. However, the tendency is passed at random. One brother may be suffering hair loss while the other still has a full head of hair.

Male-pattern baldness usually progresses as follows: (1) the hairline recedes, forming a "widow's peak"; (2) the hair on the crown also thins, eventually causing a bald spot; and (3) sometimes the receding hairline and the expanding bald spot connect, leaving only a ring of hair around the sides and back of the head.

Other Causes of Hair Loss

Temporary hair loss can be caused by serious illness, physical trauma, malnutrition, poisoning, drugs, radiation, and hormonal disorders. Scalp infections or autoimmune disorders (a disorder in which the immune system attacks the body's own tissues) can cause permanent hair loss. *Alopecia areata* is an autoimmune form of hair loss in which small, isolated clumps of hair, not necessarily from the head, fall out in patches. It can lead to *Alopecia totalis* (loss of all or nearly all hair on the head) or the rare *Alopecia universalis* (drastic loss of all body hair, including eyebrows, eyelashes, facial hair and hair on head). However, these conditions are rare.

Treatment

While male-pattern hair loss can't hurt your health, it can hurt your self-image—a problem that has lead to an excessive number of so-called hair-loss cures. Despite the Food and Drug Administration's ban on unproven hair-loss remedies, advertisements for "growing hair in just days" are just about everywhere you look. Are these concoctions miracle cures? Certainly not. In most cases, they are not even remotely effective. If you're looking for a treatment, be

COMMON MYTHS ABOUT BALDNESS

Myth: Eat right and your hair will grow.

Fact: There's no evidence that any special diet, vitamin, or mineral supplement will make hair grow thicker or faster. In fact, too much vitamin A can hinder hair growth, and gross deficiencies of iron, biotin, zinc, or even fat—all of which can be caused by crash diets—can cause temporary hair loss.

Myth: Special hair-loss shampoos can cause hair growth.

Fact: The "special" ingredients in these concoctions might cleanse the hair you have, but they're not going to produce any more. Hair-loss shampoos are nothing but suds. Don't be duped into spending the $300 to $450 a six-month supply costs.

Myth: Wash more, lose more.

Fact: The old tale that frequent shampooing increases hair loss is all fiction and no fact. However, take care when washing or drying your hair—vigorous rubbing can pull loose strands out.

Myth: Scalp massages stimulate hair growth.

Fact: No study contains evidence to support this claim. In fact, if anything, massaging too much can inflame the hair follicles and speed hair loss.

Myth: Hair loss can be caused by wearing a tight hat that prevents the scalp from "breathing."

Fact: Scalps don't need to "breathe." Hair follicles get oxygen from the blood. There is no evidence that tight hats or football helmets restrict blood flow to the point of affecting hair growth.

Myth: Shaving makes hair grow back thicker.

Fact: Hair grows in the hair follicles, not in the portion of the hair shaft above the skin. That part of the shaft is dead, and cutting it does not affect the growth rate of the live portion beneath it.

skeptical. Chances are you'll have to resign yourself to losing your hair.

Medications. The good news is that minoxidil (brand name Rogaine)—the only approved drug that's proven partially effective in hair-loss treatment—is now available over the counter. Minoxidil is the first—and, so far, the only—agent to be approved officially by the Food and Drug Administration (FDA) for the treatment of hair loss. No one is quite sure how minoxidil, developed as a blood pressure remedy, helps to prevent hair loss.

According to the FDA, one in four men shows at least a moderate reaction to minoxidil. It is not effective on the hairline, only on relatively small areas on the top of the head. Minoxidil cannot grow new hair where there is none; instead, it preserves follicles that might otherwise shrink. Hair growth resulting from minoxidil is almost never dense. And because its effects are mainly preventive, minoxidil must be applied to the scalp two times a day indefinitely (at a cost of about $30 per month), because any hair grown or preserved will fall out shortly after the treatment is stopped. The best candidates for minoxidil are men whose hair loss is relatively recent and mild—and who are willing to commit to lifelong treatment.

Another drug, finasteride (Proscar), may soon be approved for the treatment of hair loss. Finasteride works by inhibiting the enzyme that changes testosterone into dihydrotestosterone and is taken orally. It is currently approved only for treating enlargement of the prostate gland, but preliminary evidence suggests that it may stimulate hair growth as well. Preliminary studies show that more than 50 percent of men treated with the drug in a trial had moderate or greatly increased hair growth. For a small percentage of men, there are side effects that decreased with time, including erection problems, loss of sex drive, and reduced sperm count. FDA approval may come within a year.

Some doctors prescribe the acne medication tretinoin (Retin-A) and the female hormone progesterone for hair loss. Both are expensive, however, and there's no solid evidence that either boosts hair growth. Other promising medications currently are undergoing the FDA approval process. However, these drugs will not be approved any time in the near future.

If you're interested in taking a medication for hair loss, remember that they're effective in only a small number of men.

Surgery. For men whose hair follicles don't respond to minoxidil, scalp surgery is an alternative option, albeit a costly one, especially because medical insurance does not include hair-restoration treatments. The four main surgical techniques are hair transplantation, scalp reduction, scalp lifts, and hair flaps. Surgery works best for those with mild to moderate hair loss on the front of the head. Those with thick, curly hair and blond or gray hair also tend to have better results.

Hair transplantation, also known as grafting, involves moving grafts of hair from the side or back of the head to the thinning area on top or in front. If the surgery is done well, hair transplantation can be almost undetectable. If it is not, you may end up with noticeable rows of hair, like you would find on a doll's scalp. The procedure is lengthy (two to four sessions of approximately three hours each) and expensive (each session costs between $3,500 and $8,500). Furthermore, injections of anesthesia and the surgery itself can cause some pain, and there is a slight risk of infection, numbness, and excessive bleeding. The transplanted hair won't grow in fully for about a year, and further surgery may be needed in the future if hair loss persists around the treated area.

Men who have too little hair to consider grafting might consider scalp reduction, a procedure in which the size of a man's bald spot is surgically reduced by cutting out a piece of skin from the scalp, pulling the remaining edges together and stitching them shut. Sometimes, this reduction procedure must be repeated several times. When the bald spot is small enough, it is then covered with transplants.

To reduce the chance that the scalp will stretch back to its original position after surgery (postoperative "stretchback") and to decrease the need for multiple reductions, many surgeons precede scalp reduction with a procedure called scalp extension. In a scalp extension, the surgeon hooks a sheet of elastic to the underside of the scalp to stretch the skin of a large bald spot. This one-month procedure can cause infection, and it is painful. A few surgeons use balloons instead of elastic, which can result in swelling for several months. The average cost of a scalp reduction is $2,000 to $3,500, plus the transplantation fee. With a scalp extension, the price shoots to between $4,000 and $5,000. Scalp reduction is a bit riskier than transplant surgery, and the result may not be what's expected, given these possibilities: postoperative stretchback, an ugly scar that shows until the transplants grow in or grafts of newly transplanted hair that grow in different directions.

A scalp lift is a radical scalp reduction in which a surgeon separates the scalp from the skull down to the back of the head or the neck, removes a large bald spot, and pulls the loosened scalp back over the patch. Later, hair transplants are used to create a frontal hairline. The advantage of a scalp lift over a scalp reduction is the elimination of possible stretchback and visible scarring. A potential drawback is the mismatching of different hair sections. Furthermore, scalp lifts

IF YOU'RE GOING TO HAVE SURGERY

If you've decided that it's worth the risk of surgery to rid yourself of that bare patch of scalp, you should be sure to ask your practitioner the following:

- What are your credentials?

- How many operations of this type have you done? (The number should be more than one hundred.)

- What will the results of the surgery be? Will the results be permanent? Will additional surgery be required in the future?

- In transplantation, what size are the grafts? (Ideally, it should be one hair per graph on the hairline, three to four hairs per graph on top.)

- How many sessions will I need? (Watch for practitioners who promise transplantation in one session, since too many grafts may overwhelm the scalps blood supply, making the surgery less successful.)

- What are the fees? (Get a complete estimate in writing.)

- Can I meet or talk to previous patients?

require intravenous sedation or general anesthesia, and they pose a much greater risk of postsurgical complications than scalp reduction. The cost is $3,000 to $6,000, plus transplant fees.

A hair flap is a hair-bearing strip of scalp that a surgeon transplants to the front of the head.

This controversial procedure usually creates an unnaturally dense hairline; the transplanted hair may grow in odd directions; and the risk of complications, scarring, and failure are greater than those of any other hair-restoration procedures. Cost varies from $3,500 to over $10,000.

Nonmedical Alternatives

Of course, if you're not a good candidate for minoxidil and you don't want to undergo surgery but are concerned about your appearance, you might want to consider trying a wig or hairpiece. Today's hairpieces are custom made and are less bulky and awkward than older models. Hair weaves can also thicken hair by weaving a man's own hair into still-growing hair. Professional consultants, either private or national, can help you find the right look, one which doesn't look artificial; to find an expert near you, check the yellow pages of your local telephone book.

You might also want to remember that, in some men, baldness can be hidden or de-emphasized with a different hairstyle. Ask your stylist for advice. Also, keep in mind that hair loss is a natural change, and many men share your problem.

For more information:

American Hair Loss Council
P.O. Box 809313
401 N. Michigan Ave., 22nd Floor
Chicago, IL 60606-9313
800-274-8717
312-321-5128
http://www.ahlc.org

National Alopecia Areata Foundation
P.O. Box 150760
San Rafael, CA 94915
415-456-4644

HEADACHE

Headache appears to be self-defining—it's a pain in the head. But where it hurts may be the only thing any two headaches have in common. Almost all head pain is caused by one of two opposite physical occurrences—blood vessel constriction and blood vessel dilation. Constriction causes a tension headache, whereas dilation triggers a vascular headache (a migraine headache or a cluster headache). Tension headaches seem to strike both sexes equally, but women are twice as likely to develop migraines, and the overwhelming majority of cluster headache sufferers are men.

Over 90 percent of all headaches can be attributed to muscle or vascular headaches; diseases, injuries, and psychological disorders cause the rest. Anyone who suffers severe headaches should consult a doctor, not only to obtain effective prescription drug relief but also to rule out other causes of headache such as a tumor, an aneurysm (a blood clot in the brain), a hemorrhage (internal bleeding), and meningitis (an infection of the membranes that surround the spinal cord and brain).

Tension Headaches

It's usually not too hard to pinpoint the cause of a tension headache. Anything—stress, poor posture, squinting, suppressing anger—that makes you tighten up the muscles in your shoulders, neck, jaw, face, or scalp can cause head pain because the tense muscles squeeze the blood vessels around them, constricting blood flow. This constriction does several pain-producing things. It cuts oxygen flow to the muscles, which makes them tense up even more and irritates

HEADACHES: WHO GETS THEM?

Age	% Men	% Women
18–24	70	84
25–34	68	89
35–44	71	85
45–54	60	81
55–64	52	67
65–74	37	62
75–79	26	50

Source: National Center for Health Statistics

nerves in the muscles. The nerves then release a pain-inducing substance. And because the blood flow is slowed down, the circulatory system can't flush out the pain-causing substance, so it builds up and causes even more pain. More pain makes tighter muscles, which constricts blood flow and irritates nerves further, and so on and so on—a vicious cycle that has to be broken to relieve the pain.

Symptoms

Tension headaches bring moderate, steady pain felt on both sides of the head equally. The pain is generally steady and dull rather than throbbing and sharp and can last from thirty minutes to several days. Tension headaches are associated with feelings of depression or emotional stress, and they may also come on after long periods of sitting or driving. There may be a loss of appetite, but there is generally no vomiting or nausea. Physical activity does not affect the headache.

Vascular Headaches

Vascular headaches are notorious for their severe, sometimes incapacitating pain—a sharp, piercing throbbing concentrated in just one part of the skull. Vascular headaches are so named because they are caused by abnormal expansion (sometimes preceded by abnormal contraction) of blood vessels on the brain's surface and protective covering (the meninges), as well as elsewhere in the head. Migraines and cluster headaches are types of vascular headaches, as are those triggered by overexposure to the sun, overconsumption of alcohol, eating foods one is sensitive to, and even sleeping with one's head under the covers. The latter causes are easily avoided, but migraines and cluster headaches need medical care to relieve and control them. The two types of vascular headaches are migraine headaches and cluster headaches.

Migraine Headaches

Migraine headaches, which affect about 11 percent of the U.S. population, can be classic or common. The classic migraine, which occurs in one in ten migraine sufferers, is preceded by ten to thirty minutes of sensory disturbances known as an aura. The aura may involve flashing lights, distorted vision, temporary speech and hearing impairment, and loss of muscular control and balance. After the aura, the pain begins as the blood vessels in the brain expand, irritating nearby nerves. In contrast, the common migraine does not involve an aura. Migraines tend to last one to seventy-two hours.

Triggers that can initiate migraines are sudden changes in the weather, unusual physical exertion, bright or flickering lights, noxious fumes or heavily polluted air, and high altitude. Certain foods such as wine, cheese, hot dogs, chocolate, vanilla, yogurt, and soy sauce can also trigger migraines. In women (who are more than twice as likely to have migraines than men), migraines can be brought on by changes in hormone levels and are often associated with the menstrual cycle.

Migraines are most common among people between the ages of 35 and 45, and low-income people suffer 60 percent more migraines than those whose family income tops $30,000. Many people with a family history of migraines also suffer from them.

Symptoms

Migraine headaches usually occur mostly on one side of the face, and they tend to pound or throb. They are accompanied by nausea, vomiting, and a heightened sensitivity to light and noise. Migraines are made worse by physical movement, especially bending over. They often occur on weekends, holidays, vacations, or in the period following a time of excitement or stress.

Cluster Headaches

Virtually all victims of cluster headaches— 85 percent—are men. It is fortunate that cluster headaches are very rare (affecting less than 1 percent of the population) because they are so excruciatingly painful that sufferers have been known to commit suicide. Equally debilitating is their pattern—they occur several times a day, for about fifteen minutes to an hour, for several weeks ("the cluster"), then stop for long periods. Sometimes they never recur, but heavy smoking or drinking can precipitate a renewed round.

Symptoms

Cluster headaches occur in groups of four to eight a day for a period of one to three months. Attacks are accompanied by nasal congestion, discharge, and watering eyes. The pain is made worse by bending over and can be brought on by small amounts of alcohol.

Headache Medications

Medications used to treat migraines can either prevent them from occurring (prophylactic) or stop them once they do occur (abortive).

Prophylactic medications include

- Beta-blockers (acebutolol, atenolol, labetalol, nadolol, and propranolol) for migraines and cluster headaches

- Calcium channel agonists (nifedipine, niodipine, nicardipine, and diltiazem) for cluster headaches

- Tricyclic antidepressants (amitriptyline, doxepine, desipramine, and protriptyline) for migraines

- Fluoxetine (Prozac) for all types of headaches

- MAO inhibitors (Nardil and Parnate) for persistent migraines, chronic daily headaches, and headaches associated with depression and panic disorders

- Ergotamine derivatives (methysergide and methylergonovine) for migraines, chronic daily headaches, and cluster headaches

- Anticonvulsants (phenytoin and carbamazepine) for migraines, chronic headaches, and cluster headaches

HEALTHY HABITS FOR HEADACHE PREVENTION

- Get enough sleep, in a regular pattern, on a supportive mattress and pillow.

- Avoid headache triggers. Keep a diary of headache attacks to pinpoint any possible triggers—for example, foods or medications—then avoid those substances.

- Use a good chair and sit up straight. Good posture alleviates muscle and nerve problems that may contribute to headaches.

- Take regular breaks from working on computers, reading, or doing other close work. Such work often brings on eyestrain and, with it, headaches.

- Exercise regularly. Research shows that exercise can reduce the frequency and intensity of headaches. In some cases, exercise may alleviate headaches. Experiment to see if it works for you.

- Learn to manage stress. Relaxation is a strategy useful for both preventing and relieving headaches. Use time-management and stress-relieving techniques to resolve conflict in your everyday life and practice relaxation frequently. (See Relaxation Techniques, p. 124.)

- Antihistamines (cyproheptadine and hydroxyzine) for migraines in children

- Lithium carbonate for cyclical migraines and cluster headaches

Abortive medications include

- Prescription and over-the-counter analgesics such as aspirin (Bayer and Empirin), acetaminophen (Tylenol, Datril and Panadol), and analgesics with caffeine (Excedrin, Vanquish and Anacin). Aspirin should not be given to anyone under 19 years of age because of the risk of Reye's syndrome, a potentially fatal condition.

- Nonsteroidal anti-inflammatory drugs (ibuprofen and naproxen sodium)

- Ergotamine derivatives (Wigraine, Ergomarm and Cafergot) for migraine and cluster headaches

- Isometheptene for migraine sufferers who cannot take ergotamine derivatives

- Corticosteroids (prednisone and hydrocortisone) for cluster headaches and chronic migraines

- Sumatriptan (Imitrex) for migraine headaches. This relatively new drug is effective in over 70 percent of migraine sufferers and has few side effects.

Headache Self-Care

There are many drugless ways to relieve a headache:

- Get up and move around, preferably outside, if you've been sitting in one place (such as at a computer or in a car) for a while.

- Try massage. If you're suffering a tension headache, stimulating the scalp can help restore blood flow, possibly relieving pain.

Rub your scalp with your fingertips or use a hairbrush.

- Apply heat or ice. A heating pad, a hot shower, or a hot bath can also help restore blood flow to the scalp in the event of a tension headache. If you're suffering from a vascular headache, apply an ice pack to your forehead to help restrict blood flow.

- Relax. Take a two-minute relaxation break. Sit comfortably in a chair, close your eyes, and consciously tense and relax your muscles, starting with your toes and working your way up to your head. Or practice relaxation techniques such as biofeedback, visualization therapy, and meditation. (See Relaxation Therapies, p. 124.)

- Try do-it-yourself acupressure. Squeeze the web of skin between your thumb and index finger alongside the lower thumb knuckle between your other thumb and finger or press on the very base of your skull on either side of your spine.

For more information:

National Headache Foundation
428 W. St. James Pl., 2nd Floor
Chicago, IL 60614
800-843-2256
http://www.headaches.org

American Council for Headache Education
19 Mantua Rd.
Mt. Royal, NJ 08601
800-255-ACHE
609-423-0258
Http://www.achenet.org

HEARING LOSS AND RELATED DISORDERS

Hearing Loss

If you have a difficult time holding a conversation on the telephone or people tell you that the television is too loud, you are not alone. Over twenty-eight million people suffer from some degree of hearing loss.

Men account for 60 percent of those with a hearing loss, and the condition becomes more prevalent with age. Men have a higher rate of age-influenced hearing loss than women, and they begin to lose their hearing earlier in life. In fact, one estimate reveals that men are 40 percent more likely than women to develop a hearing loss as they grow older. One possible explanation for this may be that men are subject to more frequent or louder noise at work or during leisure activities.

Types of Hearing Loss

Hearing loss can be divided into two categories: conductive and sensorineural. Conductive hearing loss occurs when sound waves can't be transmitted from the outer or middle ear to the inner ear. This loss may result from a variety of causes, including excessive earwax or obstructions in the ear, ear infections, a ruptured eardrum, and problems with the bones in the ear. Conductive hearing loss also results from problems in the middle ear such as otitis media, barotrauma, otosclerosis, and cysts.

Sensorineural hearing loss, or nerve deafness, is more common than conductive hearing loss.

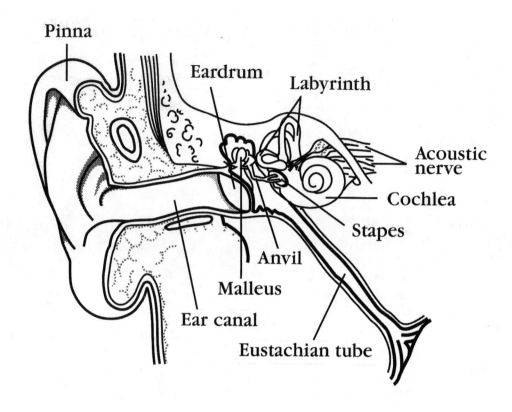

Anatomy of the Ear

This type of loss results from damage to the inner ear or the auditory nerve, and unlike many forms of conductive hearing loss, it can't be reversed. However, hearing aids and other treatments are commonly used to help people with nerve deafness. Major causes of sensorineural hearing loss include aging, exposure to noise, Ménière's disease, acoustic trauma, and congenital disorders. Other conditions causing sensorineural hearing loss include arthritis and tumors. Certain pharmaceutical products such as aspirin, diuretics, and chemotherapy drugs may also cause hearing loss in some individuals.

Around 28 percent of Americans lose their hearing as a result of natural aging, and another 23 percent have a loss created by exposure to loud or excessive noise. Combined, this accounts for over 50 percent of the people who suffer from hearing loss in the United States.

Symptoms

Although millions of Americans suffer from hearing impairments, many refuse to seek help or don't realize they have a problem. You may have impaired hearing if you

- Shout while talking

- Turn the radio or television up too loud for others

- Often think people are mumbling when they speak to you

- Have a hard time understanding others in noisy environments

- Often ask people to repeat what they have said

- Experience ringing in the ears (tinnitus)

- Have difficulty hearing on the telephone

Acoustic Trauma

Some people lose their hearing in dramatic fashion—a "pop" when jumping in the swimming pool or a substantial loss after a loud explosion. These are just two specific examples of acoustic trauma, damage to the ear drum that can cause conductive hearing loss. Ten percent of all hearing loss results from sudden loud noises. Sudden blows to the head, damage caused by an object in the ear, skull fractures, and rapid changes in pressure may also result in hearing loss, and a person's hearing may or may not return to normal, depending on the type of loss. In many cases, the eardrum repairs itself as long as the injured area is kept clean and dry. However, severe perforations that refuse to heal may require surgery. If damage to the eardrum occurs, see your practitioner immediately.

Barotrauma

Some individuals who fly or scuba dive have problems with pressure changes that cause the eustachian tube to malfunction. Barotrauma, also called *aerotitis* or "airplane ears," results when the external pressure on the eardrum suddenly becomes greater in relation to the inner pressure. Individuals who experience barotrauma suffer from pain and conductive hearing loss when flying in an airplane or diving.

To combat this problem, try chewing gum, yawning, or sucking on a piece of candy. These simple techniques help to keep the eustachian tube open, which regulates the pressure. If you're diving, rising slowly from a depth can prevent barotrauma. Also, don't fly too soon after a dive. Decongestants may also work by alleviating the congestion that blocks the eustachian tube. In most situations, the symptoms usually subside shortly after changes in pressure have ended, but see a physician if the problem persists.

Cholesteatoma

Chronic middle ear infections may lead a cholesteatoma, a benign (or noncancerous) cyst that develops in the middle ear. Although most cholesteatomas are the result of complications from ear infections, some are congenital, meaning they developed as the result of an event that occurred during pregnancy or birth. The cyst may cause conductive or sensorineural hearing loss, dizziness, or even facial paralysis if it grows large enough. Surgery is necessary to remove the cyst.

Ear Wax

One of the most common conditions that affects the outer ear is ear wax, or cerumen. The ear usually produces a small amount of wax, which gradually works its way out of the ear. However, some people produce a great deal of wax, which can build up in the outer ear and prevent sound waves from traveling to the middle ear, causing conductive hearing loss.

A TIP ON COTTON SWABS

The old saying is true—you shouldn't put anything in your ear except your elbow. Poking around in your ear with a cotton swab—or anything else—will probably force more wax deep into the ear than it removes. There's also the added danger of acoustic trauma, damage to the ear drum.

Wax usually works its way out of the ear on its own, but if you'd like to help it along, place a few drops of baby or mineral oil, with the help of an eyedropper, into your ear twice a day for several days. (Remember not to insert the dropper into your ear.) This will soften the wax. Then, fill a syringe with warm water and, with your head upright, gently squirt some of the water into your ear. Tilt your ear to allow the water to drain out. You may need to repeat this flushing several times.

If the wax remains and is interfering with your hearing, contact a health-care practitioner, who can remove it with suction or an instrument called a curette.

PREVENTING SWIMMER'S EAR

If you're often in the pool, here are a few simple steps you can take to prevent swimmer's ear:

- Put a few drops of rubbing alcohol into your ears as you're drying off. This will dry up any remaining water in the ears.

- Use a hair dryer, aimed at the ears, to dry up excess water after swimming.

- Jump around. If you can feel the water in your ears, tilt your head to one side and jump up and down until the water flows out. It may feel silly, but it's a very effective trick.

Otitis Externa

Otitis externa, commonly known as swimmer's ear, is an infection of the outer ear canal. It is caused by bacteria, allergies, or fungi and is characterized by itching, pain, swelling, and a feeling that the ear is blocked. The swelling associated with swimmer's ear can cause conductive hearing loss by blocking the ear canal. Treatment for otitis externa involves antibiotics and eardrops. People who are repeatedly exposed to cold water might develop exostosis, or surfer's ear, in which abnormal bone growth blocks the ear canal and disrupts normal hearing.

Otitis Media

Otitis media, or middle ear infection, is the most common cause of conductive hearing loss, and it's also the number one cause of hearing loss in children. Middle ear infections occur for many reasons, and the pain associated with them comes from the pressure of a fluid or pus buildup pressing against the eardrum.

Middle ear infections are often treated by prescription antibiotics such as amoxicillin, though over-the-counter painkillers, especially aspirin, can be used to relieve the pain. If medication doesn't help, a myringotomy may be done. This procedure allows the fluid to drain by making an incision in the eardrum. Tubes may be placed in the eardrum to allow further drainage and the equalization of pressure.

If proper treatment isn't sought, other complications may arise such as mastoiditis or labyrinthitis. Mastoiditis is an infection of the mastoid bone, and labyrinthitis is an inner ear infection that causes balance problems and hearing loss.

Otosclerosis

Otosclerosis is a disorder that affects the bones of the middle ear. The problem occurs when excessive bone growth within the ear prevents the tiny bones that transmit sound waves to the eardrum from vibrating so that sound waves do not reach the inner ear, causing conductive hearing loss. One out of every one hundred adults is affected by this disorder, and women are more likely to be afflicted than men. Treatment includes a hearing aid or a surgical procedure, called a stapedectomy, which involves replacing all or some of the bones of the middle ear with artificial substitutes that allow sound to enter the middle ear once again.

Noise

Noise is another factor that prompts sensorineural hearing loss. Repeated exposure to sources of high-decibel noise such as loud music (often heard through stereo headphones), firearms, airplanes, and loud engines or machinery can lead to permanent damage. Although people are aware of the problems created by loud noises, noise exposure in the workplace is often overlooked as a critical source of hearing loss. According to the National Institute for Occupational Safety and Health, you should wear ear protection if you're exposed to a noise level of 80 decibels eight hours a day; 85 decibels for four hours a day; 90 decibels for two hours; or 95 decibels for one hour. An effective and inexpensive way to combat this problem is to wear earplugs or earmuffs while in the noisy environment.

HOW MANY DECIBELS?

Here's a quick rundown of how certain noises measure up on the decibel scale:

A whisper	20 decibels
A noisy restaurant	70 decibels
Traffic	70 to 90 decibels
A snowblower	85 decibels
A rock concert	90 decibels
A shout	90 decibels
A power saw	95 decibels
Overhead plane	110 to 120 decibels

Presbycusis

As people grow older they slowly begin to lose their hearing. This progressive loss is known as presbycusis, and it results through a process where the sensory hair cells within the ear die and are not replaced. The cells that receive the high-frequency pitches usually go first, and eventually the low-frequency cells may be affected.

Natural hearing loss can begin when a person is in their thirties or forties, and by 65 one in four people has some degree of difficulty hearing. This type of loss is irreversible, but hearing aids, assistive listening devices, and aural rehabilitation help to alleviate the problems associated with it.

Tinnitus

Almost every person has experienced ringing in the ears at one time or another. But for many people, ringing or buzzing, called tinnitus, is a constant problem. Tinnitus affects approximately thirty-six million adults in the United States. It can be a symptom of hearing loss or an indicator of an underlying medical condition. Its causes

OTOTOXIC DRUGS

Some medications can be ototoxic. This means they cause problems with the inner ear such as hearing loss and tinnitus. Among these are aspirin, certain antibiotics, diuretics, and certain cancer drugs. Different medications affect people in different ways, so it's difficult to say how a particular drug will impact a certain individual. A person's condition, other medications, and the prescribed dosage are all factors that may determine if a certain drug may has a negative impact. In some cases, the condition will diminish if the drugs are discontinued.

include ear obstructions, infections, allergies, certain drugs, or injuries. Wax buildup in the ear canal is a frequent cause of tinnitus. If this is the problem then removing the excess wax (or an obstruction) will usually alleviate the ringing.

In many instances, tinnitus stems from the inner ear or unknown causes and treatment becomes more difficult. There are a number of different methods used to help people cope with tinnitus. In mild cases, shifting a person's attention away from the ringing may be enough to alleviate the problem. This might be achieved by simply focusing on other sounds or thoughts while trying to fall asleep. In more severe cases, a tinnitus masking device may be the answer. A masker works by producing a sound that will absorb or neutralize the sound resulting from tinnitus.

Certain factors such as stress, tension, or fatigue may also aggravate tinnitus. Likewise, situations that are extremely quite or really loud may also increase the perceived intensity of the tinnitus. Biofeedback, exercise, relaxation techniques, and getting an ample amount of rest may also help relieve tinnitus.

Vestibular Diseases

There are certain sensorineural auditory disorders that affect the inner ear, causing balance problems as well as hearing loss. These are known as vestibular disorders, which are characterized by dizziness and vertigo. Ménière's disease and labyrinthitis are examples of this.

Vertigo is more intense than dizziness because it involves the sensation that a person's surroundings are actually moving. This condition may also stem from central nervous system problems, diseases, and certain drugs.

Ménière's disease strikes over thirty-eight thousand people each year, and it's characterized by periods of vertigo or dizziness, tinnitus, fluctuating hearing loss, vomiting, and nausea. Although there is no known cure for the disease, there are certain treatments that can alleviate the symptoms. Medication is prescribed to control the dizziness and vomiting, and a combination of diet and diuretics may also work. Certain surgical options such as a procedure to drain the fluid may be necessary if the vertigo is intense.

Congenital Hearing Loss

In some instances, a hearing disorder is already present when a person is born. Children may be born deaf or impaired due to a genetic deficiency while congenital hearing loss often results from injury, illness, or other complications during pregnancy. Babies who are born prematurely have a greater risk of hearing impairment upon birth. Up to 4 percent of all hearing disabilities are already present at birth.

Diagnosis

If you think you have a hearing loss, the first step is to visit your family doctor or an otolaryngologist, sometimes called an otorhinolaryngologist and also referred to as an ear, nose, and throat specialist (ENT). Otolaryngologists can determine if there is a hearing loss and what type of loss it is. They will treat a person if the problem is the result of a rupture, infection, or other disorder. Medications are usually prescribed, though in certain circumstances surgery may be necessary.

If the problem can't be corrected or a hearing aid is the solution, then a visit to an audiologist is necessary. Audiologists are health professionals who can diagnose and treat hearing disabilities. The American Speech-Language-Hearing Association (ASHA) is a national organization that governs over seventy-seven thousand audiologists. Audiologists may become certified.

By conducting a battery of tests, an audiologist analyzes the high-and-low frequency levels where a person's hearing drops off as well as that person's ability to understand speech. These tests reveal the specifics of the impairment while indicating what type of hearing assistance is necessary.

Treatment

The most common hearing device is the hearing aid. Over 90 percent of those with hearing impairments can be helped with a hearing aid. The degree of benefit, of course, depends on the type and severity of the loss and the problem. There are many different shapes of aids on the market, and they range in size from those that sit behind the ear to much smaller devices that are seated in the ear canal. Aids are flesh-colored and are often hardly noticeable to others.

PREVENTING HEARING LOSS

Although you may not pay attention to how loud the stereo is playing, you should be aware that noise exposure causes you to gradually lose your hearing. There is no medical way to correct a hearing loss that stems from noise, but there are certain steps that can be taken to lessen the damage brought on by noise. For example:

- Avoid listening to music, movies, or the television at a loud level. Keep the volume on personal stereos with headphones low enough so that the music can't be heard by those around you.

- Wear earplugs when working around machines, motors, or appliances at work or home.

- Watch the types of drugs you take; some drugs such as aspirin are ototoxic and may cause hearing loss or ringing in the ears. If you suspect your medication may be causing hearing loss or ringing, consult your practitioner as soon as possible.

- If you think you have a loss, get your hearing checked. It may become worse if ignored.

There are various types of aids available, including the analog, digital, hybrid, and digitally programmable models. Each has its own benefits and drawbacks. For example, analog aids are relatively inexpensive, but they don't offer the specific programming features of a digitally programmable aid that can be set for a person

TYPES OF HEARING AIDS

1. *Analog.* Uses an amplifier to enhance sound. This is the least costly type, but it also tends to amplify without discriminating all the sounds a person hears. Certain modifications can be made to increase the performance of an analog aid.

2. *Digital.* Computer chips work to reduce background noise and improve speech perception.

3. *Hybrid.* Digital technology is meshed with analog components to create an aid that fits the needs of an individual. If digital adjustments are needed, the aid must be returned to the factory for modifications.

4. *Programmable.* These devices can be adjusted for specific situations and environments. The digital technology allows the aid to be customized for the needs of a wearer. This is the most expensive type, and many require a pencil-like remote control device to operate.

with a high-frequency loss. Ultimately, though, choosing a hearing aid depends on many factors including the severity of the loss, finances, and personal preference.

In addition to wearing a hearing aid, aural rehabilitation helps a person to make the best of the hearing that is left. Rehabilitative techniques include speech reading (lip reading), learning to discriminate among various background noises when wearing an aid, or even using body language and visual cues to improve hearing. Keep in mind that a hearing aid will not fully correct a hearing disorder, unlike the way a pair of eyeglasses corrects someone's vision.

If hearing loss is more profound, there are several assistive listening devices (ALD) that may help a person. Among these are closed captioning, telephone amplifiers, telecommunications devices, FM and loop systems, and assistive signaling and alerting devices. Recently, cochlear implants have been successful in helping those with extreme sensorineural hearing loss or deafness. An implant works by translating sounds into electrical impulses that are sent to the auditory nerve. Although this process creates certain sounds, it does not actually reproduce speech. Hence, it is currently reserved for people who are deaf in both ears or have a very profound loss.

For more information:

American Board of Otolaryngology
2211 Norfolk, Suite 800
Houston, TX 77005
713-528-6200
http://www.aboto.org

American Osteopathic Board of Ophthalmology and Otorhinolaryngology
3 MacKoil Ave.
Dayton, OH 45403
513-252-0868

Better Hearing Institute
P.O. Box 1840
Washington, DC 20013
800-EAR-WELL
703-642-0580
http://www.betterhear.org

Self Help for Hard of Hearing People, Inc.
7910 Woodmont Ave., Suite 1200
Bethesda, MD 20814
301-657-2248 (voice)
301-657-2249 (TDD)
http://www.shhh.org

Hear Now
9745 E. Hampden Ave., Suite 300
Denver, CO 80231
800-648-4327
303-695-7797
http://www.leisurelan.com/-hearnow

American Tinnitus Association
P.O. Box 5
Portland, OR 97207-0005
503-248-9985

For information on audiologists in your area, contact:

American Speech-Language-Hearing Association
10801 Rockville Pike
Rockville, MD 20852
800-638-8255 (voice/TDD)
301-897-5700 (voice)
301-897-0157 (TDD)
http://www.asha.org/asha

HEARTBURN

According to the National Institute of Diabetes and Digestive and Kidney Diseases, about 61 million of American adults experience heartburn, or acid indigestion, at least once a month, and about twenty-five million suffer from it daily. The *New England Journal of Medicine* reports that 7 to 10 percent of Americans experience heartburn daily, and 15 to 40 percent have it monthly.

Symptoms

Heartburn is usually experienced as a burning pain in the chest that begins behind the breastbone and radiates upward to the neck. Sometimes the pain is accompanied by the sensation that food is coming back up into the mouth (called acid reflux or gastroesophageal reflux) along with a bitter or acidic taste. The burning sensation can last as long as two hours, and lying down or bending over may make it worse.

Heartburn and heart attack or angina are often confused. If you have heartburn and are in a high-risk group for heart disease, see your

DIGESTIVE SYSTEM PROBLEMS

According to a Gallup survey sponsored by Janssen Pharmaceutica in 1996, 52 percent of adult Americans suffered a digestive problem in the previous months. The most common complaints included

Gas	38 percent
Indigestion	27 percent
Belching	27 percent
Heartburn	26 percent
Nighttime coughing (due to heartburn)	25 percent
Bloating after meals	17 percent

practitioner for an electrocardiogram, a diagnostic test that measures the electrical activity of the heart, to rule out a more serious condition.

Acid Reflux

At the point where the esophagus joins the stomach, the esophagus is kept closed by a muscle called the lower esophageal sphincter (LES muscle). The pressure in the stomach is usually greater than in the esophagus, so it is the LES muscle that keeps the contents of the stomach and the stomach acid out of the esophagus. When working properly, the LES muscle opens after swallowing to let the food pass through and enter the stomach, then it quickly closes to prevent the return of food and stomach juices into the esophagus.

Gastroesophageal reflux occurs when the LES muscle is not working properly; either it relaxes inappropriately or it is very weak. The pressure in the stomach then forces the stomach acid

TAKE HEARTBURN—NOT ANTACIDS—SERIOUSLY

Researchers are beginning to understand that recurrent heartburn is nothing to take lightly. In fact, one recent study from the University of Oklahoma College of Medicine, Oklahoma City, showed a startling number of people who regularly take antacids may have a serious condition.

Those in the study reported having moderate to severe heartburn on a regular basis for longer than three months, but what the researchers discovered was much more than indigestion. Of the 155 people in the study, eighty-eight were diagnosed with hiatal hernia (in which the stomach pushes through the diaphragm muscle into the chest cavity) and seventy-three had erosive esophagitis (in which the esophagus becomes inflamed by stomach acids). In addition, nine were diagnosed with Barrett's esophagus (a peptic ulcer located in the lower esophagus); four had peptic ulcer disease; one had Barrett's esophagus with cancer, and one had Barrett's esophagus with dysplasia (abnormally fast growth of healthy cells).

If you've been hitting the antacids hard, remember the following:

- Don't hide your heartburn. Antacids merely mask symptoms instead of handling the real problem, which could be a serious one.

- Take symptoms seriously. None of the individuals in the study considered symptoms such as difficulty swallowing, hoarseness, wheezing, and pain when swallowing to be important. In fact, these symptoms are known by gastroenterologists as "alarm symptoms"— signs that you may have a serious disease.

- Seek out your physician. Most people with recurrent heartburn stay away from the physician's office, afraid the doctor may tell them to cut out smoking, drinking, eating rich foods, or some other activity. Yet a trip to the doctor may be the only way to find out if you have a serious condition. Plus, chances are your heartburn can be helped, meaning you'll feel a lot better.

through the LES muscle and into the esophagus. When this happens on a chronic basis (more than twice a week), the condition is called gastroesophageal reflux disease (GERD). GERD affects men and women equally, but other more serious conditions such as esophagitis occur more frequently in men.

GERD affects up to forty million Americans and sends thousands each year to the emergency room because its symptoms closely resemble those of a heart attack. Of the six million patients who go to emergency rooms each year, experts say 10 to 20 percent have heartburn or GERD rather than heart disease.

Treatment

Most people find relief from heartburn by standing upright and taking an antacid that clears acid out of the esophagus. Nonprescription antacids provide temporary or partial relief from heartburn. Long-term use of antacids (longer than three weeks) can result in side effects, such as diarrhea, altered calcium metabolism, and magnesium retention (a problem that can be serious for kidney disease patients). Some antacids are also high in sodium, which may affect blood pressure and other conditions. If you have frequent heartburn, you should see a practitioner for diagnosis.

CONTROLLING HEARTBURN

With basic changes in lifestyle, it is possible to get heartburn under control. Here are some tips:

- Avoid eating close to bedtime; and avoid lying down after eating—gravity can cause a spill of acid into the esophagus. Also, elevate your head when sleeping or elevate the head of your bed about six inches.

- Decrease the size of meals; eat smaller meals more frequently. A full stomach is more likely to overflow.

- Make sure your pants fit comfortably. According to a report in the *Archives of Internal Medicine*, there is a condition known as "tightpants syndrome" caused by wearing trousers that are too snug. The syndrome causes heartburn, belching, and stomach discomfort after eating.

- Avoid foods that can aggravate symptoms such as fried and fatty foods, chocolate, alcohol, coffee, tomato products, highly spiced foods, and citrus fruits and juices.

- Do not smoke cigarettes; cigarette smoking dramatically decreases the pressure of the LES muscle.

- Take an antacid or alginic acid intermittently to prevent acid from building up the in esophagus.

- Lose weight if necessary.

New over-the-counter medications such as Zantac and Pepcid AC (which belong to a class of drugs called H2 blockers) are designed to prevent the stomach from overproducing pepsin, an enzyme (acid) that digests food protein; excessive acid can reflux into the esophagus, causing the burning sensation of heartburn. If nonprescription medications do not help relieve the symptoms of heartburn, see a doctor. He may refer you to a gastroenterologist, a doctor who specializes in digestive conditions and diseases. This specialist can determine if the heartburn is a symptom of a more serious digestive disease and can provide individualized treatment.

For severe cases of GERD, proton pump inhibitors such as Prilosec (omeprazole) may be prescribed. These inhibitors, which slow down the production of stomach acids even more than H2 blockers such as Zantac, are quickly becoming the world's biggest selling drugs. Prevacid (lansoprazole) is another proton pump inhibitor on the market.

For more information:

American College of Gastroenterology
4222 King St.
Alexandria, VA 22302
800-HRT-BURN

Digestive Disease National Coalition
507 Capitol Ct., N.E., Suite 200
Washington, DC 20002
202-544-7497

National Digestive Diseases Information Clearinghouse
2 Information Way
Bethesda, MD 20892-3570
301-654-3810
http://www.niddk.nih.gov

HEART DISEASE

Coronary Heart Disease

The type of heart disease most people are concerned about is coronary heart disease—those conditions in which the arteries that nourish the heart with blood become blocked, cutting off the blood and oxygen supply to the heart muscle. The heart muscle starves, causing angina pectoris—chest pain that's a warning sign of heart disease—myocardial infarction (MI), also known as heart attack.

According to the American Heart Association (AHA), coronary heart disease (CHD)—also called coronary-artery disease (CAD)—caused 487,490 deaths in 1994 and is currently the leading cause of death in America for both men and women. Some 18 percent of men ages 65 to 69 have had a heart attack, and 29.6 percent of men ages 80 to 84 have had one. Perhaps even more alarming than these statistics is the fact that 48 percent of men who suddenly die as a result of CHD had no previous indication that they had the disease.

The American Heart Association also reports that the prevalence of coronary heart disease in adults age 20 and older is 7.2 percent for the general population; 7.5 percent for Caucasians; 6.9 percent for African Americans; and 5.6 percent for Mexican Americans. In 1993, death rates from CHD were 133 per 1,000 Caucasian men and 139.3 per 1,000 for African-American men (4.7 percent higher).

Risk Factors

Men are automatically at risk for heart disease simply because of their gender. Men tend to have a greater risk of suffering heart attacks and of having them earlier in life. Other risk factors that you have little to no control over are heredity and increasing age. The American Heart Association has identified the following other risk factors:

1. *High blood pressure.* This makes the heart work and pump harder, which leads to heart failure.

2. *Smoking.* Smokers die at a 70 percent greater rate than nonsmokers.

3. *High cholesterol.* Excess cholesterol causes the formation of fatty deposits along artery walls.

4. *Inactivity.* Exercise controls cholesterol and obesity. It also lowers blood pressure.

5. *Diabetes.* More than 80 percent of diabetes patients die from some form of blood vessel or heart disease. However, studies show that women with both heart disease and diabetes are more likely to die than men with the same conditions.

6. *Obesity.* Excess weight puts strain on the heart and leads to high blood pressure and higher levels of cholesterol in the blood.

7. *Stress.* Stress causes the body's blood pressure to rise. It also increases a person's chance of engaging in other risk behaviors such as smoking and drinking.

Arteriosclerosis and Atherosclerosis

The origins of coronary heart disease often lie with arteriosclerosis and atherosclerosis. Arteriosclerosis, or "hardening of the arteries," actually describes a number of conditions in which minerals and fatty deposits collect in the arteries, causing the vessels to become rigid and inflexible. In atherosclerosis, the most common form of arteriosclerosis, the walls of the arteries become thick and irregular due to the accumulation of fats, cholesterol, and other substances, called plaque. Arteriosclerosis sets the stage for heart attack by narrowing the arteries, reducing blood flow to the heart. In addition, the rigid blood vessels cannot expand to accommodate greater blood flow when necessary. Because the buildup of plaque cannot be felt, the only symptoms of atherosclerosis may be angina or heart attack.

Angina Pectoris

The "hardening of the arteries" leads to angina pectoris, chest pain brought on by exertion. During exercise, stress, or an emotional situation—even after a big meal—the heart beats faster and works harder, which means the heart muscle must get more oxygenated blood to maintain the pace. However, because of arteriosclerosis, the arteries leading to the heart have become rigid and narrow, so not enough nutrients reach the muscle. The pain suffered during this oxygen deficiency is angina.

Angina is known as a precursor to heart attack. About half of those with angina suffer sudden death, and a third have heart attacks. About 350,000 new cases of angina are reported each year. The Cardiovascular Health Study shows that 21.1 percent of men 65 to 69 have angina pectoris, as do 27.3 percent of men ages 80 to 84. For women, those rates are 13.7 percent and 24.7 percent respectively. The angina rate is 3.4 for Caucasian men; 2.6 for African American men; and 3.4 for Mexican-American men.

Symptoms

Angina is a heavy, strangulating, suffocating pain. It seems to start under the breastbone, on the left side of the chest. It can radiate to other parts of the body, including the throat, neck, jaw, and left shoulder and arm. Occasionally, it will reach the right side of the body. Angina episodes usually last less than fifteen minutes—any longer and what is happening may be a heart attack.

Angina itself is a symptom of heart disease—one that many people actually consider beneficial. Many heart problems are symptomless and are not discovered until they're the cause of sudden death. Angina, at least, shows that something is wrong.

Diagnosis and Treatment

Angina is usually unmistakable, but there are times when it mimics other, noncardiac conditions. Diagnosis can be done through a physical examination and an electrocardiogram (EKG), a test in which electrodes attached to the chest measure the heart's electrical activity. An EKG done in combination with exercise on a treadmill or stationary bicycle, called a stress test, is also often done. Most experts agree that an angiography, an invasive test in which contrast dye is injected into the vessels and viewed with an x-ray, is unnecessary for diagnosing angina. Studies show an angiography carries with it a risk of heart attack or death (about 1 in 1,000) and costs around $3,000 to $5,000.

Treatment of angina involves learning how to remain calm in stressful or emotional situations, as well as medications and, in some cases, surgery. Medications don't resolve the problem of buildup in the arteries, but rather get around it by reducing blood pressure, slowing the heart rate, and widening blood vessels somewhat.

Calcium channel blockers (Cardizem, Procardia) are vasodilators that relax the arteries and increase blood flow. Blood-pressure-lowering medications such as diuretics and digitalis are also used to treat angina. However, nitroglycerin drugs (Isordil and Cardilate)—also vasodilators that widen vessels—are the traditional treatment for angina. Nitroglycerin drugs can be taken orally, intravenously, or transdermally (through a patch). During an angina attack, they can be placed or sprayed under the tongue to dissolve. Such drugs work very quickly.

Bypass surgery and angioplasty—discussed with heart attack—are surgical options for treating angina. However, most experts agree that they are not necessary for those with mild angina.

Heart Attack

A heart attack, or myocardial infarction (MI), takes place when a blockage—perhaps caused by a buildup of plaque—occurs in the heart artery. As a result, blood containing oxygen is cut off from the heart and the oxygen-deprived heart muscle is damaged. The area of dead or damaged tissue is known as an infarct.

Heart attack is the single largest killer of American men. There is an almost 90 percent chance of survival after a heart attack if no complications arise. If there are extenuating circumstances surrounding the attack, survival rates drop to around 40 percent. Alarmingly, 23 percent of previous heart attack victims will have another attack within six years of their first attack. According to the American Heart Association, 1.5 million Americans will have a new or recurrent heart attack this year, and one-third of these people will die.

Symptoms

A heart attacks strikes with a crushing, breathtaking pain that starts in the chest and radiates into the left arm, back, or shoulder. Victims may break out into a cold sweat or, occasionally, vomit (one reason heart attack may be confused with indigestion). Many people pass out from the pain—and never awake.

Angina is usually nothing compared with the pain from a heart attack, but those who have suffered angina may initially believe a heart attack to be another angina episode. However, if the attack lasts more than fifteen minutes or is not affected by nitroglycerin medications, it can be assumed to be a heart attack.

You can have a heart attack and not feel a thing. These are called "silent" heart attacks, and they occur for the same reason as detected attacks. However, these silent attacks go unnoticed because they are affecting a less crucial part of the heart or because the individual experiencing a silent attack might have an unusually high tolerance for pain. One of the only ways you can tell if you've had a silent attack is through an EKG.

Diagnosis

If necessary, a heart attack can be diagnosed through an electrocardiogram (EKG) or through a series of blood tests that measures enzymes in the blood.

Silent heart attacks can usually be diagnosed by using a stress test—the exercise form of the EKG—to see how the heart stands up under mild exertion. For this reason, experts recommend having an EKG done around age 40. This baseline EKG can then be used as a basis of comparison for future EKGs, making it easier to tell if a silent attack has occurred. It is recommended that a man get an EKG every three years after age 30 if he is at risk for heart attack and every three to four years after age 50 if he is not.

Cardiologists also recommend exercise stress tests to sedentary men over the age of 35 who want to begin an exercise program or who have several major risk factors for heart disease. They also recommend the test to anyone who has suffered a previous heart attack or angina even if he is symptom free.

Treatment

Immediately after the onset of a heart attack, emergency medical care should be sought. The victim should be helped into a comfortable, supine position. His collar, belt, cuffs, and shoes

---

ANOTHER REASON TO DISLIKE MONDAYS

A study in a 1996 issue of *Circulation* found that more people suffer heart attacks on Mondays than on any other day, regardless of whether they are currently working or retired.

The study looked at close to seven hundred middle-aged men with a history of arrhythmias (periods of rapid, abnormal heartbeat that may trigger heart attack) and found that the incidence of arrhythmias peaked on the first day of the workweek. The study is part of a growing body of evidence that links heart disease to psychological stress.

As for the reasons behind Monday MIs in the retired, the author of the study hypothesized that perhaps those men still felt the stress of Mondays because they had been in the workforce for so long, or perhaps because of the stress of watching other family members go to work while staying home alone.

should be loosened. If the heart and breathing has stopped, cardiopulmonary resuscitation should be started as soon as possible by someone who is properly trained.

Once the person has arrived at the hospital, thrombolytic drugs—also called "clot-busting" drugs—are given to dissolve the clot that caused the attack and restore blood flow to the heart, preventing any further damage. Eighty percent of those who are given a thrombolytic drug within two hours of a heart attack experience a restoration of blood flow to the heart. Thrombolytic drugs include streptokinase, urokinase, tissue-type plasminogen activator (tPA), and recombinant plasminogen activator (rPA). Studies have shown streptokinase, the least expensive of these drugs, to be the safest and most effective.

During a heart attack, other medications may be given depending on the circumstances. These may include injections of painkillers, blood pressure medications, or other drugs. After the person has been stabilized, the main treatment is rest to relieve any stress or anxiety that may have brought on the attack. Additional procedures and possibly surgery may be done in the days and weeks after a heart attack has passed to treat coronary heart disease.

Diagnosing Coronary Heart Disease

Following a heart attack—or, better yet, before an attack has occurred—diagnostic tests may be done to diagnose coronary heart disease and determine its extent.

When it is suspected that the heart vessels are blocked, an angiography is performed. Again, this particular procedure is effective, but costly—ranging anywhere from $3,000 to $5,000.

A form of angiography called a cardiac catheterization is also useful in diagnosing heart disease. In this procedure, a plastic tube is inserted through a blood vessel in the groin and into the patient's heart. Dye is then injected, and an x-ray is used to take detailed images of the heart's blood vessels. Through the use of this procedure, heart chamber pressure and blood samples may also be obtained in addition to showing blockages and clot formations. However, catheterization may increase the risk of death in critically ill patients, according to some studies.

Electrocardiograms (EKGs) and stress tests are also another way of diagnosing heart problems. In addition, a number of imaging techniques can also be used. Computer axial tomography (CT or CAT) scans, a computerized, three-dimensional x-ray process, and magnetic resonance imaging (MRI) scans, which creates the heart's image by using a magnetic field) are also procedures that can be performed to diagnose heart disease. In addition, x-rays may also be performed to examine the heart's structures, and so may echocardiograms, which send ultrasonic waves through the heart to create its image.

A new test called ultrafast computed tomography is now available. This x-ray procedure costs the same as the stress test and takes the same amount of time. However, it is estimated to detect 95 percent of all heart blockages, while the stress test catches only 70 percent.

Treating Coronary Heart Disease

There are a number of procedures that can be done to help restore blood flow to the heart, whether or not a person has experienced angina or heart attack.

Angioplasty

Techniques include percutaneous transluminal coronary angioplasty (PTCA), or balloon angioplasty, and direct angioplasty. In PTCA, a catheter with a balloon on the tip is inserted into a narrowed artery, where the balloon is inflated to push aside any blockages. Direct angioplasty involves the same procedure, but the balloon catheter is inserted into a totally blocked artery rather than one that is simply narrowed. One study showed direct angioplasty to be successful in restoring blood flow in 90 percent of cases. In addition, studies that compared direct angioplasty with the medication tPA found angioplasty to be safer for high-risk patients.

According to a 1992 study conducted by the American Journal of Cardiology, angioplasty is a better alternative to bypass surgery (discussed below) if the patient is considered low risk (having only one or two blocked vessels). However, if a patient is high risk (suffering from severe conditions), bypass surgery is recommended. The mortality rate for an angioplasty is only about 1 percent. However, others feel that angioplasty causes the need for further procedures. Various 1995 health reports discovered some alarming information—not only were more procedures needed after an angioplasty, but the prevalence of angina one year later is significantly higher in those who had an angioplasty as opposed to those who had bypass surgery.

Laser angioplasty may also be an option in the future. With this technique, a laser catheter would be inserted into the artery and used to burn away the blockage. The procedure is still experimental and has not been perfected, but is expected to be easier to perform, less expensive and less painful than balloon angioplasty.

Bypass Surgery

When it has been established that certain arteries are blocked and normal blood flow to the heart must be restored, coronary bypass surgery is recommended. This particular procedure requires the taking of a vessel—usually from a patient's leg or thigh—and transplanting it to the aorta and coronary artery to replace, or bypass, the clogged artery. Of the 455,000 bypasses done in 1992, 72 percent were performed on men. A mortality rate of 5 percent or less is associated with this surgery.

Again, bypass surgery is usually recommended over angioplasty for high-risk patients. While the risks associated with bypass surgery are greater, patients who have more than two blocked arteries fare better with bypass than with angioplasty. In addition, studies show that additional procedures may be needed more often after angioplasty to treat recurring symptoms.

Coronary-Stent Placement

A new technique called coronary-stent placement is also now being used to treat coronary heart disease. In this procedure, done with the aid of ultrasound, a small, stainless-steel mesh tube—called a stent—is placed on the end of a balloon catheter and threaded into the blocked artery. The balloon is then inflated, expanding the tube and lodging it firmly in place. The stent pushes the blockage out of the way and props open the artery to increase blood flow. The risks of stent placement are the same as for angioplasty, however studies show the procedure to be more effective, opening arteries wider and requiring fewer procedures in the future. Coronary-stent placement is generally more expensive than angioplasty, as well. However, stents are not appropriate for difficult-to-reach blockages since they need to be positioned carefully without puncturing the vein.

Medications

A nonsurgical alternative to treat clogged heart arteries is medication, including calcium channel blockers, nitroglycerin, aspirin, and beta blockers. If heart failure is also a factor, angiotensin-converting enzyme (ACE) inhibitors, diuretics, and digitalis may be given.

Calcium channel blockers open blood vessels wider, encouraging blood flow. They work by blocking calcium, which is used by the muscle cells to constrict the vessels. Beta blockers are used to slow blood pressure and keep heart attack damage to a minimum.

Angiotensin-converting enzyme (ACE) inhibitors work by breaking apart the fatty deposits that form along artery walls. They are successful in preventing heart failure and have been credited with preventing heart attacks in those who take them. Diuretics remove water and salt from the body by causing the patient to urinate frequently, which results in lower blood pressure. Digitalis helps keep the heart pumping more effectively by relaxing heart vessels and facilitating blood flow to the heart. It works to strengthen the heartbeat and to reduce heart size.

A low, daily dose of aspirin may also be prescribed after heart attack to prevent repeat attacks. According to a 1996 report in the *Journal of the American College of Cardiology* that monitored close to one thousand patients, 2 percent of the aspirin users died from cardiac causes, compared with 5 percent who didn't use aspirin. The benefits were greater for those who had been treated with clot-dissolving drugs, the study said.

Cholesterol-lowering drugs such as lovastatin are also often used to treat those who have had bypass surgery. The drugs help reduce the progression of atherosclerosis, the artery-clogging disease that initially causes the need for surgery.

Studies show that drug therapy is best for those at low risk for heart attack, that is, who have mild angina or who have had a heart attack with no subsequent angina. Studies show that such low-risk patients can put off bypass surgery until it may be needed in the future. However, bypass surgery relieves angina pain and other symptoms of heart disease better than medication therapy.

Preventing Heart Attacks

While there's little you can do about your age, gender, or family history, you might be able to decrease your risk for heart attack by changing your lifestyle in the following areas:

- Stop smoking. According to the AHA, smokers' risk of heart attack is more than twice that of nonsmokers. In fact, smokers who have heart attacks are more likely to die from them, and more likely to die suddenly (within an hour) than nonsmokers. But if you quit smoking, your risk almost immediately begins to decline. Within ten years of quitting, your risk will drop to close to that of a person who has never smoked.

- Control your blood pressure. High blood pressure means the heart is working harder than it should be to push blood through the system. This causes the heart to enlarge and can accelerate atherosclerosis. However, by reducing your diastolic blood pressure by only 2 mm Hg, you can substantially decrease your risk for cardiovascular disease and stroke. The average healthy blood pressure is 120/80 mm Hg. (See Hypertension, p. 307.)

- Practice relaxation. Since stress is such a factor in heart disease, eliminating it from your life can do wonders for your cardio-vascular health. Use time- and stress-management techniques or relaxation therapies to reduce your stress levels.

- Exercise. Regular exercise can help to reduce weight, stress, cholesterol levels, and high blood pressure, and it can strengthen the heart, leading to a lower pulse rate. However, too much exercise, especially isometric exercise such as weight lifting, can trigger heart attacks. Talk with your practitioner about what sort of exercise program is right for you. Choose an exercise that you will enjoy and do regularly. Start slowly, then increase this to higher levels. A good beginning regimen should be three times a week for approximately a half hour each time.

- Drink moderately. Studies show that a drink or two a day may have a protective effect on the heart. However, anything beyond that can do damage. (A drink equals 12 ounces of beer, five ounces of wine, or 1½ ounces of liquor.)

- Ask your practitioner about aspirin. Studies have shown that taking aspirin daily may reduce the risk of heart attack by thinning the blood and preventing clots from forming. It may also reduce the severity of heart attacks when they do occur. However, aspirin is not safe for everyone and may increase the risk of stroke in some people.

- Monitor your cholesterol levels. Cholesterol is a fatlike substance that plays a large role in the formation of arteriosclerosis. The famous Framingham Heart Study found that heart attack rates rise 2 percent for each 1 percent increase in blood cholesterol over 200 mg/dL. To control cholesterol, avoid saturated fat, eat fewer calories, and try to eat foods rich in fiber such as fruits and vegetables. Drugs may be an option for some people with high cholesterol. The American Heart Association recommends having your cholesterol levels checked at least once every five years. (See Cholesterol, p. 89.)

Other Forms of Heart Disease

In addition to coronary heart disease, other cardiovascular diseases exist. These include valve disorders, congestive heart failure, congenital heart defects, heartbeat irregularities, heart muscle diseases, and pericardial disease. (See Hypertension, p. 307, and Stroke, p. 359, as well.)

Valve Disorders

The heart can fall victim to various valve disorders, which affect the regulation of blood flow to the heart. Endocarditis, floppy valve syndrome, and mitral valve prolapse are three of the most common valve disorders. Endocarditis is an inflammation of the heart's inner lining, which causes scar tissue to form on the heart muscle. In turn, this scarring prevents the proper function of the valves. Floppy valve syndrome is self-explanatory. It prevents heart valves from snugly fitting together, thus causing them to "flop." As a result of this flopping, there is a leakage of blood and an unregulated amount gets

SEX AFTER HEART ATTACK

The answer is yes—it is safe to have sex after a heart attack. While it may seem as if the heavy breathing and heightened heart rate associated with sex might bring on an attack, a study in the May 8, 1996, *Journal of the American Medical Association* shows that sexual activity is only a likely contributor to the onset of heart attack in just 0.9 percent of cases. While heart attack has been triggered by sexual intercourse in rare cases, statistics show that there is a one-in-a-million chance this could happen in a healthy person. And the relative risk for those with angina or previous heart attack is no greater than those with no history of heart disease. In addition, this relative risk decreases with regular exercise.

However, while sex is safe, studies show that many men have less sex after a heart attack. While in some cases this may be due to impotence (an estimated 39 percent of men who have had a heart attack have some degree of impotence, compared with 14 percent of the general male population), experts believe the cause may be mainly psychological, triggered by fear that intercourse may be dangerous. If you have concerns about sexual activity—or if you're experiencing sexual dysfunction—talk with your practitioner about your concerns. Remember, also, that intercourse is moderate exercise and has roughly the same effect on heart and blood pressure rates as does climbing two flights of stairs.

ANGER AND HEART DISEASE

If you're likely to blow your top at the first sign of adversity, you may also be likely to suffer a heart attack. A recent study from experts at the Harvard Medical School found that older men who had high levels of anger on a personality test were at three times greater risk of developing coronary heart disease than those who had low levels of anger. Some of the best ways to manage your anger include the following:

- Look for the source of your anger. The focus of your anger is rarely what's truly behind it. For example, an argument with your partner over household chores may really be about issues of responsibility and power. By realizing what you're truly angry about, you can resolve the problem more easily.

- Try forgiveness. Even if the person you're angry with isn't apologizing, practice forgiveness and try not to dwell on how you were wronged. Many times people don't even know they've hurt or angered you.

- Let go of anger. Switching off your anger is probably not as hard as you think. Tell yourself that it's not worth wasting energy being angry—it only gets in the way of your goals. Anger actually hurts you more than it hurts anyone else.

pumped to the heart. Mitral valve prolapse is actually a common and more harmless valve disorder. It occurs when there is a backflow of blood to the heart. This condition affects women more than men, and 3 to 10 percent of all adults.

Usually, cardiac catheterization and angiography are used to determine the type and extent of the valve disorder. Valve disorders can be corrected by surgically separating the valves that are stuck together with scar tissue (commissurotomy), by cutting valves to fit more snugly (valvuloplasty), or by reconstructing the valve tissue through plastic surgery (annuloplasty). Heart valve surgeries are considered reasonably safe.

SYMPTOMS OF HEART TROUBLE

Certain indications that something may be wrong with your heart include the following:

Breathing difficulties, especially during exercise or while lying flat

Waking from sleep breathless

A dry, hacking cough

Weakness and fatigue

Dizziness/fainting

Swelling of the legs, feet, ankles or abdominal region

Nausea

Angina (chest pain)

If you experience any of these symptoms, you should undergo a complete physical exam. Some tests may be recommended, such as a chest x-ray, to determine the cause of your symptoms.

However, minor risks such as infection or blood clotting do exist.

Congestive Heart Failure

Congestive heart failure involves problems with the heart's pump, usually caused by muscle failure. When the heart does not pump efficiently, the body becomes overloaded with water and sodium, often leading to death by total heart failure. Symptoms include difficulty breathing, coughing, fluid retention, chest pain, liver pain, and diminished urination. Also with congestive heart failure, the heart often becomes enlarged in order to compensate for its inefficiency.

Treatments include use of a pacemaker to regulate the heartbeat; dietary restrictions; and medications such as digitalis, vasodilators, and diuretics. Digitalis works by strengthening the heartbeat and reducing the size of the heart. Vasodilators help improve blood flow, and diuretics speed the elimination of water and sodium from the body. Beta blockers and calcium channel blockers are also sometimes prescribed.

Congenital Heart Defects

Congenital defects are abnormalities that occur at birth, perhaps because of a developmental problem in the womb. About 32,000 babies are born each year with these abnormalities, and there are more than 35 types recognized. Congenital heart defects do not mean the death of the infant—about 925,000 Americans with heart defects are alive today.

Heart defects may be caused by a disease in the mother during pregnancy, by drugs or alcohol taken by the mother, or by genetic or environmental factors. Almost all are discovered by age 5, and can usually be heard through a stethoscope as an out-of-the-ordinary sound, or murmur. (Not all murmurs mean a heart defect. "Innocent" murmurs occur naturally in many people.) Imaging techniques such as CAT scans, MRI, and ultrasound can be used to visualize heart defects.

Common types of congenital heart defects include the following:

1. *Ventricular septal defect*—an unnatural opening in the wall between the right and left ventricle.

2. *Pulmonary stenosis*—narrowing of the right pulmonary artery.

3. *Right ventricular hypertrophy*—an increase in volume in the myocardium of the right ventricle.

4. *Dextroposition of the aorta*—arrangement in which the aorta gets blood from the right and left ventricles.

5. *Tetralogy of Fallot*—a combination of the previous four heart defects.

6. *Eisenmenger's syndrome*—a type of ventricular septal defect that includes complications.

7. *Patent ductus arteriosus*—the duct between the aorta and the pulmonary artery, which remains open in the fetus until just before birth, fails to close.

8. *Atrial septal defect*—a natural opening in the heart of the fetus that fails to close before birth.

9. *Coarctation of the aorta*—a narrowing or blockage of the aorta.

Treatment depends on the type of defect. Congenital heart defects can usually be corrected with surgery. Drugs may also be used to treat the conditions.

Heartbeat Irregularities

At times, the heart may speed up, slow down, or flutter and become out of control. While everyone's heart skips a beat now and then, conditions or abnormal heartbeat and rhythm, known as arrhythmias, may signal heart disease. In themselves, they are usually not life-threatening.

Arrhythmias can be set off by a blockage in an artery, a lack of oxygen to the heart muscle, a slow heartbeat, changes in the electrical activity of the heart, or certain drugs. The most serious form of arrhythmia is ventricular fibrillation, in which the heart muscle contracts wildly, and blood stops being pumped. Unless immediate treatment is provided, death usually occurs.

Treatment includes medications such as quinidine, lidocaine, propranolol, and procainamide. The type of drug prescribed depends on the type of arrhythmia present. In emergencies, cardiopulmonary resuscitation can help keep the heart beating during an attack. In addition, a defibrillator—a piece of equipment that provides a jolt of electricity—can also be used in emergencies to shock the heart back into rhythm.

Heart pacemakers are available to control irregularities that may exist in the heart's rhythm (called arrhythmias). Pacemakers are tiny devices (the size of a silver dollar) that weigh only two ounces. Once placed within the patient's chest, it helps regulate the heartbeat by emitting an electrical charge—sort of a scaled-down version of defibrillation. This charge is generated by batteries within the device and carried to the heart by an electrode-containing wire. Pacemakers are implanted when there is complete heart vessel blockage. Their cost ranges from $3,000 to $5,000.

Heart Muscle Diseases

There are several types of heart muscle disease, also known as cardiomyopathy, with a number of causes—some of them unknown. In this condition, the heart muscle may thicken or shrink, causing problems such as congestive heart failure, inefficient pumping action, or valve problems. Cardiomyopathy may be caused by an infection, an illness, a degenerative disease (such as muscular dystrophy), high blood pressure, and toxic substances such as chemicals, drugs, alcohol, and chemotherapy drugs. Treatment depends on the type of disease and its cause and often includes surgery or medications.

Pericardial Disease

The pericardium is the fluid-filled sac that protects the heart, and it may be affected by various types of infection.

- *Pericarditis.* Inflammation of the pericardium, due to infection. In acute pericarditis, a general infection affects the sac, causing chest pain and fever. It can be treated with antibiotics. Acute nonspecific pericarditis is a condition in which the pericardium is attacked directly by a virus.
- *Pericardial effusion.* This occurs when the sac becomes flooded with liquid. It can be caused by injury to the heart or by drugs, including radiation therapy used to treat cancer. It is not dangerous unless the fluid causes the heart to fill with blood, a condition called cardiac tamponade. In this case, a surgical procedure called pericardiocentesis is done to drain the fluid from the sac.

- *Constrictive pericarditis.* The sac becomes hard with calcium deposits and interferes with the functioning of the heart. Treatment includes surgical removal of the pericardium.

For more information:

American College of Advancement in Medicine
23121 Verdugo Dr., Suite 204
Laguna Hills, CA 92653
714-583-7666

American Heart Association
7272 Greenville Ave.
Dallas, TX 75231
800-AHA-USA1
214-373-6300
http://www.amhrt.org

Cardiac Rehabilitation
AHCPR Publications Clearinghouse
P.O. Box 8547
Silver Spring, MD 20907
800-358-9295

Coronary Club, Inc.
9500 Euclid Ave. EE37
Cleveland, OH 44195
216-444-3690

National Heart, Lung and Blood Institute
Information Center Public Health Service
P.O. Box 30105
Bethesda, MD 20824
301-251-1222

HEMORRHOIDS

About half of the country's population have experienced hemorrhoids, swollen blood vessels in and around the anus, by the age of 50, according to the National Digestive Disease Information Clearinghouse. While normally these blood vessels help to form the seal that prevents waste from leaking from the rectum, straining during bowel movements may increase the pressure surrounding the area and cause the vessels to swell. Although hemorrhoids can be painful, they are not dangerous.

Types of Hemorrhoids

There are two kinds of hemorrhoids: internal and external. Internal hemorrhoids are located inside the anus in the wall of the rectum. An internal hemorrhoid may protrude through the anus outside the body. This is called a protruding, or prolapsed, hemorrhoid, and it can become irritated and painful. External hemorrhoids are located under the skin surrounding the anus. Occasionally, a hard lump caused by a blood clot can develop. This condition is called a thrombosed external hemorrhoid.

Symptoms

The most common symptoms of hemorrhoids include

- Bright red blood covering the stool or toilet paper, or in the toilet bowl

- Discomfort or pain during a bowel movement

- Painful swelling around the anus

- A mucus discharge from the anus

- Itching around the anal opening

- A hard lump in the skin around the anus

Diagnosis

It is important to check with a doctor any time there is bleeding or blood in the stool for more than a couple of days, as these symptoms can be similar to the signs of other diseases such as colorectal cancer. Hemorrhoids are diagnosed through a physical examination. A proctoscopy, a diagnostic procedure in which a viewing scope is inserted into the rectum, is also done to rule out cancer.

Treatment

Self-care is used to treat a mild attack of hemorrhoids and is aimed at relieving the symptoms. There are a number of surgical treatments for severe hemorrhoids. Internal hemorrhoids can be treated on an outpatient basis with rubber band ligation, a nearly painless procedure that requires no anesthetic. In rubber band ligation, a proctoscope is inserted into the rectum to view the hemorrhoid. Then, through the proctoscope, a tiny band is placed around the base of the hemorrhoid. The band cuts off circulation and the hemorrhoid withers away. In a few days, the band and the hemorrhoid drop off painlessly.

In sclerotherapy, another procedure for internal hemorrhoids, a chemical solution is injected around the swollen blood vessel to shrink the hemorrhoid.

External hemorrhoids that need surgical attention may be treated in one of two ways. Electrical or laser heat can be used to vaporize the tissue in a procedure called laser coagulation. Also, infrared light, called infrared photo coagulation, can be used to burn away the hemorrhoidal tissues.

A prolapsed hemorrhoid is treated with hemorrhoidectomy, or surgical removal. In this procedure, done using a general or epidural anesthetic, the hemorrhoid is sutured and removed with a knife.

SELF-CARE FOR HEMORRHOIDS

Common and helpful self-care methods include

- *Over-the-counter medications (Preparation H)*. Applying a hemorrhoidal cream or suppository to the affected area can help relieve itching and irritation.

- *Sitz baths*. A soak in a warm bath of plain water several times a day can cleanse the area and soothe hemorrhoids.

- *Ice packs*. Swelling can be reduced by applying an ice pack wrapped in a towel to the affected area.

- *High-fiber diets*. Eating plenty of high-fiber foods—such as fruits, vegetables, beans, and whole-grain products—and drinking plenty of water can soften stool and prevent constipation, easing some of the pressure that contributes to hemorrhoid pain.

If these measures provide no relief, and the hemorrhoids become so enlarged that they become extremely painful, visit your practitioner.

Prevention

The best way to prevent hemorrhoids is to avoid constipation. Exercising, drinking plenty of fluids, and including fiber (such as fruits, vegetables, whole grains, and legumes) in your diet will help produce softer stools. Emptying the bowels as soon as the urge occurs and not sitting on the toilet for a long time help prevent straining and the pressure responsible for hemorrhoids.

If you already have hemorrhoids, gently clean the anal area after each bowel movement with a moistened towelette, then dry the area thoroughly.

For more information:

National Digestive Diseases
Information Clearinghouse
2 Information Way
Bethesda, MD 20892-3570
301-654-3810
http://www.niddk.nih.gov

HERNIA

The body's organs are held in place by a thin wall of muscle. At times, when the muscular wall becomes thin, perhaps because of an injury or congenital weakness, an organ or tissue can push through it, creating a protrusion known as a hernia. Men suffer hernias at thirty times the rate of women. Hernias can also occur in newborns.

Types of Hernia

There are several types of hernia:

1. *Inguinal hernia*. This hernia occurs when part of the intestine protrudes out of the abdomen. It can push toward the scrotum, creating a bulge in the groin area (a direct hernia) or project into the scrotum (an indirect hernia), causing pain and swelling. Eighty percent of all hernias are inguinal hernias, and 80 to 90 percent of them are suffered by men.

2. *Femoral hernia*. This hernia occurs when the intestine passes through the canal that

carries the blood vessels from the abdomen into the top of the thigh. These are most common in women—only 1 to 5 percent of femoral hernias occur in men.

3. *Incisional hernia.* This hernia occurs after surgery has left a weakness in an abdominal wall along the incision.

4. *Paraumbilical hernia.* This hernia usually occurs due to a weakness in the abdominal wall surrounding the umbilicus. It may be found in newborns.

5. *Hiatal hernia.* This hernia occurs when the stomach pushes through a small hole in the diaphragm and into the chest cavity, causing heartburn and acid indigestion.

A hernia becomes known as a strangulated hernia when an organ or tissues become trapped and the blood supply is cut off. In this case, the tissue may die, and gangrene—a life-threatening infection requiring emergency care—may set in.

Causes

A hernia may be caused by sudden stress to the abdominal wall (often the result of lifting a heavy object), by a weakening of the muscle wall caused by previous surgery, by a congenital defect, or by a combination of these factors. Constipation, extreme weight gain in the abdominal area, and heavy coughing, perhaps from smoking, can also be factors because each puts pressure on internal organs.

Symptoms

Hernia symptoms include pain or discomfort in the abdominal area while lifting an object or bending, sudden swelling of the area, and tenderness. If the hernia has become strangulated, nausea and vomiting may occur. However, in many cases there may be no symptoms at all.

Diagnosis

In some cases, a bulge of tissue in the groin or a mass in the testes may indicate the presence of a hernia. To diagnosis an inguinal hernia that is not readily visible in a male patient, a doctor will ask him to stand with his one leg flexed and with his weight resting on the other. The doctor will place a finger against the lower part of the scrotum and push the scrotal skin until the finger enters the inguinal canal. The doctor then asks the patient to cough. If he feels pressure on the fingertip or on the side of the finger, a hernia exists.

Treatment

With the exception of hiatal hernias, which can usually be treated with antacids and diet restrictions, hernias must be repaired surgically. There is no instance in which a hernia is best left untreated. While surgery can be postponed if the hernia is small enough, there is always a chance that it may become strangulated, causing tissue death and gangrene. At times, a truss—a tight-fitting device worn around the abdomen—can be used to hold a hernia in place until it is repaired; however, a truss is not a permanent solution.

Hernias are usually repaired through outpatient surgery. Common complications include hematoma (a collection of blood under the skin), infection, or injuries to the nerves and vessels of the groin. About 10 to 15 percent of all hernias recur after corrective surgery.

Through the conventional method, an incision is made over the hernia site and the protruding tissue is put back into its proper place in the abdominal cavity. The hole in the abdominal wall is then repaired by sewing strong surrounding muscles over the area. This is the most common type of hernia repair. In a few cases, the tension from the stitches may strain or tear the muscles and cause the hernia to recur. A nonstressful recovery is important to the success of the surgery.

In the tension-free mesh technique, an incision is made and the surgeon replaces the protruding tissue and repairs the abdominal wall with a piece of mesh, which is generally well accepted by the body's natural tissues. There are fewer recurrences with this method, because the introduction of the mesh prevents the strain on the newly repaired muscles.

The newest method is the laparoscopic method. The surgeon views the hernia through a laparoscope, a scope that is inserted into the abdominal cavity through an incision. At the same time, the surgeon repairs the hernia through tubes that enter the abdominal wall through other incisions. This method is still relatively new. The long-term outcomes of this procedure are unknown, but at this time it is not considered any more effective than the other methods. It may hold a greater risk of complications, and it is more expensive. If you do opt for laparoscopic repair, experts recommend choosing a practitioner who has performed the procedure before.

Prevention

Not much can be done to prevent a hernia. You can, however, try to stay fit, keeping your weight at an appropriate level. Also, use proper techniques when lifting heavy objects. To lift a heavy object, bend from the knees and keep your back straight. Hug the object close to your body and lift straight up. Do not bend at the waist, causing your back to handle the load.

You can keep a hiatal hernia from causing discomfort by wearing loose clothes, keeping your weight at an ideal level, and staying away from those foods and beverages that cause heartburn. These include coffee, fried or fatty foods, peppermint, highly spiced foods, alcoholic beverages, and chocolate. Smoking may also trigger discomfort from hiatal hernia.

For more information:

American College of Surgeons
55 E. Erie St.
Chicago, IL 60611
312-664-4050
http://www.facs.org

National Digestive Diseases
Information Clearinghouse
2 Information Way
Bethesda, MD 20892-3570
301-654-3810
http://www.niddk.nih.gov

HYPERTENSION

Blood pressure is the force your blood exerts on the walls of your blood vessels as it travels throughout the body. It's measured using two numbers, the systolic and the diastolic. The systolic, the higher number in the blood pressure fraction, represents the force of the blood at its greatest strength as the heart contracts. The diastolic, the lower number, represents the force of the blood between heartbeats, when the heart is resting.

High blood pressure, or hypertension, is diagnosed when blood pressure readings remain at more than 140 mm Hg (systolic)/90 mm Hg (diastolic) over a period of time (usually at least two readings over three days, or after several hours of rest). In contrast, the optimal blood pressure reading is 120/80 mm Hg or less.

According to the American Heart Association, approximately fifty million Americans have hypertension, or high blood pressure. Men, compared with women, have a greater risk of high blood pressure until age 55. From age 55 to 75, the risks for men and women are about equal; thereafter, more women than men develop hypertension. In 1993, some 15,306 men died from high blood pressure.

The rate of death for hypertension in 1993 was 6.5 for white men and 30 for African-American men. Caucasians and African Americans living in the Southeastern United States have higher rates of hypertension and related mortality than those from other parts of the country. High blood pressure affects 24.7 percent of Caucasians age 20 and older; 28.4 percent African Americans; and 15.1 percent Mexican-Americans. In addition, 9.7 percent of Asian men and 10.3 percent of Native American men have hypertension.

For people age 60 and older, some 60 percent of Caucasians, 71 percent of African Americans, and 61 percent of Mexican-Americans have high blood pressure. Some 73 percent of Japanese-American men between the ages of 71 and 93 have the condition.

Some 90 percent of people with hypertension—which is a disease—have no obvious causes for their elevated blood pressure levels, known as essential hypertension. For about 10 percent of people with hypertension, a definite cause or combination of causes may trigger the disease, including a genetic predisposition, kidney diseases, sleep apnea (sudden stoppage of breathing during the night), and environmental conditions. Smoking, obesity, a high-fat diet, and a sedentary lifestyle are major risk factors in the development of high blood pressure.

Symptoms

Symptoms of hypertension include headaches, heart palpitations, a flushed face, blurry vision, nosebleeds, labored breathing after moderate exertion, fatigue, a strong and frequent need to urinate, ringing or buzzing in the ears (tinnitus) or a feeling of dizziness and spinning (vertigo).

However, hypertension usually shows no symptoms in the majority of people, and for this reason, many people call it the silent killer. Most people only discover they have hypertension when they have their blood pressure checked or when life-threatening subsequent conditions occur.

Complications of Hypertension

If high blood pressure is left untreated the following conditions may result:

1. *Heart disease.* High blood pressure accelerates the development of arteriosclerosis, in which the arteries become scarred, hardened, and less elastic. This results in decreased blood flow and an increased risk of blood clots. People with high blood pressure are twice as likely to suffer heart attacks and eight times as likely to have strokes than those with normal blood pressure.

2. *Kidney damage.* High blood pressure causes kidney damage, which may eventually prevent the body from eliminating waste products from the blood efficiently.

3. *Eye damage.* Hypertension can cause retinal hemorrhaging and even blindness.

CLASSIFICATION OF BLOOD PRESSURE LEVELS

There is no such thing as a "normal" blood pressure measurement, and very few people actually have a measurement of exactly 120/80 mm Hg. Yet, guidelines have been devised to give practitioners a tool to help diagnose the stage of the disease. Below is a listing of the standards that most practitioners use to diagnose hypertension.

While it was once taken for granted that older people had higher blood pressure, studies today show that hypertension is not a natural effect of aging and, if anything, older people should be watching their blood pressure levels more carefully than younger people.

	Systolic	*Diastolic*
Optimal	<120 mm Hg	<80 mm Hg
Normal	120–129 mm Hg	80–84 mm Hg
High normal	130–139 mm Hg	85–89 mm Hg
Stage 1 hypertension	140–159 mm Hg	90–99 mm Hg
Stage 2 hypertension	160–179 mm Hg	100–109 mm Hg
Stage 3 hypertension	180–209 mm Hg	110–119 mm Hg
Stage 4 hypertension	>210 mm Hg	>120 mm Hg

Diagnosis

Blood pressure is measured using a sphygmomanometer, or blood pressure cuff, which is inflated around the upper arm to obtain a reading. Usually, blood pressure is taken by a practitioner. Experts recommend having your blood pressure checked every three years until the age of 40, and then every two years after that—an important recommendation considering that high blood pressure usually has no symptoms.

Blood pressure can also be taken at home, with a sphygmomanometer or another, automatic device. Home monitoring can be helpful in distinguishing true hypertension from white-coat hypertension, hypertension that occurs only in the doctor's office, perhaps due to nervousness. Many automatic devices can measure blood pressure several times a day and can present a more accurate overall measurement than a single, in-office test.

An examination for changes to the retina, the membrane at the back of the eye, can also help to diagnose hypertension. The retina is the only place in the body where arteries can be seen directly.

Self-Care and Prevention

While medical experts are uncertain about the specific biological reactions that cause hypertension, they do know what factors contribute to the development and progression of the disease. By taking measures to control or eliminate these factors, people with hypertension can often reduce their blood pressure, and those without hypertension can prevent its development. Most medical experts recommend the following:

- Begin a moderate exercise program under physician supervision. Aerobic exercise such as running, walking, or biking can be especially helpful. Most experts recommend against isometric exercises such as weight training for those with hypertension because it can raise blood pressure levels dramatically.

- Quit smoking. Smoking increases the heart rate and narrows the blood vessels, directly causing a rise in blood pressure.

- Avoid alcohol. Studies show that as few as two drinks a day can produce a rise in blood pressure. Men 35 years or older who drank that amount were twice as likely to have hypertension than nondrinkers.

- Reduce personal stress and anger. Stress, especially in men, can lead to significantly higher blood pressure levels. According to the Framingham Study, men who reported high levels of anxiety had more than twice the relative risk of developing hypertension than men who reported no anxiety. (See Relaxation Techniques, p. 124.)

- Lose excess weight. Obesity and high blood pressure go hand-in-hand. According to the Society of Actuaries, if you are 30 percent above average weight, your risk of coronary heart disease is 44 percent higher than someone of average weight.

- Eat a diet low in fat and salt, and high in fiber, supervised by your physician. A high-fiber, low-fat diet reduces the risk of coronary heart disease. And salt is believed to hinder the removal of water from the body and, therefore, raise blood pressure in those with hypertension. (However, salt—in moderation—probably doesn't raise blood pressure in those without risk of hypertension.)

- Monitor caffeine intake. While some studies have shown no risks from caffeine, others have seen a correlation between hypertension and higher intake of the stimulant. You might want to try going without coffee and other caffeinated foods and beverages to see how your blood pressure reacts.

Medical Treatments

If lifestyle modifications have no effect, antihypertensive drugs may be added to your treatment plan. At times, antihypertensive medication is prescribed in conjunction with lifestyle modifications right from the start, depending on the degree of hypertension and the state of overall health. Common medications for the treatment of high blood pressure include

1. *Angiotensin converting enzyme (ACE) inhibitors.* These medications block the production of angiotensin, a chemical the body produces to raise blood pressure. Angiotensin's normal role is to maintain equilibrium when blood pressure drops by tightening the arteries. ACE inhibitors include captopril (Capoten), lisinopril (Prinivil, Zestril), and enalapril (Vasotec).

2. *Beta-adrenergic blocking drugs (or beta blockers).* These drugs reduce high blood pressure by reducing the force and speed of the heartbeat. Beta blockers include propranolol (Inderal), nadolol (Corgard), and metoprolol (Lopressor).

3. *Calcium channel blockers.* Calcium channel blockers work by blocking the passage of calcium, which the muscle cells use to

WHITE-COAT HYPERTENSION

White-coat hypertension—high blood pressure that only occurs in a practitioner's presence—is generally thought to be the result of a person's nervousness during their appointment. It is usually considered harmless and is dismissed as a sign of stress. However, a new study published in *Lancet* showed that a number of people with white-coat hypertension also had abnormalities of heart function and the arteries that are usually associated with high blood pressure. This could mean that white-coat hypertension may not be completely benign.

If you have white-coat hypertension, you should be monitored regularly by your practitioner for any worsening of your condition. In some cases, treatment may be recommended.

control the size of the blood vessels. When the muscles of the arteries are prevented from constricting, blood vessels open up, allowing blood to flow more easily through them. Recent evidence also shows that calcium channel blockers may be the first known drugs to actually slightly reverse the effects of heart disease. Included in this class of drugs are nifedipine (Procardia), diltiazem (Cardizem), isradipine (DynaCirc), and verapamil (Calan).

4. *Diuretics.* Diuretics cause the body to excrete excess salt and water from the body, reducing the blood volume. As a result, the heart does not have to work as hard. Diuretics used to be the first choice in hypertension medication; however, the availability of newer drugs has changed that. Commonly prescribed diuretics include Diuril, Dyazide, and Corzide.

5. *Vasodilators.* These drugs act directly on the muscles that comprise the walls of the arteries, causing them to dilate. Some of the stronger vasodilators produce a rapid reduction in blood pressure—especially

when given by injection—and, therefore, are often used in hypertensive crisis. Hydralazine (Apresoline) is included in this class.

Antihypertensive medications may cause such minor side effects as dizziness, fainting, and stomach upset. More serious possible side effects are specific to each drug and range from disorientation, depression, and anxiety to a decrease in libido, sexual dysfunction, impaired circulation, and congestive heart failure. Discuss the possibilities with your practitioner before you begin taking a medication. Also discuss any acute or chronic conditions you have before beginning treatment. Once you begin treatment, report any side effects immediately. Never cease taking antihypertensives suddenly because this may cause a dramatic rise in blood pressure with serious consequences.

For more information:

American Heart Association
7272 Greenville Ave.
Dallas, TX 75231
800-AHA-USA1
214-373-6300
http://www.amhrt.org

HYPOTENSION

Low blood pressure, or hypotension, is one condition you may want to have. A person is considered hypotensive if blood pressure readings are less than 100/70 mm Hg. For the most part, hypotension is harmless—even beneficial—as long as you feel fine. In fact, studies show the lower your blood pressure, the longer you're likely to live.

However, there are some conditions that may spark low blood pressure. Diabetes, Addison's disease, and alcoholism are all associated with hypotension. In some people, low blood pressure can cause fainting (or syncope) after exercise or standing or sitting up suddenly. Blood-pressure-lowering medications may also be at fault, bringing blood pressure down to dangerously low levels. If low levels are causing problems, treatment may be prescribed.

Coronary Club, Inc.
9500 Euclid Ave., EE37
Cleveland, OH 44195
216-444-3690

National Heart, Lung, and Blood Institute
Public Health Service Information Center
P.O. Box 30105
Bethesda, MD 20824
301-251-1222

National Hypertension Association
324 E. 30th St.
New York, NY 10016
212-889-3557

INCONTINENCE

When the urinary system is working correctly, urine collects in the bladder and is held there by the urinary sphincter, the muscular opening of the bladder. When the bladder becomes full, a person consciously relaxes those muscles, and the urine flows through the sphincter into a tube called the urethra and out of the body.

However, problems with the bladder, the urethra, the nerves that signal the need for urination, or the muscles that surround the sphincter may result in incontinence, the involuntary leaking of urine. Urinary incontinence affects an estimated ten million Americans, according to the U.S. Department of Health and Human Services. Up to 5 percent of men between 15 and 64 years of age have experienced urinary incontinence, and some 15 percent of men older than 60 have had it. Women are twice as likely to experience incontinence than men because of hormonal factors and the stress of pregnancy and childbirth.

In 90 percent of the cases, incontinence can be successfully treated. However, many men don't seek medical care because of embarrassment or because they don't know help is available.

In men, incontinence is more likely to occur after age 60 because the bladder tends to shrink and hold less urine comfortably. An enlarged prostate, a condition known as benign prostatic hyperplasia (BPH), may also contribute to incontinence. In BPH, the prostate gland, which surrounds the urethra, gradually grows, cutting off the flow of urine. This stretches and distends the bladder, often causing problems with nerves and muscles. Surgery to correct BPH can also damage the muscles and nerves surrounding the urethra, causing incontinence, though this happens less frequently than in the past due to refinements in surgical procedures. (See Prostate Disease, p. 333.)

Use of certain medications (such as antidepressants, diuretics, tranquilizers, some blood pressure drugs, and over-the-counter cold medicine), urinary tract infection, stroke, and damage to the spinal cord can also lead to incontinence.

The main symptom of urinary incontinence is the involuntary escape of urine from the bladder. Most times only a small amount escapes, but less often there are conditions when a person loses total control of the bladder.

Types of Urinary Incontinence

There are three types of urinary incontinence: urge, stress, and overflow.

Urge incontinence is the involuntary escape of urine with little or no warning. Men with this disorder may strain when trying to empty their bladder, despite the sense of urgency, and may empty the bladder completely or incompletely. This is common among those who suffer from multiple sclerosis, spinal cord lesions, spinal disc problems, and in patients who have had a stroke.

Stress incontinence is the involuntary loss of small amounts of urine when coughing, sneezing, laughing, or performing other physical activities that increase abdominal pressure. In men, stress incontinence may occur because the urethral sphincter, the part of the urethra that holds the bladder closed, has not contracted fully, allowing drops of urine to escape.

Overflow incontinence is the involuntary loss of urine from a bladder that does not empty completely. It can be caused by nerve damage, medication side effects, a stretched or distended bladder, and an obstruction of the urethra. This is the type of incontinence often found in men who have enlarged prostates.

Diagnosis

Do not hesitate to talk with your practitioner about any problems with incontinence; it is highly treatable, and in some instances may signal a more serious disorder. Specialists who deal with incontinence are called urologists.

A practitioner will take a medical history and review any drugs being taken. Reflexes and muscle gait should be tested. Blood tests and urine tests may be done to rule out another disease or a urinary tract infection. A rectal examination may be done to determine if there are any internal problems.

Usually, these simple tests are all that are needed to diagnose the problem. However, urodynamic studies—a series of tests that include uroflowmetry, cystometry, and endoscopic procedures—may be done if the tests are inconclusive. In uroflowmetry, a practitioner records the volume of urine released, the length of urination, and the presence of any dripping after urination. In cystometry, a small, thin tube called a catheter is inserted into the bladder through the urethra to measure and monitor the bladder's functions. In endoscopic procedures, a thin viewing scope is inserted into the urethra and bladder to visualize the internal structures and spot any abnormalities.

Before visiting the doctor, it may be wise to keep track of incidents of incontinence, when they occurred, what triggered them, and what amount of urine was lost. Such a record can aid in diagnosis.

Treatment

If another condition such as a urinary tract infection is diagnosed as the cause of incontinence, that condition can be treated accordingly to resolve the problem.

In most cases, self-care techniques are all that are required to treat incontinence. (See the box, opposite, on these strategies.) Padded undergarments or catheters should not be used as a treatment for incontinence since dependence on such products should be a last resort.

Medications are often given to supplement self-care strategies. Those commonly prescribed include oxybutynin (Ditropan) to prevent spasms of the bladder muscles and phenylpropanolamine (Propagest) or pseudoephedrine (Sudafed) to tighten the muscles of the sphincter. If BPH is involved, finasteride (Proscar), or terazosin (Hytrin) may be prescribed to reduce prostate enlargement. Some evidence shows that the herb saw palmetto may also help reduce the size of the prostate.

There are several surgical treatments used when the other, less invasive, treatments fail. An artifical sphincter can be surgically implanted, or the muscles of the neck of the bladder can be suspended to improve muscle tone. The artificial sphincter treatment is reported to be successful in 90 percent of patients, while the bladder neck suspensions are effective in 80 percent.

Collagen injections may be done to firm up the area around the urethra. However, this treatment is found to be much more effective in women than in men. While it is successful for 90 percent of women, it only works in about 50 percent of men. Collagen injections may also need to be repeated to maintain results.

A new procedure, known as urethral suspension or the urethral sling, is currently being developed. This surgery involves inserting three

---

SELF-CARE FOR INCONTINENCE

- Retrain your bladder. This involves prolonging the time between urination gradually, first waiting one to two hours before a trip to the bathroom, then three to four. This stretches the bladder and can improve urge incontinence in up to 75 percent of those who try it. Talk with your practitioner about getting started.

- Avoid diuretics—substances that increase urination. These include alcohol, coffee, and tea. Also avoid liquids before going to bed at night.

- Don't smoke. Smoking can trigger coughing, which in turn triggers stress incontinence.

- Follow a proper diet. Eating well can prevent constipation (which affects urinary health) and can help fight off urinary tract infections, which can lead to incontinence.

- Check out saw palmetto. This herb has been found to be moderately successful in treating incontinence associated with benign prostatic hyperplasia. Ask your practitioner.

---

small tubes into an incision made under the scrotum. The tubes are pulled tightly against the urethra and sutured into place to help restore urinary control. In preliminary studies, it has been shown to have a cure rate of 90 percent. However, it is still considered experimental.

For more information:

American Foundation for Urologic Disease
300 W. Pratt St., Suite 401
Baltimore, MD 21201
800-242-2383
410-727-2908
http://www.acess.digex.net.~afud.org

National Association for Continence
P.O. Box 8310
Spartanburg, SC 29305-8310
864-579-7900
800-BLADDER
http://www.nafc.org

National Kidney and Urologic Diseases
Information Clearinghouse
Box NKUDIC
3 Information Way
Bethesda, MD 20892-3580
http://www.niddk.nih.gov

U.S. Department of Health and Human Services
Public Health Service
Agency for Health Care Policy and Research
Executive Office Center
5600 Fishers Ln.
Rockville, MD 20857
800-358-9295
301-443-2403

Simon Foundation for Continence
P.O. Box 815
Wilmette, IL 60091
800-237-4666
847-864-3913

KIDNEY DISEASE

The kidneys are vital organs. They filter waste products out of the body and drain excess water from your system. Chemicals in the blood are balanced, and extra amounts of acid are removed by the kidneys when they function properly. The kidneys produce a hormone that helps make red blood cells, as well. They also help regulate blood pressure by producing a chemical called resin, which excretes excess fluid from the body. Each human has two kidneys that are the size of a fist. They are located on both sides of the backbone, just above the small of the back. Each adult kidney weighs $1/4$ pound and pumps approximately 200 quarts of blood each day through 140 miles of tubes and filters that exist throughout the body.

Kidney disease is actually a catchall term that includes many different conditions, from urinary tract infections to serious malfunctions. If any form of kidney disease goes untreated, future damage may occur, possibly resulting in eventual failure of the kidneys. Many forms of kidney disease can be successfully treated if symptoms are recognized early enough. Unfortunately, if kidney disease does go untreated, the result is almost always death.

Because kidney disease takes on so many forms, it also is somewhat common—affecting one person out of twenty. Current estimates indicate that 700,000 people worldwide are suffering from kidney failure, and there are 200,000 cases of kidney disease in the United States alone.

Kidney Stones

Kidney stones, or urinary tract calculi, affect approximately 200,000 to 1,400,000 people in the United States and are the cause of one out of every one thousand hospitalizations. About 10 percent of men can expect to experience a kidney stone by the age of 70.

Also called nephrolithiasis, kidney stones form in the kidney, bladder, or ureter (the tube that connects the kidney to the bladder) when there is a buildup of salt or mineral crystals in the urine.

Small stones in the kidney usually do not cause pain until they enter the ureter. Though the passage of a stone is extremely painful, most pass out of the body through the urethra without causing any serious problems or additional damage. Most stones are less than 0.2 inches in diameter.

There are several types of stones. Calcium stones account for 75 to 85 percent of all stones and consist of calcium and carbonate. Uric acid stones account for 8 percent of all stones; these usually occur in people with gout. Struvite stones are large, rough stones that form due to a urinary tract infection. Struvite stones mainly occur in women.

Symptoms and Diagnosis

Symptoms of kidney stones include excruciating pain of the lower back or abdomen that travels toward the groin area, a frequent urge to urinate, and blood in the urine.

Stones are diagnosed through analysis of blood and urine samples. An intravenous pyelogram, in which a contrast substance that can be seen on an x-ray is injected into the bloodstream, may be done. The contrast material is filtered through the kidneys, making kidney structures visible on x-rays.

Treatment

Most kidney stones are permitted to pass out of the body naturally, and medications are prescribed to help the person through the painful process. Drinking at least six to eight glasses of water per day is also recommended.

Stones that cannot be passed can be treated with a procedure called lithotripsy. In lithotripsy, the stones are broken apart by shock waves. The waves can be administered by using a machine called a lithotripor, which is placed against the

PREVENTING KIDNEY STONES

Drinking lots of fluids can decrease your chances of forming stones by 40 percent. According to a recent study conducted by a Harvard research team, drinking even beer, wine, or coffee can be beneficial to your kidneys. Apparently, these liquids increase the flow of urine and decrease the substances within kidneys that cause formation of stones. However, intake of these beverages should be moderate, not excessive.

While at one time high calcium intake was blamed for calcium stones, cutting back on calcium is no longer recommended for those with such stones. One recent study showed that men who consumed the highest amounts of dietary calcium were actually less likely than others to get kidney stones. Experts speculate that this is because calcium may reduce the amount of urinary oxalate in the body, a substance that may contribute to stone formation.

abdomen, or while the person is seated in a tub of water, which serves to conduct the shock waves. The small pieces of the stones can then be passed out of the system during urination. Lithotripsy requires general or local anesthesia, but no incision. This procedure is used to treat approximately 10 percent of patients who have stones.

There are also surgical procedures used to remove stones. Open surgery, performed under general anesthesia, is the traditional method. Another option involves the insertion of a fiberoptic tube into the bladder or ureter. Then, another instrument is inserted to crush and remove the stone. When the tube is inserted into the bladder, the procedure is called cystoscopy. When the tube is inserted into the ureters, the procedure is called ureterorenoscopy. Although these procedures are available, over 90 percent of stones can still be treated without the use of surgical methods.

In addition to treatment to remove the stone, medications or dietary restrictions may be prescribed to prevent stones from recurring.

Other Forms of Kidney Disease

There are several other forms of kidney disease. One form is pyelonephritis. This is an inflammation of the kidney's tissues as a result of an untreated urinary tract infection. It can affect one or both kidneys, and symptoms may include fever, nausea, vomiting, burning urination, and pain. It is diagnosed through urine tests that indicate the presence of bacteria. Antibiotics are used to treat this condition. If the case is severe, hospitalization may be necessary.

Nephritis is inflammation of the kidney. It is a temporary condition that can be caused by drug reaction, another form of kidney disease, or an infection. It is indicated by retention of salt and fluid, which results in swelling, and the presence of protein in the urine. It is diagnosed through urine and blood tests. Treatment includes drugs such as penicillin and ampicillin.

Glomerulonephritis inflates the glomeruli, the areas of the kidneys that filter the blood. It is usually caused by an infection. Symptoms include discolored urine, high blood pressure, protein in the urine, anemia, extreme headaches, or possible convulsions. Treatment usually involves a low-salt diet, medications to reduce blood pressure, and measures to treat the infection. In many cases, the condition may resolve on its own. However, treatment is recommended because of the chance that glomerulonephritis may lead to total failure of the kidneys.

Polycystic kidney disease is a hereditary and progressive disorder in which cysts form around the kidneys. The symptoms include enlargement of the abdomen, pain, blood in the urine, and excessive urination. Patients may also have high blood pressure and kidney stones. There is no treatment or cure for this form of kidney disease. However, symptoms can be treated: high blood pressure can be controlled, and kidney stones can be treated. The majority of people with the condition suffer kidney failure.

Kidney Failure

The last stage of kidney disease is end-stage renal disease, or kidney failure. This occurs when the kidneys totally shut down, and it is irreversible. End-stage renal disease can result from any form of kidney disease that has been left untreated.

People can live with only one kidney and remain relatively healthy if just one of their kidneys functions at even a 20 percent capacity rate. However, if this rate falls below 20 percent, fatigue and weakness set in and medical attention becomes necessary. Two treatment options are available for those suffering kidney failure: dialysis and kidney transplant.

Dialysis

Dialysis entails using some form of machine or mechanism to filter the blood and prevent the backup of toxins in the bloodstream. It must be done on a daily basis to replace the function of the kidneys until a transplant can be performed.

The type of dialysis prescribed depends on a person's individual condition and situation.

One form of dialysis is automated peritoneal dialysis. In this procedure, an incision is made in the abdomen, and a catheter is inserted into the abdominal cavity. During each session of peritoneal dialysis, a special solution is inserted through the catheter and left inside the abdomen for several hours. During that time, waste products passing through the intestines seep through the peritoneal membrane and mix with the solution, which is then drained from the body. This form of dialysis can be done at night and, therefore, allows the patient to be treatment-free during the daytime hours. This procedure is done at a person's home and can be performed manually or by machine.

Continuous ambulatory dialysis requires no machine and cleanses the blood constantly. It uses a system of tubes and bags to flush the body of toxins. This process involves filling the abdomen with cleansing solution and then draining it. It must be done four times a day. Continuous cycling peritoneal dialysis is done by a machine that takes care of the filling and draining cleansing process. It is also given at night, usually while the patient is at home.

Hemodialysis involves filtering the blood through a machine. The blood is routed into the artificial kidney, called a dialyzer, where the wastes pass through a membrane. This procedure is done in a clinic or a hospital and takes from two to six hours per session, several times a week.

Kidney Transplant

Kidney transplants involve taking a kidney from one person and surgically implanting it into the patient. It is the most straightforward and most commonly performed type of organ transplant.

If the body accepts the kidney, the transplanted kidney successfully functions just as the original kidney did before it became diseased. However, transplanted tissue may be attacked and destroyed by the body's own immune system in some cases.

However, there are waiting lists for kidney recipients—just as there are waiting lists for almost all organ transplants. Usually, the most severe cases are tended to first, especially if there are other existing conditions that prove to be further weakening the already diseased kidneys.

For more information:

American Association of Kidney Patients
100 S. Ashley Dr., Suite 280
Tampa, FL 33602
800-749-2257

National Institute of Diabetes and Digestive and Kidney Diseases
Building 31, Room 9A-04
31 Center Dr.
Bethesda, MD 20892-2560
301-496-3583
http://www.niddk.nih.gov

National Kidney Foundation
30 E. 33rd St.
New York, NY 10016
800-622-9010
http://www.kidney.org

National Kidney and Urological Diseases Information Clearinghouse
Box NKUDIC
3 Information Way
Bethesda, MD 20892-3580
http://www.niddk.nih.gov

Transplant Recipients International Organization
1000 16th St., N.W., Suite 602
Washington, DC 20032
800-TRIO-386
http://www.primenet.com/^trio

MALE MENOPAUSE

The concept of male menopause—the idea that men undergo a drop in hormone levels as they age, just as women do at menopause—recently has been the center of media attention. It has long been known that the testosterone levels of men gradually decline as they get older and that these lowered levels result in a decrease in libido (sex drive), fatigue, depressed mood, erection problems, and osteoporosis in some men.

However, current research is now evaluating the use of supplemental testosterone to treat hypogonadism—a condition in which the body produces insufficient amounts of testosterone. This form of hormone replacement therapy is very much like estrogen replacement, used to treat symptoms of menopause in women.

Experts usually refer to male menopause as andropause or viripause because it is not the equivalent of female menopause. Menopause in women signals the end of menstruation and a slowdown in the functions of the ovaries. It is during menopause that levels of estrogen in the body decrease suddenly, causing fatigue, hot flashes, vaginal dryness, mood swings, and depression. Men, of course, don't have ovaries and don't have to deal with menstruation, and the decline of testosterone in their systems is very gradual—about 1 percent a year. The decline begins, on average, at the age of 48, but may start anytime between the ages of 40 and 50. (Some studies suggest that a man's testosterone levels may fall as much as 30 to 40 percent between the ages of 40 and 70.) An estimated 15 percent of older men have testosterone levels low enough to be considered hypogonadism.

Symptoms

Most men never feel the effects of andropause because the decline in testosterone is so slight. However, in some men, the decrease in hormones can result in loss of libido, decreased erections, loss of muscle, fatigue, and bone loss contributing to osteoporosis. While testosterone replacement therapy may be recommended for any of these conditions, its primary use is to treat erection problems and loss of libido.

Diagnosis

Testosterone replacement is not recommended for those who have not been definitively diagnosed with hypogonadism. Testosterone levels can be checked with a blood test; however, normal testosterone levels vary widely from person to person—anywhere from 200 ng/dl to 400 ng/dl—so a blood test alone can not be used for diagnosis. Any symptoms of sexual dysfunction should be evaluated to determine if their cause is lowered testosterone levels. This may include tests of the circulatory system.

Before testosterone replacement is prescribed, screening for prostate cancer must be done. Prostate cancer is not caused by hormones, but it can grow faster in their presence. A digital rectal examination, in which a gloved, lubricated finger is inserted into the rectum, should be done to check for abnormalities in the prostate. In addition, a prostate-specific antigen (PSA) test, a blood test that checks blood levels of PSA, should be done. High levels of PSA may indicate prostate cancer. If there are signs of prostate cancer or if the man is at high risk for developing the cancer, testosterone replacement should not be prescribed.

A NEW EPIDEMIC?

Testosterone replacement has long been used to treat hypogonadism (low testosterone levels) in men of all ages. However, with the advent of the new testosterone patch and increased media attention, hormone therapy for men has begun to be touted by some as a cure for the ills of midlife. Men's magazines have presented it as the fountain of youth—the key to staving off stiff joints, wrinkles, gray hairs, and a sluggish sex life—a hot issue considering all the baby-boomers now "coming of age." Men are also living longer than ever before, prompting investigation into the uses of hormone therapy for men in their 70s and 80s.

Despite the fact that it's only appropriate for a small percentage of men, some experts fear that hormone replacement therapy for men will become a popular therapy for those facing middle age—much like it is used to treat menopausal women.

But male menopause is open to interpretation. Logically, the body is going to age and change over time, and not every case of midlife fatigue, loss of libido, and decreased muscle strength can be linked to testosterone deficiency. What clouds the issue further are questions of emotional and psychological changes during middle age—perhaps triggered by thoughts of growing old and facing death—the traditional "midlife crisis."

The truth is, the gradual decline in testosterone levels in the decades after age 50 are slight—usually not enough to warrant therapy for most men. Neither is testosterone therapy recommended as a form of prevention for the problems (such as loss of libido, osteoporosis, and loss of muscle) that may come with old age. Plus, there is the risk that testosterone could fuel the growth of prostate cancer, another reason the therapy is not for everyone.

Nonetheless, don't hesitate to speak with your practitioner about any health or sexual health problems you may be having—too often, surveys show, men don't talk with their doctors about sexual health, often ignoring problems that may be easily treated.

Treatment

Testosterone replacement therapy can be provided in several different forms. An injection of testosterone into a muscle can be given; however, with this therapy hormone levels in the body are high immediately after the injection and then drop sharply and remain at low levels until the next injection is administered. Testosterone injections are usually given every two weeks. The cost may be as little as $8 a month.

The testosterone patch delivers a steady dose of the hormone through the skin. In the past, patches were worn on the scrotum, which needed to be shaved frequently. In 1996, a new, nonscrotal patch called Androderm was approved by the Food and Drug Administration. The new patch can be worn on the upper arm, thigh, abdomen, or back. The patch delivers 2.5 milligrams of testosterone per day. Two patches are worn at one time, and they last for three days each. The Androderm patch is also reported to cause fewer cases of skin irritation than the scrotal patch. The Androderm patch costs about $100 a month, compared with $80 to $90 for the scrotal patch.

There are side effects to the therapy. Because it promotes muscle growth and fluid retention, testosterone replacement can cause weight gain. In younger men and teenagers being treated for hypogonadism, acne and gynecomastia (enlargement of breast tissue) may occur. Sleep apnea, a condition in which the airways become momentarily blocked during sleep, may develop or worsen during testosterone replacement. In rare cases, liver disorders such as cysts in the liver may occur. Supplemental testosterone can also interfere with fertility.

DHEA

DHEA, short for dehydroepiandrosterone, is a naturally occurring precursor of estrogen and testosterone, meaning that DHEA is a "building block" of these hormones. DHEA is present in both men and women, and blood levels of the substance peak at age 20 and then decline. DHEA plays a role in the immune system, promotes feelings of well-being and is a component of many bodily functions.

Low levels of DHEA are linked to conditions such as arthritis, lupus, and depression. Certain cancers, diabetes, obesity, and cardiovascular disease have also been associated with low levels of DHEA. Because of its association with the development of age-related diseases, some experts feel that DHEA supplementation could decrease risk of some conditions and prevent some of the effects of aging.

DHEA may hold some promise. Lab mice given the hormone show increased muscle mass and decreased body fat and lived longer. In a study involving twenty HIV-infected people, daily doses of DHEA reduced the viral load. Another study of men older than age 50 showed that those with high levels of DHEA also had lower rates of heart disease. And in a study that looked at the antiaging benefits of the supplement, those taking DHEA reported increased psychological and physical well-being, while those taking a placebo reported no such benefits.

Despite these findings, if you're considering trying DHEA, you may want to think twice. Because of the preliminary evidence, most experts recommend against taking DHEA and consider it experimental. No effect on age or disease has been proven in humans, and because it's a food supplement, it has not undergone the clinical trials drugs go through by the Food and Drug Administration that prove safety and efficacy. To date, there have no reports of death or serious illness attributed to DHEA. Possible side effects include acne, oily skin, irritability, and aggressiveness. There is also a question of whether DHEA may fuel the growth of an already existing prostate cancer.

In addition, the synthetic version of DHEA used in the studies is not available in the United States. What is available is a natural form of DHEA that is extracted from the Mexican yam. Some pharmacies offer this form of DHEA in a compound for physicians. The DHEA found in the health food stores is made from ground Mexican yam and actually contains only a minute amount of DHEA—too little to have any effect on a human being.

MENTAL HEALTH

Mental health can be described as the ability to function in society. Difficulty shaking a blue mood, unusually paralyzing anxiety and inability to sleep are all common mental health problems that can get in the way of living day-to-day, sustaining relationships with family and friends, and carrying on with responsibilities of home and work.

While women are thought to suffer from depression more often than men, men are not exempt from depression and other mental illness—in fact, certain disorders such as paranoid, antisocial, and obsessive-compulsive personality disorders affect men more often than women. To complicate matters, men often do not seek help for mental conditions as readily as women. This is due in part to traditional male socialization, in which men are not supposed to admit weakness and are encouraged to keep their feelings hidden instead of expressing them.

Mental illness may be categorized into mainly three types: personality disorders, anxiety disorders, and mood (or affective) disorders. (For information on mood disorders, see Depression, p. 235.)

Personality Disorders

Personality is comprised of the attitudes, temperament, behavior, and thoughts that people develop in relation to their environment. Certain individuals are mentally unhealthy because of a personality disorder, an illness characterized by behavior and beliefs that are odd, emotional, erratic, anxious, or fearful. Signs of personality disorder usually arise in adolescence.

Some forms of personality disorders that men may encounter include paranoid personality disorder, schizoid personality disorder, borderline personality disorder, dependent personality disorder, and obsessive-compulsive personality disorder. Paranoid, antisocial, and obsessive-compulsive personality disorders are diagnosed more frequently in men than in women. Conversely, borderline and histrionic personality disorders occur more often in women than in men. Here are brief descriptions of each:

1. *Paranoid personality disorder.* People with this disorder refuse to confide in others. A consistent fear that other people are trying to threaten or harm them prevents them from trusting others.

2. *Schizoid personality disorder.* This disorder results in indifference to social relationships. Those with the disorder prefer to be alone, usually do not marry, rarely feel strong emotions (such as joy or anger) and have low desire for sexual experience.

3. *Schizotypal personality disorder.* People with this disorder exhibit peculiar thinking, behavior, and appearance. They often experience extreme social anxiety with people they are unfamiliar with and may hold odd beliefs, intense superstitions, and suspicions.

4. *Antisocial personality disorder.* Those with this disorder exhibit irresponsible and antisocial behavior. Characteristics include inability to follow society's rules, aggressive behavior, and lack of remorse. Before age 15, this disorder is known as conduct disorder, which is evidenced by fighting, truancy, stealing, lying, and cruelty to animals or people. People with this disorder are commonly referred to as sociopaths.

5. *Borderline personality disorder.* This disorder is characterized by unstable moods, impulsiveness (such as promiscuity, reckless driving, and shoplifting), low self-image, and erratic interpersonal relationships. These people often experience periods of anxiety, anger, depression, and self-destructive behaviors, including suicidal tendencies.

6. *Histrionic personality disorder.* Behaviors characteristic of this disorder include inappropriately seductive appearance, constant seeking of approval, and temper tantrums. Attention-seeking and being overly emotional in a given situation are also typical behaviors.

7. *Narcissistic personality disorder.* People with this disorder have an underlying fragile sense of self-esteem, resulting in a preoccupation with power and success. They require constant attention, lack empathy, and often become enraged or humiliated by negative criticism. These people usually experience poor interpersonal relationships.

8. *Avoidant personality disorder.* Due to an excessive concern with being judged inadequate and a fear of being embarrassed, those with this disorder avoid social interaction. They have few friends and avoid social situations, while still desiring to be with others.

9. *Dependent personality disorder.* This disorder is characterized by dependency and submissiveness, an excessive need for reassurance, inability to make everyday decisions, and feelings of helplessness when alone. People with this disorder often become closely attached to another person and try to please them.

10. *Obsessive-compulsive personality disorder.* People with this disorder exhibit a pattern of inflexibility and perfectionism as well as a fear of making mistakes. This results in preoccupations with details, inability to make decisions, trouble completing tasks, and extreme devotion to work at the sacrifice of leisure time.

Treatment

Personality disorders represent a lifetime pattern of being and behaving. Because of these long-standing habits, men often don't recognize how their disorders have contributed to their general unhappiness in life and interpersonal relationships. Treatment generally involves psychotherapy, medications, and cognitive-behavioral therapy.

In psychotherapy, the goal is for patients to become aware of the negative impact of their personalities on others and on their own sense of accomplishments and feelings of satisfaction. A man can learn to accept responsibility for negative traits and to understand their origins and develop adaptive behaviors.

Medications are sometimes provided to a person in order to reduce the breaks with reality and relieve the agitation, anxiety, panic, and depression of the illness, as well as stabilize impulsiveness and mood swings. Types of drugs include antipsychotics (Haldol, Thorazine), antidepressants (Prozac, Elavil), antianxiety drugs (Librium, Valium), mood-stabilizing drugs, and anticonvulsants (Lithium and Tegretol).

Cognitive-behavioral therapy is used to alter the person's set of basic assumptions that has led to the maladaptive behavior by challenging and testing the logic of these assumptions. Many times therapists use talk therapy to help the person overcome negative feelings that are the root cause of the emotional problems.

Anxiety Disorders

Some people do not have a disorder of personality, but rather they experience fear in a manner that keeps them from leading fully productive lives. Women are more likely than men to suffer from phobias and anxiety disorders. Anxiety is the result of an increase in the level of epinephrine in the nervous system. Epinephrine raises the heart and respiration rates and blood pressure levels and sends blood flow to the muscles, reactions that enable a person to react appropriately in a dangerous situation. However, in someone with an anxiety disorder, these reactions occur with little provocation.

Anxiety disorders include commonly known conditions such as panic disorder, obsessive-compulsive disorder, and posttraumatic stress disorder. Anxiety may also be a symptom of other psychiatric illness such as schizophrenia and depression.

1. *Panic disorder.* This disorder is characterized by recurring, unexpected panic attacks. Panic attacks are short periods in which a person experiences sudden, intense apprehension and fear or terror, often along with feelings of impending doom. Physical symptoms of these attacks include shortness of breath, palpitations, chest discomfort, pain, and choking or smothering sensations. Panic disorder may occur with or without agoraphobia, anxiety about or avoidance of places that might be difficult or embarrassing to escape from in the event of a panic attack, or where help may not be available for paniclike symptoms.

2. *Generalized anxiety disorder.* This condition is marked by unrealistic and excessive anxiety and worry (apprehensive expectations) about two or more life circumstances that go on for six months or more. Symptoms may include trembling, shortness of breath, heart palpitations, and trouble falling or staying asleep.

3. *Specific phobia.* This condition is characterized by intense anxiety when exposed to a particular object or situation of fear. It often leads to avoidance of that object or situation.

4. *Social phobia.* This type of phobia is characterized by significant anxiety upon exposure to certain social or performance situations. As in specific phobia, this often leads to avoidance behavior.

5. *Obsessive-compulsive disorder.* This disorder is characterized by obsessions that cause intense anxiety or distress, and/or by compulsions, which serve to relieve the anxiety. Obsessive and intrusive thoughts of violence or contamination can become persistent. As a result, the person engages in compulsive actions such as handwashing, touching, counting, and checking. Depression and anxiety often accompany this disorder. (Obsessive-compulsive disorder shouldn't be confused with obsessive-compulsive personality disorder, discussed previously.)

6. *Posttraumatic stress disorder.* Resulting from a psychologically distressing event outside

FIGHTING BACK AGAINST PANIC ATTACKS

Panic attacks may occur at any time or place and interfere with many day-to-day activities and tasks. To help prevent panic attacks and take control of your life:

- Limit intake of caffeine. Too much coffee, cola, or other foods containing caffeine can prompt anxiety attacks in panic-prone people. Also watch out for analgesics and cold medicines may contain caffeine.

- Stand your ground. Though the impulse in an anxiety attack is to escape the present situation, try to stay where you are. Tell yourself that you are not in any danger and that the attack will soon subside. The worst part of the panic usually ends within ten to twenty seconds. You will also prove to yourself that what you fear will not happen and that anxiety evaporates.

- Set goals for yourself. Choose an activity that is hindered by your anxiety—such as driving on the highway or speaking in public—then work toward that end. For example, decide that in six months you want to be able to present your newest idea to your co-workers at a conference.

- Don't dwell on the "what-ifs." If you feel a panic attack coming on, try to focus on the concrete things around you rather than on your anxiety. Sing a song, draw a picture on your notebook, or look at the design on the wallpaper.

- Try relaxation techniques. The following exercise is designed to help lower the heart rate, decrease blood pressure and develop deep, slow breathing—just the opposite of what happens during a panic attack:

  - Locate yourself in a quiet environment devoid of radio, television, or music, assume a comfortable, seated position, and close your eyes.

  - Slowly relax all of your muscles in progression, beginning with the feet.

  - Breathe naturally and easily through your nose, silently repeating a monosyllabic word such as "one" each time you exhale.

  - Concentrate on the rhythm of your breathing. If thoughts or images intrude, let them pass and return to your repetitions.

  - Try to maintain this state for ten to twenty minutes daily.

of the ordinary (such as witnessing someone being killed, knowing someone who recently was killed either by accident or by an act of violence, experiencing a violent or traumatic experience in the military, or having a serious threat to one's life), this disorder is characterized by reexperiencing the traumatic event. This is accompanied by increased arousal, an exaggerated startle response, and avoidance of stimuli associated with the event.

7. *Acute stress disorder.* Symptoms of this disorder are similar to those of posttraumatic stress disorder, but occur immediately after an extremely traumatic event.

Treatment of Anxiety Disorders and Phobias

Many practitioners now consider serotonin-specific reuptake inhibitors (SSRIs) such as Prozac, Zoloft, and Paxil the medical mainstays for treatment of anxiety disorders. Antianxiety drugs (tranquilizers) are also especially helpful in defined circumstances such as dealing with stress or handling a recent emotional upheaval.

The benzodiazepines (Librium, Valium, and Xanax) take the edge off these disorders by enhancing the actions of neurotransmitters in the brain that reduce nerve-impulse transmissions and slow down certain brain activity. However, side effects can include sleepiness, reduced coordination, and addiction.

Often medication combined with other therapies can help. For example, panic attacks are commonly treated with Xanax along with relaxation and deep breathing techniques. Systemic desensitization, in which the person is gradually exposed to the object of his or her phobia, can often alleviate the anxiety.

Mental Health and Aging

There are many mental disorders that affect the elderly. Some problems may be linked to medications, others to brain chemistry, and still others to other conditions such as Alzheimer's or stroke. While some feel that memory loss, disorientation, or depression are a result of aging, most mental disorders associated with the elderly are highly treatable. A careful diagnosis by a qualified practitioner may be the key to solving the problem.

Some common problems associated with the elderly include

1. *Delirium.* Ten to 40 percent of the hospitalized elderly develop delirium, the clouding of conscience with perceptual disturbances, incoherent speech, and disorientation. Overmedication is the biggest contributor to delirium in the elderly.

2. *Dementia syndrome.* Five percent of people aged 65 and older suffer from deterioration of the intellect, cognition, behavior, and emotions. In addition, 10 to 30 percent of these suffer from a second illness that impairs their cognitive skills.

3. *Mood disorders.* Physical illnesses that cause delirium or dementia in the elderly can bring about a secondary depression marked by mood swings. Mood disorders can also be brought on by drugs (such as antihypertensives), endocrine disorders, and structural brain lesions.

4. *Paranoid personality disorder.* Stress in the elderly can overwhelm their defenses and lead to paranoia. The stressors can include physical illness, isolation, and the deaths of family members and lifelong friends.

5. *Sleep disorders.* Depression following a heart attack often leads to sleep difficulties in the elderly. Other factors interfering with sleep are anxiety and pain. Insomnia and early morning waking are common.

For more information:

American Board of Professional Psychology
2100 E. Broadway, Suite 313
Columbia, MO 65201
513-875-1267

American Mental Health Counselors Association
801 N. Fairfax St., Suite 304
Alexandria, VA 22314
800-326-2642
703-823-9800

American Psychiatric Association
1400 K St., N.W.
Washington, DC 20005
202-682-6000
http://www.psych.org

American Psychological Association
Office of Public Affairs
750 First St. N.E.
Washington, DC 20002
202-336-5700
http://www.apa.org

Anxiety Disorders Association of America
11900 Parklawn Dr., Suite 100
Rockville, MD 20852
301-231-9350
http://www.adaa.org

Phobics Anonymous
P.O. Box 1180
Palm Springs, CA 92263
760-322-2673

National Mental Health Association
1021 Prince St.
Alexandria, VA 22314-2971
800-969-6642
703-684-7722
http://www.nmha.org

OSTEOPOROSIS

Despite the fact that most people consider osteoporosis a disease only women need to worry about, the bone-thinning disorder affects men as well. According to the National Osteoporosis Foundation, about 1.5 million men in the United States have osteoporosis, and another 3.5 million are at risk for the disease. In fact, one in every five people with osteoporosis is a man, and the figures are likely to increase as more men are living into their 80s and 90s. An American man over the age of 50 is thought to have a greater chance of suffering an osteoporosis-related fracture than developing prostate cancer. Some one hundred thousand men suffer hip fractures each year. Men are also more likely to die of an osteoporosis-related hip fracture than women, possibly because men who suffer fractures tend to be more frail than women with fractures. An estimated one-third of men with hip fractures die within a year of injury.

Bone Mass and Osteoporosis

Throughout life, bone cells called osteoclasts work to break down existing bone, while cells called osteoblasts create new bone. In a healthy person, these processes are balanced, creating proper bone density. Osteoporosis occurs when bone breaks down more quickly than it is built up.

Bone density peaks at around age 35. After that age, it either stays constant or decreases. A decrease results in brittle bones, leading to frequent fractures, a stooped stature (as the vertebrae break down and become compressed), and disability. In many cases, a hip fracture leads to death—not because of the severity of the injury but because the individual's health deteriorates while confined to bed.

The exact cause of osteoporosis is unknown. It may occur when there is a deficiency of calcium or other vitamins and minerals needed for bone growth.

Women and Osteoporosis

Osteoporosis is more common in women because women tend to have lower bone density than men—women build 10 to 25 percent less bone on their skeletons than men during development. In addition, women tend to get less weight-bearing exercise than men. Weight-bearing exercise helps to slow bone loss and prevent osteoporosis. In addition, women's levels of the hormone estrogen decline after menopause. The decreased levels make it more difficult for a woman's bones to absorb calcium and needed nutrients from the diet and result in a higher rate of bone loss directly after menopause. However, studies show that by the age of 65 or 70, the rate of bone loss in men and women is equal.

Symptoms

The symptoms of osteoporosis include the following:

- Gradual loss of height
- Rounded shoulders
- A stooped posture
- Lower-back pain
- Frequent bone fractures
- Gum disease

Risk Factors

With the exception of menopause, men and women have similar risk factors for osteoporosis. These factors include the following:

- Smoking
- Excessive consumption of alcohol
- Small stature
- Sedentary lifestyle
- Low intake of calcium
- Family history of osteoporosis
- Scoliosis (curvature of the spine)
- Testosterone deficiency
- Use of certain drugs such as steroids

Experts estimate that up to 70 percent of all cases of male osteoporosis can be traced to one or more of these factors. However, 30 percent of cases—and most cases in men under age 65, have no known cause.

Diagnosis

Diagnosis may come after the stooped stature of someone with osteoporosis becomes apparent. However, osteoporosis should be caught and treated earlier, since bone mass cannot be restored once it is lost. An early sign of osteoporosis is a fracture that occurs from a fall from standing height, rather than one that is caused by trauma.

If osteoporosis is suspected, bone-density testing may be done. In this test, the spine, wrist, or hip is placed under a scanner that measures density. Scan techniques include single-beam and dual-beam densitometers and dual-energy x-ray absorptiometry (DEXA). Of these techniques, DEXA is thought to be the more accurate.

The test produces a figure that is then compared with the measurement of peak bone mass at age 30. If the figure is more than 2.5 times lower than the peak bone mass, osteoporosis is diagnosed. However, it is important for the practitioner to keep in mind that women's bones are not as dense as men's bones when making the comparison.

Before undergoing a test, you should check with your insurance company regarding coverage. Insurance companies may not reimburse men for bone-density testing because of the belief that osteoporosis only troubles women.

PREVENTING OSTEOPOROSIS

To help prevent the breakdown of bone from osteoporosis:

- Eat foods rich in calcium, a mineral that encourages the growth of bone, throughout life. These include dairy products, kale, turnip greens, kelp, tofu, canned salmon, sardines (with bones), and soybeans. The National Osteoporosis Foundation recommends 1,000 mg daily to age 65 and 1,500 mg daily after age 65.

- Get your RDA of vitamin D. The National Osteoporosis Foundation recommends at least 400 I.U. (international units) daily, but no more than 800 I.U. daily.

- Live an active lifestyle. Exercise also helps to increase bone mass, especially weight-bearing exercise such as strength training. Experts recommend keeping the quadriceps (the thigh muscles) strong throughout life to prevent hip fractures. The quadriceps often markedly decrease in strength between the ages of 60 and 80.

- Ask about your medications. Certain medications such as steroids, anticonvulsants, and even some antacids can contribute to bone loss. Talk with your practitioner about any possible effects.

- Don't smoke or drink heavily. Smoking can contribute to the development of osteoporosis, as can excess alcohol consumption. An Indiana study showed that men who drank more than $1^1/_2$ drinks a day lost 70 percent more bone than nondrinkers.

Blood and urine tests may also be done to detect levels of calcium in the body and help diagnose osteoporosis. Digestive problems and low testosterone levels may also contribute to the disease.

Treatment

If a digestive problem is preventing the absorption of calcium, that problem should be treated to prevent further bone loss. Hormone imbalances may be treated with testosterone replacement therapy. (See Male Menopause, p. 319.)

In addition, getting the recommended dietary allowance (RDA) of calcium is necessary for those with osteoporosis. For men older than 25, the RDA is 800 mg daily. However, the National Osteoporosis Foundation recommends 1,000 mg daily for men younger than 65 and 1,500 mg daily for men 65 and older. At least 400 I.U. daily of vitamin D (but no more than 800 I.U. daily) is also recommended by the National Osteoporosis Foundation.

There are several medications available for women with osteoporosis. These include alendronate and calcitonin. While these drugs are not specifically approved for use in men—only in women—a practitioner may still prescribe them for men if necessary.

Calcitonin is a hormone that is available as a pill, an injection, and a nasal spray. It helps to slow the breakdown of bone and, in some cases, may help to increase bone density. Alendronate

(Fosamax) does not contain hormone. It works to increase bone strength and reduces the risk of fractures. However, Alendronate can cause stomach discomfort.

For more information:

U.S. Department HHS
P.O. Box 1133
Washington, DC 20013
800-336-4797
http://nhic-nt.health.org

National Osteoporosis Foundation
1150 17th St., N.W., Suite 500
Washington, DC 20036-4603
202-223-2226
http://www.nof.org

Osteoporosis and Related Bone Diseases National Resource Center
1150 17th St., N.W., Suite 500
Washington, DC 20036-4603
800-624-BONE
202-223-0344
202-466-4315 (TTY)
http://www.osteo.org

PARKINSON'S DISEASE

Parkinson's disease is a neurological disorder that affects one's ability to control the body. It is the most common form of a motor system disorder called Parkinsonism. Named for the physician James Parkinson who first described it in 1817 as "the shaking palsy," the disease initiates when neurons in an area of the brain called the substantia nigra become impaired or die and can no longer produce a needed chemical called dopamine.

The importance of dopamine lies in its ability to transmit signals to the brain, which enables smooth, intentional muscle activity to take place. When dopamine is lost, patients are unable to control their movements in a normal fashion, causing severe disability in most people who have the disease. Why the dopamine-producing neurons die is unknown. However, scientists believe it may be a result of, or a combination of, any one of the following: exposure to environmental toxins, genetics, a rapid aging process, or a damaging amount of molecules that our bodies produce from normal chemical reactions. Parkinson's affects over one million Americans, causing serious mental impairment in 15 to 30 percent of those diagnosed with the disease.

Symptoms

Early symptoms of Parkinson's include the following:

- Fatigue

- Shakiness

- Loss of train of thought

- Irritability or depression for no given reason

Major symptoms that occur as the disease progresses include the following:

- Trembling of hands, arms, legs, jaw or face

- Stiffness and rigidity of limbs

- Slowness of movement

- Impaired balance

Other possible symptoms include the following:

- Emotional changes

- Difficulty with swallowing and chewing due to loss of muscle control

- Changes in speech
- Constipation or urinary problems due to improperly functioning nervous system
- Excess oil on the skin due to improper nervous system functioning

As the existing symptoms progress, the patient may experience trouble walking, talking, or completing simple tasks. Unfortunately, all these symptoms grow worse with time. Parkinson's symptoms may also accompany other neurological disorders such as Alzheimer's disease. (See Alzheimer's Disease, and Dementia, p. 160.)

Risk Factors

According to the National Institute of Neurological Disorders and Strokes, each year an estimated fifty thousand Americans are diagnosed with Parkinson's disease. Caucasians are seemingly more at risk than African Americans or Asians. The disease strikes men and women almost equally and tends to develop after age 40, progressing for another ten to fifteen years before causing significant disabilities. People over the age of 50 are at most risk for developing the disease. Currently, the average age that Parkinson's sets in at full force is 60. However, 5 to 10 percent of current advanced Parkinson's patients are under the age 40. Although the disease is both chronic and progressive, it is not hereditary or contagious.

Diagnosis

Diagnosis is extremely difficult during the beginning stages of the disease. No advanced laboratory tests or blood work exist to help with diagnosis, but doctors do use an observation technique to determine if patients are showing signs of Parkinson's. However, experienced neurologists need to observe the suspected Parkinson's patient for a certain amount of time before a diagnosis can be made. And although observation takes time, the earliest possible diagnosis is crucial to the effective treatment of Parkinson's.

Treatment

Currently no cure exists for Parkinson's. However, symptoms can be relieved through a variety of available medications, including the drug levodopa. Found in animals and plants, levodopa enables nerve cells to produce dopamine. It has been highly successful in the treatment of Parkinson's symptoms. But levodopa does have side effects, including nausea, vomiting, low blood pressure, restlessness, and involuntary movement.

There are other options available for easing the physical effects of Parkinson's and facilitating mobility. These include a variety of available drugs besides levodopa, physical therapy, and surgery. Unfortunately, at the present time nothing is effective for preventing or slowing the mental damage that Parkinson's causes. Someone diagnosed with Parkinson's will eventually need full-time care as mobility becomes increasingly difficult and sporadic muscle movement occurs more frequently.

Self-Care

Thus far, Parkinson's disease cannot be prevented or predicted. However, scientists are working on various screening techniques that may give clues to how the disease originates. One such technique involves scanning the brain to produce pictures of chemical changes as they occur within the brain, with the hope of discovering how the disease progresses.

In order to make treatment more effective, Parkinson's patients can exercise more and eat healthy foods. Although no specific vitamin or mineral has been proven to be successful in battling the disease, those with Parkinson's are given some dietary guidelines such as a reduction in protein intake (because protein limits levodopa's positive effects).

Those with Parkinson's are told to exercise and stay physically fit so that their muscles strengthen and tone, facilitating mobility. Whereas exercising will not prevent Parkinson's from progressing, it will provide patients with more strength so that they remain as able as possible. Exercise has also been credited with improving a patient's emotional health, thus giving a feeling of well-being and accomplishment.

For more information:

American Parkinson's Disease Association
1250 Hylan Blvd., Suite 4B
Staten Island, NY 10305
800-223-2732
http://www.apdaparkinson.org

National Parkinson's Foundation
1501 N.W. Ninth Ave.
Miami, FL 33136
800-327-4545
http://www.parkinson.org

Parkinson's Disease Foundation
William Black Memorial Research Building
Columbia-Presbyterian Medical Center
650–710 W. 168th St.
New York, NY 10032
800-457-6676
212-923-4700
http://www.parkinsons-foundation.org

PENILE AND URE-THRAL DISORDERS

Aside from incontinence, urinary tract infections, and problems with the kidneys, there are a few additional health concerns that involve the penis and the urethra, the tube that carries urine from the bladder out of the body.

Balanitis

When the glans, or tip, of the penis becomes red and sore, it is known as balanitis. It can be caused by a urinary tract infection, irritation from clothing or detergents, or a yeast infection. It is more common in uncircumcised men than in those who have been circumcised because the uncircumcised foreskin may be narrow or difficult to retract, causing irritation. Those with diabetes also commonly have balanitis; those with balanitis are often tested for diabetes. Treatment involves antibiotics or antifungal medications if infection is present. Good hygienic practices—washing the penis thoroughly each day and pulling back the foreskin to wash underneath it—are also recommended.

Paraphimosis

Paraphimosis usually develops as the result of phimosis, a tight foreskin. It occurs when the foreskin retracts and becomes constricted, causing swelling and pain. Severe swelling and pain must be treated immediately to avoid permanent damage. Often, the foreskin can be gently moved back into its normal position. However, if this is not possible, treatment is circumcision or partial circumcision to release the foreskin.

Phimosis

Phimosis is defined as an abnormally tight foreskin that cannot be drawn back from the glans, the tip of the penis. While infants may have a tight foreskin until about six months of age, the condition usually disappears with age. However, in some boys, it may persist for years. It can make urination and erections difficult and painful. It may lead to balanitis and paraphimosis. It can be treated with circumcision.

Peyronie's Disease

In some men, the penis becomes curved during an erection, a condition known as Peyronie's disease, or curvature of the penis. This progressive condition, caused by the formation of scar tissue within the penis, makes it difficult or impossible to have sexual intercourse. It is not known why the scar tissue forms in some men, though some studies suggest it can be the result of genetic inheritance or trauma to the penis. Peyronie's disease can be diagnosed by feeling the penis for the telltale ridge of scar tissue. There is no specific treatment for Peyronie's disease, although treatment is usually not necessary in mild cases. In some cases, the disease disappears on its own.

Priapism

This rare condition is marked by a prolonged, painful erection that continues without sexual stimulation. Priapism is caused by a problem within the spinal cord, leukemia, or inflammation of the urethra. Symptoms include an erection in which the tip of the penis is soft and the shaft is hard, and the erection does not disappear after sexual activity ends. Immediate treatment is necessary to prevent permanent damage to the penis. The erection can be alleviated by administering spinal anesthesia or by drawing blood through a wide needle to help relieve pressure.

Urethral Stricture

In this rare condition, the urethra narrows because of scar tissued caused by injury or infection. At times, the urethra may become completely blocked. Symptoms include difficult and painful urination. If infection is involved, diagnosis includes testing the urine or any discharge to identify the organism. A cystoscopy— a thin, flexible, fiberoptic tube—may be inserted into the penis to view the inside of the urethra for diagnosis. Urethral stricture is treated by administering a local anesthetic and inserting a thin instrument into the urethra to stretch the tube. The procedure may need to be repeated several times. If opening the urethra in this way is not successful, surgery is necessary.

Urethritis

Urethritis is inflammation of the urethra. It is often caused by sexually transmitted disease, though at times the cause remains unknown. Symptoms include pain during urination, an urge to urinate frequently, and discharge from the penis. It is diagnosed through examination of the discharge. It is usually treated with antibiotics, and treatment for a sexual partner may be necessary as well.

For more information:

American Foundation for Urologic Disease
300 W. Pratt St., Suite 401
Baltimore, MD 21201
800-242-2383
410-727-2908
http://www.acess.digex.net.~afud.org

PROSTATE DISEASE

The prostate is a walnut-shaped gland of the male reproductive system located in front of the rectum and at the base of the bladder. The prostate surrounds the urethra, the tube that carries urine out of the bladder through the penis. The gland weighs a little less than an ounce. Its outer surface is covered with a layer of muscle, called the prostatic capsule, which encases the glandular tissue.

The prostate is not a sex organ, though its main role does concern reproduction. The prostate produces seminal fluid, the secretion that supports the sperm in the semen. A problem with the prostate will not affect the ability to have an erection, contrary to popular belief. However, it can affect the possibility of conception and interfere with urination.

Common problems of the prostate gland include prostatitis, or inflammation of the prostate, and benign prostatic hyperplasia, noncancerous enlargement of the prostate. In addition, prostate cancer affects one in eight American men in his lifetime. (For more information on prostate cancer, its diagnosis, and its treatment, see Prostate Cancer, p. 214.)

Prostatitis

Prostatitis, inflammation of the prostate, can affect a man at any age. In fact, most men will visit the doctor for this problem at least once during their lifetime. There are two main types of prostatitis: nonbacterial and bacterial.

Nonbacterial Prostatitis

Nonbacterial prostatitis, the most common form of prostatitis, describes two separate conditions: congestive prostatitis and prostatodynia.

Congestive prostatitis occurs when prostatic fluid collects in the gland instead of being ejaculated out of the body. The prostate routinely produces prostatic fluid, according to how often ejaculation occurs. However, if a man's sexual habits change and his rate of ejaculation drops, that fluid builds up in the prostate, causing it to swell.

Prostatodynia (which means "painful prostate") indicates a condition in which pain seems to be coming from the prostate gland, though usually it is coming from surrounding muscles or inflammation in the pelvic bones. In most cases of prostatodynia, the prostate is normal. Experts are not sure what causes prostatodynia, although there is evidence that it is stress related.

Bacterial Prostatitis

Bacterial prostatitis, which is sometimes referred to as infectious prostatitis, can be acute or chronic. Acute bacterial prostatitis is a rare and serious disease caused by bacteria in the prostate gland. Swimming in or drinking unclean water can expose a man to the bacteria. The bacteria may also come from an infection in another part of the body such as a sinus infection or ear infection. Bacterial prostatitis may also occur in men who have enlarged prostates. It is not contagious and cannot be sexually transmitted.

Chronic bacterial prostatitis is a recurring prostate infection that usually results when invading bacteria are not eradicated for various reasons.

Symptoms

The symptoms for nonbacterial and bacterial prostatitis are similar. They include the following:

- Discharge of fluid from the penis

- Pain or itching deep within the penis

- Discomfort during urination

- Difficulty urinating

- A fever, aches and pains, and lower-back pain (acute bacterial prostatitis)

Many of these symptoms are also symptoms of sexually transmitted diseases.

Diagnosis

A visit to a family physician or urologist, a specialist who deals with problems of the urinary and reproductive systems, is necessary for prostatitis. Proper testing and diagnosis are necessary to ensure that a prostate problem is dealt with correctly.

Diagnosis is done through a series of tests and examinations, as well as a person's medical history and a physical examination. A urinalysis, a laboratory analysis of the urine, may be done to check for signs of infection, which would indicate bacterial prostatitis. Also, a digital rectal exam (DRE) is performed to examine the size of the prostate. In this test, a gloved, lubricated finger is inserted into the rectum to feel the prostate. An enlarged, spongy prostate may indicate nonbacterial prostatitis. If there are symptoms of acute bacterial infection, the DRE should be done delicately (if at all) because the prostate will be highly inflamed or irritated. Too much probing may force the infection into other parts of the reproductive system.

To diagnose chronic bacterial prostatitis, a segmented urine culture may be done. In this test, the practitioner takes one routine urine sample and one from the midstream of the urine. Then a DRE will be performed, and the prostate will be massaged to release prostatic fluid. Then another urine sample, which contains the released prostatic fluid, is taken. The samples are then compared to determine if the infection lies in the prostate or in the urethra.

A cystoscopy, in which a flexible, lighted, viewing tube is inserted into the urethra, may be used to confirm a diagnosis. However, this procedure is usually not necessary.

Proper diagnosis is essential in treating prostatitis because the various forms are handled differently. A diagnosis of prostatitis does not

---

SELF-CARE FOR NON-BACTERIAL PROSTATITIS

Although there is no clear-cut treatment for nonbacterial prostatitis, you can lessen the symptoms by taking the following steps:

- Avoid coffee, alcohol, and spicy foods. Evidence suggests that these aggravate the prostate gland.

- Consider your activities. Excessive driving, cycling, heavy lifting, and vigorous exercise are thought to worsen symptoms.

- Practice relaxation. Stress has been linked to prostatodynia, so relaxation therapy may be helpful. (See Relaxation Techniques, p. 124.)

- Try a hot sitz bath. The warm water increases blood flow, which causes the prostate to loosen up.

---

indicate any greater risk of benign prostatic hyperplasia or prostate cancer.

Treatment

Bacterial prostatitis is treated with a regimen of antibiotics. If symptoms are severe, painkillers and bed rest may be prescribed. If the urethra becomes blocked, if fever leads to dehydration, or if there is a risk the bacteria may spread throughout the body, hospitalization may be necessary.

Antibiotic treatment must be thorough and complete to eradicate all the bacteria.

The prostate is a tough area to rid of infection, and although the symptoms of bacterial infections often disappear shortly after treatment begins, the bacteria often remain hidden within the prostate. Therefore, antibiotic therapy may last up to a month. For chronic infection, antibiotics such as trimethoprim and sulfa may be prescribed for an extended period of time covering many months.

Surgical removal of the prostate, or prostatectomy, is a last resort for those with chronic bacterial prostatitis. If the condition is causing complications such as urinary retention or kidney problems, prostatectomy may be considered.

Antibiotics are not effective for nonbacterial prostatitis. For congestive prostatitis, regular ejaculation (through intercourse or masturbation) is often prescribed. Prostatodynia can be treated with over-the-counter medications such as ibuprofen or aspirin. Muscle relaxants may be prescribed for prostatodynia because it is considered to be stress-related.

Benign Prostatic Hyperplasia

Benign prostatic hyperplasia (BPH) is a noncancerous enlargement of the prostate gland, which surrounds the urethra, the tube that carries urine from the body. In BPH, the prostate slowly becomes larger, squeezing the urethra and hindering, if not obstructing, urination. BPH can lead to bladder problems, frequent urinary tract infections, and possibly, urinary retention, in which a man becomes unable to urinate.

BPH, also called enlarged prostate, affects over 50 percent of men over the age of 50 and approximately 80 to 90 percent of men over the age of 80.

Risk

No one is sure what causes BPH, but researchers feel that its development is somehow linked to the production of testosterone: BPH does not occur in men who have had their testicles surgically removed or in men with low levels of an enzyme known as 5-alpha-reductase, which converts the hormone testosterone into another hormone, called dihydrotestosterone (DHT).

Some recent studies point to a high-fat and high-cholesterol diet as a risk factor of BPH, since the body converts cholesterol into male hormones. In addition, studies have shown that Asian men who eat lower fat diets than American men have a lower rate of BPH. Obesity is also being eyed as a risk factor of prostate enlargement. Men with a waist size of more than 43 inches are twice as likely as those with a size 35 or smaller to develop BPH, one source reports. However, there is no conclusive evidence of a link between obesity and BPH.

Symptoms

The symptoms of BPH are often described as either irritative or obstructive. Irritative symptoms, which result from the inability to completely empty the bladder, include the frequent need to urinate, numerous trips to the bathroom at night (nocturia), and urgency (the frequent or constant feeling of the need to urinate). These are generally the first symptoms of a prostate problem, even though they might not be noticeable until years after the prostate has begun to grow.

Obstructive symptoms are related to problems with urine flow. They include the inability to urinate (urinary retention), trouble starting or stopping the flow of urine, a weak flow, and dribbling after urination.

Other symptoms include frequent urinary infections, marked by a burning feeling during urination and strong-smelling urine. There may also be blood in the urine (hematuria), which occurs when blood vessels are stretched and broken by growing prostate tissue.

If you have any of these warning signs, you should consult your family physician or a urologist. Although BPH isn't cancerous, in advanced cases, kidney damage or failure may occur.

Diagnosis

BPH is diagnosed through a series of tests from a practitioner, usually beginning with a physical examination that includes a medical history and a review of urinary habits. A urinalysis and urine culture will also be done to rule out an infection. The practitioner may press down on the bladder to tell if it's distended (enlarged or swollen) or may perform a digital rectal examination (DRE), in which a gloved, lubricated finger is inserted into the rectum to feel the prostate. A DRE indicates whether the gland is enlarged. However, the part of the prostate that usually obstructs urine flow is the middle lobe, which cannot be felt during a rectal exam. For this reason, a DRE may be of limited use in diagnosing BPH.

A practitioner may also do a series of tests known as a urodynamic evaluation to measure

HOW SEVERE ARE YOUR SYMPTOMS?

The American Urological Association has put together a questionnaire to help you and your practitioner gauge the severity of BPH. Give yourself a 0 for never; 1 for less than one time in five; 2 for less than half the time; 4 for more than half the time; and 5 for almost always.

- Over the past month, how often have you had a sensation of not emptying your bladder completely after you have finished urinating?

- Over the past month, how often have you had to urinate again less than two hours after you finished urinating?

- Over the past month, how often have you found you stopped and started again several times when you urinated?

- Over the past month, how often have you found it difficult to postpone urination?

- Over the past month, how often have you had a weak urinary stream?

- Over the past month, how often have you had to strain to begin urination?

- Over the past month, how often have you typically had to get up to urinate from the time you went to bed at night until the time you got up in the morning?

A score of 7 or less may indicate, at the most, a mild problem; 8 to 19 may indicate a moderate problem; and 20 to 35 may indicate a severe problem. Talk with your doctor about your symptoms and your score.

urine flow and residual urine (the amount of urine left in the bladder after urination). The amount of residual urine can also be measured using a catheter (a thin tube that drains the bladder) inserted though the penis.

Blood tests may be done to rule out kidney disease and cancer. In addition, a practitioner may take x-rays or do an ultrasound—a noninvasive test in which sound waves are used to create an image of the prostate. A cystoscopy, a procedure in which a lighted viewing tube is passed through the urethra into the bladder, may also be done to allow visual examination of the urinary tract.

While none of these tests alone can definitively diagnose BPH, as a group they can confirm a diagnosis.

Treatment

Treatment of BPH depends upon the severity of the symptoms, the health risks involved, and the individual. For example, some people are bothered or inconvenienced by milder symptoms, while other men can handle the more severe problems.

There are various treatment methods for an enlarged prostate. One option for men with slightly enlarged prostates and minimal symptoms is called watchful waiting. This requires careful monitoring of a patient without administering any treatment. During observation, the symptoms sometimes decline or stabilize on their own. Studies have shown that 30 to 50 percent of those with BPH exhibit some improvement on their own.

But as the problems associated with BPH become less tolerable, more aggressive treatment is needed. Medication and surgery are then used to treat an enlarged prostate.

Medication

There are two major types of medication used to treat an enlarged prostate: alpha blockers (also called antihypertensives) and drugs that shrink the prostate. Because symptoms return if medication is stopped, these drugs must be taken daily indefinitely.

According to the American Academy of Family Physicians, alpha blockers have a positive effect for about 75 percent of the men who try them. Alpha blockers such as terazosin (Hytrin) work by relaxing the muscles of the prostate, which allows urine to flow more freely. But like most medications, Hytrin may have side effects for certain individuals. These include low blood pressure and dizziness.

Proscar (finasteride) is a drug that relieves symptoms by reducing the size of the prostate. Proscar takes approximately three to six months to produce results, but it has been shown to reduce prostate size by up to 30 percent. Sixty percent of the men who use Proscar have some relief of their symptoms. However, the relief may not be substantial. In some cases, sexual problems such as a decreased interest in sex or erection problems may result from taking Proscar. Additionally, evidence reveals that finasteride reduces PSA levels in the bloodstream by approximately one-half. This, in turn, must be taken into account when screening for prostate cancer.

As far as which drug is more effective, a 1996 study that compared Hytrin to Proscar found that Hytrin reduced prostate symptoms by one-third, while Proscar was only slightly more effective than a placebo. Though that study points to Hytrin as the more effective, another analysis shows Proscar to be effective in men with prostates larger than 40 cc. In other words, the larger the prostate, the better Proscar might work. However, even in those men with exceptionally large prostates, Hytrin probably will work better. In addition, it is less expensive than Proscar.

Surgery

Surgical procedures center around removing or reducing prostate tissue in a prostatectomy or partial prostatectomy. A prostatectomy can be open or closed. In an open prostatectomy, the gland is removed through an abdominal incision. Closed prostatectomies involve surgery performed through the urethra or a small incision. Open prostatectomies have been largely replaced by closed procedures, though they are still used if the prostate is very large, if other procedures need to be done at the same time, or if an open procedure is preferred to the more technically difficult closed procedures.

One closed procedure, a transurethral resection of the prostate (TURP), involves inserting an instrument into the urethra to remove excess prostate tissue from the area. The major benefit of this procedure is a reduction in the urinary troubles that accompany BPH. It is one of the most commonly performed surgical procedures, with 300,000 to 400,000 TURPs done each year. Approximately 90 percent of those who opt for this surgery show improvement, although an estimated 10 percent report erection problems and 3 percent report incontinence. In addition, a second prostatectomy is needed for roughly 10 percent of men who have TURPs because the glandular tissue continues to grow.

The other closed procedure is transurethral incision of the prostate (TUIP or TULIP). This differs from the TURP in that the procedure requires a surgeon to make slices in the prostate to lessen the stranglehold the gland has created on the urethra. This method reduces the chances of erection problems and other sexual dysfunction. Again, a repeat procedure may be necessary.

One procedure that provides temporary results is balloon dilation. Here, a balloon is inserted into the urethra and inflated in the area where the prostate is restricting the flow of urine. By expanding the balloon, the area within the urethra is enlarged to allow a stronger flow.

Recently, several new surgical methods have been developed. Among these are microwave thermotherapy, intraurethral stents, and transurethral needle ablation (TUNA). Microwave thermotherapy, also known as hyperthermia, uses heat to eliminate some of the prostate tissue. Intraurethral stents are small, tubelike structures inserted into the urethra that enlarge it to provide relief from urinary problems. Transurethral needle ablation (TUNA) uses lasers to cut away excess prostate tissue. The long-term effects of these procedures are not known at this time.

For some men, surgery may not be necessary. Studies show that surgery for BPH can safely be delayed for years—if not indefinitely—with watchful waiting if you feel you can handle the symptoms and no dangerous complications develop. This approach to treatment requires regular checkups and monitoring to keep track of the progress of the condition. If surgery is recommended—as with all invasive procedures—seek a second opinion before agreeing to the procedure.

Complementary Therapies

In addition to surgery and medication, a number of herbal remedies have been reported to be helpful in treating BPH. Ask your practitioner's advice before using herbal remedies as well as vitamins and minerals as part of your treatment. Herbs are essentially drugs and should be treated as such.

Self-Care and Prevention

Although an enlarged prostate may seem to be out of your control, there are certain issues to investigate that may reduce problems associated with BPH (or other prostate problems):

- Stick to a low-fat, low-cholesterol diet. Research shows men who follow such a diet have a lower risk of BPH.

- Eat more vegetables. Men who do so have a lower rate of BPH than those who do not.

- Limit your fluid intake. To lessen the number of trips to the bathroom, don't drink too much before bed.

- Avoid caffeine and alcohol. They can irritate the prostate and increase the need for nighttime urination if consumed before bed.

- Monitor your medications. Certain drugs aggravate urinary problems, including oral bronchodilators, diuretics, tranquilizers, and antidepressants. Over-the-counter cold remedies such as antihistamines and decongestants can also worsen urinary conditions.

1. *Zinc.* Some experts believe zinc sulfate can improve prostate health and suggest a supplement of 50 mg of zinc sulfate daily. Other sources of zinc include pumpkin seeds, nuts, oysters, milk, eggs, chicken, lentils, and beef liver. Check with your practitioner about the proper dosage for you.

2. *Saw palmetto.* This plant—specifically the berry it produces—is one of the best known natural remedies for BPH. The herb has been found to shrink prostate tissue in some men, making urination less painful and reducing the number of nighttime trips to the bathroom. Recommended dosage is 320 mg a day; it is rare that side effects are reported. Keep in mind that saw palmetto doesn't treat BPH; it only relieves its symptoms.

3. *Pygeum africanum.* This natural substance, derived from the bark of a tropical African evergreen tree, has gotten mixed reviews. While some experts swear by its benefits, studies have shown that daily use for six to eight weeks results, on average, in one fewer nighttime trip to the bathroom every three nights, which may not even be worth the trouble and expense of taking the supplement.

Other treatments that have been reported to be helpful include lecithin, calcium, and magnesium tablets and a combination of the amino acids glycine, alanine, and glutamate. Ask your practitioner for more information.

For more information:

American Urological Association
1120 N. Charles St.
Baltimore, MD 21201
410-727-1100

National Kidney and Urological Diseases
Information Clearinghouse
Box NKUDIC
3 Information Way
Bethesda, MD 20892-3580
http://www.niddk.nih.gov

Prostate Health Council
American Foundation for Urologic Disease
300 W. Pratt St., Suite 401
Baltimore, MD 21201
800-242-2383
410-727-2908
http://www.acess.digex.net.~afud.org

SKIN CONDITIONS

The skin is the largest and most visible organ in the body. It protects you from the sun's rays, bacteria, and infection. It also regulates body temperature, stores fat and water, senses the environment, excretes sweat, and aids in the body's synthesis of vitamin D. Men's skin tends to be thicker and less sensitive than the skin of women, and it is also less prone to wrinkles. Skin disorders can be caused by cell and follicle dysfunction, parasites, allergens and irritants, infection, heredity, and excessive sunlight exposure. (See Skin Cancer, p. 221.)

Anatomy of the Skin

The skin is composed of the epidermis, dermis, and subcutaneous tissue. The epidermis, the outermost layer of the skin, is composed of flat squamous cells, round basal cells, and a stratum corneum (a nonliving layer of keratin, a tough, fibrous substance). Also found in the epidermis are keratinocytes (producers of keratin), melanocytes (producers of melanin, the pigment of the skin), and Langerhans' cells (linked with immune system surveillance). The epidermis not only regulates bodily water loss (through openings called pores), produces melanin and keratin, and serves as the barrier between the environment and the internal organs, but also produces new skin cells.

The dermis, made up of an upper section called the papillary dermis and a lower section called the reticular dermis, contains reticuloendothelial cells, fibrous connective tissue, follicles, blood and lymph vessels, sweat and sebaceous glands, sensory nerves, and muscle. The subcutaneous tissue is composed mainly of fat that protects against injury, insulates the body, and is a reserve for calories, which fuel the body.

Acne

Acne, characterized by an eruption of pimples on the skin, affects most teenagers, and especially boys. (Acne, however, is not restricted to any age group; even men in their 40s can develop it.) Rising hormone levels cause sebaceous (oil) glands found in the dermis to secrete an excess of oil, called sebum. Sebum, skin cells, and bacteria can build up in the follicles of the skin. If the sebum ruptures the follicle walls, whiteheads (closed pores), blackheads (open pores), or pimples (inflamed pores) appear on the skin's surface.

In severe forms of acne, the blocked sebum forms lumps under the skin known as sebaceous cysts. Secondary infection from bacteria and other microorganisms can exacerbate acne, and scarring of the skin in varying degrees may occur. Acne usually occurs on the face and neck, but in more severe cases it may also appear on the shoulders, chest, and upper back. Although androgens (hormones that stimulate the development of male sex characteristics) play an important role in the development of acne, heredity also contributes.

Treatment

Mild acne can be alleviated by thoroughly washing your face with soap and warm water two to three times daily, taking care not to irritate the skin by rubbing too vigorously. Don't overdo it, though; washing too often could aggravate the acne. Your dermatologist may break open pimples or remove blackheads and whiteheads. You should *not* try to do this yourself. Squeezing the pimples may result in more redness, swelling, inflammation, and scarring.

Further treatment involves the application of an over-the-counter topical antibacterial product such as benzoyl peroxide or tretinoin (Retin-A). For severe cases of acne, a dermatologist can prescribe antibiotics, both topical and oral form, including tetracycline, erythromycin, and topical clindamycin. An increasingly popular but controversial oral antibiotic is isotretinoin (Accutane), a derivative of vitamin A. This agent has been proven potent and effective for the treatment of cystic acne, but it can cause side effects such as dry skin, chapped lips, and nosebleeds. Minor surgery and dermabrasion may be used to remove sebaceous cysts and restore a more normal appearance to the skin's surface.

Shampooing your hair frequently will help to decrease the amount of oil on the skin, thus

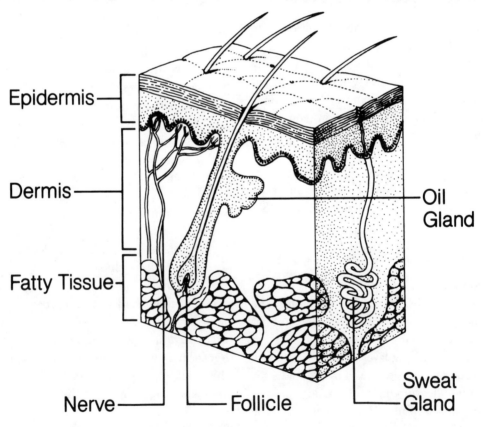

Epidermis

Dermis

Oil Gland

Fatty Tissue

Nerve — Follicle

Sweat Gland

Source: National Cancer Institute

TAKING CARE OF YOUR SKIN

- Drink eight glasses of water each day. Plenty of water helps keep the skin flexible and elastic.

- Eat right. A balanced, low-fat diet ensures that you're getting all the substances your body needs to build healthy skin. In addition, high-fat intake has been associated with an increase in risk for precancerous lesions.

- Use a mild, moisturizing soap. Harsh deodorant soaps can dry skin and make it more vulnerable to disease by removing protective outer layers. A moisturizer applied after a shower can help to minimize dry skin. Avoid scented products, which can be drying or irritating to the skin.

- Don't be hard on yourself. Avoid rubbing your skin vigorously while washing and try not to dry off too roughly after a shower. This can stretch and damage skin. Wash gently—especially your face, where skin is most delicate—and pat yourself dry.

- Forego the long, hot shower. Hot water (as well as excessively cold water) harms the skin, and long showers can remove protective oils from the surface of the skin. Stick to a temperature of about 95° to 100° F, and don't stay in longer than ten minutes. Be careful, as well, in a hot tub, bathtub, or sauna.

- Fight wrinkles. The amount of collagen in the skin begins to decrease at the rate of 1 percent a year beginning in the 20s, leading to crow's feet and other small wrinkles in the 30s and full-blown wrinkles in most men by their 50s. To help prevent wrinkles, don't smoke. Smoking deprives the skin of blood and much needed nutrients. By some estimates, smokers are likely to have five times as many premature wrinkles as nonsmokers. Also, try to sleep on your back. If you sleep on your side, with your face pressed against a pillow, you'll be more likely to develop wrinkles than someone who sleeps on his back.

- Get your vitamins and minerals. Certain vitamins can benefit the skin and help protect it against bacteria and other damaging forces. For example, a B-vitamin deficiency can lead to cracks at the corners of the mouth and large pores on the nose; too little vitamin C is associated with bruising; and vitamin A deficiency leads to dry, rough skin. Other necessary nutrients include the following:

    Essential fatty acids to prevent dryness

    Magnesium to promote strong skin

    Zinc to aid healing and help maintain healthy skin

    Vitamin E, an antioxidant, to neutralize free radicals that may contribute to the development of wrinkles, to aid healing and to maintain elasticity

continues

- Protect yourself against the sun every day. Ultraviolet rays are damaging to the skin, and sunburn reduces elasticity of skin and increases the risk of wrinkles and skin cancer. The American Academy of Dermatology and the Skin Cancer Foundation recommend that a sunscreen with a sun protection factor (SPF) of at least 15 be used on all bare areas when you are outside. If you have dry skin, avoid using a product that contains alcohol.

- Conduct a monthly skin examination, using a mirror to be aware of any changes in your skin. See your doctor immediately if you find a suspicious mole, growth, or lump on your skin or if there has been a change in size, shape, or color of an existing mole. (See Watch Out for Skin Cancer, p. 346.)

- If you have a skin condition or infection, avoid using a washcloth. Washcloths can harbor germs.

helping to prevent acne development. If you have acne and you shave, try both an electric and a safety razor to see which is more comfortable. When using a safety razor, you should first soften the beard with warm soap and water and then shave as lightly as possible over the skin. Always use a sharp blade.

Dermatitis (Eczema)

Dermatitis, or eczema, is a general term used to describe any inflammation of the skin. Examples of eczema include atopic eczema, allergic contact dermatitis, and seborrheic eczema.

An itching, blistering, sometimes crusting rash, combined with a family history of allergies, may indicate atopic eczema. The skin eruptions can accompany allergies such as hay fever and asthma. Atopic eczema can occur at any age, but it most often affects infants and young adults. It can be treated with topical cortisone or tar creams, oral antibiotics, and in severe cases, ultraviolet light therapy.

Allergic contact dermatitis, in which the skin swells and blisters, can be caused by almost anything that touches the skin. Common allergens include nickel, rubber, dyes, poison ivy, poison oak, poison sumac, and related plants. Allergic contact dermatitis can be treated and prevented by identifying and removing the offending allergen. (See Allergies, p. 156.)

Seborrheic eczema causes patches of yellow-pinkish-brownish, greasy scales to erupt on the skin, most commonly on the scalp (dandruff) and face. The itching and discomfort of seborrheic dermatitis can be relieved with hydrocortisone creams for the face and dandruff shampoos for the scalp.

Fungal Nail Disorders

Nails are made of the protein keratin, and they grow from the lunula, the white area at the base of the nail. Fungal nail disorders can affect fingernails and toenails. Nails may become brittle or thickened or may be completely destroyed.

Nails become susceptible to fungus when they are traumatized. When the nail is repeatedly injured, it can become dislodged from the nail bed. In this case, it has no contact with the skin and loses its only blood supply. The nail turns white. Without blood, the nail becomes food for fungus. It will yellow, thicken, and change color. A partial coloring of the nail is called mild onychomycosis. When the entire nail is thick and yellow or when much of the nail is damaged, the condition is called severe chronic onychomycosis. To diagnose the condition, a doctor takes clippings of the nail and examines them microscopically.

To treat the condition, a doctor may prescribe an oral antifungal medication. Griseofulvin, which takes six to twelve months to be effective, is commonly prescribed, although two new oral drugs, Sporanox (itraconazole) and Lamisil (terbinafine), that are available work in three to four months. However, these new drugs are more expensive than griseofulvin and have more side effects.

Another treatment includes grinding the surface of the nail to make it porous, then applying an antifungal cream. At home, the cream is applied daily, and the nail is filed every two or three weeks with an emery board.

Jock Itch

Jock itch, or *tinea cruris*, is a contagious skin infection of the groin. It is caused by a group of fungi called dermatophytes, and is often called ringworm. It can be passed by a person, an animal, soil, or an object such as a shower stall. Because the fungus thrives in warm, moist environments such as those created by perspiration, jock itch is common among male athletes, especially those who wear jockstraps. (Athlete's foot is caused by the same fungi that cause jock itch. For more information on this condition, see Foot Conditions, p. 264.)

Its symptoms include burning, itching, and red, scaly lesions or rings on the genitals and the inner thighs. Usually, jock itch can be identified by its appearance. However, if confirmation of diagnosis is necessary, the fungus can be cultured in a laboratory to identify its type.

Although jock itch can be irritating and annoying, it is usually not difficult to treat or prevent. To get rid of jock itch, apply a topical over-the-counter antifungal ointment, such as Micatin, Cruex, Desenex, Lotrimin, or Tinactin, to the affected area for two weeks after the symptoms disappear to ensure that the fungus is gone for good. Oral antifungal medications such as griseofulvin may be prescribed for widespread infection that affects other parts of the body, such as the scalp and the nails.

To prevent future infections, make the groin area inhospitable for the fungus by keeping the skin dry and clean and by wearing absorbent cotton underwear. If necessary, use drying powders and products that reduce sweating. Change out of sweaty or wet gear as soon as possible after athletic activity. Also, bring a clean towel from home if you plan on showering at the gym—a breeding ground for fungi and other germs—and dry off from head to toe, not vice versa.

Moles

Moles appear in many shapes and sizes, on all parts of the body, alone or in groups. At first, they are flat and brown or black, not much different from a freckle. Over the years—each mole has its own growth pattern—moles usually change, becoming raised and lighter in color. Some seem to just fade away, some hardly change a bit, and some become so raised that they eventually fall off or are rubbed off. Exposure to the sun and certain steroid drugs used in therapy can cause moles to darken. The average mole "lives" for about fifty years.

WATCH OUT FOR SKIN CANCER

When examining moles or other skin changes, look for these warning signs. If one or more are present in a mole or a growth, see a dermatologist immediately.

1. *Asymmetry.* The halves of a mole do not match up.

2. *Border.* A mole is ragged, blurred, or irregular.

3. *Colors.* A single mole is not uniform in color.

4. *Diameter.* The mole is larger than the eraser of a pencil.

Studies have shown that some moles have a higher-than-average risk of developing into a form of skin cancer known as malignant melanoma. Large moles that appear at birth, known as congenital nevi, are more likely to become cancerous than those that appear later in life. Moles called dysplastic nevi or atypical moles are usually larger than a pencil eraser, irregularly shaped, and unevenly colored. People with these moles, which tend to be hereditary, may have an above-average chance of developing malignant melanoma.

The majority of moles and other blemishes, like freckles, are not cancerous and are nothing to worry about. Only those that suddenly change size, shape, or color, or those that bleed, itch, become painful, or first appear when a person is over 30 warrant medical concerns. If a mole does not follow the normal pattern (see box), see a dermatologist. For diagnosis, the dermatologist may want to remove all or part of a mole in order to examine it under a microscope. Most mole removal procedures are quick and can be done in the dermatologist's office. You may also want to have a mole removed simply because you don't like it. (Moles in the beard area can be quite annoying.) The most common methods of removal are shave excision or cutting out the mole and stitching the area closed.

Shaving over a mole will not cause it to become cancerous. Hairs that grow out of moles can be clipped close to the surface of the skin, or a dermatologist can remove them permanently.

Psoriasis

In psoriasis, an overproduction of skin cells causes scaly red patches of skin, most often on the elbows, knees, groin and genitals, arms, legs, scalp, and nails. Two out of every one hundred people in the United States have psoriasis, and approximately 150,000 new cases occur each year. The cause of psoriasis is unknown, though there could be a genetic link. It usually occurs in those between the ages of 10 and 30.

The severity and form of psoriasis differ from case to case. Usually, it begins with little red bumps that slowly grow and form scales. It usually does not itch. Although the silverish scales on the skin's surface flake off easily, those beneath adhere to each other, and bleeding usually occurs when they are removed. Nails infected by psoriasis have pits on them and may thicken or crumble. Inverse psoriasis occurs in the armpits and in skin folds around the groin, buttocks, and genitals.

Treatment of psoriasis depends on the affected individual's health, age, and lifestyle, as well as the severity of the psoriasis. The scales can be loosened with moisturizers and then scrubbed away. A dermatologist may prescribe topical medications containing cortisone or cortisone-like compounds, synthetic vitamin D, tar, or anthralin. These may be combined with light therapy, either from the sun or ultraviolet light rays, both of which slow the growth of skin cells. Because of the dangers associated with ultraviolet rays, light therapy must be used cautiously. In extreme cases, oral medications may be required to control psoriasis. As of yet, no treatment offers a permanent "cure" for psoriasis; however, many treatments, either alone or in combination, can clear or greatly improve its nagging symptoms.

Rosacea

Rosacea (rose-AY-sha) afflicts approximately one in twenty people in the United States. Often wrongly labeled "adult acne," it begins with redness in the center of the face and slowly spreads, causing the cheeks and chin to flush and swell. As rosacea progresses, tiny pimples—both solid and pus-filled—may appear, and enlarged blood vessels may be visible (a condition called telangiectasia). Although it can afflict adults of any age and skin color, it is more prevalent among 30- to 50-year-old, fair-skinned people. It is more common in women but usually more severe in men.

Advanced rosacea may develop into rhinophyma, characterized by a bulbous nose, puffy cheeks, and thick bumps and lines on the skin's surface. About half of all rosacea patients also develop conjunctivitis, which causes burning and grittiness of the eyes. Conjunctivitis must be treated, or it could threaten vision.

Although the exact cause of rosacea is not known, most cases are thought to be inherited. Research suggests that repressing anger, fear, or other strong emotions can increase facial flushing associated with the condition. Certain drugs, including strong steroid-containing creams, may cause or aggravate rosacea.

Rosacea is a chronic condition that may recur from anywhere from five to ten years. However, after that time it usually disappears. To help relieve the symptoms of rosacea, stay out of the sun as much as possible, and avoid extreme hot and cold temperatures. Also avoid rubbing or massaging the face, which can irritate the skin. Consumption of too much alcohol, spicy foods, hot drinks, and smoking will aggravate the redness of rosacea. The condition has been wrongly linked to alcoholism (in part because comedian W. C. Fields, a heavy drinker, had a severe case of rosacea and resulting rhinophyma). While alcohol may worsen rosacea, symptoms can be just as bad in someone who abstains from drinking.

Prompt treatment is best since rosacea rarely heals itself, and without treatment it will become worse over the years. Over-the-counter skin creams and ointments may aggravate rosacea. A dermatologist may prescribe a topical medication in gel or cream form, which should create a noticeable improvement within two months. Steroid creams are also available to heal bumps and reduce redness, but they should not be used for an extended period.

Rosacea patients should be careful to avoid skin irritants. Choose facial products that are free of alcohol or other irritating ingredients. Moisturizers should be applied gently only after topical medication has dried. Protect your face from ultraviolet sunlight by always using sunscreens, which should have an SPF of 15 or higher.

Dilated blood vessels (telangiectasia) may be closed off with a small electric needle, a laser, or surgery. Rhinophyma is usually treated with laser or scalpel surgery and dermabrasion to help improve the scar's appearance.

Warts

A wart is a contagious growth on the skin or a mucous membrane caused by the human papilloma virus (called HPV), of which there are 30 types (some of which do not cause warts at all). These rough, flesh-colored growths develop several months after exposure to HPV. Warts can be passed from person to person, but they are harmless and are not painful. They do not have roots or branches, and they can be located anywhere on the body. Some warts appear to be speckled with black dots, which are capillaries that have been clotted. Some people are more susceptible to warts, than others.

Types of Warts

For the most part, warts are similar with the exception of their location on the body. If you've never had a wart before, it's important to see a dermatologist for diagnosis and treatment, because what appears to be a wart may be something else, possibly a sign of skin cancer. There are several types of warts: common hand warts, foot warts, flat warts, and genital warts.

Common warts are rough, flesh-colored growths that are usually found on the hands, face, knees, and scalp. These warts can grow up to 1/4 inch in diameter. They commonly occur where skin has been broken, because the broken skin allows an acquired virus access into the body.

Also called foot warts, plantar warts are common warts found on the soles of the feet. They tend to grow in a group the size of a quarter or larger, and they do not stick up above the skin's surface. While plantar warts themselves are harmless, many times the pressure from walking on

the warts may cause pain. Plantar warts are more common in people whose feet sweat a lot and in people who do a lot of walking and exercising.

Flat warts are tiny, flesh-colored warts that grow in multiples, sometimes as many as one hundred at a time. They are not as rough as common warts, and they generally occur on the wrists, the hands, and the face. On men, they most often grow in the beard area; skin irritation may account for their appearance.

Genital warts can occur in both genders on the genitalia, around the anus, and within the rectum, and they can appear within the vagina and the cervix in women. Genital warts tend to be soft, pink, cauliflower-like bumps that grow extensively. These are caused by HPV and are transmitted by sexual contact. (See Sexually Transmitted Diseases, p. 387.)

Treatment

About 50 percent of all warts disappear on their own in 6 to 12 months. While genital warts and some plantar warts require treatment, other types do not need to be removed except for cosmetic reasons.

Over-the-counter medications, which contain salicylic acid, are available to treat warts. Alternative remedies recommended for warts include applying the contents of a vitamin A capsule each day, or applying a paste of a crushed vitamin C tablet and water. Do not treat a wart without a practitioner's advice unless it has been definitively diagnosed.

Warts can also be treated by a dermatologist. Cryotherapy, freezing and removing the wart, is a painless procedure that results in very little scarring. Repeat treatments may be necessary as the growths caused by the virus continue to become noticeable. Electrosurgical destruction, or burning away the wart, is also an option. This treatment often can be done in only one office visit, but it is associated with pain and some scarring. Warts can also be surgically removed under local anesthesia.

Genital warts are the most difficult to treat, as they are often difficult to locate. Sometimes a rectal exam is required to locate all the genital warts so they can be treated effectively. Genital warts are treated with the drug podophyllin, along with a topical application. A practitioner can also remove genital warts with acid or by freezing, and periodic office visits may be necessary.

Prompt treatment is necessary for genital warts, which can occur up to eighteen months after infection. According to the American Academy of Dermatology, there seems to be some increased possibility of skin cancer at the site of long-standing genital warts. Women with genital warts also have an increased risk of cancer of the cervix. For this reason, a man who has been diagnosed with genital warts should inform his sexual partner so she can seek effective treatment immediately. Those with genital warts also have an increased risk of contracting the AIDS virus because warts provide a vulnerable point through which the virus can enter.

Sometimes warts recur as fast as they are cured. This often happens for two reasons: reinfection from an infected person or the old warts have shed the virus to other areas of the skin before they were treated. To avoid this, treat new warts as soon as they are noticed, before they have time to shed the virus to new areas.

For more information:

American Academy of Dermatology
930 N. Meacham Rd.
P.O. Box 4014
Schaumburg, IL 60173
847-330-0230
http://www.derm-infonet.com

Dermatology Foundation
1560 Sherman Ave., Room 302
Evanston, IL 60201-4802
847-328-2256

National Psoriasis Foundation
P.O. Box 9009
Portland, OR 97207
800-723-9166
503-244-7404
http://www.psoriasis.org

National Rosacea Society
800 S. Northwest Hwy., Suite 200
Barrington, IL 60010
847-382-8971
http://www.rosacea.org

American Skin Association
150 E. 58th St., 32nd Fl.
New York, NY 10155-0002
212-753-8260

SLEEP DISORDERS

Everyone has been affected by a sleep problem at some time in his life, whether it's a night of restless sleep before a big meeting or game, complaints about snoring, or a bout of daytime sleepiness. There are some 222 known sleep disorders, among them insomnia, snoring, sleep apnea, narcolepsy, parasomnias, and REM behavior disorder, which are detailed below. Even though sleep disorder medicine is a relatively new field, there are growing numbers of sleep clinics and practitioners who concern themselves with sleep research and study.

The Mechanics of Sleep

New insights into what sleep is and why and how people sleep has lead to greater understanding of sleep disorders. To start with, sleep is a period during which the body repairs itself, consolidates memory, removes wastes from its systems, and collects energy for the next day. The average person spends about one-third of his life asleep—about 205,000 hours in a 70-year lifetime.

NREM and REM Sleep

More specifically, sleep is made up of the REM (rapid eye movement) period and the NREM (nonrapid eye movement) period, which alternate in ninety-minute cycles throughout the night.

Up to 25 percent of the night's sleep is spent in REM sleep. This is a shallow sleep cycle that is thought to restore memory function. It is during REM sleep that most dreams—at least those that can be remembered—occur. Most REM sleep occurs in the last third of a night's sleep.

Eighty percent of the average adult's night's sleep is spent in NREM sleep, a deep sleep period during which the body's functions are restored, rejuvenated, and revitalized. Most NREM sleep occurs during the early sleep cycles in the first part of the night.

The Body's Clocks

Two complex, clocklike systems—the circadian clock and the homeostatic clock—keep time for the body, together determining when a person wakes and sleeps.

The circadian clock, also called the circadian rhythm, works on a cycle of about twenty-four hours—the length of a day. Essentially, it controls body temperature. Alertness comes with a high body temperature, while low temperatures mean sleepiness. Most adults' temperatures peak at midmorning and midevening.

The homeostatic clock works on a cycle of twenty-eight hours, which synchronizes with the twenty-four-hour circadian pattern. Experts

How Much Sleep Do You Need?

According to the National Commission on Sleep Disorders and Research:

Babies need eighteen hours of sleep a day, which they receive.

Young children (preteen) need and receive ten to twelve hours of sleep a day.

Teenagers need up to ten hours, but usually get six.

Adults need an average of seven to nine hours, but get fewer than seven.

Older people need about eight hours, and get five to seven.

believe that the homeostatic clock prompts us to go to bed in the evening, while the circadian clock keeps us asleep throughout the night.

These clocks keep the body on a somewhat regular schedule, although this schedule does change throughout life. Younger people, for example, run on a cycle that is longer than the twenty-four-hour average. Older people tend to run on a shorter cycle—the reason many older sleepers wake early in the morning. Most people also supplement their body's clock with alarm clocks and predetermined bedtimes that help keep them on schedule.

Brain Chemicals

A great deal of sleep research is now being focused on the brain chemicals that aid sleep. These chemicals, called neurotransmitters, are hormonelike substances that conduct nerve impulses among brain cells.

Cortisol levels in the body increase in the early morning and decrease around midnight, in correlation with the body's energy levels. Melatonin and serotonin also help to induce sleep, while epinephrine, norepinephrine, and dopamine promote alertness and activity. Increases and decreases in the levels of these chemicals in the system are key parts of the body's sleep-wake cycle.

Insomnia

Insomnia, the most common sleep disorder, is the inability to fall asleep or stay asleep. At least 40 million Americans suffer from chronic sleep disorders—lasting for months or even years—and twenty to thirty million more suffer from intermittent insomnia.

Why is that so alarming? Because sleep is a highly complex activity that is an important part of physical and mental health. A recent study at the University of California at San Diego found that some immune-system activities decrease as much as 30 percent after nights when people miss three or more hours of sleep. And while you sleep, the brain consolidates the day's learning into the memory, which helps make your thought processes sharper when you're awake.

Some of the most common causes of insomnia are stress; anxiety; medical conditions; allergies; excess alcohol; nicotine; excessive intake of caffeine; poor sleeping conditions (noise, light, cold, etc.); pain; urinary problems; depression; biorhythm disturbances (shift work, jet lag, etc.); and prescription and over-the-counter drugs.

Diagnosis

Before doing anything else, determine whether your sleep problem is insomnia or a sign of a more serious medical and/or psychological condition. Many medical conditions—intestinal malabsorption problems, heart disease, diabetes, anemia, and chronic sinus infections, just to name a few—include insomnia as a secondary effect. See your doctor for a full exam to rule out a medical condition.

Be sure to tell your doctor about all the prescription and over-the-counter (OTC) medications you're using since dozens of medicines contain ingredients that preclude sleep. Drugs that can keep you awake at night include those containing caffeine (including some OTC painkillers like Excedrin and Anacin); diet aids that contain amphetamines; alertness pills such as NoDoz and Vivarin; some allergy medications, especially those containing the stimulant hormone ACTH;

INSOMNIA INSIGHT

- One in three Americans—36 percent—doesn't get enough sleep. The average adult needs seven to nine hours a sleep each day.

- Twenty percent of middle-aged men and 60 percent of elderly men snore enough to disturb their own sleep.

- Serious sleep deprivation directly cost the U.S. economy $15.83 billion in 1990, a figure that was higher than the costs of AIDS and cigarette damage for the same year.

- Some forty thousand persons a year die and another 250,000 are injured after falling asleep at the wheel, according to the Highway Safety Commission. The Department of Transportation estimates that 200,000 highway accidents a year are sleep-related.

nasal decongestants such as Sudafed and Sinutab; blood pressure medications; many asthma drugs; steroid preparations; thyroid hormones; various beta blockers taken for heart disease and high blood pressure; some antidepressants; and some antimetabolites used in cancer treatments. Herbal remedies should also be treated like drugs.

If you suspect that an OTC drug may be keeping you awake, change the time you take it or reduce the dosage. For prescription medications, your doctor may change the dosage and time taken or switch you to a related drug that doesn't affect sleep.

MELATONIN—MIRACLE CURE FOR INSOMNIA?

Melatonin, a hormone produced in the brain's pineal gland, is released into the bloodstream at night and sends the message to the rest of the body that it is time for sleep. Melatonin is plentiful in young people but decreases with age, which may explain why elderly people often find it hard to fall asleep. Because melatonin naturally regulates our sleep-wake cycles, supplements of the hormone are being looked at as a cure for insomnia.

Some researchers believe that taking a supplement of melatonin in the evening can regulate the biological clock disturbances associated with insomnia, jet lag, and shift work. Melatonin may also be useful for "phase lag syndrome" in which a person's body clock is hours behind what it needs to be, resulting in trouble falling asleep at night and awakening in the early morning.

But there are concerns about melatonin, especially since it is not a drug and is, therefore, not regulated by the Food and Drug Administration. Possible side effects include nausea, headaches, and nightmares. Melatonin may also contribute to depression.

The effectiveness of melatonin is also uncertain. A survey of more than four hundred people found that one in eight tried the substance for insomnia, but only 25 percent of those found melatonin helpful. Almost 50 percent said melatonin did nothing for their symptoms.

Melatonin dosage is also a concern. Melatonin, sold in health-food stores nationwide, comes in doses from 0.25 mg to 3 mg. But again, no standards exist for recommended dosages, and there is no solid research on harmful effects from large doses. In addition, if people take a dose at the wrong time in their sleep cycle, melatonin may throw off the body's clock even further.

It's believed that melatonin works as a natural contraceptive and, therefore, may decrease fertility. And it's been suggested that melatonin may boost the immune system so much that people with allergies, autoimmune diseases, and immune-system cancers should not take the hormone because it may exacerbate their conditions.

Researchers and doctors caution that not enough is known about melatonin and its long-term effects to be recommended as a cure for insomnia. The American Sleep Disorders Association regards melatonin treatments experimental and does not recommend self-administered doses of the hormone.

Treatment

Insomnia can often be treated by adopting good sleep habits and self-care techniques. (See Self-Care for Sleep Disorders, p. 357.) Yet some medical causes of insomnia may require care by a specialist. An ear, nose, and throat (ENT) specialist or an internist with a background in breathing disorders or in pulmonary diseases can treat problems related to snoring or sleep apnea, while a neurologist can treat sleep problems related to the central nervous system.

More than three-quarters of America's chronic insomnia problems have a psychological basis, and many are curable with professional attention. If your doctor concludes that depression or psychological problems are the root of your insomnia, counseling or behavior-modification treatment may be recommended. You also may consider seeing a psychiatrist with experience in treating sleeping disorders.

Sleeping pills are intended to be used for short periods only to reestablish good sleep, either in association with self-help measures or after other causes of insomnia have been ruled out. OTC sleeping remedies usually contain antihistamines, drugs mainly used to relieve allergies that have sedative side effects. While the Food and Drug Administration (FDA) has ruled these substances safe, few doctors find them to be effective as sleep inducers. In addition, they can have side effects.

Prescription sleep medications work by suppressing nerve-cell activity within the brain. They include two major classes of drugs: benzodiazepines and tricyclic antidepressants.

Benzodiazepines are prescribed to treat short-term insomnia caused by emotional stress or travel. They relieve anxiety, promote sleep, and are effective for short periods—about two weeks. Side effects include sweating, nausea, rapid pulse, and depression. Benzodiazepines, which include Valium and Halcion, can be addictive.

Tricyclic antidepressants are prescribed for insomnia related to chronic pain or nonrestorative sleep. They are effective in very small doses, and therefore, their side effects are usually mild—dry mouth, constipation, urinary problems, and tremors. Common tricyclic antidepressants are Elavil and Tofranil.

Some alternative therapies have also been shown to be effective in treating insomnia, including acupuncture, chiropractic care, massage, yoga, self-hypnosis, and relaxation techniques. Herbal teas containing sleep-inducing herbs such as valerian, hops, and wildflowers may help. And melatonin—the neurotransmitter that induces sleep by helping to control circadian (light-dark) rhythm—has been touted as sleep-regulating supplement that can help reset body clocks.

Snoring

Snoring is the noise that occurs during sleep when a partial obstruction of the nasal airway causes the rear, fleshy part of the roof of the mouth, called the soft palate, to vibrate. Such obstructions usually occur as the muscles of the throat and tongue relax during sleep.

An estimated twenty million Americans habitually snore. Perhaps because they tend to have more tissue in their neck and throat areas, men are more likely to snore than women. In fact, the American Sleep Disorders Association estimates that 60 percent of all adults who snore are men.

While snoring is usually nothing more than a nuisance—one that may bother your roommate or partner more than it bothers you—it may signal more significant problems such as high blood pressure and sleep apnea, a condition in which breathing may actually stop during sleep. (See Sleep Apnea, p. 354.)

Causes of Snoring

There are many factors that contribute to snoring. Enlarged tonsils or adenoids, a large soft palate or a large uvula (the piece of soft tissue that hangs down at back of the throat) may constrict the nasal passage and cause snoring. If you sleep on your back, you're more likely to snore as your tongue relaxes and falls back over the airway. Older people are more likely to snore as well, as the throat tissues lose their tone with age. Use of alcohol and some medications such as sleeping pills may also relax the throat muscles and cause snoring.

Obesity also increases the chances of snoring: People who weigh 20 percent more than their ideal weight are three times more likely to snore than those who are not obese. This is because people with weight problems have a tendency to deposit extra fatty tissue in the neck area, and the extra mass often causes snoring.

Nasal blockage is another cause of snoring. The nose may be blocked by a deviated septum (a bend in the cartilage that separates the nasal cavities), a nasal polyp (a growth within the nose), or inflammation of mucous membranes within the nose caused by smoking, allergies, an infection (such as a cold), or medication.

Conditions Associated With Snoring

Some 85 percent of those who snore also suffer from sleep apnea, a condition in which the muscles of the throat relax during sleep partially or totally obstructing breathing. Loud snoring, marked with pauses and gasps, is often a sign of sleep apnea, which can result in daytime drowsiness, difficulty concentrating, depression, and irritability. In men, apnea and snoring may result in erectile failure because of changes in the blood flow to the penis.

Heavy or habitual snoring has also been associated with cardiovascular problems such as high blood pressure, though experts are not sure of the exact cause-and-effect relationship. One Canadian study found high blood pressure to be twice as common among snorers than as nonsnorers. In addition, some 14 percent of snorers suffer from heart disease, while only 8 percent of nonsnorers do. For the most part, high blood pressure is attributed to sleep apnea: The heart pumps harder and faster when breathing stops, an effect that lasts even after the person is awake. However, even among those who snore but do not have apnea, blood pressure rises and falls markedly.

Treatment

Snoring is most commonly treated with self-help techniques. (See Self-Care for Sleep Disorders, p. 357.) However, some medical treatments are available.

If your snoring is caused by allergies, for example, a physician can help pinpoint what is causing the allergy and prescribe medication such as a decongestant to help alleviate symptoms. Remember, however, that decongestants provide only temporary relief from congestion and snoring.

If snoring stems from physical obstructions of the nasal passage or the upper airway, a variety of mouthpieces are available to keep the tongue from blocking the airway during sleep. If the nose is stuffy from a cold, an infection, or a deviated septum, some say a nasal strip may help. These adhesive strips, available over-the-counter, are taped across the bridge of the nose.

A spring within the strip gently pulls the nasal passage open.

Unless sleep apnea is diagnosed, surgery is rarely used to treat snoring. (For information on surgical treatments, see Sleep Apnea, below.)

Sleep Apnea

Sleep apnea, a potentially life-threatening sleeping disorder, affects millions of people often totally unaware of the problem. The American Sleep Disorders Association (ASDA) estimates that five out of every one hundred people suffer from obstructive sleep apnea. It is more common in men than women—most often middle age, overweight men. One study in the *New England Journal of Medicine* suggested that 9 percent of the men between the ages of 30 and 60 have sleep apnea.

Sleep apnea is a brief absence of breathing during sleep that occurs when the airway becomes blocked and collapses, disrupting the normal breathing pattern. Each period where breathing stops—called an apnea—may last ten seconds or more. When oxygen levels become too low, the body's inherent safety mechanism kicks in, rousing the sleeper from sleep until the breathing process begins again.

The disruption of sleep is often so short that a person is often unaware of what has happened, yet people who suffer from sleep apnea may stop breathing hundreds of times a night. Experts estimate these disruptions may number as high as two hundred to four hundred times during an eight-hour sleep period.

Symptoms

Sleep apnea manifests itself in a variety of ways. Warning signs include:

- Daytime tiredness or fatigue
- Restless sleep
- Snoring
- Gasping or pauses in snoring during sleep
- Morning headaches
- Night sweats
- Memory problems
- Difficulty concentrating

Uncommon symptoms include depression and impotence (as sleep disorders disrupt blood flow to the penis).

Types of Sleep Apnea

There are two major types of sleep apnea—obstructive and central. Obstructive sleep apnea is the most common. It results from a narrowing or total collapse of the airway during sleep that occurs when the muscles around the pharynx relax and interrupt breathing. Before apnea becomes a problem, there is usually a history of snoring.

A second form of sleep apnea, called central sleep apnea, is the result of a failure of the respiratory system instead of an obstruction. This occurs when the diaphragm stops functioning. It is more common in older people, and the ASDA estimates that one in four people over the age of 60 experiences a certain degree of disrupted breathing during sleep. Occasionally, central and obstructive sleep apnea occur together.

Causes

Certain factors such as obesity, allergies, enlarged tonsils and adenoids, alcohol, and sleeping pills may all lead to or increase the severity of sleep apnea. Obesity, defined as greater than 20 percent of a person's ideal weight, is a factor because of the increase in fatty tissue in the neck and throat area.

Another factor that may affect the rate of sleep apnea is alcohol consumption. Not only does alcohol consumption cause throat muscles to relax, it may also delay waking in people who already suffer from apnea. Sleeping pills and other drugs may have the same effect.

Risks

If left untreated, other problems may arise from this condition. Among these are high blood pressure (hypertension), heart disease, and stroke. Studies have shown that there is a correlation between high blood pressure and sleep apnea. Research suggests that blood pressure rises enough during the apnea episodes to prevent it from returning to average levels during normal breathing or waking hours. In fact, some estimates show that 40 to 60 percent of those suffering from sleep apnea also have hypertension, and 30 percent of those with hypertension have sleep apnea.

Sleep apnea also seems to have an influence on the likelihood of a person being involved in a car accident. Studies show that people suffering from sleep apnea are two to five times more likely to be involved in a collision than the general population. This fact may be attributed to the daytime tiredness that results from the disorder.

Sleep apnea can be life-threatening. If a person doesn't wake when breathing stops or if the heart beats irregularly or stops, death may occur. In preliminary research, sleep apnea has been linked to sudden infant death syndrome as well as implicated in certain instances where apparently healthy people died in their sleep.

Diagnosis

A person may be aroused often enough or hard enough to notice gasping or snorting, but it is usually a partner or family member who notices a problem and suggests that the person go for help. The first step is to consult the family physician. The physician will study the patient's medical history, conduct a physical exam while checking for indicative symptoms, and possibly consult a partner or family members.

If apnea or another sleep disorder is suspected once other conditions are ruled out, you may be referred to a sleep disorder center. By studying various physiological characteristics that occur when a person sleeps (polysomnography) a proper diagnosis can be obtained.

Treatment

Mild sleep apnea may be helped by using self-care techniques. (See Self-Care for Sleeping Disorders, opposite.) There are a variety of treatments available that depend upon the severity of the sleep apnea. One nonsurgical option is continuous positive airway pressure (CPAP), in which a mask connected to a compressor is worn during sleep. The mask forces air through the nasal passages and into the airway, keeping it open. Recent research has focused on developing self-adjusting CPAP machines that automatically change air flow and pressure in response to feedback. While a reported 60 to 70 percent of people who try CPAP are able to continue this type of treatment, some find the system is too troublesome and confining to use.

Oral appliances, which include tongue retainers and jaw-advancement devices, are sometimes used to treat mild cases of sleep apnea. Tongue retainers hold the tongue in place so that it does not block the airway, while jaw advancement appliances alter the position of the lower jaw.

Protriptyline, an antidepressant medication, may also be prescribed. This drug works by reducing or inhibiting REM (rapid eye movement) sleep, the phase when sleep apnea is most likely to occur. It may also help to increase the tone of the throat muscles.

If these treatments are not effective or if a physical abnormality such as enlarged tonsils or a deviated septum is the cause of the apnea, there are many surgical options. As always, be sure to seek a second opinion before making a decision on surgery.

Laser-assisted uvulopalatoplasty (LAUP) is a new procedure that uses a laser to remove part of the soft palate and uvula. LAUP is done in a practitioner's office in several sessions. Because it is a new procedure, its effectiveness has not yet been determined. In fact, studies to date have shown conflicting results, with some predicting a success rate of 93 percent while others predict a rate as low as 44 percent. Side effects may include a dry throat, heightened gag reflex, and moderate pain as the area heals.

Uvulopalatopharyngoplasty (UPPP) surgery involves removing the uvula, tonsils, and part of the soft palate. According to the ASDA, 50 percent of patients are helped by this procedure. Temporary side effects include mild to severe throat pain. Side effects that may become permanent include nasal sounding speech and the possibility that liquids may be regurgitated through the nose when swallowing.

Other procedures to open the airway include inferior sagittal mandibular osteotomy (ISO) and geniohyoid advancement with hyoid myotomy (GAHM). In ISO, the lower bone of the jaw is brought forward. In GAHM, the hyoid bone (the u-shaped bone that holds your lower teeth) is attached to the windpipe. The success rates of these surgeries depends upon a person's weight and jaw structure.

Another procedure, maxillomandibular advancement (MMO) involves moving both the upper and lower jaw forward. After surgery, the jaw is wired shut for four weeks, necessitating a liquids-only diet. Orthodontic work may be necessary after the procedure to realign the teeth. Those with a small jaw or a jaw that is set too far back benefit most from this procedure.

Uncommon surgical procedures for sleep apnea include laser midline glossectomy (LMG) and lingualplasty, in which the throat is enlarged by removing portion of the back of the tongue. A tracheostomy may be necessary in patients with life-threatening sleep apnea. This process involves making an opening in the trachea and inserting a tube that bypasses the obstruction.

Self-Care for Sleep Disorders

Sleep disorders can often be treated with simple lifestyle changes. Try these tips to help you get a good night's sleep:

- Stick to a regular sleep time. Going to bed and getting up at the same time every day will set your body's inner clock. Don't sleep late on your days off and avoid napping during the day.

- Make your sleeping conditions as ideal as possible. Your bed should be comfortable and the room should be warm, dark, and quiet.

- Avoid substances—especially in the evening—that interfere with sleep: caffeine, nicotine, alcohol, and rich and heavy foods.

- Exercise. Active people sleep better and more easily; but don't do strenuous exercise right before bedtime.

- Don't drink an excessive amount of fluid in the evening so that a full bladder disturbs your sleep.

- Set aside quiet time an hour or so before you go to bed each night. Reflect on the day and clear your mind before problems and details keep you awake all night.

- Use your bed only for sleeping and sex. Don't watch television, read, talk on the phone, do paperwork, work on a laptop computer, or hold discussions in bed.

- Learn a relaxation technique and use it before you go to bed. Slow down your breathing and think about the air moving in and out of your body. Listen to soothing music. Take a warm bath.

- Snack on complex carbohydrates (bread, cereal, crackers) one or two hours before bedtime to promote deeper sleep. Avoid foods with protein and sugars, which stimulate the body.

- Drink a glass of warm milk if it helps you sleep. In some people, the amino acid L tryptophan in milk acts as a sedative. But note that the amino acid tyrosine, also in milk, will energize other people.

To help silence your snores and prevent sleep apnea:

- Quit smoking. Smoking irritates and inflames the nasal passages, promoting snoring.

- Avoid alcohol or medication such as sleeping pills. These items cause the upper airway muscles to relax and lose their tone.

- Lose weight. Slimming down can reduce fatty tissue in the neck and throat area which may be constricting the airway.

- Avoid eating a heavy meal before bedtime. A heavy meal causes the body's muscles—including those of the throat—to relax.

Eating late may also increase your weight (and your tendency to snore). Dinner should be three to four hours before bed.

- Get into position. Snoring and apnea is usually worse when you sleep on your back, so try sleeping on your side. Many experts recommend sewing a pocket containing a tennis ball to the back of your pajamas as a reminder to stay on your side. Commercial alarms are also available to help you stay on your side.

- Elevate your head. Raising the head of your bed a few inches—easily done by putting bricks under two of the legs of the bed—can help open the airway and stop snoring. Specially designed pillows are also available to help snorers.

- Get more sleep. A study from Stanford University's Sleep Research Center showed that sleep deprivation can increase the amount of time a person spends snoring.

- Use a humidifier. Keeping your sleeping environment moist helps prevents mucus from building up in the throat.

For more information:

American Sleep Disorders Association
1610 14th St., N.W., Suite 300
Rochester, MN 55901-2200
507-287-6006
http://www.asda.org

Better Sleep Council
P.O. Box 19534
Alexandria, VA 22320
703-683-8371

National Sleep Foundation
729 15th St., N.W., 4th Floor
Washington, DC 20005
202-347-3471

STROKE

A stroke, or cerebrovascular accident, is often called a "brain attack." The brain, which consists of more than ten billion cells, uses 25 percent of the oxygen you breathe in order to function. Oxygen is supplied to the brain through the blood. When the blood supply is interrupted and the oxygen can no longer be delivered, these cells, which run the various functions of the brain, begin to die. This injury, which can affect any part of the brain, is called a stroke.

Each year more than 500,000 Americans have a stroke and 150,000 die from stroke-related causes, according to the American Heart Association. On the average, someone in the United States suffers a stroke every minute—and every 3.4 minutes someone dies as the result of stroke. Some 28 percent of those who have a stroke each year are under age 65. The incidence of stroke is 19 percent higher for men than for women.

The estimated prevalence of stroke is 2.2 percent for white men; 1.8 percent for African-American men; and 1.1 percent for Mexican-American men. Yet the death rates for stroke are 26.8 per 100,000 for white men and 52 per 100,000 for African-American men (94 percent higher). Compared with whites, young African Americans have a two- to threefold greater risk of stroke. African-American men are also 2.5 times more likely to die from stroke than white men are.

The effects of a stroke are determined by the part of the brain affected and the extent of the damage. A stroke may be mild, with few permanent or serious effects. However, a stroke may be severely debilitating, leaving an individual weak or paralyzed, uncoordinated, off-balance, and unable to use language.

Types of Strokes

There are two ways blood flow, and thus oxygen supply, can be interrupted: through a blockage or through bleeding. A blockage of a blood vessel in the neck or in the brain is called an ischemic stroke. A rupture of a blood vessel in or near the brain causes the second type of stroke, called hemorrhagic stroke.

Ischemic stroke is the most common type of stroke, accounting for 80 percent. In ischemic stroke, a blood vessel may become blocked by a thrombosis, an embolism, or stenosis, cutting off the oxygen supply to the brain. A thrombosis is a blood clot that forms within a blood vessel of the brain or neck. An embolism is a clot that forms in another part of the body, then moves through the bloodstream to lodge in a vessel of the brain or neck. Stenosis indicates severe narrowing of an artery in or leading to the brain.

A hemorrhagic stoke can be caused by a head injury, by the rupture of an aneurysm (a bulge in the wall of a blood vessel), or by a weak or abnormal blood vessel.

A transient ischemic stroke (TIA), or ministroke, occurs when a blood clot temporarily clogs an artery. In a TIA, the blood flow returns to normal quickly, and stroke symptoms usually disappear within twenty-four hours. More than one-third of those who suffer TIAs eventually have a stroke. In about 20 percent of the cases, the stroke occurs within a year.

Symptoms

If you observe one or more of these signs of a stroke or a TIA, seek emergency care immediately.

- Sudden weakness or numbness of the face, arm, or leg

- Sudden dimness or loss of vision, particularly in one eye

- Sudden difficulty understanding speech or speaking

- Sudden severe headache with no known cause

- Unexplained dizziness, unsteadiness, or sudden falls, especially with any of the other signs.

Risk Factors

There are a number of risk factors for stroke—some are preventable, while others cannot be changed. Your risk of stroke increases as the number and severity of the known risk factors increase. Having a risk factor doesn't mean you will have a stroke, but it does increase the chances of one. On the other hand, not having a risk factor doesn't mean you will never have a stroke, though it dramatically reduces the possibilities.

Risk factors that can be modified include the following:

1. *High blood pressure.* Stroke risk corresponds directly with blood pressure.

2. *Heart disease.* People with heart problems have more than twice the stroke risk of those with normally functioning hearts. Those with atrial fibrillation, a type of irregular heartbeat in which the upper chambers of the heart are affected, are especially at high risk.

3. *Smoking.* Smoking damages the cardiovascular system, reduces the amount of oxygen in the blood, and encourages the development of blood clots.

4. *Transient ischemic attacks (TIAs).* About 10 percent of strokes are preceded by TIAs.

5. *High red blood cell count.* A high blood count encourages the development of blood clots, increasing the risk of stroke.

Risk factors that cannot be changed include the following:

1. *Age.* Older people have a higher risk of stroke than younger people. The risk of stroke in people aged 65 to 74 is 1 percent a year.

2. *Gender.* The incidence of stroke is about 30 percent higher in men than in women.

3. *Heredity.* The risk is higher for people who have a family history of stroke.

4. *Race.* Deaths attributed to stroke are 3 to 4 times more common in African Americans than in whites. This may be due to the greater incidence of high blood pressure among African Americans. Hispanics and Asian-Pacific Islanders also have a higher risk of stroke than Caucasians.

5. *Diabetes.* Having diabetes—even controlled diabetes—increases stroke risk. High blood pressure is also common in those with diabetes.

The Effects of Stroke

Each stroke has different effects, depending on what part of the brain is injured, how bad the injury is, and the person's overall health. Some of the effects of stroke include the following:

- Weakness or paralysis on one side of the body. The side of the body opposite of the side of the brain that had been injured is affected. The whole side may be affected or just the arm or the leg.

Score Your Stroke Risk
for the Next Ten Years

Key: **SBP** = systolic blood pressure (score one line only, untreated or treated); **Diabetes** = history or diabetes; **Cigarettes** = smokes cigarettes; **CVD (cardiovascular disease)** = history of heart disease; **AF** = history of atrial fibrillation; **LVH** = diagnosis of left ventricular hypertrophy

A

Points	0	+1	+2	+3	+4	+5	+6	+7	+8	+9	+10
Age	55–56	57–59	60–62	63–65	66–68	69–72	73–75	76–78	79–81	83–84	85
SBP-untrtd	97–105	106–115	116–125	126–135	136–145	146–155	156–165	166–175	176–185	186–195	196–205
or SBP-trtd	97–105	106–112	113–117	118–123	124–129	130–135	136–142	143–150	151–161	162–176	177–205
Diabetes	No		Yes								
Cigarettes	No			Yes							
CVD	No				Yes						
AF	No				Yes						
LVH	No					Yes					

B

Your Points	10-Year Probability	Your Points	10-Year Probability	Your Points	10-Year Probability
1	3%	11	11%	21	42%
2	3%	12	13%	22	47%
3	4%	13	15%	23	52%
4	4%	14	17%	24	57%
5	5%	15	20%	25	63%
6	5%	16	22%	26	68%
7	6%	17	26%	27	74%
8	7%	18	29%	28	79%
9	8%	19	33%	29	84%
10	10%	20	37%	30	88%

C

Compare with Your Age Group	Average 10-Year Probability of Stroke
55–59	5.9%
60–64	7.8%
65–69	11.0%
70–74	13.7%
75–79	18.0%
80–84	22.3%

Source: National Institutes of Health.

- Problems with balance or coordination. A person may find it hard to coordinate movements in order to sit, stand, or walk even if the muscles are strong enough.

- Problems using language. A person with aphasia may have trouble understanding speech or writing, or can understand but cannot think of the words to speak or write. A person with dysarthria knows the right words but has trouble saying them clearly.

- Being unaware or ignoring things on one side of the body. Often the person will not look toward the injured side of the body.

- Pain, numbness, or odd sensations. These can make it hard for the person to relax and get comfortable.

- Problems with memory, thinking, attention, or learning. A person may have trouble with mental activities, such as following directions or keeping track of the date or time.

- Being unaware of the effects of the stroke. The person may try to do things that are unsafe as a result of the stroke.

- Trouble swallowing, called dysphagia.

- Problems with bowel or bladder control.

- Fatigue.

- Sudden bursts of emotion such as laughing, crying, or anger. These emotions may indicate that a person needs help, understanding, and support in trying to adjust to the effects of the stroke.

- Depression. It is common for a person to feel sad over the problems caused by a stroke, but some experience a major depressive disorder that should be diagnosed and treated.

Treatment

Emergency treatment after the onset of a stroke involves stabilizing the individual and preventing any additional damage to the brain. While at one time it was thought that the timing of treatment would not affect the severity of a stroke, it has now been shown that immediate treatment may help to reduce the effects of the stroke and prevent permanent damage in some cases.

In the case of ischemic stroke, treatment focuses on improving blood and oxygen flow to the brain, which is done by using anticoagulants, or blood-thinning drugs. Anticoagulants help prevent the formation of clots in arteries that have narrowed. Surgery may be done to open an artery and restore blood flow to the brain. Researchers are investigating how clot-busting agents, called thrombolytics and commonly used to prevent heart attacks, can dissolve blood clots that cause stroke.

Hemorrhagic strokes are treated with blood-pressure-lowering medications to slow the flow of blood. A leaking artery may be injected with a substance to stop the flow of blood. Surgery may also be done to close ruptured blood vessels.

Treatment after a stroke may also include a change in lifestyle and diet, designed to reduce the risk of another stroke.

Rehabilitation

The type of rehabilitation a patient requires depends on the severity of the brain injury and the patient's overall health before the stroke. Rehabilitation is usually physical therapy

PREVENTING A STROKE

To help prevent stroke, you need to take steps to reduce your risk. Many risk factors can be managed, and although the risk of stroke is never zero at any age, by starting early and controlling your risk factors you can lower your risk of death or disability by stroke. In fact, experts at the National Institutes of Health predict that, with continued attention to reducing the risks of stroke and by using currently available therapies and developing new ones, Americans should be able to prevent 80 percent of all strokes by the end of this decade.

- Eat a low-fat, high-fiber diet. A balanced diet with less that 30 percent of calories from fat reduces the risk of heart disease, high cholesterol, and high blood pressure.

- Eat at least five servings of fruits and vegetables every day. A 1995 study by the Harvard Community Health Plan in Boston found that for every three servings of fruits and vegetables a man ate per day, his stroke risk decreased by 22 percent.

- Control your blood pressure. In addition to lifestyle changes, have regular medical exams and consult your doctor regarding medication if you do have high blood pressure. This is by far the most dangerous condition linked to stroke.

- If you smoke, quit. Not only does smoking increase your risk of stroke, it is also directly linked to cancer. Help in quitting is available. (See Smoking, p. 95.)

- Be active. A regular program of physical fitness helps to reduce blood pressure and the risk of heart disease and keeps off excess pounds that may contribute to stroke risk.

- Maintain a healthy weight. Obesity increases the risk of stroke by contributing to risk factors such as heart disease and high blood pressure.

- Diabetes. Treatment of the disease can delay complications that increase the risk of stroke. Those with diabetes should also monitor blood pressure carefully.

designed to retrain the brain: Unlike other body tissue, the brain does not regenerate. Once a brain cell that controls a particular function is dead, another brain cell must learn the new role and take over that function.

Rehabilitation often involves speech therapy, psychological therapy, occupational therapy, and physical therapy. Generally, a person who has had a stroke is evaluated to determine in which combination these therapies should be used.

Rehabilitation may take place at a home, hospital, nursing facility, or outpatient clinic. Those requiring extensive therapy are usually treated at a hospital or nursing facility. If mobility and daily functioning are not greatly affected, rehabilitation may take place at home.

While some patients improve slowly over a long period, most recovery takes place within six to nine months of the stroke. Long after formal rehabilitation has ended, however, family, friends, and other supporters contribute to the healing process. Medical equipment, such as wheelchairs, braces, and computers are available to aid those who have suffered stroke.

For more information:

American Heart Association
7272 Greenville Ave.
Dallas, TX 75231
800-553-6321
214-373-6300
http://www.amhrt.org

American Dietetic Association
216 W. Jackson Blvd., Suite 800
Chicago, IL 60606
800-366-1655
312-899-0040

National Aphasia Association
P.O. Box 1887
Murray Hill Station
New York, NY 10156
800-922-4622

NIH Neurological Institute
P.O. Box 5801
Bethesda, MD 20824
301-496-5751
http://www.ninds.nih.gov

National Stroke Association
96 Inverness Dr., E., Suite 1
Englewood, CO 80112-5112
800-STROKES
303-771-1700
http://www.stroke.org

Strokes Club International
805 12th St.
Galveston, TX 77550
409-762-1022

National Rehabilitation Information Center
8455 Colesville Rd., Suite 935
Silver Spring, MD 20910-3319
800-346-2742
http://www.nric.com/nric

SUICIDE

Suicide, the deliberate taking of one's life, accounts for approximately thirty thousand deaths each year in the United States. Though more women than men attempt suicide, men are more likely to complete suicide because of their choice of more lethal means: Men are more likely to use guns, while women often use pills or other methods than are slower, making intervention and treatment possible. (For information on assisted suicide, see Death and Dying, p. 138.)

Risk Factors

Suicide is a growing problem among older adults. A recent study of suicides in Nevada (the state with the highest rate of suicide) found that total (male and female) suicide rates were highest among adults over 65. According to the Senate Special Committee on Aging, white men over the age of 80 are six times more likely to commit suicide than any other segment of the population. While older adults make up about 13 percent of the population of the United States, they account for 20 percent of all suicides.

The primary motivation for suicide among people of this age group was deteriorating health. Other reasons included depression, loss of control, and changes in financial, marital, social, or work status. According to the National Institute of Mental Health, 6 million older adults suffer from depression, and over 75 percent of those people are not treated for the condition.

Suicide is the third leading cause of death among adolescents aged 15 to 19 years in the United States. Teenaged lesbians and gay men are two to three times more likely to attempt suicide than straight teens. The majority of teen suicides involve the ingestion of drugs.

Suicide and Depression

Depression affects 11.5 percent of men and is closely related to suicide attempts. By conservative estimates, at least 50 percent of suicides can be attributed to major depressive disorder. Practitioners consider thoughts and talk of suicide as symptoms of a depressive disorder. Recurrent thoughts of death or suicide without a specific plan, a suicide attempt, or a specific plan for committing suicide are part of the nine criteria that the American Psychiatric Association uses to diagnose depression. (See Depression, p. 235.)

Warning Signs

The warning signs that someone may be contemplating suicide include the following:

- Statements such as "I wish I were dead," "I don't want to go on living," or "Soon you won't have to worry about me." The common belief that "if he talks about it, he won't do it" is a myth. Talk of suicide must be taken seriously.

- Depression. Symptoms include sleep disturbances, loss or increase in appetite, lack of energy, abrupt behavior changes, and feelings of hopelessness, low esteem, and despair.

- Sudden settling of affairs, including the giving away of prized possessions.

- Erratic behavior such as excessive irritability, crying, guilt, and inability to concentrate.

- Any previous suicide attempt. No matter how weakly it may have been undertaken, any suicide attempt must be regarded as a cry for help that, if ignored, might become more lethal in the future.

If you or someone you know is suffering from depression or is considering (or has already attempted) suicide, seek professional counseling. Hot lines for local agencies can be found in the phone book. In addition, there are a number of national organizations that may be able to provide assistance or a referral.

For more information:

Suicide Hotline
800-367-6274

The Samaritans
500 Commonwealth Ave.
Boston, MA 02215
617-536-2460

American Association of Suicidology
2459 S. Ash St.
Denver, CO 80222
303-692-0985

TEMPOROMANDIBULAR DISORDERS

Temporomandibular disorder (TMD or TMJ) is a catchall phrase used to describe a variety of head and neck pains and other symptoms related to the temporomandibular joints that connect the jawbone to the skull near the ear and that allow the mouth to move. Though TMD can be a disruptive condition, in all but a small percentage of those who have it, TMD is rarely serious and eventually disappears. However, because it is not a well-defined condition, TMD is difficult to treat.

The National Institutes of Health estimate that more than 10 million Americans have symptoms associated with TMD. Signs often appear between the ages of 15 and 45. Although a significant number of men suffer from the disorders, they appear to be more prevalent in females. The majority of sufferers are women in their 20s and 30s.

Causes

The most common cause of TMD is spasm of the chewing muscles. The spasms can be triggered by clinching or grinding of the teeth, usually under periods of emotional stress. Research indicates that during periods of stress, an oversecretion of the hormone norepinephrine occurs, causing the trigeminal nerve that controls the jaw reflex to become overexcited, which results in pain. In some cases, muscle spasm is caused by myositis, an inflammatory condition of the muscles.

An incorrect alignment of the teeth, or bite, may place additional pressure on the muscles and contribute to the disorder. Dislocation or fracture of the joint as a result of jaw, head, or neck injuries and joint disease such as arthritis may also cause TMD. There is some evidence that TMD may have a genetic link.

In some cases, TMD may be caused by a nerve that transmits pain signals, even though there is no underlying cause of pain. Psychosocial factors such as negative self-image and social isolation have also been associated with TMD. The prevalence of the disorders in women of child-bearing age suggests the possible influence of additional hormonal factors, as well.

Symptoms

Common symptoms include headaches, tenderness of the jaw muscles, and dull, aching facial pain, including intense sensitivity in or around the ear. Other manifestations include clicking or popping noises when the mouth is opened or closed, difficulty opening the mouth and jaws

that lock when opened. The resulting pain—which may range from minor discomfort to debilitating dysfunction—is a result of the muscles and ligaments that control and support the joints failing to work together correctly.

Diagnosis

Diagnosis of TMD calls for a detailed medical history and a thorough medical examination. The nerves, muscles, and joints of the jaw should be examined, and the teeth should be checked to see how the lower and upper teeth fit and function together. X-rays; computer axial tomography (a CT or CAT scan), which creates a three-dimensional image of the joints and tissues; and magnetic resonance imaging (MRI), in which magnetic rays are used to create an image of tissue, may also be used for diagnosis.

Treatment

Treatment of the disorder falls into two main categories: conservative/reversible and irreversible.

Conservative Treatment

Conservative treatments, which do not invade the tissues of the face, jaw, or joint, are applied to people who do not have severe symptoms. These treatments include self-care practices and use of a dental device, called a bite splint or plate, that prevents clenching or grinding and holds the mouth and jaw in place. A dentist or orthodontist may also correct the alignment of the teeth to be sure that they all engage at the same time and pressure. This approach, called equilibration, is a long-term process.

Nonsteroidal anti-inflammatory drugs such as aspirin and ibuprofen can be used to relieve pain. Chiropractic treatment may also be helpful since misalignment of the spine and poor posture can trigger headaches and contribute to TMD. Counseling and relaxation exercises may also help patients cope with the pain associated with TMD disorders and may help to relieve stress that may be triggering the condition.

Irreversible Treatments

Irreversible treatments are appropriate for only a small percentage of people with TMD and should be undergone only as.a last resort. Such treatments result in permanent changes in the structure or position of the jaw and teeth. Surgery to permanently alter the jaw structure may be indicated in severe cases.

The treatments are very controversial; in many instances, people who have undergone surgery for TMJ have faced destructive results, and forms of these treatments lack research showing that they are superior to noninvasive therapies. If any practitioner recommends an invasive procedure, be sure to seek a second opinion.

For more information:

American Association of Oral and Maxillofacial Surgeons
9700 Bryn Mawr Ave.
Rosemont, IL 60018
800-467-5268

American Dental Association
Bureau of Communications
211 E. Chicago Ave.
Chicago, IL 60611
312-440-2806

SELF-CARE FOR TMD

Though TMD is ongoing and can be annoying, it does not usually progress. However, many people with the condition have found themselves undergoing severe, invasive—and expensive— treatment. Because there is no specific treatment program for the condition, the National Institutes of Health recommends that those who have it explore the least expensive and least invasive treatment options first. In 1996, the NIH recommended the following:

- Practice a healthy lifestyle. In some cases, getting enough sleep, exercising regularly, and eating a healthy diet may help TMD symptoms.

- Eat right. Soft, nonchewy foods are best for those with TMD. Avoid eating foods that require opening the jaw wide, such as large sandwiches or apples. A diet of only soft foods may be used for a few weeks to see if it helps alleviate symptoms.

- Avoid severe jaw movements, such as gum chewing, wide yawning, and singing.

- Try an ice pack or a heating pad at the site of the joint to help relieve pain.

- Exercise your jaw. A doctor or physical therapist may be able to recommend simple exercises that can be performed at home.

- When you feel stressed, practice a relaxation technique, such as meditation, imagery, or progressive relaxation. (See Relaxation Techniques, p. 124.)

TESTICULAR DISORDERS

The testicles are two small, oval organs that are suspended within the scrotum, a sac that hangs outside the body below the abdomen. Within these organs, sperm are produced. The location of the testicles outside of the body helps to regulate the temperature and keep the sperm viable. In cold temperatures, the scrotum draws close to the body to preserve heat, and in hot weather it drops away from the body to cool the testicles.

In addition to sperm production, the testicles secrete the hormone testosterone into the bloodstream. This hormone helps to maintain a man's sex characteristics—facial hair, a deep voice, and muscle mass and strength.

The following is a brief list of conditions that may affect the testicles and the scrotum.

Epididymitis

Epididymitis is an inflammation of the epididymis, a tube that transports sperm from a testicle to the vas deferens, another tube that carries the sperm to the urethra and out of the body. Symptoms include severe pain in the scrotum, fever, and a swollen area that may feel hot to the touch. It can be diagnosed with a urine sample. It is treated with antibiotics if the infection is of bacterial origin. Bed rest, over-the-counter pain relievers, and application of an ice pack to the scrotum may also be prescribed. This condition does not cause permanent damage.

Hydrocele

A hydrocele is a buildup of fluid within the sacs that house the testicles. This harmless swelling is soft and usually painless. It can be diagnosed by a practitioner by manual examination. A practitioner may also shine a light through the scrotum: If the light shines through the swelling, it is a hydrocele. Treatment is usually not required unless the swelling has become exceptionally large or uncomfortable. If the hydrocele must be removed, it is done surgically.

Orchitis

This condition is an inflammation of the testicle. It is usually caused by the mumps, though it can also result from an infection in the prostate or epididymis. Symptoms include pain in the scrotum, swelling (usually only on one side of the scrotum), and a feeling of weight in the scrotum. Diagnosis is through a manual examination and analysis of a urine sample. If the infection is bacterial, antibiotics are prescribed as treatment. For a viral infection, bed rest and pain relievers are prescribed. Orchitis can result in permanent damage to one or both testicles and may cause infertility.

Testicular Torsion

The testicles are each suspended within the scrotum by a structure known as the spermatic cord. Rarely, the cord becomes twisted, cutting off the blood supply to a testicle. This condition, called torsion, may occur after physical activity, though often there is no known cause. Symptoms include sudden, severe pain in a testicle; one testicle higher within the scrotum; nausea and vomiting; swelling; and fever. Torsion is diagnosed through a manual examination. Surgery is required to untwist the cord and possibly stitch the cord into place to prevent it from twisting again. Prompt treatment is required because, if the cord remains twisted for more than a few

TESTICULAR INJURY

For most men, just the thought of a blow to the testicles is enough to make them squirm. But though a blow can cause a lingering, agonizing pain, permanent injury to the testicles is rare. The tissues within the scrotum are spongy and flexible and can absorb a great deal of shock without suffering permanent damage.

The pain felt after an injury is caused by the swelling of the testicle within its protective sac. The pressure caused by the swelling inflamed surrounding nerves, causing pain to spread throughout the lower abdomen. An ice pack applied to the scrotum and anti-inflammatory medications can be used to reduce swelling and pain after an accident.

If swelling and pain persist for longer than an hour or the scrotum is bruised, quickly seek medical care. Too much pressure within the scrotum can cause tissue damage that might lead to infertility, blood clots, or even the loss of a testicle.

hours, the testicle will die due to lack of blood and will have to be removed.

Undescended Testicle

Before birth, the testicles are housed in the abdomen. About one month before birth, they descend into the scrotum. Rarely, in 1 percent of males, one or both testicles remain in the abdomen after birth. This can be diagnosed through manual examination. Usually, the condition does not require treatment and corrects itself. However, if the testicle does not descend within a year, medications or surgery may be prescribed to bring it into position. The best age for surgery is twelve to eigtheen months. If a testicle remains undescended in a child over the age of 5, infertility may result. A testicle that was previously undescended is more vulnerable to cancer than a normal testicle and is also more likely to contribute to infertility. (See Testicular Cancer, p. 224, and Infertility, p. 412.)

Varicocele

A varicocele is a collection of varicose veins within the scrotum. It is caused by a malfunction of the valves within the veins that causes blood to collect in the area. It is characterized by a painless swelling that usually occurs on the left side. Diagnosis is through manual examination. The practitioner will also shine a light through the testicle—the light will not shine through the veins. While the varicocele itself is not harmful, the collection of blood in the testicles may cause infertility. If infertility occurs, surgery can be done to tie off the varicose vein and restore fertility. Otherwise, treatment is not necessary.

ULCERS

An ulcer is an open sore or lesion that forms in the lining of the esophagus, stomach, or the duodenum (the upper part of the small intestine). Ulcers in the stomach are known as gastric ulcers. Those in the duodenum are called duodenal ulcers. All types of gastrointestinal ulcers are known as peptic ulcers.

About four million Americans each year are afflicted by ulcers, and 20 million Americans—10 percent—have an ulcer at some time in their lives. Usually, stomach ulcers occur in those over age 60, while duodenal ulcers occur for the first time in people between the ages of 30 and 50. Duodenal ulcers occur more frequently in men than in women, while gastric ulcers occur more frequently in women than in men.

Symptoms

An ulcer may cause no symptoms at all. However, a gnawing or burning pain in the abdomen between the breastbone and the navel is the most common symptom of an ulcer. The pain often occurs between meals and in the early morning, lasting anywhere from a few minutes to a few hours. Often, eating or taking antacids relieves the pain.

Less common symptoms include nausea, vomiting, loss of appetite, a bloated feeling, loss of weight, fatigue, and blood in the stool. If an ulcer is bleeding heavily, blood will appear in vomit or in tarlike, black stool.

Causes

Ulcers are caused by a variety of factors. If the stomach, for any reason, is unable to protect itself from its own digestive fluids (hydrochloric acid and the enzyme pepsin), an ulcer can occur. Ulcers are often triggered by bacteria called Helicobacter pylori (H. pylori), which infect the lining of the stomach and make it vulnerable to damage from stomach acids and pepsin. (Infection usually occurs when infected stool comes in contact with hands, water, or food.) In addition, lifestyle factors—such as smoking or a high caffeine intake—are also linked to the

development of ulcers. Overuse of nonsteroidal anti-inflammatory drugs such as aspirin and ibuprofen also make the stomach vulnerable to the effects of acid.

Stress is no longer thought to be a cause of ulcers, although it is thought to aggravate ulcer symptoms. There is also no proof that alcohol consumption causes ulcers, although, like stress, it is an irritant.

Diagnosis

If symptoms of an ulcer are present, a practitioner may recommend an upper gastrointestinal (GI) series. In this test, the individual swallows a chalky liquid called barium and then has an x-ray taken of the abdomen. The barium coats the digestive tract and makes its structures—as well as any ulcers that are present—visible on an x-ray.

In another procedure called endoscopy, a small flexible fiberoptic tube is inserted through the mouth into the esophagus, stomach, and duodenum. The tube allows the practitioner a direct view of the digestive tract. Samples of the stomach lining or ulcers can also be collected for analysis during this procedure. An endoscopy is usually done, using a local anesthetic and a mild sedative.

Once an ulcer is diagnosed, tests are done to detect the presence of H. pylori. A blood test may be done, or a sample of tissue removed during endoscopy can be analyzed for the bacteria. Researchers are currently looking at a breath test to help detect H. pylori; however, this test has not yet been approved by the Food and Drug Administration.

Treatment

Ulcers are treated with medications that block the production of stomach acids or protect the mucosal stomach lining. Acid-suppressing drugs include H2-blockers, such as cimetidine (Tagamet), ranitidine (Zantac) and famotidine (Pepcid), and acid pump inhibitors such as omeprazole. Protective drugs include sucralfate (Carafate) and misoprostol (Cytotec) as well as antacids. If H. pylori are found to exist, antibiotics are prescribed in combination with these drugs. Medical treatment of ulcers is usually ongoing; though most ulcers heal within eight weeks, the chance of recurrence is between 60 and 70 percent without a maintenance dose of ulcer medications.

A few lifestyle changes are also recommended. Though practitioners no longer recommend a bland diet, someone with an ulcer should avoid smoking, which slows healing, and caffeine, which stimulates the production of stomach acid.

COMPLICATIONS OF ULCERS

Left untreated, ulcers can cause serious complications, such as bleeding, perforation of the walls of the stomach or small intestine, and narrowing and obstruction of digestive tract passages.

1. *Bleeding.* An ulcer erodes the muscles of the stomach or the duodenal wall, sometimes damaging blood vessels. Blood will seep slowly into the digestive tract if the affected vessels are small. Anemia, weakness, dizziness, and fatigue will result if bleeding continues over time.

   If a large vessel is damaged, the individual will feel weak and dizzy when standing and may vomit blood or faint. The stool may turn a black color from the blood. These are signs of a serious problem and require prompt medical attention.

   Most bleeding ulcers are treated endoscopically—the damaged blood vessel is cauterized with a heating device or injected with material to stop the bleeding. Traditional surgery in which the abdomen is opened with an incision may be required if endoscopic treatment is unsuccessful.

2. *Perforation.* When an ulcer creates a hole in the wall of the stomach or duodenum, bacteria and partially digested food may enter the opening into the abdominal cavity, or peritoneum. The result is peritonitis, an inflammation of the abdominal cavity and wall. Sudden, sharp, and severe pain are the usual symptoms of peritonitis, which requires immediate treatment because it is potentially fatal. Surgery may be required to repair the wall and treat the infection.

3. *Narrowing and obstruction.* Ulcers located where the duodenum attaches to the stomach often cause swelling and scarring. This may narrow or close the intestinal opening, preventing food from leaving the stomach and entering the small intestine. The main symptom is vomiting. Endoscopic balloon dilation, a procedure that uses a small balloon to force open a narrow passage, or another form of surgery may be necessary.

Medications are usually all that are needed to treat ulcers. However, in some cases when ulcers persist, surgery may be necessary. In surgery, the ulcer is removed and the lining of the digestive tract is repaired. In some cases, the nerve that controls acid production in the stomach may be severed to decrease the levels of acid.

For more information:

National Digestive Diseases
Information Clearinghouse
2 Information Way
Bethesda, MD 20892-3570
301-654-3810
http://www.niddk.nih.gov

URINARY TRACT INFECTIONS

A urinary tract infection (UTI) is an overgrowth of bacteria in the bladder, kidney, or urethra, the small tube that drains urine from the bladder. UTIs, which account for eight million doctor visits each year, are less common in men than in women, because the male urethra is longer than the female urethra, making it more difficult for bacteria to ascend the urinary tract. In addition, the prostate gland produces secretions that slow bacterial growth.

Yet men must often deal with UTIs. While they are rare in young men, men over age 50 may get them as a result of a urinary stone, enlarged prostate, an obstruction of the urinary tract, or a medical procedure involving a catheter. UTIs can also be sexually transmitted. In addition, some experts say uncircumcised men are more prone to UTIs because bacteria can be trapped more easily beneath the foreskin.

Causes

Urine is normally free of bacteria, viruses, and fungi. Infections occur when bacteria and other microorganisms from the digestive tract enter the urinary tract and then multiply. Most infections are from the Escherichia coli (E. coli) bacteria, which usually is found in the colon.

Sexually transmitted diseases (STDs) such as chlamydia, gonorrhea, and herpes and nonsexually transmitted infections may cause urethritis, inflammation of the urethra, in men. UTIs from sexually transmitted diseases usually occur in younger men, while nonsexually transmitted infections are more common in older men.

Some people are more prone to getting UTIs, and a kidney stone or any other obstruction of the flow of urine increases the risk of infection. Disorders that suppress the immune system, such as diabetes, also raise the risk of UTIs.

A UTI can lead to prostatitis (inflammation of the prostate gland); urethritis (inflammation of the urethra usually caused by STDs); cystitis (infection of the bladder); and pyelonephritis (rare but serious infection of the kidney).

Symptoms

Symptoms of urinary tract infections include

- Pain and discomfort (burning, itching) when urinating

- Pain during intercourse and ejaculation

- Frequent and urgent need to urinate (especially at night)

- Cloudy or milky urine

- Urethral discharge (clear fluid or pus from the penis)

- Abdominal pain

- Full feeling in rectum

- Fever

- Blood in the urine

- Back pain (lower-back pain is usually associated with prostatitis, high back pain with pyelonephritis)

- Prostatic tenderness

- Fatigue

UTIs can last a long time and, if left untreated, can cause damage to the kidneys, bladder, or prostate.

Diagnosis

To diagnose a UTI, a practitioner reviews your medical history, examines you, and tests a sample of your urine for pus and bacteria. This test is called a urinalysis. Samples of any discharge from the urethra may also be sent for lab analysis. A prostate and rectal exam should be included in the exam as well. Self-tests for urinary tract infection are available over-the-counter. However, these are neither very sensitive nor reliable.

If a UTI does not respond to treatment, the doctor may order a test to take images of the urinary tract. One of these tests is an intravenous pyelogram (IVP), which gives x-ray images of the bladder, kidneys, and ureters. Other testing includes ultrasound, which produces pictures from the echo patterns of sound waves from internal organs, and cystoscopy, a procedure in which the urethra and bladder are viewed through a tube inserted into the urethra. These tests may be done on an outpatient setting in a hospital or in a clinic. Some practitioners may

DOES CRANBERRY JUICE HELP UTIs?

You've probably heard that cranberry juice is a natural cure for UTIs. But by itself, cranberry juice probably won't cure or safeguard against UTIs.

While cranberry juice breaks down into hippuric acid, a compound that has natural bacteria-destroying properties, you would have to consume an outrageous amount each day to prevent an infection. Plus, the juice you buy in grocery stores is usually only 10 to 25 percent cranberry juice with a lot of added sugar.

Drinking large quantities of cranberry juice can help flush the bladder of impurities. And cranberry juice's acidity will increase the effectiveness of some medications used to treat UTIs. On the other hand, that same acidity will counter the effects of certain antibiotics.

have the equipment to perform these procedures in their offices.

Treatment

If bacteria are present in the urinary tract, they will be grown in a laboratory in a test called a culture. The culture is then tested with what's called a sensitivity test to identify the bacteria and which antibiotic destroys them most effectively. This test, along with the man's history, is used to determine which antibiotic is prescribed—although often practitioners will prescribe a broad-spectrum antibiotic (one that combats a wide range of bacteria) without

SELF-CARE AND PREVENTION FOR URINARY TRACT INFECTIONS

To prevent UTIs:

• Drink plenty of fluids. This helps flush the urinary tract of bacteria.

• Empty your bladder often and completely.

• Protect yourself against sexually transmitted diseases by using a condom during intercourse.

If you have a UTI:

• Avoid coffee, alcohol, and spicy foods. These can make UTIs worse.

• Try a warm bath or a heating pad on the lower abdomen to help relieve pain.

doing a culture first. Common drugs used to treat UTIs include trimethoprim (Trimpex), trimethoprim/sulfamethoxazole (Bactrim, Septra, and Cotrim), and amoxicillin (Amoxil, Trimox, and Wymox).

While UTIs that have affected the prostate or kidney usually need several weeks of antibiotic treatment, most common UTIs often disappear about twent-four hours after the drugs are taken. But it's important to finish taking the full course of antibiotics prescribed since infection may recur otherwise. Once the treatment is over, a follow-up urinalysis should be performed to confirm that the urinary tract is infection-free. The length of the treatment in men is usually longer than in women to help prevent prostate

infections. Prostatitis is harder to cure because antibiotics don't battle infected prostate tissue effectively.

For more information:

American Foundation for Urologic Disease
300 W. Pratt St., Suite 401
Baltimore, MD 21201
800-242-2383
410-727-2908
http://www.acess.digex.net.~afud.org

National Digestive Diseases
Information Clearinghouse
2 Information Way
Bethesda, MD 20892-3570
301-654-3810
http://www.niddk.nih.gov

PART IV

Sexual Health

Though it is rarely discussed and often taken for granted, sexual health is an important part of the overall health and well-being of any man. Sexual health plays a role in much more than just reproduction and intercourse, affecting mental health as well as physical. And while sexual health concerns may appear trivial next to threats such as heart disease and prostate cancer, some diseases—such as AIDS—can be deadly.

Still, surveys show that men and their medical practitioners are reluctant to talk about matters of sexual health. According to a 1996 Gallup poll, 90 percent of physicians said they believe discussions about sexual function to be important; however, only 43 percent said they ever have such discussions. In another Gallup poll, only 28 percent of men reported ever being asked about sexual function by their doctors. Both polls also found that only 26 percent of college-educated men would see a physician about a loss of sex drive and only 19 percent would visit a doctor for a change in sexual performance.

Today, sexual health problems are widely recognized and treatable. While at one time most erection problems were attributed to psychological difficulties, today it is known that 75 to 80 percent of such problems are physical and highly treatable. Progress is being made in the treatment of male infertility, as well as in the treatment of sexual dysfunction and the development of more contraceptive options for men. There is also focus on sexually transmitted diseases, which are more of a public health concern now than ever before.

In this section, you'll find discussions of sexual development and sexual orientation, as well as information on topics such as circumcision and vasectomy. There are complete, straightforward discussions of erection problems and other forms of sexual dysfunction and their causes, diagnoses, and treatments. Infertility problems in men are also discussed. We also cover safe sex, sexually transmitted diseases, and contraception.

SEXUAL DEVELOPMENT

What makes a man? While some might ponder the philosophical implications of that question, the truth lies in the genes: Gender is determined the moment the sperm fertilizes the egg, delivering its half of the genetic material necessary for development of a new person.

Although gender is determined from the first moment, the development of male characteristics does not happen all at once. The testicles of a male fetus form around the sixth week of pregnancy, and the fetus does not take on the appearance of a male until eight weeks later, when the testicles begin producing male hormones. It is at this point that the penis, scrotum, and prostate begin to form. Then, usually shortly before the birth of the child, the testicles descend into their place within the scrotum. Once these changes have occurred, the levels of hormones in the body remain stable for about ten years.

Puberty

The next phase of sexual development occurs during a period known as puberty. Puberty usually begins around the age of 11 and may last until age 17.

Puberty begins in the brain, even before a boy starts to show any signs of sexual development. When a boy is around the age of 9 or 10, his hypothalamus, the area of the brain that controls hormone production, stimulates his pituitary gland, the gland located at the base of the brain that regulates the function of the rest of the endocrine system. In response, the pituitary gland begins secreting hormones—follicle stimulating hormones (FSH) and luteinizing hormone (LH)—into his bloodstream that trigger the production of testosterone in his testicles. This first phase of adolescence is known as the "Tanner stage one" stage of puberty after the British physician who categorized the physical changes of sexual development.

Tanner stage two, which occurs around the age of 12 or 13, marks the visible onset of puberty. Because of the hormones FSH and LH, the boy's testicles begin to enlarge, and fine, straight pubic hair sprouts at the base of his penis. The hormones may also kick off a growth spurt. Because rapid growth may occur at different rates in different parts of the skeleton, the spurt may result in awkward growth— for example, the hands and feet may grow larger before the arms and legs catch up. In general, the body grows taller and heavier, and the shoulders widen, resulting in a stronger upper body. This stage lasts, on the average, thirteen months, though it can be as brief as five months and as long as twenty-six.

Though Tanner stage three is usually the briefest stage of puberty, lasting, on the average, ten months, it produces the most striking physical changes in the maturing boy. Around the age of 13 or 14 (although it can happen as early as 11 or as late as 16), a boy's penis begins to lengthen and his pubic hair becomes thicker and coarser. One testicle (usually the left) will begin to hang lower than the other. His voice begins to deepen as his larynx enlarges (though that process is punctuated by a "cracking" voice), he continues to gain height (sometimes as much as five inches in a year), weight, and muscle, and he begins to grow hair on his upper lip, arms, and legs.

Most boys experience their first ejaculation (almost always during sleep—the involuntary nocturnal emission) during Tanner stage four. This is a sign that the testicles are beginning to produce sperm (the male equivalent of a girl's menstrual periods beginning) and that the libido, or sex drive, is beginning to awaken. Spontaneous erections may also occur frequently, triggered by hormones in the system. However, the frequency of both nocturnal emissions and spontaneous erections diminish over time.

Also during stage four, which usually begins around the ages 14 or 15, the penis begins to widen as well as lengthen, and the testicles continue to grow. The skin on the boy's genitals darkens, and his pubic hair spreads across his groin area. Body and facial hair also become more apparent, perspiration gets heavier, and often his skin and hair will become oilier. The latter often leads to acne and dandruff. This often-awkward period can last for as few as five months, though it usually lasts two years and can hang on for up to three years.

Probably the most troubling physical symptom of puberty for boys is breast enlargement, known in medical terms as adolescent gynecomastia. Between 50 and 85 percent of all boys have some degree of this in early puberty, due to hormone production and imbalance; they may also experience some pain and/or small lumps in the breasts. However, gynecomastia is rarely a sign of a hormonal disorder. These problems usually disappear in twelve to sixteen months; boys should be warned, however, that drugs such as amphetamines or steroids can cause breast enlargement at any age. (See Breast Cancer, p. 194, for more information on gynecomastia.)

Once he has reached Tanner stage five, the teenage male is sexually mature—his genitals have reached their full size, though he may still gain a few more inches in height until the age of 21. By this time, usually between the ages of 15 and 18, he has the physique of a man and has begun to shave; however, many teenagers continue to develop body hair, especially on the chest, until their early 20s.

MASTURBATION

While a male of any age—even an infant—is capable of having an erection, it is not until puberty that ejaculation can occur. Masturbation, or the stimulation of one's own genitals, is an activity that often begins during adolescence because of the onslaught of hormones that suddenly boost the sex drive. However, it does not begin and end in adolescence. According to a 1993 survey, 55 percent of men and 38 percent of women masturbate regularly. A 1950s sex survey by expert Alfred Kinsey reported that 92 percent of men had masturbated to orgasm at some time in their lives.

Masturbation may be a way of relieving sexual tension without inappropriate behavior, and it often involves sexual fantasy. In addition, couples may masturbate together as an alternative to intercourse. There are also some health reasons for masturbation. It helps maintain sperm quality, for example. If you have not ejaculated in several days, stored sperm lose their speed and may not function well—regular masturbation helps to keep sperm production at its highest and the sperm at their healthiest. Regular ejaculation also promotes prostate health. If a man who is used to regular ejaculation suddenly has a "dry spell," prostatic fluid can build up in the system, creating inflammation and congestion called congestive prostatitis. If this condition occurs, masturbation may be prescribed as treatment. Masturbation is also used as therapy for both men and women dealing with sexual dysfunction.

There are quite a few myths surrounding masturbation—that it will make you go blind, cause hair to grow on your palms, or cause warts to grow on your genitals. While some discourage masturbation, it is a normal, harmless activity—it is not dangerous or shameful.

Rates of Development

Few things contribute more to the angst of the male teenage years than the rate and progress of physical development, particularly when it seems to be "slow." Though there are average ages at which each stage generally commences, the range of ages at which they can occur in healthy, normal boys is fairly large. Thus it is not uncommon to find 15-year-old, 185-lb. varsity linemen who shave every morning in the same high school classroom as reedy, peach-fuzzed boys of the same age. "Late bloomers" may have parents who were also late at reaching or completing puberty, though heredity is not the only factor. Boys who lag very much behind their peers in physical development should be examined by a physician; others just need reassurance from a trusted adult that they will, in fact, mature.

APHRODISIACS

An aphrodisiac is any food, drink, or other substance that is believed to stimulate sexual desire. For centuries, men have been looking for a magic potion that will fuel the libido, or sex drive, and boost performance in the bedroom. Suspected aphrodisiacs range from common items such as tomatoes, chocolate, and honey to the unusual—rhinoceros horn, deer sperm, and Spanish fly.

According to the Food and Drug Administration (FDA), there is no such thing as an aphrodisiac. In fact, in 1990 the FDA banned interstate commerce and over-the-counter sale of any product whose label implies that it will enhance libido or sexual ability. The ruling is designed to protect consumers from fraud as well as from dangerous substances.

The concern is not unwarranted. In 1996, the Centers for Disease Control and Prevention released a report on a brown, rocklike substance that was sold illegally in major cities under the names "Love Stone" and "Rock Hard." The substance, which contained natural steroids, caused four deaths from cardiac failure and severe vomiting and heart palpitations in another person.

Research on Aphrodisiacs

There have been few studies on the effects of supposed aphrodisiacs, and those that have been done face criticism because of the question of the placebo effect—the idea that an inactive substance will affect those who believe it has an effect. While it is possible to observe sexual response in animals, scientifically measuring sexual stimulation in humans would require laboratory observation. According to the FDA, a study would need to compare a placebo (an inert drug with no active ingredient) with the aphrodisiac, with neither the researchers nor the patients knowing who was getting the test substance. However, because of cultural taboos, few studies have been undertaken.

There is also controversy regarding testing because certain drugs have effects that may seem to be sexual, but may actually relate to mood changes. An example would be alcohol, which seems to be an aphrodisiac because it lowers inhibitions, but actually depresses the sex drive and the ability to gain an erection.

The Search for the Love Drug

Still, the search goes on for effective aphrodisiacs. The following is a quick list of some of the foods and other substances once thought—or still thought—to be associated with sex, along with some information on their reported effects.

- *Alcohol.* Alcohol has long been thought to be an aphrodisiac because it lowers inhibitions. However, it is a depressant drug, and significant amounts of alcohol reduce the sex drive, cause erection problems, and impair the ability to have an orgasm.

- *Chocolate.* The reputation of chocolate as an aphrodisiac was especially strong centuries ago when it was difficult to obtain. Since it has become commonplace, that reputation has faded. However, experts report that chocolate contains a substance that stimulates the pleasure centers of the brain, which increases feelings of well-being and boosts the sex drive.

- *Oysters and rhinoceros horns.* Foods and substances that resemble the male genitalia have long been associated with sex. However, there is no evidence that eating such substances increases your sex drive.

- *Chili, hot peppers, curries and spicy foods.* These are considered aphrodisiacs because they increase heart rate and cause sweating. However, they have no true effect on libido.

- *Ginseng.* Ginseng is another substance that gained its reputation by its shape. In fact, the word "ginseng" means "man's root." Ginseng is known to be a stimulant, and it does reduce the effects of extreme temperatures, stress, and strenuous exercise, which may create a feeling of well-being and health. This, in turn, may lead to a greater libido. Studies that involved giving ginseng to rats showed a sexual response in the animals. However, there is no evidence that ginseng has an aphrodisiac effect on humans.

- *Yohimbe.* This substance is derived from the bark of the African yohimbe tree and is thought to be a sex drug and stimulant. Clinical studies have shown that yohimbe restores erections in one-third of men who take it. While some attribute the success of yohimbe to the placebo effect, others believe that it is truly effective.

  While medical treatments for erection problems are much more effective than yohimbe is thought to be, yohimbe is inexpensive and has few side effects. (It can cause an increase in blood pressure, so those with high blood pressure or heart disease should not take it.) Because the ingredients in over-the-counter preparations available in health food stores vary greatly, you may consider getting a prescription from your practitioner if you're interested in trying yohimbe. That way, you are guaranteed a standardized substance and can be monitored by a health-care professional. You should talk with your practitioner before taking any herbal preparation.

- *Spanish fly.* Spanish fly is actually crushed, dried beetle remains. It causes irritation in the urinary and genital tract, creating a rush of blood to the sex organs—the origin of its reputation as an aphrodisiac. Spanish fly, however, is a poison. It can burn the mouth and throat and can lead to urinary tract infections, scarring of the urethra, and even death.

Use of Aphrodisiacs

Again, the FDA maintains that there are no effective aphrodisiacs. If you have a problem with erections or a loss of libido, talk with your practitioner. Sexual dysfunction and erection problems are highly treatable, and new therapies such as testosterone therapy might be helpful for some men with a lowered desire for sex. (See Male Menopause, p. 319.)

CONTRACEPTION

Put simply, a contraceptive is a device or method that prevents pregnancy. And unless you want to play proud papa, contraception is something you need to think about if you're sexually active. Statistics show that of one hundred women who do not use birth control, 85 percent will become pregnant within a year. In addition, certain forms of contraception also protect against sexually transmitted diseases (STDs) such as human immunodeficiency virus (HIV), the virus that causes AIDS. (See Safe Sex, p. 398.)

For men, the temporary, reversible options in contraception are limited, and include abstinence and periodic abstinence (not having sex or refraining from sex during a partner's fertile period), the condom (a sheath worn over the penis to catch the semen), and the withdrawal method (removing the penis from the vagina before ejaculation). A permanent method of birth control for men is the vasectomy, a surgical procedure that blocks sperm from entering the ejaculate. (See Vasectomy, p. 385.)

It's not a long list to choose from, and for that reason many men count on their partners to provide birth control. However, whether you're taking the precautions against pregnancy or your partner is, it's important to remember that both of you need to take responsibility. In addition, both partners' preferences and needs should be taken into account when choosing a method of birth control. Religious or medical concerns may dictate a choice in contraception. For this reason, information about contraceptives used by women is also included here.

Effectiveness

Each method of birth control has a failure rate stated in terms of how many pregnancies occur per one hundred women each year. There are two different failure rates—one for typical use and one for perfect use. Typical use indicates the number of pregnancies that will occur when the method is not always used correctly or consistently—the way most people typically use birth control. Perfect use indicates the number of pregnancies that will occur when the method is used correctly and consistently—for example, using a condom exactly right each and every time you have sex.

To increase your chances of preventing pregnancy, choose the form of contraception with the lowest failure rate and follow your physician's or package instructions.

Methods of Contraception

The common methods of reversible contraception for both men and women are listed below, in order of most effective to least effective, along with their advantages and disadvantages. Keep in mind that some forms of contraception can be used in combination to increase protection against pregnancy and protect against STDs.

Abstinence

Abstinence—not having vaginal intercourse— is 100 percent effective in preventing pregnancy

COMPARISON OF EFFECTIVENESS

Number of Pregnancies per One Hundred Women During One Year of Use

Method	Typical Use*	Perfect Use**
Continuous Abstinence	0.00	0.00
Outercourse	N/A	N/A
Norplant	0.09	0.09
Sterilization		
Men	0.15	0.1
Women	0.4	0.4
Depo-Provera	0.3	0.3
IUD	0.8	0.6 ParaGard (copper T-380A)
	2.6	1.5 Progestasert
The Pill	3.0	0.1 combination pills
		0.5 progestin only mini-pills
Emergency Contraception (per use)	2.0	2.0 hormonal
	0.1	0.1 IUD insertion
Condom	12.0	3.0
Diaphragm	18.0	6.0
Cervical Cap		
Women who have not given birth	18.0	9.0
Women who have given birth	36.0	26.0
Withdrawal	19.0	4.0
Periodic Abstinence	20.0	1.0 postovulation method
		2.0 symptothermal method
		3.0 cervical mucus method
		9.0 calendar method
Fertility Awareness Methods	N/A	N/A
Contraceptive Foam and Suppositories	21.0	3.0
Vaginal Pouch ("Female Condom")	21.0	5.0
No Method	85.0	85.0

Effectiveness rates updated from Trussell et al. (1990) as published in *Contraceptive Technology*, Irvington Press: New York, 1994.

*"Typical Use": refers to failure rates for women and men whose use is not consistent or always correct.

**"Perfect Use": refers to failure rates for those whose use is consistent and always correct.

N/A: Failure rates not available.

Source: Planned Parenthood Federation of America, 1997.

and sexually transmitted diseases when it is practiced without fail.

Periodic abstinence involves refraining from sex during a woman's fertile period. This period can be determined through several methods, including monitoring a woman's temperature (basal body temperature method), observing changes in her cervical mucus (cervical mucus method), charting her menstrual cycle on a calendar (the calendar or rhythm method), combining these three methods (symptothermal method), or refraining from intercourse until several days after ovulation (postovulation method). Kits are available to help teach these methods.

Many religious groups recommend abstinence to unmarried people and periodic abstinence to those who are married. Abstinence has no medical side effects, though periodic abstinence does not prevent against STDs.

Norplant

With Norplant, six soft capsules are implanted in the upper arm of the woman. These matchstick-size implants release synthetic hormones that prevent the ovaries from releasing eggs (ovulation) and thicken the cervical mucus at the opening of the uterus to prevent sperm from joining with the egg. It protects against pregnancy for five years and is reversible. Advantages include an extremely low risk of pregnancy and contraceptive benefits that last for years. However, it does require minor surgery and has a number of side effects (though it contains no estrogen). In some women, the capsules can cause scarring and be difficult to remove. It also does not protect against STDs. Norplant is available by prescription only and may cost between $500 and $750 for insertion.

Depo-Provera

Depo-Provera provides contraception through an injection given to a woman every twelve weeks. It works by preventing ovulation and thickening cervical mucus. While it doesn't offer protection against STDs and may have side effects for some women, it removes the burden of day-to-day contraception and may reduce menstrual cramps (some women have no periods after one year while using this method). Depo-Provera is reversible. It is available with a prescription, and costs range from $20 to $40 per injection.

The Pill

Oral contraceptives, or the Pill, are taken daily by a woman to prevent ovulation and, therefore, pregnancy. The pills contain estrogen and progestin (combination pills) or only progestin (minipills). Women who use the Pill tend to have regular periods with a lighter menstrual flow. The Pill may also help prevent endometrial cancer, ovarian cancer, noncancerous breast cysts, and ovarian cysts. However, a woman needs to remember to take the Pill at roughly the same time each day, and there are side effects and some risks associated with the Pill. Women with a risk of heart disease, blood clots, stroke, and liver disease should not take the Pill. In addition, women who smoke and who are over 35 should not take the Pill. It does not protect against STDs. The Pill is reversible and is available by prescription. Costs range from $15 to $25 per month.

IUD

An IUD, or intrauterine device, is a plastic device placed within the uterus to prevent fertilization of the egg and to alter the uterine lining to prevent an egg from implanting. It is best used by women who have had a child. It is a reversible, long-term form of contraception (the ParaGard brand lasts for ten years while the Progestasert must be replaced every year) and does not interfere with spontaneity during sex. There is no pill to remember to take every day. Again, there are side effects, and the IUD offers no protection against STDs. While in the 1970s IUDs were taken off of the market because of safety concerns, today's IUDs are considered to be one of the safest and most effective forms of birth control available. A prescription is required for an IUD. Insertion may cost between $150 and $300.

Condom

A condom is a sheath of latex or animal tissue that is worn over the penis during intercourse to catch semen and prevent pregnancy. Latex condoms also help protect against the spread of STDs. Latex provides an effective barrier to even small viruses such as human immunodeficiency virus (which causes AIDS) and hepatitis B. (For information on proper condom use, see Safe Sex, p. 398.)

Condoms are available in many different styles and even a few different sizes. Condoms may be lubricated or dry or may have a spermicide—a chemical that immobilizes sperm—added for extra protection against pregnancy. Spermicides and lubricants can also be added during intercourse. Avoid oil-based lubricants such as petroleum jelly or baby oil—they can damage the condom and cause it to break. Instead, use water-based lubricants such as KY-Jelly. (See Safe Sex, p. 398, for instructions on condom use.)

Advantages of condoms include low cost (about thirty cents each), no side effects (unless there is an allergy to latex), and protection against STDs. However, condoms can break (though

usually this only occurs during improper use or after improper storage), and semen may spill out. In addition, some couples feel using a condom interrupts intercourse and reduces sensation for the man. (See Allergies, p. 156, for more information on latex allergies.)

Condoms are available without a prescription at drugstores, supermarkets, vending machines, and health clinics. Condoms can be used in combination with other forms of birth control to increase protection against pregnancy or help prevent STDs.

Diaphragm and Cervical Cap

A diaphragm is a soft, rubber cup with a flexible rim that is worn over the woman's cervix to prevent the entrance of sperm into the uterus. A cervical cap, also rubber, is a thimble-shaped cup that is worn over the cervix. These devices are used with spermicides to immobilize the sperm and increase protection against pregnancy. Because they contain no hormones, neither the diaphragm nor cervical cap has any side effects, though women who use them may be more prone to urinary tract infections. Some women may not be able to use them because of the shape of the cervix—a practitioner must fit each device to the particular women. Diaphragms and cervical caps must be inserted before intercourse and must remain in place for eight hours after sex. Some partners feel that insertion interrupts intercourse. The spermicide used with these devices may offer some protection against STDs. The devices cost between $13 and $25, on the average.

Withdrawal

The withdrawal method involves removing the penis from the vagina before ejaculation. It is usually used when no other form of birth control is available, although it is unreliable because small amounts of semen are released prior to ejaculation, which can result in pregnancy. To practice withdrawal effectively, a great deal of self-control and experience is necessary; for this reason, it is especially not recommended for teenagers. While it has no side effects and is free, the withdrawal method does not protect against STDs.

Contraceptive Foam and Suppositories

These over-the-counter contraceptives work by creating a barrier of bubbles that block the entrance of the uterus and contain a spermicide that immobilizes sperm. After the foam or suppository is inserted into the vagina, a couple needs to wait ten minutes before intercourse to allow the method to take effect. Effectiveness lasts up to one hour after insertion. More of the product must be inserted each time sex is repeated. Foams and suppositories are available without a prescription in most drugstores and supermarkets. These methods do not protect against STDs. Side effects include vaginal irritation, and the method may interrupt intercourse and get messy because of the liquid involved. Applicator kits cost about $8, and refills cost $2 to $5.

Vaginal Pouch

Also known as the female condom, the vaginal pouch is a polyurethane sheath that is worn in the vagina. Like the condom, the vaginal pouch collects semen to prevent fertilization from occurring. It also allows a woman to take responsibility for STD prevention. The pouch may slip during intercourse, and it may squeak. In addition, the rings that hold the pouch in place may irritate the penis or vagina. Some people say

sensitivity is reduced. Vaginal pouches are available at most stores and cost about $2.50 each.

On the Horizon

Science is working on putting together more contraceptive options designed specifically for men. One possibility is a contraceptive injection of testosterone that would halt sperm production. A study that investigated this reversible method of contraception found that of 399 normal men, only 12 failed to respond to the therapy—meaning that the injections were effective contraception in 98.6 percent of cases. After four to seven months after the injections ended, sperm output was back to normal.

However, about 106 men dropped out of the study because of side effects, including decreased testicle size and weight gain or because they didn't like getting the injections, which were given intramuscularly on a weekly basis.

An oral contraceptive for men is also in development. An Italian research study gave pills of testosterone and the progestin/antiandrogen cyproterone acetate to four men twice daily. At the beginning of the study, all men had sperm counts between twenty-five million and fifty million sperm per milliliter. Eight weeks into the study, sperm counts were down to 1, 2, and 5 million/ml. in three subjects and had disappeared in the other—enough to prevent conception. Sperm counts returned to normal after the study ended, though it took several months. However, one side effect of the drug was a decreased sex drive.

For more information:

National Family Planning and Reproductive Health Association
122 C St., N.W., Suite 380
Washington, DC 20001-2109
202-628-3535

National Organization of Adolescent Pregnancy
and Parenting and Prevention
1319 F St., N.W., Suite 401
Washington, DC 20004
202-783-5770
noappp@aol.com

Planned Parenthood Federation of America
810 Seventh Ave.
New York, NY 10019
800-230-PLAN
http://www.ppfa.org/ppfa

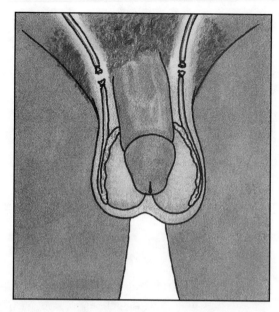

Vasectomy

VASECTOMY

Vasectomy is a permanent method of birth control for men. Each year about half a million American men have a vasectomy, and at least fifteen million men have already undergone the procedure. (For information on reversible forms of birth control, see Contraception, p. 380.)

Procedure

The vas deferens are small tubes through which sperm travel from the testicles, past the prostate, and into the urethra. In the urethra, the sperm are mixed with seminal fluid from the prostate to form semen.

A vasectomy, also called sterilization for men, is a surgical procedure in which the vas deferens are blocked. This obstruction keeps the sperm out of the ejaculate—instead of being mixed with seminal fluid and sent on their way to cause fertilization, the sperm are absorbed into the body. There is no difference in the amount of ejaculate or the ability to have an erection after a vasectomy, and the procedure has no effect on hormone production. The only difference is that the small amount sperm will be missing from the semen.

Most vasectomies are performed on an outpatient basis by a urologist, a specialist in men's reproductive health. In the traditional vasectomy, the doctor administers a local anesthetic into the groin area and makes an incision on each side of the scrotum to reach the vas deferens. Once the tubes are located, a small section of each tube is removed. The ends of the cut tubes may be tied off, cauterized, or blocked with surgical clips. Finally, the small incisions in the scrotum are stitched closed. The procedure takes fifteen to twenty minutes.

While the area may be sore for a few days, side effects are rare. Possible effects include swelling, pain, infection of the wound, and skin discoloration.

An alternative to the traditional vasectomy is the no-scalpel vasectomy (NSV). This procedure, developed in China in 1974, was first introduced to the United States in 1985.

With a NSV, the surgeon punches one tiny hole in the center of the scrotum and draws the tubes out, instead of making two half-inch cuts in the scrotum to reach the vas deferens. Unlike

NO-SCALPEL VASECTOMY— CHOOSING A PRACTITIONER

A no-scalpel vasectomy (NSV) is a delicate procedure. While it is less painful and less invasive than the traditional procedure, it requires more skill to perform, so it is best to find someone who has been trained in the procedure. Here are some questions to ask your doctor:

- Do you do NSVs?

- If so, how many have you done in the past year? (Since practice makes perfect with this delicate procedure, fifty or more is a good answer.)

- If not, could you refer me to another urologist who can?

If your practitioner is not aware of any physicians who perform NSVs near you, you can contact Access to Voluntary and Safe Contraception International for a referral.

the traditional vasectomy, no stitches are required with the NSV, and there is very little bleeding. In addition, there is little risk of infection and swelling—and there is less pain and discomfort than with a traditional procedure.

Both the traditional and NSV procedures are not effective immediately because sperm are stored in the vas deferens beyond the area of the blockage. It takes about fifteen ejaculations before the sperm are cleared from the tubes. Another form of birth control should be used after vasectomy until two sperm analyses show the semen to be free of sperm.

Advantages and Disadvantages

A vasectomy may be a good choice if you know that you and your partner do not want to have any children in the future. This may be because you're afraid of passing on a genetic disease, because of health concerns of a partner, or simply because you've decided your family is complete.

Vasectomy is a highly effective form of birth control, with a failure rate of less than 1 percent. (Very rarely, the tubes may reconnect by themselves, making it possible that a pregnancy may occur.) The safe, simple procedure takes about twenty minutes to perform, and recovery is quick.

The procedure has a one-time cost of about $1,000—much less than the cost of a tubal ligation, the equivalent procedure for a woman that requires major surgery, general anesthesia, and a longer recovery period. In addition, there are no hormonal side effects or regimens to worry about.

However, vasectomy cannot protect against sexually transmitted disease. In addition, it should be considered permanent (though surgical reversal may be possible in some cases). Your decision to have the procedure should be well thought-out and discussed with your partner.

As with any surgery, complications can occur during vasectomy. However, the good news is that major complications are rare. Possible temporary side effects include blood clots, infection, and swelling or tenderness near the testicles.

Vasectomy Reversal

It is possible to reverse a vasectomy—that is, surgically reconnect the vas deferens to allow the sperm back into the semen. The procedure is an option for men who have had a vasectomy and then decided they want to have a child. Most often, studies show, men change their minds because of a change in their situation; they've divorced and remarried, for example, and now want children. Each year, about 6 percent of American men who have had a vasectomy undergo vasectomy reversal.

A vasectomy reversal is a difficult operation that carries no guarantees. Using microsurgery, the surgeon must reconnect the vas deferens, structures that are only .3 millimeters in diameter. The procedure is done under general or epidural anesthesia, and it can take up to four hours. The cost of a vasectomy reversal ranges from $1,600 to $5,000.

In 90 percent of men, sperm can be returned to the ejaculate with vasectomy reversal. About half of those men can father children. Studies show that the more recently the vasectomy was done, the better the chances of a successful reversal.

Despite the fact that a vasectomy can be reversed in some cases, it is not 100 percent reversible. For this reason, a man thinking about having a vasectomy should consider the procedure permanent for all intents and purposes.

For more information:

Access to Voluntary and Safe Contraception International (AVSC International)
79 Madison Ave., 7th Floor
New York, NY 10016
212-561-8000
. http://www.avsc.org

Planned Parenthood Federation of America
810 Seventh Ave.
New York, NY 10019
800-230-PLAN
http://www.ppfa.org/ppfa

THE CANCER CONTROVERSY

In 1993, a study published in the *Journal of the American Medical Association* provided evidence suggesting vasectomy increases risk of prostate cancer. However, recent studies have yet to confirm those results. In a 1995 *Journal of the National Cancer Institute* article, researchers who studied men in both the United States and Canada failed to find an association between vasectomy and prostate cancer. A second study, conducted by the same researchers who found a link earlier, found "little support for an association of vasectomy with the risk of prostatic cancer."

Since the jury is still out on this issue, more research is needed. The American Urological Association, the American Cancer Society, and the National Institutes of Health have all issued statements saying that the evidence for a link between vasectomy and prostate cancer is very weak.

If you are considering a vasectomy, the possible cancer connections should not deter you. If you have already had a vasectomy, there's little reason to worry.

SEXUALLY TRANSMITTED DISEASES

Sexually transmitted diseases (STDs), also called sexually transmitted infections (STIs) affect twelve million Americans each year. At least one in four Americans and, according to some reports, as many as one in two Americans will be infected with an STD at some point in his or her life.

STDs are usually transmitted through sexual contact—oral, anal, and vaginal intercourse. However, some STDs can be transmitted through intimate contact—such as kissing and touching—as well. STDs are caused by viruses, bacteria, and parasites, which thrive in warm, moist surroundings such as the mouth, urethra, anus, and a woman's vagina. All STDs, including HIV (the virus that causes AIDS), die when they are outside the body. Therefore, STDs cannot be caught from toilet seats, door handles, water fountains, and other public facilities.

Symptoms

STDs are often not accompanied by symptoms, or if symptoms are present, they are often mistaken for another condition. STD symptoms men might experience are the following:

- A white or clear discharge from the penis

- A discharge from the rectum

- Genital sores, bumps, or lumps

- A genital or anal rash

- A burning sensation or pain in the penis, especially while urinating

- Itching around the genitals

It's important to see a doctor for treatment if any of these symptoms are present or if a partner is experiencing STD symptoms. STDs that are left untreated can lead to serious and irreversible damage such as sterility, liver damage, and, in the case of syphilis, brain damage. STDs are preventable and treatable. If an STD is diagnosed, any sexual partners should also see a physician for possible diagnosis and treatment.

Types of STDs

There are more than thirty different kinds of STDs. Here are some of the most common types of STDs that affect men.

Chancroid

There are some 1,500 cases of chancroid reported each year in the United States, and men are infected more often than women. Chancroid is an especially dangerous STD because the sores it causes (which eventually become open) increase the chance of getting HIV. Symptoms of chancroid first appear about a week after infection. First, a small boil (called a bubo) appears on the genitals. The bubo then becomes an open sore and may produce pus and pain. Untreated chancroid can infect and swell the glands located in the groin.

Chancroid is spread through vaginal, anal, and oral intercourse. The sores from chancroid can be confused with other STDs; only a microscopic examination of the discharge can diagnose chancroid. Chancroid is caused by a bacteria and can be successfully treated with antibiotics. Condoms can provide protection.

Chlamydia

The most common STD in the United States, chlamydia affects four million American men and women each year. Symptoms include discharge from the penis or anus, burning during urination, and painful intercourse. In 25 percent of men with the disease, chlamydia is symptomless. Left untreated, it could lead to sterility as well as urinary tract infection, pneumonia, eye infections, and blindness.

Chlamydia is spread through vaginal and anal intercourse, and, rarely, from the hand to the eye. A tissue analysis and urine sample are necessary for diagnosis. Its transmission may be prevented by using a condom. Chlamydia is caused by a bacteria and can be cured with antibiotics.

Cytomegalovirus (CMV)

CMV is the most common STD passed from a woman to her child; a baby can contract the disease from its mother before birth or during breast-feeding. Symptoms of CMV include swollen glands, fever, fatigue, gastrointestinal irritation, and loss of vision. While there are usually no symptoms with the first occurrence of CMV, they often occur during subsequent flare-ups.

CMV can be transmitted through contact with saliva, semen, blood, vaginal secretions, urine, and breast milk. Some 40 to 80 percent of Americans with CMV contract the disease before adolescence from close contact with an infected person. Adults usually get CMV through sexual activity. Condoms provide some protection during intercourse, although kissing and intimate touching can also spread the virus. There is no cure for CMV—the virus remains in the body for life. Symptoms can be controlled with intravenous drugs.

Gonorrhea

More than one million new cases of gonorrhea are reported in the United States every year. Symptoms include a puslike discharge from the penis and painful urination. Ten percent of men with gonorrhea have no symptoms. Left untreated, gonorrhea can cause sterility, arthritis, heart problems, and disorders of the central nervous system.

Gonorrhea is spread through vaginal, anal, and oral intercourse. Diagnosis is done through microscopic examination of discharge. Condoms may help prevent gonorrhea from being spread through intercourse. Gonorrhea is caused by a bacteria and is treatable with antibiotics.

Hepatitis B Virus (HBV)

Some 200,000 Americans acquire HBV each year, despite the fact that a vaccine is available to prevent it. There are about 1.5 million people in the United States with the disease. Symptoms include fatigue, headache, fever, nausea, vomiting, and stomach pain. Later, dark urine and jaundice (yellowing of the eyes and skin) may occur. Symptoms may not be present through the disease's most contagious stages.

Hepatitis B is very contagious and can be transmitted through kissing; vaginal, anal, or oral sex; or a puncture with a contaminated needle. A blood test is done for diagnosis. Hepatitis B can be prevented with an HBV vaccine. Condoms offer protection during intercourse, but the condition can still be passed through kissing and intimate contact. There is no cure for HBV, though the active infection usually passes within eight weeks. Some people may remain contagious indefinitely.

Herpes

Herpes simplex-1 is associated with cold sores and fever blisters, while herpes simplex-2 tends to affect the genitals. Herpes simplex-2 currently affects thirty million Americans. Possible symptoms include a recurring rash and blisters on the penis, mouth, anus, buttocks, or other places on the body, as well as pain in the affected area. There is no cure for herpes, although the sores and symptoms may come and go.

Herpes is spread through intimate contact, including kissing and vaginal, anal, and oral intercourse. It is usually only contagious from when the sores are present until they are completely healed, though some people are contagious when they have no symptoms. Condoms offer some protection. Diagnosis is done through examination of the discharge from the sores. Symptoms can be treated with a prescription medication called acyclovir.

Human Immunodeficiency Virus (HIV)

About one million Americans have HIV, the virus that causes acquired immune deficiency syndrome (AIDS). This disease weakens the body's immune system and eventually causes death. There may be no symptoms for as many as ten years after infection. Possible symptoms include weight loss, diarrhea, fatigue, fever, night sweats, headaches, dizziness, a yeast infection of the tongue or mouth or purple growths on the skin. About 5 percent of those with HIV never develop symptoms.

HIV is spread through contact with infected blood, semen, vaginal fluids, and breast milk. It can be diagnosed with a blood test or a test that samples saliva, and condoms can help prevent its spread. There is no cure for HIV, though some treatments are available to slow the progression of the disease. (See AIDS/HIV, opposite.)

Human Papillomavirus (HPV)

About forty million men and women are currently infected with human papillomavirus (HPV). There are sixty different kinds of human papillomavirus. While some types of HPV have no symptoms, other types cause small, cauliflower-shaped warts on the genitals, the urethra, and the anus to develop a few weeks after infection. Untreated genital warts can eventually grow to block the opening of the urethra and can be painful.

HPV is transmitted through vaginal and anal intercourse and may be prevented with the use of condoms. Diagnosis is done by identifying the warts. HPV cannot be cured. A drug called podophyllin, along with a topical medication called trichloracetic acid, can be used to shrink the warts. Also, the warts can be removed with surgery, laser surgery (burning the warts away with a concentrated beam of light), or cryosurgery (freezing the warts). The warts may recur. It is important to see a doctor to be examined for warts regularly.

Molluscum Contagiosum

This virus affects hundreds of thousands of Americans each year. A disease of the skin and mucous membranes, molluscum contagiosum involves small, round pimples on the genitals and thighs.

The condition is spread through oral, anal, and vaginal intercourse and other intimate contact. Condoms may offer some protection, but often the virus comes in contact with areas not protected by the condom. It is not always sexually transmitted. The virus is identified through analysis of tissue taken from a sore. Growths can be removed surgically, with laser surgery, or with cryosurgery.

Syphilis

There is currently a total of 120,000 reported cases of syphilis in the United States. Syphilis, caused by a bacterium called a spirochete, does not always produce symptoms. If left untreated, it goes through a series of phases. In the first phase, sores appear on the genitals, lips, mouth, or anus and last for three to six weeks. Symptoms in the second phase include body rashes on the soles of the feet and palms of the hands, as well as fever, fatigue, sort throat, hair loss, weight loss, swollen glands, and muscle aches. These symptoms may come and go for up to two years. Then, a latent phase without any symptoms occurs. In the final phase, the nervous system becomes damaged, along with the heart, brain, and other organs. Death can result.

Syphilis can be spread through vaginal, oral, and anal intercourse, as well as through kissing. It is very contagious when sores are present early in the disease because the liquid that oozes from them is very infectious. It is usually not contagious during the latent phase. Condoms offer protection during vaginal, anal, and oral intercourse. The disease is diagnosed with microscopic examination of the fluid from the sores, blood tests, and examination of spinal fluid. Syphilis is caused by bacterium and, therefore, may be cured with antibiotics. The damage that can be caused by syphilis, however, cannot be reversed.

Prevention

Because STDs are passed through contaminated bodily fluids such as blood, semen, and vaginal secretions, their transmission be prevented by not having sex and not sharing intravenous drug equipment. When both partners have never had sex with anyone else, sex can also be considered safe.

However, because so many STDs have no symptoms—and because many people are embarrassed, unknowing, or dishonest about their sexual histories—it is impossible to tell without testing whether a person who has had more than one partner is free of infection. Therefore, it's necessary to take precautions against STDs by practicing safe sex, namely, wearing a condom during intercourse. (See Safe Sex, p. 398.) However, there are some STDs that may be transmitted through touching or kissing. If you are at risk for a sexually transmitted disease or if you

are experiencing any symptoms, talk with your practitioner.

For more information:

American Social Health Association
P.O. Box 13827
Research Triangle Park, NC 27709
919-361-8400
National STD Hotline
800-227-8922
http://sunsite.unc.edu/asha

Centers for Disease Control and Prevention
National AIDS Hotline
800-342-AIDS
800-344-SIDA (Spanish)
800-AIDS-TYY (deaf access)

National Herpes Hotline
Herpes Resource Center
P.O. Box 13827
Research Triangle Park, NC 27709
800-230-6039
919-361-8488

National Institute of Allergy and Infectious Diseases
National Institutes of Health
Bldg. 31, Room 7A50
31 Center Dr., MSC 2520
Bethesda, MD 20892-2520
301-496-5717
http://www.naid.nih.gov

Planned Parenthood Federation of America, Inc.
810 Seventh Ave.
New York, NY 10019
800-230-PLAN
http://www.ppfa.org/ppfa

AIDS/HIV

Acquired immune deficiency syndrome (AIDS) is the final stage of a progressive disease in which the body's immune system is gradually destroyed by the human immunodeficiency virus (HIV).

If your life has not yet been touched in some way by AIDS, you should consider yourself lucky. Though this modern plague crosses all lines of race, gender, and sexual orientation, men are possibly the most likely to be affected by it. AIDS is a leading cause of death in men 25 to 44 years old in the United States, and young women are the fastest-growing group of people with AIDS. In 1996, the number of people in the United States who died from AIDS declined by 12 percent, the first decline since the epidemic began in 1981. The decline in deaths was greatest for whites (down 21 percent). There were 2 percent fewer AIDS-related deaths among African Americans and 10 percent fewer among Hispanics.

To date, there is no cure for HIV infection or AIDS, though some new treatments can slow the progress of the disease, making it more manageable. Specifically, protease inhibitors, a new class of drugs, have proved effective in preventing the development of AIDS in those with HIV. In addition, you can protect yourself against HIV and AIDS by avoiding activities that put you at risk.

According to the Centers for Disease Control and Prevention:

- 581,429 cases of AIDS were reported as of the end of 1996 in the United States; 488,300 of those people were adult males.

- As of 1992, between 650,000 and 900,000 Americans were infected with HIV. Of those, between 550,000 and 750,000 were men.

- The World Health Organization (WHO) reported that as of December 1996 there were 1.5 million reported cases of AIDS worldwide. However, WHO estimates the actual number of AIDS cases worldwide to be 8.4 million.

Progression of the Disease

Despite the fact that HIV affects and progresses in each individual in different ways and at different rates, there are general stages of HIV infection.

In the first stage, the body produces infection-fighting substances known as antibodies in response to HIV infection. Usually within six months of infection, these antibodies can be detected in the blood. However, HIV may lie dormant for years—usually somewhere between eight and ten years—before noticeable symptoms develop. However, during this time an HIV-positive individual can still pass along the infection. Through the early stage of HIV infection (called seroconversion), symptoms include fatigue, malaise, swollen lymph glands, rash, night sweats, and diarrhea.

In the second stage of the disease, the HIV virus becomes active. Once it does, it attacks and cripples the immune system. The immune system usually protects the body against invaders (called antigens) such as bacteria, viruses, toxins, and foreign tissues by producing antibodies. However, HIV attacks the antibodies known as T cells, the cells responsible for attacking and destroying antigens. When T cells are destroyed by HIV, the immune system cannot function and becomes vulnerable to a variety of infections and diseases. These infections—called opportunistic infections because they take advantage of the weakened immune system—are usually fatal.

Until recently, it was unknown how HIV attacks the T cells. In early 1996, researchers from the National Institute of Allergy and Infectious Diseases reported the discovery of a protein called fusin that must be present on a cell's surface in order for HIV to invade. The discovery may lead to the development of new drugs and vaccines to combat HIV. It also may help explain why some people are less susceptible to HIV infection than others and why some infected people stay healthy for longer periods.

The third stage of the disease is marked by the development of AIDS-related complex (ARC). As HIV infection progresses and the immune system has sustained considerable damage, symptoms of ARC can appear, including fever, weight loss, severe diarrhea, swollen lymph glands, and night sweats. Also at this stage, characteristic disorders of ARC are recognized. These disorders include severe rash, arthritis, intellectual impairment, pneumonia, kidney infection, personality changes, yeast infections of the mouth, and neurological disorders.

In the final stage, full-blown AIDS occurs as the immune system is severely impaired and diseases and infections plague the body, eventually causing death. The most common diseases are *Pneumocystis carinii* pneumonia, HIV-wasting syndrome (acute HIV infection), yeast infection of the mouth and esophagus (called thrush), Kaposi's sarcoma (a form of cancer that affects the skin and internal organs), tuberculosis, and other respiratory infections.

Other diseases include various other cancers, viruses, and infections: toxoplasmosis, a condition that damages the brain, heart, and lungs, causing pneumonia; hepatitis and other diseases; chronic herpes infections of the mouth, esophagus, and lung; various forms of lymphoma (a cancer); eye diseases; and cryptosporidiosis infection of the intestine, which causes diarrhea.

Transmission

The HIV virus can be found in the blood, semen, vaginal secretions, and breast milk of an infected person. It is transmitted when one of these infected fluids comes in contact with a cut or sore or the moist lining of the vagina, penis, rectum, or mouth. Most commonly, HIV is transmitted through unprotected vaginal and anal intercourse or through the sharing of contaminated drug needles. At one time, HIV was transmitted through blood transfusions. However, blood is now routinely screened for HIV in the United States, making the probability of contracting HIV from blood products extremely low.

Although scientists have found small amounts of HIV in body fluids such as saliva, feces, urine, tears, and sweat, there is no evidence that the virus can be spread through contact with these substances. HIV cannot be transmitted through hugging, touching, nonsexual contact, or sharing of food utensils, towels and bedding, swimming pools, telephones, or toilet seats.

Experts report that men are at lower risk than women for contracting HIV during vaginal intercourse, possibly because the urethral opening of the man is much smaller than the vaginal opening of the woman. However, though the risk is statistically smaller, there is still a definite risk that the virus will be passed from the woman to the man.

Prevention

Because many people who have HIV have no symptoms and may not know they are infected, there is no way you can know for sure whether a potential sexual partner is infected, unless he or she has been repeatedly tested for the virus or has never engaged in any risky behavior. Abstinence is the best protection against HIV and all sexually transmitted diseases (STDs).

If you are sexually active, you can help protect yourself against HIV by refraining from risky behaviors. Use a latex condom or vaginal pouch

THE LINK BETWEEN SEXUALLY TRANSMITTED DISEASES AND HIV

According to research presented at the 11th International AIDS Conference in 1996 in Vancouver, British Columbia, the treatment of other STDs is significant in reducing the spread of HIV. Researchers have known for some time of the link between HIV infection and other STDs, but new evidence presented showed for the first time the impact of STD treatment on the rate at which people become infected with HIV.

STDs are believed to increase the risk of HIV infection in two ways. STDs such as chancroid, syphilis, and herpes can cause genital sores, or ulcers, which may provide an easy point of entry for HIV. Even when ulcers are not present, untreated STDs cause inflammation of the genital tract that may also increase the risk of infection during sexual contact.

whenever having oral, anal, or vaginal sex with someone you are uncertain is free of HIV or other STDs. Although condoms cannot give 100 percent protection from HIV, studies show that using latex condoms substantially reduces the risk for HIV transmission. Use of a "female" condom (also called a vaginal pouch), a lubricated polyurethane sheath that is inserted into the vagina, is another barrier to the HIV virus.

According to the Public Health Service, laboratory studies have shown that spermicides (such as nonoxynol-9) may inactivate HIV and other STDs; however, spermicides offer less protection than condoms and are more effective when used in conjunction with condoms, rather than in place of them. (See Safe Sex, p. 398.)

Diagnosis

Because early HIV infection often has no symptoms, a blood test is done to check for the presence of antibodies to HIV. HIV antibodies generally do not reach detectable levels until one to three months following infection, and it may take as long as six months following infection for the body to produce enough to show up in HIV-antibody test.

HIV testing is done in most health-care providers' offices, laboratories, and clinics. Many sites offer anonymous or confidential testing, and counseling before and after the test may be available if needed. Check your phone book or contact one of the AIDS hotlines listed on page 397 to find out the location of a testing site near you.

Two different blood tests are used to diagnose HIV: ELISA (enzyme-linked immunosorbent assay) and the Western blot test. In addition, an oral HIV test called Orasure, in which a treated cotton pad is placed between the gum and the cheek to collect antibodies, was approved by the Food and Drug Administration (FDA) in June 1996. Clinical trials showed the test to be as accurate as the traditional blood tests. The oral test is also considered safer for health-care workers to perform: because there are no sharp needles or blood involved, there is no risk of accidental HIV transmission.

Home-screening tests for HIV became available in early 1997. A person using the test kit draws blood from a finger, puts it on a special laboratory paper, and mails the sample to a certified testing laboratory. The results, which remain anonymous, are provided a week later by telephone. If needed, the service provides local medical referrals. The tests are available over-the-counter in drugstores or by mail order.

HIV-POSITIVE—WHAT TO DO AFTER YOU'RE DIAGNOSED

If you've been diagnosed with HIV, remember that a positive test does not mean you have AIDS—it can take up to ten years for the symptoms of AIDS to develop. And in the meantime, there are steps you can take to help yourself stay well longer:

- Visit a practitioner or clinic right away. An immediate checkup and a regular schedule of doctor visits can help you keep track of the progress of the disease and treat any problems that do arise. You should also be tested for tuberculosis, because some people with HIV also have TB, which needs to be treated right away. Medications to slow the progress of the virus may also be prescribed. Take all medications according to your practitioner's instructions.

- Learn all you can about your condition. Ask your practitioner about the effects of HIV and AIDS, available treatments (including experimental or new treatments), and types of health-care services you may need. Ask about how much treatment will cost. (In some cases, financial assistance may be available to help pay for treatment.) By being informed, you can make better decisions about your health and participate in your own care.

- Know how to prevent the spread of AIDS. If you have HIV, that means you can infect another person. If you have intercourse, practice safe sex. Also, don't share intravenous drug needles if you're infected. Ask your practitioner for more information on how you can keep from spreading AIDS.

- Live a healthy lifestyle. Eat well, exercise, get plenty of rest and don't drink, smoke, or use drugs. All of these things help to strengthen your immune system, making it easier for your body to fight off illness.

- Share your feelings when you're ready. Telling friends or family about your HIV status can help a lot. You may also want to join a support group in your area. Ask your practitioner or local health department about how to find a group that suits you.

The CDC's National AIDS Hotline (listed on p. 397) can provide additional information as well as referrals to a number of counseling and service organizations in your area.

Source: National Institutes of Health

People who have been exposed to HIV should be tested for HIV infection as soon as they are likely to develop antibodies to the virus—three to six months after infection may have occurred. Early testing will allow them to receive appropriate treatment at a time when they are most able to combat HIV and stop the emergence of opportunistic infections. Early testing also allows people with HIV to help stop the spread of the virus by notifying sexual partners. If preferred, public health officials will notify an individual's sexual partners. People infected with the disease should not donate blood, share drug needles, or engage in unprotected sexual activity.

Treatment

Because of varied immune responses, the mutable and unstable nature of the AIDS virus, and lack of understanding on the part of researchers, there is no cure or vaccine available.

Traditional treatment of AIDS focuses on the following three areas:

- Arresting the progression of the virus through the use of drugs called nucleoside analogues, which prevent the replication of HIV. Initially, the drug AZT is used. Other similar drugs, such as ddI, ddC, and d4T, are added to the regimen when AZT loses its effectiveness.

- Treating the opportunistic infections and disease through antimicrobial drug therapy

- Attempting to restore the health of the immune system through such methods as bone marrow transplants and immunoglobulin therapy

In the past, the number of helper T cells in the blood was measured regularly in order to gauge the progression of the HIV infection and determine proper treatment. However, a recently developed test called viral load measures the actual amount of viral RNA (HIV's strand of genetic information) circulating in a person's bloodstream in a milliliter of blood. To date, this appears to be the best way of predicting the course that HIV will take in an individual, helping a practitioner predict whether a person's immune system will fight the virus for a few years or up to fifteen years or more, for example. This knowledge allows healthcare providers to decide with greater confidence when to begin a patient on drug treatment and how aggressive that treatment should be.

In July 1996, researchers announced that more than a dozen clinical trials had shown that a new class of drugs called protease inhibitors in combination with nucleoside analogues could reduce levels of HIV in blood to below detectable levels. Specifically, the clinical trials tested drug combinations of nucleosides such as AZT and 3TC—which prevent the replication of HIV—with the newly developed protease inhibitors (marketed as Crixivan, Invirase, and Norvir), which appear to "cut" the protein of replicating HIV. In addition to slowing virus production, the drugs also proved to increase T cell numbers.

Many AIDS experts, however, caution that the clinical data are not conclusive and that the combination treatment should not be considered a cure. The findings do not necessarily mean that the drugs can rid the body of HIV; the virus could still lurk somewhere in the body such as in the dense tissue of the lymph nodes. In addition, because participants in the clinical trials had been taking the combination of drugs for less than two years, it is unknown how long the effect of the drugs will last. Controversy also surrounds the affordability of the drug treatment. At $10,000 to $15,000 per year, the drug combinations may not be accessible to the majority of people infected with HIV.

There are also alternative therapies that may help HIV/AIDS patients. Alternative methods of treatment include acupuncture, use of herbal medicine, massage, dietary modification, chiropractic therapy, homeopathic medicine, and body and mind relaxation exercises. These therapies are used in combination with traditional drug therapies and are intended to strengthen the immune system, remove impurities from the body, relieve pain, and promote relaxation, among other things.

Although some physicians are skeptical concerning their overall value of effectiveness, alternative methods offer little or no side effects and may be a more comforting mode of treatment than drug therapy. Therapy can be sought from an alternative practitioner (See Complementary Therapies, p. 436.) In addition, organizations that provide alternative therapy for those with HIV and AIDS include the AIDS Alternative Health Project in Chicago; Bastyr University's Natural Health Clinic in Seattle, Washington; the Northwest Naturopathic Clinic in Portland, Oregon; and Lincoln Hospital in Bronx, New York. Bastyr University is currently conducting studies on the effect of alternative therapies on the course of the disease.

For more information:

AIDS Clinical Trials Information Service (ACTIS)
800-874-2572
800-243-7012 (deaf access)

American Social Health Association
P.O. Box 13827
Research Triangle Park, NC 27709
919-361-8400
National STD Hotline
800-227-8922
http://sunsite.unc.edu/asha

Centers for Disease Control and Prevention
National AIDS Hotline
800-342-AIDS
800-344-7432 SIDA (Spanish)
800-243-7889 (TTY)

Center for Disease Control and Prevention
National AIDS Clearinghouse
P.O. Box 6003
Rockville, MD 20849-6003
800-458-5231
800-243-7012 (deaf access)

CLINICAL TRIALS—ARE THEY FOR YOU?

If people with HIV or AIDS want to try experimental treatments, they may participate in clinical drug trials—studies done to test the effectiveness and safety of new drugs. There are a number of benefits and risks to participating in a drug trial. If you participate, you'll have access to top medical care, and you may be one of the first helped by a new drug. Some treatment costs may be paid. In addition, you'll have the satisfaction of knowing you're helping others. On the other hand, the treatment may not be effective—it might even have harmful side effects. There may be a lot of tests, requirements, or other inconveniences that go along with the study.

Studies are designed to protect the privacy of those who participate, so you may join without others knowing you have HIV or AIDS. There are several other safeguards. First, all participants must be fully informed of all the possible risks and benefits of the study before entering it (this is known as informed consent). Also, the trial is reviewed by the National Institutes of Allergy and Infectious Diseases, the hospital or clinic that is sponsoring it, and a special safety board. Finally, people involved in the study have the right to stop treatment at any time.

If you're interested in taking part in a clinical trail, contact the AIDS Clinical Trials Information Service at 800-TRIALS-A for more information.

Lesbian and Gay Rights AIDS Project
American Civil Liberties Union
132 W. 43 St.
New York, NY 10036
212-944-9800 ext. 545

National Institute of Allergy and Infectious
Diseases
National Institutes of Health
Bldg. 31, Room 7A50
31 Center Dr., MSC 2520
Bethesda, MD 20892-2520
301-496-5717
http://www.naid.nih.gov

Project Inform National Hotline
AIDS Treatment Information
800-822-7422

SAFE SEX

Having safe sex means taking precautions during sexual activity to help prevent the transmission of sexually transmitted disease (STDs), including the human immunodeficiency virus (HIV). HIV is the virus that causes acquired immune deficiency syndrome (AIDS), which is the leading cause of death in males 25 to 44 years of age. There are more than thirty STDs, including syphilis, gonorrhea, human papillomavirus, and chlamydia. STDs that are left untreated may lead to serious and irreversible damage such as sterility, liver damage, and in the case of syphilis, brain damage. (See Sexually Transmitted Diseases, p. 387.)

Practicing safe sex not only means protecting your own health against sexually transmitted disease; it also means protecting the health of your partner as well as any future partners—and even the health of any children that may come along (as some STDs can be passed from a woman to her child or can contribute to birth defects). For these reasons, discuss safe sex with

any potential partner and be honest about your sexual history. Though it may be uncomfortable to talk about such issues with a partner, don't let your embarrassment become a threat to your health and your life.

Transmission of STDs

STDs can be passed through contact with an infected partner's bodily fluids—blood, semen, preejaculate (the few drops of semen that are released before ejaculation), and vaginal secretions. Contact with sores caused by STDs can also transmit a condition. A few types of STDs can be passed through intimate contact, including kissing and touching. STDs can also be passed by infected needles used to inject drugs.

Diseases that can be passed during vaginal or anal intercourse include gonorrhea, chlamydia, syphilis, chancroid, human papillomavirus, HIV, herpes, hepatitis B, and cytomegalovirus. Gonorrhea, syphilis, chancroid, herpes, hepatitis B, HIV, and cytomegalovirus can also be transmitted through oral sex. Herpes and cytomegalovirus can be transmitted through intimate contact without intercourse. (See AIDS/HIV, p. 391, and Sexually Transmitted Diseases, p. 387.)

Men have a lower risk of acquiring sexually transmitted diseases they are exposed to than women because the penis is less vulnerable to infection than the vagina. For example, a woman is twice as likely to be infected with HIV by a man than a man is likely to be infected by a woman.

Preventing STDs

The way to avoid STDs is to avoid behaviors that put you at risk. One guarantee against STDs is to not be sexually active and to not use intravenous drugs. Also, if you have never had sex and your partner has also never had sex, sex with that partner can be considered safe.

HOW TO USE A CONDOM CORRECTLY

For condoms to provide maximum protection, you must use them consistently and correctly. Consistent use means using a condom from start to finish every time you have sex. The Food and Drug Administration provides the following instructions for using a condom correctly.

- Use a new condom for every act of vaginal, anal, and oral (penis-mouth contact) sex. Do not unroll the condom before placing it on the penis.
- Put the condom on after the penis is erect and before any contact is made between the penis and any part of the partner's body.
- If the condom does not have a reservoir top, pinch the tip enough to leave a half-inch space for semen to collect. Always make sure to eliminate any air in the tip to help keep the condom from breaking.
- Holding the condom rim (and pinching a half-inch space if necessary), place the condom on the top of the penis. Then, continuing to hold it by the rim, unroll it all the way to the base of the penis. If you are also using a water-based lubricant, you can put more on the outside of the condom.
- If you feel the condom break, stop immediately, withdraw, and put on a new condom.
- After ejaculation and before the penis gets soft, grip the rim of the condom and carefully withdraw.
- To remove the condom, gently pull it off the penis, being careful that semen doesn't spill out.
- Wrap the condom in a tissue and throw it in the trash where others won't handle it. (Don't flush condoms down the toilet because they may cause sewer problems.) Wash your hands with soap and hot water.
- Store condoms in a cool, dry place that is out of direct sunlight.

Using the right kind of condom also is important in preventing the passage of the viruses and bacteria. When purchasing condoms, look for the following on the package label:

- The condoms should be latex. Natural condoms (such as lambskin condoms) contain natural pores that microscopic germs can pass through; they do not provide an effective barrier against STDs.
- The condoms should be made specifically for preventing disease. Novelty condoms or those that do not cover the entire penis are meant only for sexual stimulation, not protection. Even if they are the most expensive ones available, if the condom package does not say that they are made for disease prevention, the will provide no protection against STDs.
- The condom should have an expiration or manufacture date. Do not use a condom after its expiration date or if it has been damaged in any way. Condoms can be used up to five years after their manufacture date.

However, many people have more than one partner in a lifetime. Because many people who have STDs—especially HIV—have no symptoms and may not even know that they are infected, there is no way of knowing with certainty whether a sexual partner is infected unless he or she has been repeatedly tested for STDs or hasn't engaged in any risky behavior. Therefore, it is important to protect yourself against STDs. Keep in mind that practicing safe sex during intercourse does not guarantee against the transmission of an STD—it simply lowers the risk of transmission to help prevent infection.

Because many sexually transmitted diseases are spread though blood, semen, and vaginal secretions, practicing mutual masturbation and caresses without penetration is one way to have safe sex. Some infections such as herpes simplex, however, may be transmitted via genital to genital, or skin to skin, contact with or without penetration.

Latex condoms are possibly the best protection for those who are sexually active. The Public Health Service recommends that people use latex condoms whenever having oral, anal, or vaginal sex with someone they are uncertain is free of HIV or other sexually transmitted diseases. A condom is a sheath worn over the penis that catches the semen and prevents contact with a partner's bodily fluids. A condom or a device called a dental dam can be held over the genitals during oral sex to prevent contact as well. Although condoms cannot give 100 percent protection from STDs, they offer good protection against gonorrhea, chlamydia, chancroid, HIV, and syphilis. They also offer some protection against human papillomavirus, herpes, and hepatitis B. Women may use a vaginal pouch, or female condom, which also offers some protection against STDs. A vaginal pouch is a lubricated polyurethane sheath with a ring on each end that is inserted into the vagina.

According to the Public Health Service, laboratory studies have shown that spermicides such as nonoxynol-9 can offer some protection against chlamydia and gonorrhea. However, they should not be relied upon to protect against diseases such as HIV or herpes. Spermicides may be used with condoms to increase protection against both STDs and pregnancy.

For more information:

American Social Health Association
P.O. Box 13827
Research Triangle Park, NC 27709
919-361-8400
National STD Hotline
800-227-8922
http://sunsite.unc.edu/asha

National Institute of Allergy and Infectious Diseases
National Institutes of Health
Bldg. 31, Room 7A50
31 Center Dr., MSC 2520
Bethesda, MD 20892-2520
301-496-5717
http://www.naid.nih.gov

Planned Parenthood Federation of America, Inc.
810 Seventh Ave.
New York, NY 10019
800-230-PLAN
http://www.ppfa.org/ppfa

SEXUAL ORIENTATION AND HEALTH

Sexual orientation is defined according to the gender of sex partner a man or women desires. Men who are sexually attracted to men are homosexual, or gay, while heterosexual, or straight, men are attracted to women. A homosexual woman, one who is attracted to other women, is a lesbian. However, sexual orientation may not be definite, and preferences may change throughout life. Bisexuality, for example, is the attraction to people of both genders. People may also choose to refrain from sex or may not consider themselves to have any sexual orientation.

When it comes to the importance of health, all men are alike, regardless of their sexual preferences. Whether a person is straight, bisexual, asexual, or gay, the same concerns about conditions such as heart disease, high blood pressure, diabetes, and prostate cancer exist. However, men who are bisexual or homosexual are at increased risk for a few conditions such as sexually transmitted conditions and urinary tract infections. For the most part, these higher risks occur because of sexual practices. However, there are also some social aspects such as discrimination within the health-care system that may affect the health of gay and bisexual men.

Homosexuality

Though it is hard to determine the number of gay men in the United States, a 1996 survey reports that 2.4 percent of men define themselves as homosexual, have male partners, and experience homosexual desire. In the same study, 10.1 percent of men define themselves as having at least one of those three aspects.

No one is sure what determines homosexuality; some experts theorize that genetics play a role in sexual orientation, and others believe that society and family life create a tendency in some toward homosexuality. Still others believe homosexuality to be an individual lifestyle choice. Most gay men realize their orientation during adolescence.

However, some may not realize it until they are older—possibly even after they are married.

Homophobia, the irrational fear and hatred of homosexuality that exists in society, often keeps gay men from "coming out of the closet" and being open with friends, family, and co-workers about their sexual orientation. Men who reveal their homosexuality often face insults and embarrassment, and many lose their jobs, support of family members, or even custody of their children.

While being homosexual within a predominantly heterosexual society is stressful, many gay individuals and communities enjoy a great deal of pride. More and more, informal and formal organizations of gay men are forming to provide each other with support and to celebrate their lifestyles.

Bisexuality

Bisexual men and women have sex with partners of both genders at some point in their lives. The relationships may occur at the same time, or they may be spread out over the years as a series of relationships with partners of alternating genders. The patterns of bisexual behavior vary greatly and occur for different reasons. In fact, many people who have relationships with people of both genders describe themselves as either heterosexual or homosexual.

Bisexuality has not been studied as extensively as homosexuality, and, therefore, not much is known about it. However, one survey shows that some 20 percent of men report sexual contact with men during their lifetime, while 6 to 7 percent report such activity during adulthood. As with homosexuality, the factors that determine bisexuality are unknown.

Health Concerns of Gay and Bisexual Men

The sexual behaviors of gay and bisexual men, as well as a number of social factors, put them at higher risk for some health conditions.

Perhaps the biggest health concern among sexually active gay men is human immunodeficiency virus (HIV), the virus that causes acquired immune deficiency syndrome (AIDS). Men who have sex with men make up the largest category of people affected by the disease. In 1994, 34,974 cases of AIDS were reported among men whose only exposure to HIV was through sexual contact with other men. (See AIDS/HIV, p. 391.) The risk of HIV transmission is greater during anal sex than during vaginal sex because the lining of the rectum is delicate and may be easily torn, allowing the virus easy entrance into the body. Condoms are essential in the prevention of the spread of HIV. (See Safe Sex, p. 398.)

Sexually active gay men are also at high risk for hepatitis B. This sexually transmitted disease—which is passed through intimate contact such as kissing as well as through intercourse—can cause fatigue, headache, stomach pain, and jaundice. While condoms can provide some protection, the best way to avoid hepatitis B is to receive a vaccine, which is recommended for all sexually active gay and bisexual men. (See Sexually Transmitted Diseases, p. 387.)

Gay men are also more likely to get anal cancer than heterosexual men. One study found that men who reported homosexual behavior were twenty-five to fifty times more likely to get anal cancer than straight men. The increased risk may be related to a higher risk of human papillomavirus, a sexually transmitted disease that often causes precancerous skin changes, HIV infection and smoking among gay men. Men who are at risk for anal cancer can be monitored by a physician with tests designed to diagnose the earliest signs of cancer.

There are also a number of sexually transmitted diseases for which gay men are at high risk. These include herpes, syphilis, chlamydia, and gonorrhea. Gay men are also likely to suffer gastrointestinal and urinary tract infections if they participate in anal sex. This is because bacteria from the rectum can affect the urethra, and infection transmitted from the urethra can make its way up the digestive tract and affect the intestines.

Drug and alcohol abuse are also health problems that affect a number of gay men. Studies show that some 28 to 35 percent of gay men and women abuse drugs or alcohol, while only 10 to 12 percent of the heterosexual population suffer substance abuse. Not only does use of drugs—ranging from drinking to abusing illegal drugs such as cocaine and marijuana—directly endanger a person's health by increasing the risk for disease, it also increases the chances that a person will engage in risky behavior, such as unprotected sex.

Bisexual men who are sexually active share the health concerns of gay men. For the most part, bisexual men fall somewhere between heterosexual and homosexual men as far as risk is concerned, having lower rates of sexually transmitted diseases than gay men and higher rates than straight men. Again, however, there is little information available about bisexual behavior and health risk due to the lack of surveys and studies.

Emotional Well-Being

A lack of emotional support, societal discrimination and issues such as AIDS can make being a gay or bisexual man a difficult emotional experience. Even though being openly gay today is more accepted than it has ever been in the United States, some state and federal laws ban homosexual relationships and marriage, and physical and verbal abuse—"gay bashing"—is a reality for gay men.

Many teenagers who are struggling with their sexual orientation may feel confused, isolated from friends and family, and may fear rejection. Without support, such boys may become depressed, turn to drugs, or run away from home. A study from the Secretary's Task Force on Youth Suicide found that gay teenagers were two to three times more likely to commit suicide than heterosexual teenagers. Another study showed that 76 percent of gay and bisexual teens used alcohol, 42 percent used marijuana, and 25 percent used cocaine and crack. Again, this drug abuse not only harms the individual directly but also increases the risk of unsafe sex and consequent HIV infection.

Homosexual men also often deal with the stress of living in an unaccepting society—or with the stress of hiding their sexual identity from those around them. Homosexuals often have difficulty finding partners and meaningful relationships and often face loneliness. The threat of AIDS also takes its toll on the emotional health of gays in the United States. Not only must gay men deal with the deaths of partners and friends from the disease, but they also face the pressure of a society that often associates or blames the deadly disease on the gay community. All of these issues contribute to a high incidence of depression, suicide, and drug abuse among gay men.

Health Care for Gay and Bisexual Men

In the early 1970s, homosexuality was still listed as a category of mental disorders by the American Psychiatric Association. Today, though some still consider homosexuality a form of dysfunctional behavior, most practitioners recognize homosexuality as normal. However, this does not mean that health-care practitioners are comfortable with it. One 1989 study of general practitioners showed that only 32.7 percent of those surveyed felt comfortable with gay men. In a 1994 survey conducted by the Gay and Lesbian Medical Association, 98 percent of respondents felt that gay patients should tell their practitioners their sexual orientation, though 64 percent also believed that doing so might result in substandard care.

In 1995, the American Medical Association adopted a policy on gay and lesbian health care, calling for "nonjudgemental recognition of sexual orientation" and pledging that the AMA will "work with the gay and lesbian community." The twenty-page report specifically rejects therapy to change sexual orientation and covers issues such as HIV, access to health care, substance abuse, negative attitudes from health-care providers, and the need for doctors to remain unbiased about the sexual histories of their patients.

Some men may be afraid to seek medical care because of the risk of rejection, poor care, or prejudice—or perhaps the fear that a practitioner may try to "treat" their sexual preferences. A gay or bisexual man should search for a practitioner who is comfortable with all types of sexual orientation and understands the needs of patients. If a man is not comfortable revealing his sexual orientation, he should find another practitioner with whom he is comfortable. Otherwise, important medical problems and health risks might be overlooked.

The best way to find such a practitioner is simply to ask the practitioner about his or her attitude regarding homosexuality when making the appointment or at a first meeting. Friends and local and national organizations and resource groups may be able to provide referrals to practitioners who are comfortable and knowledgeable about the needs of homosexuals.

Some medical schools are beginning to put together programs designed to teach future practitioners about the needs of gay men and lesbians and help the practitioners feel more comfortable and confident about treating gay patients.

For more information:

Gay and Lesbian Advocates and Defenders
294 Washington St., #740
Boston, MA 02180
617-426-1350

National Gay and Lesbian Task Force
2320 17th St., N.W.
Washington, DC 20009
202-332-6483
http://www.ngltf.org

Office of Lesbian and Gay Concerns
Unitarian Universalist Association
25 Beacon St.
Boston, MA 02108
617-742-2100 ext. 470
http://www.uua.org

P-FLAG (Parents, Families and Friends of Lesbians and Gays)
1101 14th St., N.W., Suite 1030
Washington, DC 20005
202-638-4200
http://www.pflag.org

ERECTION PROBLEMS

An erection problem is the health problem (and it is most likely a *physical* health problem, not a mental one) that men fear most and are least likely to admit having. In fact, most doctors and therapists prefer the term *erection problems* to "impotence." They're not just being politically correct—it's really a more accurate description of what's going on. At least half of all men between 40 and 72 have at least occasional problems either getting or keeping an erection, or both. While nearly all men have experienced erection problems, at least twenty million American men are chronic sufferers. Men who have high blood pressure, diabetes, or heart disease are four times more likely to suffer erection problems than men without these conditions. Smoking increases the risk of problems even more.

Physiologic Erection Problems

Until about twenty years ago, erection problems were always labeled psychosomatic—that is, mentally or emotionally induced. Now, doctors and therapists know that most of the reasons are physical; the most common estimates are that 75 to 80 percent of all cases of chronic erection problems have a physiologic—physical—cause. This means the problem is probably treatable. But it also means that persistent erection problems should send you to a qualified physician right away, because it's possible that a serious problem such as diabetes or circulatory disease exists. Treating that ailment may well relieve erection difficulties. Causes of physical erection problems include the following:

1. *Medications.* Many over-the-counter and prescription medications, especially antidepressants and blood pressure drugs, list erection problems as a possible side effect. If you experience an erection problem that you think is a result of the drug, talk with your doctor about

changing your prescription—don't just stop taking the medication.

2. *Circulatory problems.* Heart disease and cholesterol buildup in the arteries can restrict blood flow to the penis, making erections difficult.

3. *Nerve disorders.* Brain or spinal cord problems can cause erection problems in rare cases. Damage to nerves may also occur with alcoholism or diabetes or during surgery to the bladder, prostate, or rectum. However, refined procedures and skilled surgeons have now made surgical injury to the nerves less common.

4. *Hormone imbalances.* Testosterone, the primary male hormone, is usually not to blame for erection problems—more often a testosterone deficiency will result in a drop in libido, or sex drive. However, imbalances in the hormone insulin can cause problems.

5. *Trauma.* Pelvic trauma can be caused by some seemingly innocuous things: a fall during sports, for instance, or even long rides on an uncomfortable bike seat.

The Psychological Factor

Though most erection problems have physical causes, there's often a strong psychological component as well. It's not difficult to see how the physical and the mental get tied together. For example, a single experience with an erection problem can lead to a fear of recurrence—that apprehension can, in itself, cause the problem to happen again. In addition, men are often reluctant to see a doctor about their difficulties—

one survey found that 64 percent of men who were having erection problems waited a year to go to the doctor.

Erection problems can often be a symptom of stressful living. Everyday stress and pressure can take their toll on the body, interfering with circulation, increasing blood pressure, and contributing to heart disease. These effects of stress can hinder the ability to get or sustain an erection as well. Stressed-out men often rationalize recurrent erection problems by telling themselves they're just tired—and if the problems occur just once in a while, that's probably true. However, long-term stress that interferes with sexual function should be treated with relaxation techniques and time management strategies.

Age and Erection Problems

Researchers from the New England Research Institute who conducted the Massachusetts Male Aging Study in 1994 found that the risk of erection problems increased with age. Though these results may make it seem that erection difficulties are an effect of aging, in truth they reflect the fact that older men tend to suffer illnesses such as heart disease, high blood pressure, and diabetes more than younger men. And all of these conditions are known to affect the ability to have an erection—as are many of the drugs used to treat them. In other words, it's illness, not age, that often causes erection problems in older men. In fact, it appears that healthy older men are much less likely to have erection problems than those who are not healthy, especially if they continue to have sex. If you're facing an erection problem as an older adult, don't just accept your problem as a natural part of growing older—talk to your practitioner about possible causes and treatments.

Diagnosis

Too many men wait too long to seek medical help for chronic or recurrent erection problems. How long should you wait? Five weeks, say Bruce and Eileen MacKenzie, founders of Impotents Anonymous, an organization that provides support and information to men with erection problems and to their partners.

The specialist who treats erection problems is the urologist. You may ask your general practitioner for a referral, or check with a local medical society for a reputable urologist in your area. Remember that any doctor may practice a specialty regardless of whether he or she has obtained additional specialized training—look for board certification.

When you see a doctor, he or she will take a thorough medical history, looking for signs of problems such as heart disease and diabetes. The blood pressure in the penis might be measured to evaluate blood flow and determine if a circulation problem is the cause of erection difficulties. The doctor will also ask a lot of detailed questions about your sex life. It is best to be completely open and honest. For example, if you have more than one sex partner and experience problems only with one, it's likely that your problem is psychogenic, not physical. That's probably also the case if you have morning erections or erections during sleep (both common occurrences), but not when you want to have sex. Erection failure that starts suddenly is also most likely psychogenic, whereas problems due to physiologic causes usually build slowly.

Depending on your history, the doctor will order tests. One common, noninvasive test is the stamp test (or nocturnal penile tumescence—NPT—test), in which a strip of perforated stamps is glued around the penis before sleep. If the perforations are broken the next morning, you'll know you had an erection during the night, meaning your problems are probably psychogenic rather than physical. Another test is biothesiometry, in which a device similar to a tuning fork is held against the penis to indicate nerve damage. Ultrasound, which uses sound waves to create an image of the tissues of the penis, may also be used. The doctor may also give you a trial injection of an erection-producing drug: If it takes a high dose to produce an erection, that indicates a physical problem.

Treatment

In the past decade, great strides have been made in treating physiological erection failure. If there is an underlying condition causing a problem, it can be treated to help relieve impotence, although in many cases (such as with diabetes) the damage may be irreversible.

There are now several treatment options available, which is another reason for consulting a qualified urologist who can review all of them with you and your partner and help you decide which is most appropriate for you. In most cases, the least invasive treatment should be tried first.

1. *Oral medications.* At this time, there are no oral medications that stimulate an erection. The closest things to appear to be yohimbe (a prescription drug derived from a kind of Africa tree bark) and an antidepressant called Desyrel. However, most researchers believe yohimbe to be ineffective, having only a placebo effect, and Desyrel may cause fatigue and dangerously prolonged erections.

   The Food and Drug Administration is in the process of reviewing a possible oral drug called sildenafil (Viagra) for erection problems. The drug promotes natural erections by blocking an enzyme that causes erections to fade. In early studies, the drug was shown to be effective and well tolerated, improving sexual function in close to 50 percent in those who took it. Reported side effects included headache, backache, and indigestion.

2. *Hormonal treatments.* About 5 percent of erection problems can be attributed to low testosterone levels. In those cases, testosterone replacement—either through monthly injections or a patch worn on the skin—may sometimes solve erection problems. However, this treatment should be limited to those with genuinely low testosterone levels and should not be used in men with a high risk of prostate cancer.

3. *Vacuum devices.* This is the cheapest and least invasive way to artificially induce an erection. The flaccid penis is placed inside a hard plastic tube attached to a small, sealed vacuum pump. When the pump is activated, air pressure inside the tube is reduced, drawing blood into the penis. Once the penis is engorged, a rubber band is slipped around its base to maintain the erection. A study from the University of Texas Health Science Center at Houston reported that 85 percent of the men in the study reported that they and their partners were satisfied with the device. The pumps are available through a practitioner. Some physicians will loan pumps to patients for a trial period.

4. *Topical drugs.* Creams that are applied to the penis may become a treatment option. Italian researchers have found that minoxidil (a drug famous for preventing hair loss), applied to the penis before insertion into a vacuum device, reduced the length of time it took men to achieve an erection. In some cases, they did not need the elastic ring to sustain their erections. Early tests of a three-drug cream that is applied to the penis to create an erection also have been promising. The cream was more effective for men with psychological causes of impotence than for impotence caused by another medical condition. Additional testing must be done before the drug becomes available.

5. *Injection therapy.* Five to fifteen minutes before intercourse, a prescription vasodilator is self-injected into the base of the penis, which results in an erection that lasts one to four hours. There are currently three drugs used for this procedure: papaverine, phentolamine, and prostaglandin E1 (alprostadil or Caverject); sometimes doctors prescribe a mix of the latter two.

Apart from the problems most men have with injecting themselves in the penis, injection therapy cannot be used by anyone with heart or liver disease. Side effects may include pain in the penis, prolonged erections, and, rarely, scarring and hematoma (pockets of blood). Injection therapy can also cost as much as $200 a month.

In November 1996, a pellet form of alprostadil was approved by the Food and Drug Administration. The pellet is placed into the urethra, using a special applicator. While some men may prefer this method over an injection, not everyone responds to this form of treatment.

6. *Implants.* There are two kinds of surgical implants: semirigid, bendable rods or

inflatable tubes. With a rod implant, the penis is always rigid; it is simply bent into an upright position for intercourse. The implant is noticeable. Possible complications include infection, formation of scar tissue, and migration—the implant shifting or moving within the penis.

With an inflatable device, a pump is surgically placed in the scrotum and inflatable tubes are placed in the penis. When an erection is desired, the pump is squeezed and the tubes are filled with gel, creating an erection. When the release valve is squeezed, the gel drains from the tubes back into the pump. Possibly complications include mechanical failure, and there may be problems with infection, migration, and formation of scar tissue.

Studies show a 70 percent satisfaction rate among patients with implants ten years after surgery. In many men, implants will need to be replaced at some time because of a malfunction or other problem.

7. *Bypass surgery.* In cases where the blood flow to the penis has become blocked, surgery may be done to reroute the vessels in the pelvic area around the blockage. Surgery may also be done to seal off veins in the penis that are leaking blood. Often, this procedure is combined with bypass surgery.

Psychogenic Erection Problems

Though the majority of erection problems can be blamed on a physical cause, 20 to 25 percent are psychological, or psychogenic. But this doesn't mean that you're problem is "all in your head" or imaginary—it means that what's going on in your mind is causing a real problem that affects your penis. One of the most striking things that distinguishes a psychogenic problem from one caused by physical problems is that it usually starts suddenly, rather than beginning as the occasional episode of erectile failure that becomes more and more common.

Fear of performance failure is probably the most common cause of psychogenic erection problems, say Bruce and Eileen MacKenzie of Impotents Anonymous. This performance anxiety can trigger a vicious circle: A man has a temporary erection problem, which makes him feel self-conscious and worried about the possibility of permanent impotence, which in turn causes further problems. Lack of self-esteem, depression, premature ejaculation, marital difficulties, and a history of sexual abuse may also trigger psychogenic erection problems.

PREVENTING ERECTION PROBLEMS

It is possible to preserve your potency in both your middle and retirement years by doing all the good things that also preserve your heart: Don't smoke, cut down on fat in your diet, eat plenty of fruits, vegetables, and fiber, get regular aerobic exercise, and learn to manage stress. Two other factors to consider if you are having erection difficulties are your alcohol intake (remember Shakespeare's line about its boosting desire while taking away performance?), which you can do something about, and any prescription drugs you may be taking, which you should discuss with your doctor.

It's best to get a diagnosis of psychogenic impotence from a qualified urologist, say the MacKenzies; such a specialist should be able to refer you and your partner to an expert mental health professional who can help you get to the cause of your problem.

Counseling Options

Counseling is an option for men with psychogenic erection problems, as well as those with physical problems. Even in cases of purely physiologic erectile failure, couples counseling is virtually mandatory, say the MacKenzies of Impotents Anonymous. After successful treatment such as injection therapy or penile implants has restored the man's ability to have intercourse, the relationship with a partner needs to be restored as well. Even the most loving couple will have experienced great stress during their intercourse-less period, and they must understand that resuming sexual relations is also going to be rather stressful, especially if it involves the use of injections or devices.

Counseling focuses on communication between partners. Men and their partners are taught how to talk with each other about sexual and nonsexual problems and how to express their needs and feelings to each other. Exercises in communication can help solve relationship problems, restore self-esteem, and relieve negative emotions that may be contributing to erection problems.

Therapy may also include exercises in lovemaking designed to improve sexual function. For example, sensate focus exercises developed by sex experts William Masters and Virginia Johnson begin with sessions of simple touching and caressing. The reactions to the sessions are then discussed with the therapist. The couple eventually graduates to sessions of genital stimulation and gradually builds up over several weeks to sexual intercourse. The program helps to relieve performance anxiety and improves sexual communication.

For more information:

American Association of Sex Educators, Counselors and Therapists
P.O. Box 238
Mount Vernon, IA 52314-0238

Impotence Information Center
10700 Bren Rd., W.
Minnetonka, MN 55343
800-328-3881

Impotents Anonymous
10400 Little Patuxent Pkwy., Suite 485
Columbia, MD 21044-3502
800-669-1603
410-715-9605

Osbon Foundation
Impotence Information Center
1246 Jones St.
Augusta, GA 30903
800-433-4215

SEXUAL DYSFUNCTION

Sexual dysfunction is a term used to describe a group of disorders that prevent men and women from enjoying sex. Sexual dysfunction affects just about every man at some point in his lifetime for any number of reasons, including stress, effects of prescription drugs, psychological issues, and physical illness. Stress and psychological factors are the most common reasons for a disorder. Sometimes the disorder requires treatment, but many times help from a partner and understanding and intimacy between a couple, in a loving and caring relationship, resolves the problem. If sexual dysfunction persists, it's important to discuss it with a doctor so that the possibility of a physical problem can be ruled out.

Common Sexual Dysfunctions

The most common sexual dysfunctions among men are premature ejaculation, retarded ejaculation, erection problems, and decrease in sexual desire. Discomfort during intercourse is another, although less common, sexual dysfunction. (For more information on erection problems, see Erection Problems, p. 404.)

Premature Ejaculation

Any ejaculation that happens before it's desired is considered premature. For example, ejaculation may occur during foreplay, during penetration, or just after penetration, though there is no specific guideline other than an individual's own perception. Premature ejaculation is most common among younger men, and it's often caused by either overeagerness or anxiety about sexual performance—rarely is it due to a physical problem. Rather, it is a matter of timing.

Medications such as antidepressants and antipsychotics are sometimes prescribed for premature ejaculation, though these are not very reliable. However, there are a number of non-medical techniques that may be more successful.

A condom may be worn to decrease sensitivity and prolong orgasm. Another option is to masturbate to orgasm before a sexual encounter, since a second erection usually lasts longer than a first.

Another solution is the pinch or squeeze technique, which can be done during masturbation or during intercourse with a partner. When a man feels he is about to ejaculate—called "the moment of inevitability"—he or his partner reacts by firmly squeezing the tip of the penis, called the glans, and holding the squeeze for several seconds. Some experts recommend firmly squeezing the base of the penis. Either approach causes the erection to soften slightly, after which sexual stimulation is continued and the process is repeated. By practicing this technique, perhaps for a few dozen sessions, a man can gradually learn how to control his orgasms and delay ejaculation for as long as fifteen to twenty minutes. The same techniques can also be used without the squeeze; stimulation is simply stopped whenever the man feels ejaculation coming on.

A sex therapist may also be able to teach a man techniques that may be used to delay ejaculation.

Retarded Ejaculation

Retarded ejaculation refers to an inability to achieve orgasm once it is desired. The condition results in delayed ejaculation and, at times, no ejaculation at all. It results in frustration, physical discomfort, and a loss of interest in sex. It is just as much a problem of timing as is premature ejaculation.

Men with retarded ejaculation often brag about their prolonged erections and ability to sustain intercourse. However, if a man is not able to have an orgasm when he wishes—which is different from refraining from orgasm in order to please a partner—he may want to visit a sex therapist for treatment.

Decrease in Sexual Desire

Sexual desire, or libido, is defined as one's interest in having sexual activity. Decreased sexual desire is defined as diminished or no sexual desire, or not enough sexual desire to sustain interest in sexual activity. It's important to note that desire is not the same as participation. One can participate in sexual activity without actually having the desire. In addition, a loss of desire does not mean a loss of affection for a partner.

There is no appropriate or normal amount of sexual desire; how little is too little and how much is too much is a personal assessment. If a person feels that he would like to have more sexual desire, then he may have a sexual desire problem. However, having less sexual desire than a partner does not mean there is problem with sexual desire. There is only a discrepancy between how much each person desires sex.

A loss of libido can occur for many reasons— stress, fatigue, the birth of a child, or relationship problems, for example. Sexual abuse as a child may lead to loss of desire in an adult, as can problems with intimacy and commitment. Problems may also stem from a medical condition such as kidney or liver disease or from a prescription drug. High blood pressure and depression medications include loss of libido as a side effect.

A drop in the male sex hormone, testosterone, which stimulates the male sex drive, may affect a man's libido and capacity for arousal and an erection. In a small percentage of men, hormone levels drop with age, making libido drop. Hormone therapy for men, while it is relatively new, is becoming more widely used. However, for most men, hormone levels drop only slightly with age; two-thirds of men over 65 produce as much or more testosterone than healthy 20-year-old men. (See Male Menopause, p. 319.)

A decrease in sexual desire often passes with time and open communication with a partner, and changes in sexual desire are common as a man ages. However, if you believe you have a libido problem, visit your practitioner for a medical examination to rule out any medical conditions. Simple exercises such as sensate focus, in which partners touch each other without the goal of sex in mind, may be recommended to help boost libido and reduce stress. If a problem continues for more than three months, a sex therapist may be enlisted for treatment. If left untreated, loss of libido usually gradually grows worse over time and may lead to depression and other disorders.

CHANGES OF SEXUAL FUNCTIONING THAT COME WITH AGE

Most older people are able to lead a healthy and satisfying sex life. Older women do not lose their capacity for experiencing orgasms and older men are capable of having erections.

There are, however, a few changes that occur with age. Older men notice that it may take them longer to attain an erection, although it is usually a matter of only a few more minutes after stimulation. And he may find that the erection may not be as large or as firm as in his younger years. He may also experience a shorter sensation that an ejaculation is about to occur. The loss of erection after ejaculation may be more rapid, and it may take more time to achieve another erection.

When problems with sexual ability occur, they should not be considered normal. Talk with a doctor. Medical attention can help preserve a sexual life well into old age. He can also provide advice about sex and medical conditions such as heart disease and diabetes.

FINDING HELP

If your sexual dysfunction cannot be traced to a physical cause, your practitioner might suggest a sex therapist. This professional, trained to treat individuals or partners, reviews the partners' sexual history and provides an explanation of reproductive anatomy. The therapist will also assign exercises for an individual or couple to practice at home. These exercises are designed to increase communication, lessen anxiety, and increase sexual pleasure.

The American Association of Sex Education Counselors and Therapists can be contacted for a referral to a qualified therapist. Remember that a professional therapist will never engage in sexual activity with clients or encourage practices such as observed sex, group sex, partner switching, or other questionable situations.

Discomfort During Intercourse

Discomfort or pain during intercourse may be a sign of a physical disorder. Intercourse should not be painful; if it is, see a physician or urologist, a physician who specializes in the male reproductive organs. Painful intercourse for men may be caused by the following:

- Sexually transmitted infections such as herpes

- Irritation of the skin of the penis from allergic reactions to substances such as spermicides

- Infections of the prostate, urethra, and testicles

- Cancer of the testicles and penis

- Physical disabilities, arthritis, and lower-back pain

For more information:

American Association of Sex Educators, Counselors, and Therapists
P.O. Box 238
Mount Vernon, IA 52314-0238

INFERTILITY

According to the American Society for Reproductive Medicine, 5.3 million Americans are affected by infertility, defined as an inability to conceive after a year of unprotected intercourse. In roughly 40 percent of the cases, the cause of infertility lies within either the man or the woman. In 20 percent of cases of infertility, problems are found in both partners. An estimated 25 percent of infertile couples have more than one factor causing infertility.

When it comes to infertility in men, the cause can usually be traced to the sperm, the microscopic cells contained in the semen that penetrate the woman's egg to cause pregnancy. In a fertile man, the sperm count (number of sperm per milliliter of semen) may be anywhere from fifty to one hundred million sperm per milliliter of semen. A man with less than fifty million sperm per ejaculate is said to have oligospermia—a low sperm count.

Causes

Infertility problems in men are usually linked to problems with the sperm—either there are not enough active sperm, the sperm are damaged or weak, or they can't make its way to the egg to cause pregnancy, perhaps because of a blockage within the male reproductive system or sexual dysfunction such as an erection problem.

Causes of infertility in men include the following:

1. *Injury to the testicles.* Damage to sperm-producing cells can lower the number of sperm present in the semen.

2. *Infections.* Illness and infections such as the flu can slow sperm production and lower sperm counts. In rare cases, fertility is permanently affected. The testes may be damaged by diseases such as syphilis, the mumps, and tuberculosis, while sexually transmitted diseases such as gonorrhea and chlamydia may result in blockage and damage to the spermatic ducts.

3. *Hormonal imbalances.* Problems with testosterone production in the testicles or diseases that affect the pituitary gland (which controls puberty) can result in infertility. Hormone disorders cause a reported 5 to 10 percent of male infertility.

4. *Undescended testicles.* This condition in which the testicles do not descend from within the abdomen just before birth may cause problems with the functioning of the testicles even when it is corrected early. Undescended testicles occur in 1 percent of newborn boys.

5. *Congenital problems.* In a few men, infertility may be caused by a disorder present from birth. Disorders include cystic fibrosis, sickle cell anemia, underdeveloped testicles, and the absence of a spermatic duct.

DECLINING SPERM COUNTS?

A 1996 Paris study that reported that sperm counts were declining among healthy men throughout the world brought to the surface worries that today's environment and pollution is taking its toll on the fertility of men. However, a number of conflicting studies have failed to support or deny the Parisian study's conclusions.

For example, a study done in the French countryside found no decline in sperm counts in three hundred men between 1977 and 1992. In a Scottish study of close to six hundred donors, researchers found that 25 percent of the volunteers had less healthy sperm than men born in the 1950s. And a study of 1,283 sperm donors in New York City and in a Minnesota city found that there had been an increase in sperm counts over the past twenty-five years.

6. *A chromosomal problem.* Kleinfelter's syndrome, in which a man has an extra X chromosome, results in small testicles and infertility.

7. *Drug and alcohol use.* These cause a decrease in sperm production and may result in damaged or malformed sperm. Some activities that lower fertility include cigarette smoking, alcohol abuse, and use of such illegal drugs as cocaine, marijuana, and anabolic steroids.

8. *Varicocele.* This enlargement of the veins that surround the spermatic cord can lower sperm counts, possibly because the collection

of veins increases the temperature around the testicles. This condition occurs in 10 to 15 percent of men, though not every man with a varicocele will suffer infertility.

9. *Antibodies to sperm.* In 3 to 7 percent of men, the immune system produces antibodies to sperm, considering them invading cells. The presence of antibodies does not always cause infertility, but may cause the sperm to swim more slowly and clump together.

10. *Retrograde ejaculation.* This condition occurs when semen is forced into the bladder during ejaculation rather then through the urethra and out of the penis. It is caused by diabetes, prostate surgery, and other disorders that may damage the nerves around the bladder. It occurs in 10 percent of men with no sperm in their semen.

Infertility in Women

There are many causes for infertility in women. There may be a blockage in the fallopian tubes that prevents the sperm from reaching the egg. (The fallopian tubes connect the uterus, the female organ also known as the womb, to the ovaries, the female organs that store and release eggs. It's within the fallopian tubes that fertilization usually occurs.) Obstructions can also be caused by scarring from surgery, damage from sexually transmitted diseases, or endometriosis (abnormal growth of the lining of the uterus).

Hormonal problems can also affect ovulation (the time the eggs are released from the ovaries and can be fertilized) and fertility, as can thyroid disorders and chronic diseases such as diabetes. The uterus may be shaped incorrectly

for implantation or may contain tissue that interferes with implantation. In some women, the cervical mucus (mucus that covers the cervix, the opening of the uterus, and helps to prevent infection) contains antibodies that attack the sperm and prevent it from entering the uterus.

Diagnosis

A physical examination and medical history are initially done to determine any secondary causes of infertility—for example, a sexually transmitted disease, diabetes, or sexual dysfunction.

Before any extensive or costly testing for the woman begins, experts recommend that a man undergo a semen analysis, a simple, noninvasive procedure. A sample of the semen is collected by masturbation after two to three days of abstinence and is analyzed within two hours. At least two semen analyses are done to ensure accuracy.

The semen is examined for volume, appearance, sperm count, sperm motility (the percentage of sperm moving rapidly), and sperm morphology (shape of the sperm). The semen is also analyzed for sugar content (to check for diabetes) and to determine whether antibodies and infection are present.

Usually a semen analysis is enough for diagnosis. Blood tests also may be done to check for hormone problems. In rare cases, tests such as a chromosome analysis (in which a man's cells are grown in a tissue culture and the chromosomes are counted), a testicular biopsy (a diagnostic test for testicular cancer), or a vasogram (a test in which dye is injected into the spermatic tube to make any obstructions or abnormalities visible) may be done.

If all other tests are negative, a test known as a hamster assay may be done to see if there are any hidden abnormalities within the sperm. This diagnostic test mixes a treated hamster egg with human sperm to determine the percentage of

KEEP YOUR SPERM HEALTHY

As we've seen, most infertility problems in men involve the sperm—perhaps there aren't enough of them or perhaps the ones produced are weak or malformed. However, you can probably do more to keep your sperm healthy than you think. And keep in mind that what you do today can affect your sperm production for up to three months—the time it takes for the body to produce new sperm.

- Don't smoke, drink heavily, or use drugs. Nicotine, alcohol, and illegal substances all have a toxic effect on sperm, lowering sperm counts and possibly contributing to birth defects. One study showed that smoking was associated with a 15 percent drop in sperm counts.

- Regulate the thermostat. Sperm do best when they're kept about 4° below body temperature—the reason the scrotum adjusts itself to hang closer or farther away from the body. For sperm health, avoid hot baths, saunas, and hot tubs. You may consider wearing cotton boxer shorts rather than briefs as well, since they don't hug the testicles close to the warm body. Excessive exercise and sports such as bicycling and running may also reduce sperm counts.

- Beat stress. Stress has been linked to lower sperm counts, though experts aren't sure what the connection is. Practicing time management techniques and relaxation therapies can help reduce stress. (See Relaxation Techniques, p. 124.)

- Get your antioxidants. The antioxidant vitamins C and E and beta carotene neutralize damaging molecules known as free radicals. Free radicals are known to interfere with sperm production.

- Have some zinc. Zinc has been linked to good prostate health as well as to healthy sperm. Sources of zinc include oysters, pumpkin seeds, beef, and crabmeat. However, don't take more than the recommended dietary allowance (RDA) without a doctor's advice. The RDA for men is 15 mg daily.

- Protect yourself against dangerous substances. Some metals such as lead, pesticides, and the chemicals in glue and paint can reduce sperm counts. If you work in an environment with dangerous chemicals, use safety precautions to protect yourself. You can contact the National Institute for Occupational Safety and Health (listed at the end of this topic) with any questions about your work environment.

eggs that are penetrated by the sperm. If less than 10 percent of the eggs are penetrated, infertility is diagnosed.

Common tests for women include a pelvic examination and urine and blood tests. A more invasive test is the hysterosalpingogram, in which dye is injected into the uterus and fallopian tubes. Then, the area is visualized, using x-rays in order to diagnose any blockages. A laparoscopy, a procedure in which a thin, lighted scope is inserted through an incision in the abdomen, may also be used to diagnose infertility in women.

Treatment

In some cases, treating an underlying condition can reverse infertility. If the problem is an infection, antibiotics can be used to treat infertility. In those with erection problems, treatment for sexual dysfunction can remedy infertility problems.

Medication

If infertility can be traced to a hormonal deficiency, regular injections of hormones such as testosterone, luteinizing hormone (LH), follicle-stimulating hormone (FSH), and human chorionic gonadotrophin (hCG) can be used to regulate levels. These are the same hormones that are used to treat women with infertility, though they are used in different amounts to treat men.

Decongestants such as Sudafed can be used to treat retrograde ejaculation because they stimulate the nerves that control the bladder neck. Antidepressants may also be used for this condition.

Surgery

A varicocele can be corrected through a varicocelectomy, in which the varicose vein is tied. The traditional procedure can be done through an incision in the groin made under local or regional anesthesia. Microsurgery, in which the procedure is done through a much smaller incision with the aid of a microscope, is another option. Microsurgery is less invasive than the traditional procedure and results in fewer complications such as nerve disturbance. The traditional procedure also requires a few days in the hospital, whereas microsurgery can be done on an outpatient basis.

Another surgical treatment for a varicocele is balloon occlusion. In this procedure, a long, flexible tube with a balloon on the tip is threaded through a vein in the thigh into the enlarged testicular vein. The balloon is then inflated and lodged permanently in the vein, blocking the blood flow and shrinking the vein. This surgical procedure usually takes more time than traditional surgery, and it should be performed by a specialist who does such procedures regularly. In rare cases, the balloon may break loose and lodge somewhere else in the body, such as the heart, lung, or brain, causing serious complications or possibly death.

If a blockage exists in the epididymis or vas deferens, microsurgery can be used to open the offending duct, though it does not guarantee fertility. Some 15 to 20 percent of men who have suffered an infection become fertile after this surgery.

Advanced Treatments for Infertility

Artificial Insemination

When a man's sperm count is low or when sperm is not available because of a blockage or sexual dysfunction, artificial insemination may be used. This procedure involves the placement of sperm near the cervix (the entrance to the uterus) at the most fertile times of a woman's menstrual cycle. Artificial insemination has an average pregnancy success rate of 10 percent per cycle, according to the American Society for Reproductive Medicine. Most women who get pregnant by this method do so in the first three to five cycles.

A woman's partner or an anonymous donor may be the source of the sperm. The sperm is usually collected by masturbation. In men with an obstruction, retrograde ejaculation, or sexual dysfunction, sperm can be collected surgically for insemination.

The quality of the sperm can be improved through several techniques. In sperm enhancement, the sperm are placed in a test tube and the strongest swimmers swim to the surface, where they are collected for insemination. The sperm may also be washed to remove chemicals, blood cells, dead sperm, and other contaminants that may hinder fertilization. Antibodies may be temporarily suppressed with a course of medications to decrease immune system function.

The semen with the sperm may be placed in a small cup under the cervix and left in place for six to twelve hours to allow the sperm to swim up the cervix and enter the uterus. Also, a sample may be inserted through the cervix into the uterus, using a small tubing and a syringe, a procedure called intrauterine insemination.

In Vitro Fertilization

For women who have an obstruction within the fallopian tubes but who have healthy ovaries, in vitro fertilization (IVF) is an option. In this procedure, whose name means "fertilization in glass," fertility drugs are used to prompt the ovaries into ripening several eggs. These eggs are then surgically removed before they are released in ovulation. After the eggs are collected, they are fertilized in a glass dish, using prepared sperm collected from a partner or donor. The chances of fertilization may be increased through microinsemination, a process that concentrates sperm near the eggs in the dish. When the eggs are fertilized, they are transplanted into the uterus, where it is hoped that at least one will develop into a pregnancy. Multiple births can occur when several eggs are successfully transplanted.

THE MAN'S INFERTILITY SPECIALIST

The urologist is a physician who specializes in the treatment of reproductive and urinary health problems in men. While the first steps of diagnosing infertility can be taken by a general physician, this specialist may be recommended for more invasive tests, procedures, and surgeries. Lists of fertility specialists and information on infertility and treatment are available from RESOLVE (a self-help group for individuals and couples) and the American Society for Reproductive Medicine. (Contact information is listed at the end of this topic.)

According to the American Society for Reproductive Medicine, the rate of pregnancies resulting in live births for women undergoing IVF in the United States was approximately 18.3 percent in 1993. For women undergoing three trials of IVF, the rate rose to 50 percent.

GIFT and ZIFT

Gamete intrafallopian transfer (GIFT) is a variation of IVF. In GIFT, eggs are collected, mixed with sperm, and transferred to the fallopian tubes (rather than the uterus) during a single procedure in the hopes that fertilization may occur within the body. The American Society for Reproductive Medicine reports that pregnancy rates are 23 to 28 percent for GIFT—5 to 10 percent higher than for IVF.

Zygote intrafallopian transfer (ZIFT) is another variation. In ZIFT, the egg is collected and fertilized outside of the body. The fertilized egg is then surgically placed into a fallopian tube. In

SPERM BANKING

A sperm bank is a facility that preserves and stores sperm for future use by using cryopreservation—freezing at extremely low temperatures (–196° C). It is done by freezing a sample of sperm in liquid nitrogen. The sperm must be preserved within a few hours of when it was ejaculated in order for it to remain viable.

A sperm bank may be used by men who wish to save their sperm in the event they become infertile. For example, a man may bank sperm before chemotherapy or radiation treatments that may threaten his fertility. He may also use a sperm bank if he has low sperm counts. In this way, he's able to store multiple samples of sperm that may be used in *in vitro* insemination and other assisted fertility procedures. (However, assisted fertility procedures that use previously frozen sperm tend to be less effective than others that use sperm that has not been banked.)

Sperm banks also serve as a storage facility for sperm that has been anonymously donated. The sperm can then be used in artifical insemination procedures where there is no sperm available, for example, when a man's sperm count is too low or a woman has no male partner. Many sperm banks will pay donors for their sperm. However, donors usually must meet strict criteria before they are allowed to donate sperm. All donor sperm is screened for sexually transmitted diseases before it is used.

some cases, the egg is allowed to divide several times before it is transferred to the fallopian tube in a slightly different procedure known as tubal embryo transfer (TET).

ZIFT or TET has an advantage over GIFT because fertilization is assured. These two procedures are often used for infertility in men, especially if the ability of the sperm to penetrate and fertilize the egg is questionable.

Intercytoplasmic Sperm Injection (ICSI)

Intercytoplasmic sperm injection (ICSI) is the newest treatment for male infertility. In this procedure, doctors isolate a single sperm, which can be collected from the epididymis or the testicles. The sperm is then injected directly into an egg, using a microscopic needle. The egg is then transplanted into the woman. The success rate of the procedure is estimated at 35 percent.

Because it requires only one sperm, ICSI may be used for men who are essentially infertile, with very low sperm counts, or with vasectomies that cannot be reversed. Previously, no treatment was available for these men. Some experts say that the procedure carries genetic risks, since men with low sperm counts often have a chromosomal abnormality that may be passed on to the child. Studies to date, however, have shown that ICSI does not lead to any more abnormalities than standard IVF.

In addition, some experts oppose the procedure because they feel it can be used for genetic selection—for example, if a sperm were chosen for its chromosomal characteristics in order to create a certain gender baby.

For more information:

American Society for Reproductive Medicine [formerly the American Fertility Society]
1209 Montgomery Hwy.
Birmingham, AL 35216-2809
205-978-5000
http://www.asrm.com

National Institute for Occupational Safety and Health
4676 Columbia Parkway
Cincinnati, OH 45226-1998
800-35-NIOSH

RESOLVE
1310 Broadway
Somerville, MA 02144
617-623-1156
http://www.resolve.org

CIRCUMCISION

Circumcision—not the nose job or liposuction—is the most common form of surgery in the United States. It's also possibly the world's oldest surgical procedure, first described in the Bible some three thousand years ago.

Circumcision is the surgical removal of the foreskin, the shaft of skin that covers the glans, or the tip, of the penis. The procedure—performed on some 60 percent of male newborns in the United States—is done for religious and hygienic reasons. The fifteen-minute procedure is done by placing a bell-shaped device over the penis and then cutting away the foreskin, exposing the glans. The incision is then stitched closed, and a waterproof dressing is applied. It is usually done on boys about a week old, though adults may undergo the procedure as well.

Circumcision is often done without an anesthetic in infants, though a local anesthetic such as lidocaine may be provided. Some experts believe that infants who undergo the procedure without anesthesia are more sensitive to pain in the months following the procedure. In adults, a general anesthetic is often used.

Despite circumcision's history and the fact that it is commonplace in the United States,

QUESTIONS TO ASK

As with any physician, a fertility specialist should be chosen carefully. Some questions to ask include the following:

- Are you board-certified in your specialty?

- What is your training? Where and when were you trained?

- What is your success rate for my type of fertility problem? How many of the related procedures have you done?

- What definition of success is being used? Is it based on fertilizations? Pregnancies? Live births?

- Do you have any restrictions on treatment? Is there an age limitation or limit to number of treatments?

- What will this cost? Many insurance companies do not cover infertility testing, procedures, and surgery.

controversy surrounds the procedure: whether it should be routinely performed; whether it has any health benefits or risks; and whether it's fair to remove the foreskin of a child too young to make his own decision.

According to the American Academy of Pediatrics, there is no need for routine circumcision of all male infants. However, the organization acknowledges that the procedure carries both benefits and drawbacks. The group advocates allowing the parents to make their own decision after all of the information has been considered.

Health Issues

Many experts believe that circumcision has a number of health benefits such as prevention of infection and penile cancer. However, some researchers have found little or no relationship between circumcision and these benefits.

A 1996 study shows that uncircumcised boys were more likely to get urinary tract infections than those who were circumcised. It is thought that the foreskin tends to trap bacteria, which then infect the urethra. In addition, in young boys who are not circumcised, the foreskin may not be fully separated from the glans, creating an additional risk for urinary tract infection. Young, uncircumcised boys are also thought to be at higher risk for balanitis, infection of the foreskin and glans. Again, it might occur because of bacteria trapped beneath the foreskin.

There is also evidence that those who are not circumcised may acquire sexually transmitted diseases more easily than those who are circumcised. Several studies have shown that uncircumcised men are twice as likely as circumcised men to catch syphilis, herpes, human papillomavirus, and HIV during unsafe sex.

Yet, despite studies that find benefits to circumcision, other studies have not found any benefit to circumcision or any evidence that it lowers the risk of contracting a sexually transmitted disease. For example, a 1997 study that looked at the data from the National Health and Social Life Survey found that there is no preventive benefit to circumcision.

A risk of penile cancer is associated with a lack of circumcision. The belief is that if the penis is not kept clean, smegma, a buildup of mucus and other secretions, can collect under the foreskin and cause irritation and inflammation of the glans and contribute to the development of cancer. Almost all cases of penile cancer occur in men who are not circumcised at birth, and areas of the world where circumcision is uncommon have higher rates than countries where boys are regularly circumcised. Studies have also shown that cleanliness is a factor in penile cancer because in Sweden, where circumcision is rare but cleanliness is high, there are few cases of penile cancer.

A rare condition that may affect the uncircumcised is phimosis. In this condition, the foreskin is too small, causing painful erections. Phimosis can lead to paraphimosis, in which the tip of the penis becomes constricted by the foreskin, causing pain and swelling. It can be treated with circumcision.

Those who oppose routine circumcision in infants argue that simple hygienic measures such as regularly pulling back the foreskin and washing the penis thoroughly with soap and water can negate risks of infection and penile cancer. The main risk associated with the surgical procedure for circumcision is infection, which affects one child in every one hundred. The risk of death for the procedure is one per 500,000.

Circumcision in Adults

Although most circumcisions are performed on infants, some adult men undergo the procedure as a treatment for a health condition such as paraphimosis, phimosis, recurrent infections, or obstruction of urine flow.

In adults, circumcision is usually done by using general anesthetic. It is an outpatient procedure, with the man allowed to return home once he has urinated successfully. Discomfort usually persists for a few days. Rare complications include bleeding, infection, and injury to the penis. Keeping the area clean, according to a practitioner's advice, can help reduce the chance of infection.

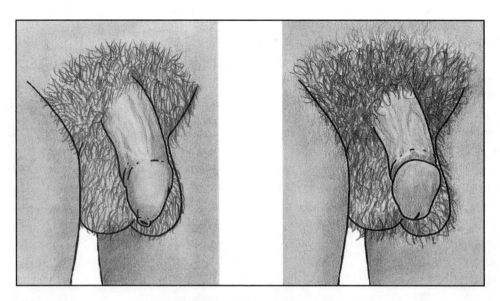

Uncircumcised/Circumcised Penis

Circumcision and Sexual Pleasure

Removal of the nerve-rich foreskin is thought by many to reduce sexual pleasure and lead to a loss of sensitivity in the penis. Opponents of the practice also maintain that men who have been circumcised have less control over ejaculation than men who still have a foreskin.

However, according to a landmark survey by sex experts William Masters, M.D., and Virginia Johnson, Ph.D., no difference could be found between the two groups of men. In fact, they observed that in most uncircumcised men, the foreskin pulled completely away from the glans during intercourse and had a limited effect on sexual pleasure or ejaculation.

Circumcision and Legal Rights

In addition to the question of pain for the newborn and the sexual health of an older man, there are a number of issues regarding rights. For example, female circumcision (a procedure in which the clitoris, the female equivalent to the penis, and labia, the surrounding folds of skin, are removed) is illegal in the United States, while male circumcision is routine and rarely given a second thought. Then there is the question of whether a man should have the opportunity to choose to keep his foreskin rather than have it removed before he's old enough to exercise choice.

Treatment

A form of treatment is available for adult circumcised men who would like to have a foreskin. The procedure, which is called foreskin restoration, epispasm, or decircumcision, involves fastening the remaining skin around the glans, gradually stretching it over the course of years until it becomes large enough to replace the foreskin. While this treatment, known as stretching, cannot add sensitivity (since nerve endings that were removed cannot grow back), the stretched skin can provide protection for the glans.

For more information:

American Academy of Pediatrics
P.O. Box 927
141 Northwest Point Rd.
Elk Grove Village, IL 60007
800-433-9016
800-421-0589 (Illinois)
708-228-5005

National Organization of Circumcision
Information Resource Centers (NOCIRC)
P.O. Box 2512
San Anselmo, CA 94979-2512
415-488-9883

PART V

The Wise Medical Consumer

Finding your way through the medical system can be a confusing, difficult endeavor, yet it is one worth mastering if you intend to take control of your health. After all, your doctor, your pharmacist, and your insurance company form a network of support for *your* benefit—to maintain your health when you're feeling good and take care of you when you're under the weather.

But there are times when the health-care system can seem overwhelming—when you're facing surgery, for example, or trying to get a simple explanation of your diagnosis from professionals who seem to speak a different language. While no one wants to find himself in the hospital or in the midst of a crisis with an insurance company (or, worse, in the midst of a malpractice suit), knowing your rights and knowing the system can mean the difference between getting the best care and getting the short end of the stick.

By understanding and feeling comfortable with the way the health-care system works, you can be sure you're making the right decisions and receiving the best of care—in other words, being a smart medical consumer.

This section of the book is designed to help you in your dealings with the health-care system and its components. You'll learn how to choose the practitioner who is right for you and how to use medications wisely. If surgery is in your future, you'll understand how to weigh the advantages and disadvantages of the procedure, decide on the right surgeon, and minimize your risk of complications. The important issues of patient rights, medical records, and informed consent are discussed. A primer on insurance is included, providing information on the different types of policies available as well as a glossary of terms. A number of valuable lists and charts also help you navigate the system by giving you the tools you need to decipher prescriptions, your medical chart, and unfamiliar medical language.

CHOOSING A PRACTITIONER

Primary-Care Physicians

Knowing and understanding the education and medical viewpoints of different health-care professionals can help you to make choices that may ultimately ensure better health care for you and your family.

Finding a primary-care physician—a doctor who will take care of any common health concerns and provide you with preventive care—is much more difficult than it used to be. First of all, there are many more specialists and alternative practitioners available. While at one time a general practitioner handled all that was wrong with you, the medical landscape is now filled with practitioners who specialize, some who subspecialize, and some who only consult with subspecialists.

A primary-care physician is the practitioner you use for most—if not all—of your initial health-care needs. This is the doctor you call when you come down with the flu, sprain your ankle, or throw your back out. Ideally, you should have a long-term relationship with your primary-care physician—he or she should know you and be familiar with your medical history and lifestyle, both factors that can help with diagnosis.

Most people visit an allopathic physician (doctor of medicine, or M.D.) or an osteopathic physician (doctor of osteopathy, or D.O.) for primary care. Except for a difference in philosophy, these practitioners are essentially the same. M.D.'s focus their attention on the condition or disease being treated, while D.O.'s hold that the body is an interrelated system. D.O.'s emphasize the role of bones, muscles, and joints in a person's well-being, and often practice a more hands-on form of treatment than M.D.'s do. Other than this distinction, M.D.'s and D.O.'s undergo the same type of training, hold the same unlimited practice rights, and have roughly the same specialized fields. M.D.'s may belong to the American Medical Association, while D.O.'s may belong to the American Osteopathic Association.

There are three types of primary-care physicians from which to choose.

1. *General practitioners.* These are physicians who have completed medical school and have one year of internship experience—supervised on-the-job training. While at one time most doctors were generalists, since the 1950s general practice has begun to decline, with more and more physicians turning toward specialization.

2. *Family practitioners.* These doctors are specialists who have completed three years of supervised specialty training (called a residency) that covers internal medicine, minor surgery, psychiatry, preventive medicine, orthopedics, pediatrics, obstetrics, and gynecology.

3. *Internists.* Internists are specialists in internal medicine who have advanced training in diagnosing and treating problems involving the heart, lungs, kidneys, gastrointestinal system, and endocrine system. They usually have no training in pediatrics, obstetrics, or orthopedics.

Criteria for Selecting a Doctor

The time to find the right practitioner is *before* you need one. Don't wait until you have a

CHOOSING A DOCTOR WITHIN A HEALTH MAINTENANCE ORGANIZATION

If you're involved with a health maintenance organization (HMO), a form of managed care, you might also have to face the problem of a limited choice of doctors. These health insurance programs contract with specific physicians, who provide care for a set fee per patient per month. As a result, you must seek care only from selected doctors in order to be covered under the plan, and in most cases, a referral is necessary if you need to see a specialist.

Even before you join a HMO, check the list of practitioners to be sure that you'll be satisfied with your choices. When you enter a managed care program, you basically agree to use its doctors and facilities for a set monthly premium. If you go outside its network of providers, you will either pay a significant portion of the cost or all of it. Therefore, it is essential that you are comfortable with the doctors and facilities in the program.

Before you decide to join:

- Make sure all primary-care doctors and specialists are board certified in their specialties.

- Make sure the managed care program has no fewer than three doctors in any specialty and no fewer than ten primary-care physicians.

- Be sure you can pick any doctor on the list. Sometimes, physicians limit the number of patients they take from any given managed care program. Check to see that the practice(s) you're interested in using is open to new patients.

- Find out what happens when your doctor is unable to see you or is on vacation. Who is the backup practitioner?

medical problem or, worse yet, a medical emergency. Friends, neighbors, and family members are good sources of recommendations—word of mouth is still one of the best methods of finding a doctor. The old adage of "If you want to find a good doctor, ask a nurse" is probably a good one, but not always practical. Here are some other suggestions:

- Your present doctor

- Doctor referral services

- Newspaper advertisements of doctors announcing the opening of a new practice

- Telephone directory listings

- Your company personnel office

- Your health insurance company

- Senior centers

When Should You Switch Doctors?

You should change doctors when you are no longer getting the best care for your dollar, but that's not always easy to evaluate. First, you should know the legal aspects of the doctor-patient relationship. Once established, this relationship becomes a legal arrangement, which only four conditions can end:

- If both parties agree to end the relationship

- If it is ended by the patient

- If the doctor is no longer needed

- If the doctor gives reasonable notice that he/she is withdrawing from the relationship

If these procedures are not followed, a patient could make a case for abandonment by the doctor.

When things are going wrong with the doctor-patient relationship, certain signs should serve as warnings to you that all is not well.

1. *Overcrowded waiting rooms.* The doctor who crowds too many appointments into the day is going to leave at least one person waiting too long and/or have to whisk people in and out of examinations/consultations.

2. *Excessive waiting time.* You should be willing to accept the explanation that the doctor had an emergency, but not if it happens every time. To save time and money, try telephoning ahead to ask if the doctor is on schedule or what the approximate wait is.

3. *A rushed appointment.* A doctor who does not permit you sufficient time to explain your symptoms or complaints and ask questions may not be providing the best of care.

4. *Unavailability.* A doctor should be available to speak with you over the phone if you have a question or a problem. Be aware, however, that it is not uncommon—or even unreasonable—for a doctor to charge for a telephone consultation, but the fee should be less than that of a regular office visit.

5. *Lack of communication.* How well does the doctor explain the medical problem and any proposed tests and/or treatments? If the doctor does not engage in effective dialogue with you, preferring instead to issue orders or pronouncements and if he/she shows little interest in what you have to say or shows annoyance when you raise questions, then you may want to shop around.

6. *Fee increases.* If you're like most people, you can accept an increase in fees when the increase is justified by better service or a legitimate claim of higher overhead. But paying more money for the same old service does not set well with you. The problem may be compounded by your insurance company's unwillingness to pay the higher fee, meaning you're stuck with an out-of-pocket expense.

7. *Refuses access to medical records.* Treating your medical record with confidentiality is one thing; denying you rightful access is another. How can you develop an equal partnership with a doctor who does not trust you enough to share copies of *your own* health history and medical record with you? (See Medical Records, p. 479.)

The Get-Acquainted Visit

Doctor-shopping should include a get-acquainted visit, a short, fifteen-minute meeting, the object of which is to determine if you and the doctor are right for each other.

When you telephone for an appointment, be sure to tell the receptionist that you want to arrange a get-acquainted visit. If the doctor refuses, go on to the next doctor on your list. You should be aware that some doctors charge a fee for a get-acquainted visit and some do not.

The first thing you want to notice is the doctor's office and staff. Most offices will have a receptionist who will greet you and ask you to complete a few forms for their records. Ask the receptionist to orient you to the particulars regarding making appointments, telephoning the doctor, getting prescription refills, and obtaining copies of your medical records. Be sure to let them know, especially the doctor, that you have not yet decided on becoming a patient.

A first-time visit will probably run ten to fifteen minutes, so you need to have your questions ready and make the minutes count. When you meet the doctor, concentrate on credentials—medical degree, board certification, and other specialized and/or postgraduate education—and hospital affiliations. If the doctor is not on the staff of any hospital, or at least the hospital of your choosing, then the doctor may not be able to serve you when your needs are the greatest. Ask about the doctor's fee schedule and payment plans. A doctor who will openly discuss fees may be more willing to discuss other aspects of your medical care. If you are on Medicare, find out if the doctor accepts assignment. If not, ask if an exception can be made in your case; it's negotiable.

Determine what importance the doctor places on preventive health measures and what the doctor's philosophy of practice is—especially whether the patient is seen as a full partner in health care. An excellent point of reference is the People's Medical Society Code of Practice, which immediately follows this topic.

Pay particular attention to the doctor's manner and attitude as he or she answers your questions. Is the doctor addressing the heart of your questions and answering in a forthright manner?

You should also notice a few other things.

- Is the practice solo or group? While a group practice offers the advantage of someone always covering the office even during weekends, the possible downside is an overcrowded waiting room and the feeling that you are receiving assembly-line medical care. The doctor may be a part of a one-specialty group or a multispecialty group where there is a mix of primary-care doctors and specialists. The latter can be helpful when, needing a second opinion and having to find a specialist, you can be referred to another doctor in the group. But the multispecialty group works against your best interests when the doctors refer only to the specialists in the group and not necessarily to the best specialist for you.

- Does the office appear neat and clean?

- Is the office staff professional and friendly?

- Is your insurance coverage accepted?

- Was your appointment kept on time?

Specialists and Board Certification

A specialist is a doctor who concentrates on a specific body system, age group, or disorder. After obtaining an M.D. (doctor of medicine) or D.O. (doctor of osteopathy) degree, a doctor then undergoes two to three years of supervised specialty training (called a residency) to become a specialist. Many specialists also take one or more years of additional training (called a fellowship) in a specific area of their specialty, called a subspecialty.

Board Certification

How can you tell if a doctor is a trained specialist? A doctor who has taken extra training in his or her field often chooses to become what is called board certified. In addition to the extra training, the doctor must pass a rigorous examination administered by a specialty board, a national board of professionals in that specialty field. A doctor who passes the board examination is given the status of Diplomate. Plus, most board-certified doctors become members of their medical specialty societies, and any doctor who meets the full requirements for membership is called a "Fellow" of the society and may use the designation. For instance, the title "FACOG" after a doctor's name denotes that he or she is a Fellow of the American College of Obstetricians.

In its most basic sense, board certification indicates that a physician has completed a course of study in accordance with the established educational standards. Board certification has been called a minimum standard of excellence and nothing more. Paper certification does not produce professional excellence. On the other hand, although there are some inferior doctors who somehow manage to become board certified and some excellent doctors without board certification, board certification is a good sign that the person is up to date on the procedures, theories, and success-failure rates in the specialty.

The training requirements are similar for D.O.'s (doctors of osteopathy, or osteopathic physicians) and M.D.'s (doctors of medicine, or allopathic physicians), though they are certified by different boards. Allopaths are certified by one or more of the twenty-four member boards of the American Board of Medical Specialties (ABMS); board-certified osteopathic physicians are designated by the department of certification of the American Osteopathic Association (AOA). The training programs for ABMS-recognized specialties are only offered at accredited medical schools with approved programs. There are also self-designated medical specialty boards, which are not recognized by the ABMS or the AOA and may not have the same standards and training requirements as the national boards.

The Official ABMS Directory of Board-Certified Medical Specialists (published by Marquis Who's Who and available at most local libraries) lists ABMS board-certified specialists in the country who wish to be included. The entries include information on education, state, specialty, membership in professional organizations of his or her specialty, and training. It also lists where practitioners did their residency training and how long they've been practicing as doctors.

Another directory is the *American Medical Directory: Physicians in the United States*, again usually found in most local libraries. This lists every doctor who is a member of the American Medical Association, year of license, primary/secondary specialty, type of practice, board certification, and premedical and medical school education.

The People's Medical Society Code of Practice

In 1983, the People's Medical Society created the Code of Practice as a statement we believe each doctor should subscribe to. Ask your doctor to review it and tell you whether he or she will apply it to your care.

I will assist you in finding information resources, support groups and health-care providers to help you maintain and improve your health. When you seek my care for specific problems, I will abide by the following Code of Practice:

Office Procedures

1. I will post or provide a printed schedule of my fees for office visits, procedures, tests and surgery and provide itemized bills.

2. I will provide certain hours each week when I will be available for nonemergency telephone consultation.

3. I will schedule appointments to allow the necessary time to see you with minimal waiting. I will promptly report test results to you and return phone calls.

4. I will allow and encourage you to bring a friend or relative into the examining room with you.

5. I will facilitate your getting your medical and hospital records and will provide you with copies of your test results.

Choice in Diagnosis and Treatment

6. I will let you know your prognosis, including whether your condition is terminal or will cause disability or pain, and will explain why I believe further diagnostic activity or treatment is necessary.

7. I will discuss with you diagnostic, treatment and medication options for your particular problem (including the option of no treatment) and describe in understandable terms the risk of each alternative, the chances of success, the possibility of pain, the effect on your functioning, the number of visits each would entail, and the cost of each alternative.

8. I will describe my qualifications to perform the proposed diagnostic measures or treatments.

9. I will let you know of organizations, support groups and medical and lay publications that can assist you in understanding, monitoring, and treating your problem.

10. I will not proceed until you are satisfied that you understand the benefits and risks of each alternative and I have your agreement on a particular course of action.

QUESTIONS TO ASK BEFORE VISITING A SPECIALIST

You usually encounter a specialist when your primary-care doctor wants to confirm a diagnosis or wants a second opinion. If your family physician recommends a specialist or you seek one on your own, then here are questions that need to be answered:

- "Why do I have to see a specialist?" Ask your doctor to furnish you a complete and understandable, point-by-point diagnostic portrait. Going to a specialist should not be a casual next step routinely taken in every medical situation.

- "Why this kind of specialist?" You need to know about the specialist's areas of expertise and what is involved with the performance of that specialty. Knowing this will help you determine whether you want to see the specialist at all. That is an option. You don't have to see a specialist (or see that particular specialist) immediately if you are not convinced that consultation is justified.

- "Why this particular specialist?" Why Dr. Jones and not Dr. Smith? Are you being sent to Dr. Jones because she is an excellent representative of her profession? Or is it because Dr. Jones and your doctor are friends who have an arrangement, each recommending the other? While there is nothing wrong with friends referring patients to each other, you want to feel confident that competence is the basic reason for the referral.

If you wish to call to verify the credentials of a specialist, you can contact the American Board of Medical Specialties at 800-776-CERT. For more information on osteopathic certification, contact the American Osteopathic Association, Department of Certification, 142 East Ontario Street, Chicago, IL 60611; 800-621-1773 or 312-280-5845.

GLOSSARY OF MEDICAL SPECIALTIES

Below is the list of what the American Medical Association calls "self-designated [medical] specialty classifications." Translated, this means that these specialties are those the physicians use to describe themselves and their primary and secondary fields of practice. The American Medical Association is quick to point out that this list does not imply "endorsement" or "recognition" [quotes theirs] by the AMA; it is merely a catalog of the myriad of possible areas of "expertise" a physician may claim.

You should be aware that a licensed physician may practice any specialty and call himself/herself a specialist in a particular field, whether or not the physician is actually board certified in that specialty.

Abdominal surgery. Subspecialty of surgery involving the abdominal organs.

Adolescent medicine. Subspecialty of pediatrics dealing with the medical needs of young people between the ages of 14 and 19.

Allergy and immunology. Subspecialty of internal medicine or pediatrics involving the diagnosis and treatment of all forms of allergy and allergic disease and other disorders potentially involving the immune system.

Anesthesiology. Involves the administration of drugs (anesthetics) to prevent pain or induce unconsciousness during surgical operations or diagnostic procedures. Anesthesiologists may further specialize in critical care medicine as practiced in critical care and intensive care units, postanesthesia recovery rooms, and other settings.

Cardiovascular diseases (cardiology). Subspecialty of internal medicine that deals with the heart and blood vessels.

Cardiovascular surgery. Subspecialty of cardiology involving surgery on the heart and associated vascular system. Cardiovascular surgeons perform open-heart surgery, which may include heart transplants.

Colon and rectal surgery (proctology). Diagnosis and treatment of diseases of the intestinal tract, rectum and anus.

Cosmetic surgery. Surgery to reshape normal structures of the body in order to improve a person's appearance and self-esteem.

Dermatology. Diagnosis and treatment of benign and malignant disorders of the skin and related tissues. The dermatologist also diagnoses and treats a number of diseases transmitted through sexual activity.

Diagnostic radiology. Subspecialty of radiology employing the use of ionizing, electromagnetic, or sound wave imaging devices to diagnose medical problems.

Emergency medicine. Focuses on the immediate decision making and action necessary to prevent death or further disability. It is primarily based in the hospital emergency department.

Endocrinology. Subspecialty of internal medicine that deals with disorders of the internal (or endocrine) glands such as the thyroid and adrenal glands. Endocrinology also deals with disorders such as diabetes, pituitary diseases, and hormonal problems.

Family practice/general practice. Concerned with total health care of the individual and the family. The scope of family practice is not limited by age, sex, organ system, or type of disease.

Gastroenterology. Subspecialty of internal medicine that involves disorders of the digestive tract: stomach, bowels, liver, gallbladder and related organs.

General surgery. Surgery of the parts of the body that are not in the domain of specific surgical specialties (some areas do overlap, however).

Geriatrics. Subspecialty of family practice and internal medicine that deals with the diseases of the elderly and problems associated with aging.

Gynecology. Diagnosis and treatment of problems associated with the female reproductive organs.

Hand surgery. Subspecialty of orthopedic surgery, general surgery, or plastic surgery that is limited to the musculoskeletal structure of the hands, including bone, muscle, and ligaments.

Head and neck surgery. Subspecialty of otolaryngology that deals with surgery of the head and neck, excluding the brain and eyes.

Hematology. Diagnosis and treatment of diseases and disorders of the blood and blood-forming parts of the body.

Immunology. Study and treatment of problems of the body's immune system, which may include allergies, infections and life-threatening diseases such as AIDS (acquired immune deficiency syndrome).

Infectious diseases. Subspecialty of internal medicine involving the diagnosis and treatment of life-threatening infectious illnesses.

Internal medicine. Diagnosis and nonsurgical treatment of diseases, especially those of adults. While internists may set up practices in which they act as highly trained family doctors, they often subspecialize in many other areas.

Laryngology. Branch of medicine that involves the throat, pharynx, larynx, nasopharynx, and tracheobronchial tree.

Maxillofacial surgery. Subspecialty of dentistry that deals with problems of the mouth and jaw.

Neonatal-perinatal medicine. Subspecialty of pediatrics that deals with disorders of newborn infants, including premature ones.

Nephrology. Subspecialty of internal medicine concerned with disorders of the kidney.

Neurology. Diagnosis and nonsurgical treatment of diseases of the brain, spinal cord, and nerves.

Neurological surgery (neurosurgery). Diagnosis and surgical treatment of diseases of the brain, spinal cord, and nerves.

Nuclear medicine. Use of radioactive substances for diagnosis and treatment.

Nuclear radiology. Subspecialty of radiology that involves the use of radioactive materials in the diagnosis and treatment of disease.

Obstetrics and gynecology. Care of pregnant women and treatment of disorders of the female reproductive system.

Occupational medicine. Subspecialty of preventive medicine that deals with the special physical and psychological risks in industry.

Oncology. Subspecialty of internal medicine concerned with the diagnosis and treatment of all types of cancer and other benign and malignant tumors.

Ophthalmology. Diagnosis, monitoring, and medical/surgical treatment of vision problems and other disorders of the eye, including the prescription of glasses/contact lenses.

Orthopedic surgery (orthopedics). Care of diseases of the muscles and diseases, fractures, and deformities of the bones and joints.

Otolaryngology. Medical and surgical care of patients with diseases and disorders that affect the ears, respiratory, and upper alimentary systems and related structures: in general, the head and neck.

Otology. Subspecialty of otolaryngology that deals with the medical treatment of and surgery on the ear.

Pathology. Examination and diagnosis of organs, tissues, body fluids, and excrement.

Pediatrics. Concerned with the physical, emotional, and social health of children from birth to young adulthood.

Physical medicine and rehabilitation (physiatry). Diagnosis, evaluation, and treatment of patients with impairments and/or disabilities involving musculoskeletal, neurologic, cardiovascular, or other body systems.

Preventive medicine. Focuses on the health of individuals and the prevention of disease through immunization, good health practices, and concern with environmental and occupational factors.

Psychiatry. Diagnosis, treatment and prevention of mental, emotional and/or behavioral disorders. (Do not confuse the psychiatrist with the nonphysician psychologist.)

Psychosomatic medicine. More a way of practicing medicine than a specialty as such; a concept of total medical care that considers the emotional needs of the patient by taking into account the mind-and-body interactions of the patient.

Public health. Branch of medicine that deals with the protection and improvement of community health by organized community effort and includes the monitoring and screening of populations to prevent the spread of communicable diseases. Many consider public health to be allied with, if not actually a subspecialty of, preventive medicine.

Pulmonary diseases. Subspecialty of internal medicine concerned with diseases of the lungs and other chest tissues, including pneumonia, cancer, occupational diseases, bronchitis, emphysema, and other complex disorders of the lungs.

Radiology. Study and use of various types of radiation, including x-rays, in the diagnosis and treatment of disease.

Reconstructive surgery. Surgery on abnormal structures of the body, caused by congenital defects, developmental abnormalities, trauma, infection, tumors, and disease. It is generally performed to improve function but may also be done to approximate a normal appearance.

Rheumatology. Subspecialty of internal medicine that deals with diseases of the joints, muscles and tendons, including arthritis.

Rhinology. See otolaryngology.

Surgical critical care (traumatic surgery). Subspecialty of surgery that deals with the treatment of the critically ill patient, particularly the trauma victim and the postoperative patient in the emergency department, intensive care unit, trauma unit, burn unit, and other similar settings.

Therapeutic radiology (radiation oncology). Subspecialty of radiology that deals with the therapeutic applications of radiant energy, especially in the treatment of malignant tumors.

Thoracic surgery. Operative, peri-operative, and critical care of patients with disease-causing conditions within the chest, including coronary-artery disease, cancers of the lung, esophagus, and chest wall, abnormalities of the great vessels and heart valves, and injuries to the airway and chest.

Urology. Diagnosis and treatment of diseases of the urinary system, as well as the organs of reproduction in men, such as the prostate.

Urological surgery. Subspecialty of urology that deals with the surgical treatments of the adrenal gland and genitourinary system.

Vascular surgery. Subspecialty of surgery that deals with medical disorders affecting the blood vessels, excluding those of the heart, lungs, and brain.

DENTISTS

Dentistry is concerned with the care and treatment of teeth and the surrounding tissue and bone structure of the oral cavity. Dentists treat problems with a wide array of materials and techniques and emphasize prevention of tooth and mouth problems as well as restorative procedures such as crowns.

The Education of Dentists

Some dentists affix the initials D.D.S. after their names and others have D.M.D. Currently, the majority of dental schools in the United States award their graduates the D.D.S. (doctor of dental surgery) degree, but more and more schools are adopting the other designation—the D.M.D. (doctor of medical dentistry) degree. The schools that award the D.M.D. degree claim that their curriculums are more "medically oriented," but, in actuality, there is no difference between the two designations. According to the American Dental Association, all dental schools in the United States are accredited, with clearly stated requirements, and there is no difference in what is taught.

Dental Specialties

According to the American Dental Association (ADA), a specialist in a field of dentistry must have two years of education beyond the general degree at an accredited dental school and/or certification by an ADA-recognized certifying organization. To be granted board certification, a dentist must pass qualifying examinations administered by a specialty board. Certification is not necessarily an indicator of higher quality or skill, but it does indicate additional education.

The American Dental Association has approved eight special areas of dental practice: endodontics (root canals); oral and maxillofacial surgery (surgery on mouth, jaw, and related structures; oral pathology (diagnosis of mouth disease); orthodontics (correction of malocclusion, or improper position of the teeth); pedontics (children's teeth); periodontics (gum disease); prosthodontics (prosthetic teeth—caps, bridges, and dentures); and dental public health (community education and care). Cosmetic dentisty, although not a recognized specialty, is also a growing field of specialty dentistry.

Dental Hygienists

The dentist is not the only professional found in most dental offices. Another is the dental hygienist, a specialist in oral hygiene. Hygienists clean your teeth and make notes on the general health status of your mouth, gums, and teeth. They also take x-rays, apply fluoride, administer topical anesthesia and apply tooth sealants. The duties of the hygienist vary according to the licensing laws in the state where they are practicing.

To become a dental hygienist, a person must complete a two-year program (for a certificate or associate degree); a four-year program (for a baccalaureate degree); or a master's level program (for those interested in research, education, and administration). After graduating from an accredited program, a person takes a national board examination and a regional and state board examination before becoming licensed

COMMON DENTAL TERMS

Amalgam. Silver/mercury alloy used to fill teeth.

Anteriors. Front teeth.

Bitewing x-rays. X-rays of upper and lower back teeth.

Bonding. New tooth restoring process in which the tooth surface is mildly etched to create microscopic voids for receiving a plastic material that will change the tooth shape or improve its appearance.

Bridge. A replacement for a missing tooth or missing teeth, to "bridge" the gap. A bridge can be fixed or removable.

Calculus (tartar). Plaque hardened into crusty deposits.

Caries. The disease that causes cavities.

Crown. (1) The part of the tooth above the gum line; (2) Also called cap for jacket: An artificial tooth-shaped cap put over the natural crown of a tooth after some of it has been ground away to make space, as a cover for a broken tooth, a way to save a tooth so full of filling that it's crumbling away or a necessary support for a fixed bridge.

continues

Fluoride. Mineral that protects teeth from decay.

Full mouth x-rays. A series of sixteen to eighteen x-rays.

Gingiva. Gum tissue.

Gingivitis. Inflammation of the gums, an early form of gum disease.

Malocclusion. A bad bite caused by the upper and lower teeth not meeting properly when they are brought together.

Nitrous oxide (laughing gas). Used as a dental analgesic to reduce anxiety.

Novocain. A local anesthetic.

Operatory. Dental treatment room.

Periodontitis (pyorrhea). An advanced form of gum disease in which the underlying bone is attacked.

Plaque. Bacterial substance that caused dental decay.

Pocket. A space between the tooth and the gum where food can be trapped, usually associated with gum disease.

Posteriors. Back teeth.

Primary teeth (baby teeth). A child's first teeth.

Prophylaxis. Professional teeth cleaning.

Root. Part of the tooth anchored to the jaw.

Root canal therapy. A process involving drilling down to the nerve of the tooth, removing it and other dead material, then sealing up the tooth. A root canal serves to save the tooth rather than extract it.

Scaling. The removal of calculus, stains, and other deposits from the tooth surface by dental instruments, including ultrasonic scaling machines.

Sealant. Plastic coating to protect teeth from decay.

There are five surfaces to a tooth:

Occlusal. The biting side.

Mesial. The side toward the midline.

Distal. The side away from the midline.

Facial. The side toward the face.

Lingual. The side toward the tongue.

Temporomandibular joints. The joints that connect the jawbone to the skull near the ear and that allow the mouth to move.

Temporomandibular disorder (TMD; or myofascial pain dysfunction). A catchall phrase to describe a variety of head and neck pains and other symptoms related to the temporomandibular joints.

Third molars. Wisdom teeth.

by the state. Those who are licensed use the designation R.D.H. or L.D.H. to indicate that they are registered (or licensed) dental hygienists.

For more information:

American Dental Association
Bureau of Communications
211 E. Chicago Ave.
Chicago, IL 60611
312-440-2806

American Dental Hygienist Association
444 N. Michigan Ave., Suite 3400
Chicago, IL 60611
800-243-ADHA
312-440-8900

COMPLEMENTARY THERAPIES

It's no secret that modern medicine doesn't have all the answers. With that truth in mind, millions of Americans are turning to complementary, or alternative, therapies. More and more, these therapies are being found effective and useful in managing conditions ranging from headaches and stroke to muscle soreness and stress.

Complementary therapies—for example, herbal therapy, biofeedback, and acupuncture—are usually considered to be outside the realm of mainstream medicine. However, conventional practitioners are starting to recommend some forms of these therapies along with traditional medical care. While these nontraditional treatments are often called *alternative*, today the preferred term is *complementary*. The change in terminology is intended to emphasize the fact that these therapies work hand in hand with traditional medical regimens, not instead of them.

What follows is a discussion of some of the most common complementary therapies—where they originated, what they involve, what they treat, and how to find a practitioner in your community. Many of these therapies can also be used for self-care for common conditions at home. Remember, however, to talk with your regular practitioner before starting any other therapy and keep him or her abreast of your progress; while most complementary therapies have no side effects, there are some—such as herbal therapy—that may be inappropriate or even dangerous for some people. In addition, some therapies may not be appropriate for use in treating some conditions.

Acupressure

In acupressure, a practitioner known as an acupressurist applies pressure at specific points on the body to stimulate the body's healing powers. As with acupuncture, it involves an acceptance of opposites of yin and yang (expressed as day and night, male and female, negative and positive) and a flow of a life force called ch'i. Chinese medicine teaches that in a healthy person the yin and yang forces must be balanced and that the ch'i must be flowing through the body smoothly along a set of invisible pathways known as meridians. When the flow is disrupted, illness occurs. Shiatsu is the Japanese equivalent of Chinese acupressure and is based upon these same principles.

The acupressurist examines the meridians, then rubs or massages specific acupressure points along the meridians with the fingers (rather than with needles, as in acupuncture) in order to promote an even flow of ch'i, restoring health and energy. Acupressure can be easily learned, perhaps from a practitioner, a book, or a class, and used at home for self-care.

For more information:

Acupressure Institute
1533 Shattuck Ave.
Berkeley, CA 94709
510-845-1059

Acupuncture

Acupuncture is an ancient Chinese healing art that reportedly dates from 1600 B.C. In this therapy, a practitioner, called an acupuncturist, inserts very thin needles under the skin to treat illness and restore good health. Acupuncture has attracted renewed attention in the West since the reopening of China in the early 1970s. New studies are showing acupuncture to be effective for a number of conditions such as asthma, nausea, bronchitis, and stroke. It is also effective for treating addictions, chronic pain, and sports injuries. Acupuncture may be used in conjunction with herbal medicine, massage, relaxation techniques, and other therapies.

A key element in understanding acupuncture is acceptance of the Eastern belief in the opposites of yin and yang (expressed as day and night, male and female, negative and positive) and a flow of a life force called ch'i. Chinese medicine teaches that in a healthy person the yin and yang forces must be balanced and the ch'i must be flowing through the body smoothly along a set of invisible pathways known as meridians.

When illness occurs, it's thought to be because the ch'i is blocked or is not flowing smoothly. The acupuncturist then examines the meridians, feeling for the specific pulse of that meridian, and selects acupuncture sites. The acupuncturist then places extremely thin needles of gold, silver, or copper in the sites just below the skin to stimulate the flow of the ch'i and correct the imbalance. The needles may be left in place for a few seconds or for an hour or more. After successful treatment, the ch'i circulates freely and balance is restored.

To date, acupuncture is licensed in more than twenty-five states. In states where there is no licensing board, only licensed medical and osteopathic physicians may practice acupuncture, or the acupuncturist must operate under physician supervision or referral. Contact one of the following organizations for help in finding a practitioner near you.

For more information:

American Association of Acupuncture and Oriental Medicine
433 Front St.
Catasauqua, PA 18032
610-433-2448
http://www.aaom.org

National Commission for Certification of Acupuncturists
P.O. Box 97075
Washington, DC 20090-7075
202-232-1404

Traditional Acupuncture Institute
American City Building
10227 Wincopin Circle, Suite 100
Columbia, MD 21044
301-596-6006

Alexander Technique

The Alexander technique is a manipulative therapy that attempts to correct a range of disorders by improving posture. The technique was developed in the late 1800s by F. Matthias Alexander, an Australian actor who had experienced problems with his voice. He found the solution to his problem was to change his posture, and he concluded that by misusing our bodies—slouching, tensing, and slumping—

we bring on illness and stress. As a result, he developed a technique to maintain proper use of the body.

The Alexander technique teaches what *not* to do with your body. There are no formal exercises, and technique varies according to the individual. In most cases, a teacher does an evaluation to determine where changes are needed and where reconditioning must begin. Then the teacher manipulates various parts of the body such as the head, neck, limbs, and pelvis, and instructions are given on how to correct any problems. The technique is repeated until the problem is corrected.

To learn the Alexander technique, you should find a qualified instructor.

For more information:

American Center for the Alexander Technique
Abraham Goodman House
129 W. 67th St.
New York, NY 10023
212-799-0468

North American Society of Teachers of the Alexander Technique
P.O. Box 517
St. Petersburg, FL 33733
813-343-4811

Applied Kinesiology

Applied kinesiology, also called touch for health, is a form of healing that uses therapeutic touch to correct imbalances in the body's energy system and to restore health. In the system, developed by George Goodheart, certain muscle groups are thought to be related to the major internal systems of the body. By testing muscle strength and examining posture, a kinesiologist (a practitioner of applied kinesiology) can determine the state of the related internal

system. Food or nutritional supplements may also be given to determine its effect on muscle strength. The technique is helpful in diagnosing, for example, allergies and problems of an emotional nature, which can then be treated.

This method is complicated because detecting the subtle differences in muscle strength in a person can be difficult, but it can be learned from a qualified practitioner and practiced in the home.

For more information:

International College of Applied Kinesiology
6405 Metcalf Ave., Suite 503
Shawnee Mission, KS 66202
913-384-5336
icak@aol.com

Ayurvedic Medicine

Ayurveda is a system of holistic medicine that originated in India. It is among the oldest of the healing arts, founded on the mysticism of Eastern religion. Through the centuries, ayurvedic medicine has grown to be more scientific, and much of modern ayurvedic practice follows Western practice. Branches of ayurvedic medicine include surgery, pediatrics, and psychology.

Ayurveda views the person in terms of body, mind, and spirit. Ayurvedic physicians believe that disease is caused by imbalances in the body's five basic elements (earth, fire, water, air, and ether) and the forces in those elements.

The elements combine into three principles, or humors, known as the *tridosha*. The first of these humors is *vata*, which is formed by air and ether, and the second is *pitta*, formed by fire and water. The third and last is *kapha*, formed by earth and water. These elements govern all the biological, psychological, and physiological functions of the individual. When these elements are out of balance, disease occurs.

An ayurvedic physician will take a complete history from the patient and conduct a thorough physical examination before determining what caused the particular imbalance. Fasting, baths, diets, and applications to the skin are used to cleanse the body before a specific treatment is recommended. A complete collection of medications is available, and drugs to restore normal health and balance are given in the form of jellies, tinctures, powders, pills, and oils.

For more information:

Ayurvedic Institute
P.O. Box 23445
Albuquerque, NM 87192-1445
505-291-9698

Educational Service of Marharishi Ayurvda International
P.O. Box 49667
Colorado Springs, CO 80949
800-843-8332

Bach Flower Remedies

These remedies, devised in the early 1930s by Edward Bach, M.D., a British bacteriologist who later became a pathologist, are derived from trees and plants and used to heal emotional states that he believed were the cause of many diseases. The remedies have been found to be useful in treating stress-related conditions.

The remedies are created by collecting the flowering heads of wild plants, placing them in spring water to extract their essence and then filtering the solution before bottling. He believed that the solutions he prepared contained the properties, as he saw them, of the derivative plants. He chose essences by holding his hand over a flowering plant to determine its emotional

"aura." Bach's remedies are divided into seven groups that cover the negative states of mind that affect most people: depression, despair, fear, uncertainty, indecision, overconcern for others, and lack of interest in the present. The remedies are intended to stimulate the body's healing mechanisms and quiet the disharmonies within the person, restoring health.

Bach's remedies are available at most health food stores and are best taken for emotional, rather than physical symptoms. Usually, a drop or two of the remedy is taken in a glass of water or juice, or the drops can be placed on the tongue. Bach flower remedies have no side effects because the solutions contain no plant material.

For more information:

Westbrook University
112 S. Church St.
Aztec, NM 87410
800-447-6496
http:\\www.westbrooku.edu

Biofeedback

Biofeedback is a therapy used to train the conscious mind to control involuntary bodily functions such as respiration, heartbeat, and body temperature. This psychological therapy, taught with the aid of a monitor or other device, can be learned by anyone and is helpful in treating conditions such as stress, headaches, back pain, and nerve damage.

For example, thermal biofeedback teaches how to direct blood flow away from the head and into the fingers, allowing a person to consciously raise the temperature of the hand. To learn thermal biofeedback, one wears a heat-sensitive device that transmits the temperature of the finger or hand to a monitor. An instructor can show a person how to get started; however, no one can teach another exactly how to raise the hand's temperature; you must use your imagination—and concentration—to accomplish this. Any change brought about will be registered on the monitor's gauge. A second type of biofeedback, electromyographic (EMG) biofeedback, teaches how to control muscle tension in the face, neck, and shoulders. It also uses a device that measures muscle tension.

Biofeedback may be combined with relaxation methods. Ultimately, you are weaned from the monitor so you can perform biofeedback anywhere, whenever you feel stress, headache, or another condition coming on. Once you learn biofeedback, you will not need a monitor to guide you; you will be capable of raising body temperature and other involuntary functions just by concentrating on the task.

Training in biofeedback is available through several centers in the United States and through complementary practitioners in your area.

For more information:

Association for Applied Psychophysiology and Biofeedback
(formerly the Biofeedback Society of America)
10200 W. 44th Ave., Suite 304
Wheat Ridge, CO 80033
303-422-8436
http://www.aapb.org

Chinese Medicine

Chinese medicine is a combination of acupuncture, massage and herbal medicine. It involves an acceptance of opposites of yin and yang (expressed as day and night, male and female, negative and positive) and a flow of a life force called ch'i. Chinese medicine teaches that, to be healthy, the yin and yang forces must be balanced and the ch'i must be flowing through the body smoothly along a set of invisible pathways known as meridians.

In place of highly technological diagnostic and treatment equipment, practitioners of Chinese medicine rely upon looking, listening, smelling, asking and touching to make their diagnoses, which is done according to a theory called Five Elements. The five elements are fire, wood, earth, metal and water, which practitioners of Chinese medicine use when evaluating bodily functions, organs, acupuncture meridians, emotions and external influences to discover some disturbance in the flow of ch'i throughout the body.

Touch is an important aspect of Chinese medicine, much more so than in Western medicine. By carefully taking the pulses of the body, which flow along the meridians, the practitioner can detect slight imbalances that may indicate a condition or disease.

When a diagnosis is made, the practitioner will decide upon one or all of the treatment methods available, specifically acupuncture, acupressure or herbs.

For more information:

American Association of Acupuncture and Oriental Medicine
433 Front St.
Catasauqua, PA 18032
610-433-2448
http://www.aaom.org

Christian Healing

Christian healing is a therapy centered on the belief that God has the power to cure physical illnesses through a healer by the laying-on of hands. It is also called faith healing or therapeutic touch.

Healing without medicines and surgery has always been viewed with skepticism, not only by traditional medicine but also by mainstream religions. Miracles were always the province of religion, and their occurrences have been recorded in scripture. It was believed that only simple-minded people with limited education would have any interest in healing, and it was not until parapsychologists began investigating the claims of healers that serious attention was paid to this practice. Recent research now shows that prayer and healing do play a role in healing those who are sick. Christian healing does not require any spiritual faith on the part of the patient; in fact, it can be performed without the patient's knowledge.

For further information:

Healing Light Center Church
261 E. Alegria Ave., #12
Siera Madre, CA 91024
818-306-2170

New Life Clinic
Mt. Washington United Methodist Church
Falls Road
Baltimore, MD 21209
410-561-0428

Chiropractic

Chiropractic is a therapy that emphasizes manipulation of the spinal vertebrae to restore health. It was developed in 1895 after Daniel David Palmer manipulated the spine of a deaf man and restored his hearing. Chiropractic is based upon the principle that the spinal column is central to a person's entire sense of well-being because it is instrumental in maintaining the health of the nervous system. It is especially helpful in treating back pain that is not accompanied by nerve involvement. However,

chiropractic is not helpful in treating systemic diseases such as arthritis or infection.

Chiropractic is considered a drugless therapy since chiropractors generally believe the body's own healing forces can be used to combat disease. Diagnostic procedures used by chiropractors include treadmills, measurement of temperature, stationary bicycles, and devices to measure the distribution of the body weight. The x-ray remains the staple for examination of the spinal column.

Chiropractic treatment generally consists of spinal adjustments in which the chiropractor pushes on the vertebrae to reposition them. When a chiropractor is making an adjustment, the patient may hear a "pop" or "click" sound as the vertebra goes back into place. (Remember, however, that the sound, or absence of it, does not indicate whether the appropriate adjustment has been made.) Other areas such as the neck or shoulders may also be manipulated.

There are two main schools of thought in the practice of chiropractic today. The straight school emphasizes traditional spinal manipulation. Chiropractors from this school adhere to the principles first set down by Palmer and, as such, do not use any adjunctive therapies such as heat, ultrasound, traction, vitamins, minerals, and exercise. Chiropractors who supplement traditional spinal manipulation with adjunctive therapies are said to be from the mixed school, which accounts for the majority of chiropractors in practice today.

Chiropractors hold the degree of doctor of chiropractic (D.C.) and are licensed to provide treatment. While they are not medical doctors, chiropractors are becoming more and more mainstream. Chiropractic adjustments have been successful for a number of people; however, chiropractors point out that adjustments may not work in every case. When a chiropractor detects a condition that is beyond his or her scope of practice, a referral should be made to the proper medical specialists.

For more information:

American Chiropractic Association ["mixed school"]
1701 Clarendon Blvd.
Arlington, VA 22209
703-276-8800
http://www.amerchiro.org.aca

International Chiropractors Association ["straight school"]
1110 N. Glebe Rd., Suite 1000
Arlington, VA 22201
800-423-4690
http://www.chiropractic.org

Feldenkrais Technique

The Feldenkrais technique was designed by Dr. Moshe Feldenkrais for the purpose of improving posture and general health. In some respects, Feldenkrais owes his concept to the work done by F. Matthias Alexander in the development of the Alexander technique. Like the Alexander technique, the Feldenkrais technique strives to correct posture and break bad habits that lead to muscular and joint discomfort.

There are two facets to the Feldenkrais technique: awareness through movement and private manipulative treatment. The first involves group-based classes where various exercises are performed while lying down in order to lessen the effects of gravity on the body. The purpose is to gently exercise the muscles and joints with as little strain as possible. A Feldenkrais teacher instructs pupils on the proper way to completely relax until they feel "that the body is hanging lightly from the head, the feet do not stomp on the ground and the body glides when moving."

The second foundation of the Feldenkrais technique is private manipulative therapy, referred to as "functional integration." This is a person-to-person phase of the technique in which the teacher works with the pupil by using a series of gentle manipulative movements, but does not work directly on a problem in the belief that this could add to the pain and discomfort. For example, the legs and pelvis may be manipulated in order to relieve a problem in the shoulders.

While there are Feldenkrais teachers, the most likely place to find the technique practiced is in other types of massage therapy.

For more information:

Feldenkrais Center for Learning
1616 Center St., Suite 527
Northampton, MA 01060
413-584-1414

Feldenkrais Guild of North America
P.O. Box 489
Albany, OR 97321
800-775-2118

Herbal Therapy

Herbal therapy uses compounds made from various plants to prevent and cure illnesses. Herbology, the use of plants as medicine, was practiced by many ancient peoples, including the Chinese, Egyptians, Babylonians, and Aztecs. Humans probably learned how to use herbs to treat illness by observing which plants animals ate when they were sick. The modern word *drug*, in fact, is derived from the German word *droge*, meaning "to dry"—the process herbs undergo before being used. While at one time herbal therapy was relegated to the status of folk medicine or quackery, today it is recognized as an effective treatment for many conditions—for example, enlarged prostate (saw palmetto),

HERBS AND THEIR USES

Herbal remedies can be very effective in the treatment of symptoms. This list gives just a few of the many remedies available.

1. *Chamomile.* Diarrhea, migraine, gastritis, colitis, overindulgence in food or drink, insomnia, nightmares.

2. *Valerian.* Insomnia, anxiety, tension.

3. *Sage.* Insomnia, depression; increased perspiration, bad breath.

4. *Garlic.* High blood pressure, reduced resistance to infection.

5. *Lemon balm.* Anxiety, stress, palpitations.

6. *Peppermint.* Indigestion, colic, anxiety.

7. *Ginseng.* Stress, lack of energy, tiredness.

8. *Rosemary.* Nervous tension, headaches.

fatigue (ginseng), and insomnia (chamomile, passionflower).

Herbs can be found in many different forms in health food stores, and they can be prepared in many different ways. An infusion, a kind of tea, can be made of herbs by steeping them in hot water. The roots, bark, and seeds of plants are often boiled or simmered to release their properties, creating a decoction. A tincture is made by adding powdered herbs to an alcohol solution and steeping for several weeks; tinctures are then taken by the spoonful in water or tea. Finally, herbs can be used in a poultice, a mixture of crushed herbs, water, and flour or cornmeal that is applied externally and covered with a cloth.

Herbs are drugs. You should talk with an herbalist, a practitioner who specializes in treatment involving herbs, or a medical practitioner before using herbs for self-care as some may have harmful side effects (for example, licorice may have harmful effects in people with heart disease or high blood pressure). As with medications, the key to using herbs is to carefully research the claims for each one. Libraries and health food stores usually have books on herbal medicine.

For more information:

American Botanical Council
P.O. Box 201660
Austin, TX 78720-1660
512-331-8868
http://www.herbalgram.org

American Herbalists Guild
P.O. Box 746555
Arvada, CO 80006
303-423-8800

Association of Natural Medicine Pharmacists
8369 Champs de Elysses
Forestville, CA 95436
415-453-3534

Homeopathy

Homeopathy, developed by Samuel Christian Hahnemann in the late eighteenth century, is a system of medicine founded on the principle that "like cures like." Hahnemann observed that quinine, a malaria drug, produced symptoms of malaria when taken by healthy individuals. He concluded through research and testing that in some cases substances that cause symptoms of diseases in healthy people will bring about cures in sick people. Those who practice homeopathy are called homeopathic physicians—they are often mainstream medical practitioners with special training in homeopathy.

Homeopathic remedies are taken from naturally occurring substances such as plants, animal materials, and natural chemicals. Only one medication is ever taken at a time, doses are small to prevent reaction or rejection by the body, and the remedies are repeatedly diluted from the original material, which is believed to increase its potency, according to homeopathic theory. These remedies can be found in most health food stores. Labels on the products indicate its uses and how often it has been diluted. The preparations are taken by mouth and are usually tasteless. Because they have been diluted so many times, homeopathic remedies do not produce side effects. (However, the substances within homeopathic remedies may be dangerous, so large doses of remedies are not recommended.) Because they are safe, they are ideal for home care. However, a homeopathic physician may be needed to determine which of the remedies is most appropriate for the condition.

For more information:

National Center for Homeopathy
801 N. Fairfax St., Suite 306
Alexandria, VA 22314
703-548-7790
http://www.homeopathic.org

International Foundation for Homeopathy
P.O. Box 7
Edmonds, WA 98020
206-776-4147
http://www.ish.nwlink.com

Hydrotherapy

Hydrotherapy is the use of water internally or externally to treat certain illnesses and conditions.

Archaeological records suggest that ancient civilizations made great use of water as a healing therapy. Public baths were commonplace in the Roman Empire, with most early baths located adjacent to hot mineral springs with widely known therapeutic powers. Hydrotherapy is especially useful in treating injuries and stress-related conditions. Hydrotherapy is also considered a relaxation technique.

Hydrotherapy comes in many different forms—the water can be any temperature and in any form (liquid, ice, or steam). Examples of hydrotherapy include applying ice to an injury to prevent swelling, soaking in a hot tub to relieve muscle soreness, using a humidifier to relieve congestion from a cold, having a colonic (an internal application of water to flush out the lower digestive tract), and swimming for physical fitness. Hydrotherapy, in the form of a hot tub or sauna, is also used as a relaxation technique to relieve stress. Chances are you've used hydrotherapy many times in your life, even though you may not have called it by that name.

Hypnotherapy

Hypnotherapy is the use of hypnosis, the induction of a trancelike state, to treat physical and mental disorders, for example, pain from migraine headaches, chronic pain, stress, stomach problems, arthritis, and colitis. Some evidence suggests that hypnosis was known in ancient times, when the Druids were said to be able to induce a "magic sleep." Certain Egyptian writings also refer to hypnosis.

Although not exactly asleep, a person in a hypnotic state is not fully awake either. The state is, if nothing else, an altered one wherein the subject is more responsive to the power of suggestion. A person who is hypnotized may have incredible powers of concentration and be able to accomplish things not necessarily possible in a more conscious state.

Contrary to popular myth, you cannot be hypnotized against your will or forced to do something you do not want to do. If you can be hypnotized, you may be able to use the power of your subconscious to focus all your mind's energy on one problem. The ability to focus on one problem is a result of being insulated from the distractions of the outside world.

Hypnosis may also be self-administered. Learning to break an old habit or establish a new healthy habit can be accomplished through hypnosis. People wishing to quit smoking often use hypnosis, and there have been reports of success in helping people to lose weight and adhere to a new diet. Some therapists, especially those in pediatric hospitals, use hypnosis to help patients overcome their fears of hospitalization.

For more information:

American Institute of Hypnotherapy
16842 Von Karman Ave., Suite 475
Irvine, CA 92606
800-872-9996
714-261-6400

American Society of Clinical Hypnosis
2200 E. Devon St., Suite 301
Des Plaines, IL 60018
847-297-3317

Massage

Massage therapy is an alternative therapy as well as a means of relaxation. Rooted in Eastern medicine and based on the balance points of the human body, massage is employed to create a feeling of relaxation, ease mental and physical tensions, alleviate aches and pains, improve circulation, and generally reinvigorate and stimulate the body's systems. Forms of massage therapy include Swedish massage, acupressure, shiatsu, reflexology, and bioenergetics.

In the past, massage therapy in the United States has been limited to the conditioning of athletes—used to limber up joints or relieve aches and pains. Today, however, massage is used for a wide range of health-care problems, including stress, fatigue, headaches, insomnia, lower-back pain, and muscle fatigue, as well as an aid to digestion and circulation. Studies show massage to be helpful in treating the symptoms of diabetes, asthma, and arthritis. Plus, massage, to put it simply, feels good.

Most massages begin at the head or feet, then gradually work toward the heart, since this is the body's natural circulatory path. Each massage is composed of a series of strokes (such as kneading, tapping, or striking and gliding) and movements done with a different pressure. Swedish massage uses vibration and friction as well.

Massage therapy involves no drugs and can be performed by professionals or amateurs. Self-massage of the feet and hands is also possible.

For more information:

American Massage Therapy Association
820 Davis St., Suite 100
Evanston, IL 60201-4444
847-864-0123

Associated Bodywork and Massage Professionals
28677 Buffalo Park Rd.
Evergreen, CO 80439
303-647-8478

Myotherapy

Myotherapy is a method of pain relief that is based upon locating "trigger points" within the muscles that cause the muscles to go into spasm.

Many physical therapists, chiropractors, osteopaths, and massage therapists practice myotherapy techniques. Myotherapists can also become certified through special training programs.

Trigger points are sensitive spots that contribute to pain. The pain occurs when these points "fire," causing the muscles to react. Trigger points come about because muscles are subjected to bumps, sprains, blows, and strains. Many of these points can be located in a single muscle, and during a lifetime it's possible to accumulate a large number of them. Not limited only to the large muscles of the body—legs, back, shoulders, chest, and so on—trigger points also occur in the muscles of the face, hands, and feet.

Very familiar with anatomy and the complete muscle structure of the body, a myotherapist searches for trigger points by pushing on or putting pressure on the muscles. Since myotherapy is a drugless therapy, the only tools are fingers, knuckles, and elbows, and a bodo, a wooden dowel used to apply pressure.

Once located, trigger points are released or neutralized by applying pressure for a least seven seconds, a rule that works fine for most muscles; however, smaller muscles respond to as little as four seconds of pressure. (This is also a basic tenet of acupressure.) Myotherapists also go easier when working with children or the elderly.

While there is no scientific basis per se for myotherapy, it has received favorable notice from the media and is looked upon as a form of physical therapy.

For more information:

Bonnie Prudden Pain Erasure
8700 Speedway
Tucson, AZ 85710
800-221-4634

Naturopathy

Naturopathy emphasizes the body's natural healing forces and makes use of massage, hydrotherapy, herbal therapy, homeopathy, and a number of other complementary therapies to treat a range of conditions. A person schooled in naturopathy has earned the degree of doctor of naturopathic medicine (N.D.) and is known as a naturopathic physician or naturopath. Students enrolled in naturopathic medical schools complete courses that are a balance of traditional naturopathic philosophy, medical science, and the effectiveness of natural therapeutics. Naturopaths are often conventional medical doctors with naturopathic training.

Naturopathic medicine in rooted in the concept of *vis mediatrix naturae*, the healing power of nature. To the naturopath, a person's medical history is the most important piece of information used to make a diagnosis. Naturopaths also rely on laboratory tests and other diagnostic techniques such as x-rays, scans, and physical examinations. Once the diagnosis is made, the naturopath sets about restoring health by taking the whole person and not just the symptoms into account.

Naturopaths consider diet and nutrition essential to good health and advise patients on proper nutrition, including the types of food to eat as well as those to avoid. In some cases, naturopaths recommend fasting as one method for detoxifying the body before beginning a new regimen of diet and nutrition. The fasting process is not designed to be starvation; rather, it is an attempt to permit the body's metabolic functions to rest, thus enabling the body to eliminate waste and toxic products, and thereby cleanse itself.

While naturopathy may not be the choice for someone with a serious condition, it may be ideal for someone who wants to improve their overall health and well-being.

For more information:

American Association of Naturopathic Physicians
2366 Eastlake Ave., E., Suite 322
Seattle, WA 98102
206-323-9700

John Bastyr College of Naturopathic Medicine
14500 Juniata Dr., N.E.
Bothell, WA 98011
206-523-9585
http://www.bastyr.edu

National College of Naturopathic Medicine
049 S.W. Porter St.
Portland, OR 97201
503-499-4343
http://www.ncnm.edu

Reflexology

Reflexology is the practice of using the hands to stimulate certain areas of the feet that are thought to correspond to various organs and other parts of the body. Reflexology has its origins in Chinese medicine and is considered a cousin of acupuncture. Both of these therapies focus on the flow of ch'i, the life force, throughout the body, believing that an imbalance in the flow can lead to illness. Some sources indicate that reflexology can be effective in helping to relieve headaches, stress, sinus problems, constipation, and other conditions.

In reflexology, the muscles and toes of the feet are kneaded and rubbed by a practitioner called a reflexologist to improve circulation of ch'i to the organs and joints in the body. A reflexologist examines the foot for symptoms of illness, indicated by a gritty or sandy feeling. These gritty areas, referred to as crystals, represent waste products that are impeding normal circulation. The reflexologist uses the thumbs and fingers to break up the crystals and restore normal circulation.

Reflexology can be learned and practiced at home, and many instructional books are available on the subject.

For more information:

International Institute of Reflexology
P.O. Box 12642
St. Petersburg, FL 33733
813-343-4811

Rolfing

Rolfing is a therapy in which very deep massage is used to correct improper structural or postural positions. A practitioner skilled in the use of this deep muscle massage to bring about structural balances is called a rolfer.

Rolfing was developed in the 1930s by Ida Rolf and involves the manipulation of muscles and fascia (connective tissue of the body, including tendons, lymph nodes, and ligaments) to permit freer movement of the body. As the muscles and fascia are manipulated, the body returns to its natural posture. Rolfing usually consists of ten sessions conducted over a five- or ten-week period. These sessions are divided into three distinct parts in which the rolfer has very specific objectives to achieve.

Rolfers are interested in freeing the body from the constraints imposed by stress, poor living habits, and bad posture. Since part of the problem is related to breathing, the rolfer works to loosen the chest and pelvic muscles during the first sessions. The second group of sessions concentrates on the ankles and feet. The final sessions concentrate on establishing new patterns of movement, and once these are developed, the person should notice an improvement in both physical and mental energies.

Some massage therapists, kinesiologists, and chiropractors may be familiar with the technique of rolfing.

For more information:

Rolf Institute
205 Canyon Blvd.
Boulder, CO 80302
303-449-5903

Yoga

Yoga is a philosophy of life that originated in India that espouses the uniting of body, mind, and spirit in order to achieve a higher self-realization; it has been practiced for some six thousand years. According to legend, yoga exercises were designed by Lord Shiva at the beginning of time and have remained the same since then. The first codified yoga system is believed to have been written in the second century B.C. by the Indian sage Pantanjali. To this day yoga, utilizes eighty-four of the postures handed down by Pantanjali.

Yoga is deeply rooted in Eastern mysticism and the belief in some formless god who creates and arranges all matter. The yogi, a person who practices or teaches yoga, attempts to unite with this force and reach a state of consciousness and awareness in which harmony exists. But before reaching this state, the yogi must perform a series of exercises involving breathing and posture. This is hatha yoga.

Other forms of yoga include

1. *Mantra yoga.* A mantra is a word or phrase that is repeated thousands of times. The mind focuses on the vibrations of the mantra and thus increases concentration.

2. *Bhakti yoga.* This is the yoga of faith, devotion, and worship. Yogis chant to help increase their spiritual bliss.

3. *Jnana yoga.* This is the yoga of knowledge or intellect. It requires the yogi to focus on those things that have occurred and to learn from them.

4. *Karma yoga.* This is cause and effect, with good deeds producing good karma and bad deeds producing bad karma.

5. *Raja yoga.* This is the ultimate state of superconsciousness, or deep meditation, that yogis strive to attain. This form of perfect mind control permits the yogi to control all thought processes and remain free from distractions.

6. *Laya yoga.* This yoga explores the seven energy centers of the body known as the chakras. It requires a person to still the mind and awaken the inner force called kundalini.

The practice of yoga in the West has been increasing as more people seek alternative methods for achieving a feeling of well-being and seek to improve their self-discipline, concentration, and positive thinking.

For more information:

Integral Yoga Institute
227 W. 13th St.
New York, NY 10011
212-929-0585

Himalayan International Institute of Yoga Science and Philosophy
R.R. 1, P.O. Box 400
Honesdale, PA 18431
717-253-5551

MEDICATIONS

Prescription and Over-the-Counter Medications

More than 80 percent of all office visits end with at least one prescription being written. Medications are an important part of a person's medical care. In some cases, the benefits are the difference between life and death.

Yet most people know little about the medications they take. Studies suggest that almost half of all prescriptions filled are never fully used. Consumers report confusion about side effects, shelf life, and even how to read the instructions given to them by a doctor or pharmacist.

Prescription Medications

Prescription medications are powerful substances that work to alter the function of the body. Different people react differently to drugs, and medications may react with other drugs or even with food or vitamins and minerals to create harmful side effects. The dosage for drugs being taken over the long term should be adjusted regularly as well.

Before writing a prescription, a health-care practitioner should find out your medical history, including the following:

- Have you ever had an allergic reaction to any drug?

- Are you currently taking any other prescription or over-the-counter medications? Any vitamin or mineral supplements?

- Do you have any medical conditions (such as heart disease or diabetes)?

- Are you on a special diet?

- How much alcohol do you consume?

You should ask your practitioner the following before taking the prescription:

- What is the name of the drug? What are its effects?

- How much should I take? When should I take it? For how long?

- Are there any foods, drinks, other medications or activities I should avoid?

- What are the possible side effects? If they occur, what should I do?

- Where can I find out more about the medication? Check *The Physician's Desk Reference* (Medical Economics Data, 1996) and *The Complete Drug Reference* (Consumer Reports Books, 1996) for information about specific medications.

Over-the-Counter Medications

You might think the fact that over-the-counter (OTC) drugs are available without a prescription is enough to guarantee their safety. But no drug is harmless and completely safe. Each one is a chemical designed to alter the body's function in some way. Compared with prescription drugs, OTCs are relatively safe. Nonetheless, OTCs must be used with caution. Some nonprescription drugs are as strong as the medications your doctor prescribes. And keep in mind that—even despite approval from the Food and Drug Administration—ineffective and marginally effective drugs do exist.

With more than 300,000 OTC products on the market, the choices can be confusing. Don't

DRUG ERRORS IN A HOSPITAL SETTING

When you're in a hospital, it can be difficult to keep tabs on what medications you should be taking. In addition to your usual medications, you may be prescribed several new drugs at one time while in the hospital. In addition, doctors and nurses have many patients to care for. For these reasons, medication errors often occur in hospitals. A medication error can be defined as (1) being given the wrong medications; (2) being given the wrong dosage or missing a dose; and (3) being given medication at the wrong time.

Surveys have shown medication errors to be common in hospitals across the United States. Some $76.6 billion a year is spent on drug errors. Adverse drug events occur at a rate of .2 per one hundred admissions to ten per one hundred admissions.

You can prevent dangerous medication errors while at home or at the hospital by being alert about the medications you take. The following guidelines from the American Society of Hospital Pharmacists (ASHP) can be used to avoid medication errors during a hospital stay:

- Inform all your health-care providers (physicians, nurses, and pharmacists) of your known allergies, sensitivities, and current medications.

- Ask questions about any recommended procedures and treatments.

- Learn the names of all drug products that are prescribed and administered to you.

- Keep track of the medications. Record all drug therapy, including prescribed drugs, nonprescription drugs, home remedies, and special diets.

- Be assertive if something seems incorrect or different from the norm. For example, if you receive a different pill than the one you were expecting (for example, a red pill instead of a green pill), ask why. Also ask if you have not been given medication you are expecting.

- Take prescription medication as prescribed. If possible, bring your prescription medications to the hospital with you and make arrangements with your doctor and the nursing station to take them according to schedule. The hospital may request that you sign a release form.

rely on television and other advertising to help you make your decision. Instead, talk with your pharmacist about which medication would be best for your symptoms. Also, ask if there are any equivalent drugs that may cost less. OTC drug sales are big business. In 1997, U.S. manufacturers' sales were around $18 billion, according to the Food and Drug Administration. All

the more reason to choose a pharmacist who knows the business.

A word of warning regarding OTCs: In the interest of health, be sure to consult a pharmacist and possibly a physician before buying any OTC preparation for babies, young children, elderly persons, debilitated patients, or pregnant or breast-feeding women.

MEDICATIONS AND SAFETY

Just as medications ae not always foolproof cures or effective treatments, neither are they always safe to use. To help prevent medication problems:

- Keep an eye out for tampering. If the seal of a medication is disturbed in any way, do not purchase the product or return it to the store where it was purchased.

- Store medications in a cool, dry place. Extreme temperatures can alter the chemical composition of drugs.

- Store medications in their original containers to avoid mix-ups. Labels also list important dosing information.

- Always check the expiration date on the medications in your home medicine cabinet. After that date, the product could begin to deteriorate or lose its effective. Replace any drugs that are old, appear strange or discolored, or give off an unusual odor.

- Check the label before taking or giving any medication.

Generic Drugs

A generic drug (the name of which is usually a condensed version of the drug's original chemical name) is one whose active ingredients duplicate those of the brand name product.

After a drug is created by a pharmaceutical company, that company has a patent for the drug for twenty years, which ensures it a monopoly on the sale, marketing, and advertisement of the drug itself. When the drug comes off patent, generic drug companies may manufacture generic versions of the pioneer drug. About fifteen drugs a year come off patent.

The generic drug manufacturer must prove that the generic version is bioequivalent to the brand name drug. A generic drug is termed bioequivalent if the active ingredient of the drug is absorbed into the bloodstream at the same rate and at the same extent as the brand name drug's absorption rate. Inert fillers, preservatives, coloring agents, and binders are added to further distinguish the generic version. Because generic drug manufacturers are at liberty to choose the fillers they ultimately use in their drug, it is not always known what kind of side effects or allergic reactions are possible due to the inclusion of these fillers.

Generic drugs are usually less expensive than their brand name equivalents—on the average, 30 percent cheaper than brand name drugs, even 50 to 70 percent cheaper than the more expensive medicines—because their manufacturers do not go to the expense of advertising them, nor do they sink money into inventing new products.

With the ever-climbing costs of health care and of prescription drugs, more and more consumers are choosing to purchase generic drugs.

Safety of Generic Drugs

Because of the subtle differences between generics, issues regarding the safety and substitution of generics for brand name drugs have arisen. While in the late 1980s the Food and Drug Administration was criticized for not keeping a close eye on new generic products, extensive measure have since been undertaken to ensure the overall safety of generic drugs. Most states have repealed their antisubstitution laws, under which if a doctor prescribed a certain brand of a drug, the pharmacist could not substitute the generic version, even if it cost less and was the chemical twin of the prescribed brand.

Now, pharmacists nearly everywhere can fill a prescription with a generic, but the process varies, depending on state law. Some require the doctor to write "dispense as written," "brand necessary," or similar words to that effect, and in most of the other states the doctor must sign on either one of two signature lines—one line allows the pharmacist to substitute, the other to dispense only as written. Find out what your state's law is concerning the substitution of a generic drug. These laws strengthen the role—and responsibility—of the consumer *and* the pharmacist in decision making.

For more information:

American Pharmaceutical Association
2215 Constitution Ave., N.W.
Washington, DC 20037
202-628-4410
http://www.aphanet.org

Pharmaceutical Research and Manufacturers of America
1100 15th St., N.W., Suite 900
Washington, DC 20005
202-835-3400
http://www.phrma.org

Nonprescription Drug Manufacturers Association
1150 Connecticut Ave., N.W., Suite 1200
Washington, DC 20036
202-429-9260

Choosing a Pharmacist

Though you may only think of a pharmacist as the clerk who fills your practitioner's prescriptions, a pharmacist is actually an important part of your health-care team. A good pharmacist does more than simply measure out drugs and ring up your order. A good pharmacist should be available to give advice about prescription and over-the-counter medications, answer questions about drugs, make sure you understand your own prescription, and serve as a final check against drug errors and other problems.

The Making of a Pharmacist

To be a pharmacist, a person must train at an accredited school of pharmacy, of which there are seventy-two in the United States and Puerto Rico. Basically, there are two professional degrees awarded in pharmacy: the bachelor of science (B.S. Pharmacy) and the doctor of pharmacy (Pharm. D.). The pharmacist must also hold a valid license—it is illegal to practice without a license. In order to receive one, a graduate in pharmacy must pass an examination given by the board of pharmacy in the state where he or she plans to practice. In order to retain the license, many states require the pharmacist to take continuing-education courses. And in the event of misconduct or incompetence, the pharmacist is subject to disciplinary action by the state board.

If you wish to verify that the pharmacist has complied with state licensing requirements, ask him or her to show you the license. It's usually posted on the wall behind the pharmacy counter. You can also contact the state licensing board to verify credentials.

The Patient Medication Profile

The patient medication profile, or simply "patient profile," is a system that aids the pharmacist in preventing medication errors and

WHAT A GOOD PHARMACIST DOES: A CHECKLIST

- DOES more than merely read a doctor's prescription, fill it, label it, and charge for it. Instead, a good pharmacist is willing and eager to expand the pharmacist's role, beyond that of a "pill-counter," to a recognized member of the health-care team and a drug-information specialist.

- KEEPS important family medication records called patient medication profiles and uses them to help prevent allergic reactions to drugs, dangerous interactions, duplicate medications, and drug abuse.

- ADVISES how to use prescription and nonprescription medication: how and when to take it; what the possible side effects are; what the shelf life is; how to store the medication; and whether there is potential for dangerous interactions with foods and/or other medications.

- ANSWERS your questions about the staggering variety of medicines, remedies, tonics, pills, elixirs, lotions, salves, capsules, and powders on the market.

- ADVISES you, when it seems necessary, to seek a medical practitioner's help.

harmful drug interactions. The system contains basic patient information such as drug allergies, other prescription drugs used or being used, and any pertinent medical information. The pharmacist reviews the profile when dispensing a prescription as a double-check against drug interactions and other potential problems. These profiles range from the simple—a card file—to the highly technological—a computerized system that will store and retrieve new and old information and even type labels. The American Pharmaceutical Association recommends that a patient medication profile contain the following:

- Your name, address, and phone number

- Your birthday (The pharmacist has to know this to check if the dosage is appropriate to the age of the user.)

- Any allergies, reactions, and adverse effects you've demonstrated

- Any drugs that have proved ineffective for you

- A concise health history, including any conditions or diseases that would preclude the use of certain drugs (for example, diabetes, hypertension, and ulcers)

- The over-the-counter, or nonprescription, medicines you take

- The date and number of each prescription filled for you, the name of the drug, its dosage and strength, quantity, directions for use and price. Also, the prescriber and dispenser of each medication.

Keep in mind that this service will only be useful if you buy all your medicine from the same pharmacy.

How to Read Prescriptions

A standard prescription, written by a health professional and subsequently filled by a pharmacist, contains several basic facts: the practitioner's name and address; the patient's name and address; the name of the drug, its strength and its dosage; special instructions that the patient must be aware of (for example, whether the drug should be taken with food or at bedtime); the practitioner's signature; and authorization for or against any generic substitutions of a brand name drug.

The information on most prescriptions, however, is usually coded and may be puzzling to the untrained eye. Here are some phrases and terms that are frequently noted on prescription sheets:

a.c. = before meals

ad lib. = freely; as needed

AM = morning

b.i.d. = twice a day

c = with

cap(s) = capsule(s)

cc = cubic centimeter

cm = centimeter

disp. = dispense (number of tablets or amount of medicine to dispense)

ext = for external use

gtt = drops

h.s. = at bedtime, before retiring

mg = milligrams

ml = milliliters

noct. = at night

non repetat = no refill

OD = right eye

OS = left eye

OU = both eyes

pc = after meals

PM = evening

p.o. = per os (by mouth)

prn = as needed

qd = once a day

qh = every hour

q.i.d. = four times a day

rep = repeat

s = without

sig = write; let it be imprinted; label; directions

sig ut dict = take as directed

stat = at once

tab = tablet

t.i.d. = three times a day

top = apply topically

X = times

MEDICAL ABBREVIATIONS

Doctors, nurses, and other health-care professionals have a long-established habit of using abbreviated medical terms and everyday words, especially in charts and medical records. They have been trained to think that no one except another doctor or nurse will look at what is scribbled there, and they have all learned the code in the course of their training. But patients do not know it, and when you look at your chart and records (something you ought to do regularly), you are at a loss and have no hint of what your doctor is thinking about you, about your condition, and about your prognosis. It is a major obstacle blocking your participation in your own care.

The following list can change that. It is a collection from many sources of abbreviations frequently used in records, on forms and prescriptions, and even in everyday conversation. If something you see or hear doesn't appear on this list, ask your doctor, nurse, hospital patients' representative, or some other person to translate.

One reason doctors or hospital personnel might not want you to know what they've written may be that they fear that the message could be misunderstood and even be embarrassing for them if interpreted accurately. Sometimes descriptive terms medical people use in referring to their patients and their patients' conditions are derogatory and couched in a colorful code purposely indecipherable for the uninitiated. For example, if you hear that the patient next door "boxed," that means he or she died. A "gork" is a brain-damaged person, a vegetable. A "gomer" is the acronym for "Get Out of My Emergency Room"—a patient whom no one wants to treat.

And what about the abbreviations that pertain directly to your state of health or medical care? If you see "FBS," followed by numbers, this is the results of your test for "fasting blood sugar." Same with "B.M.R." That means "basal metabolic rate."

In medicode, a "delightful" patient is one who does anything anybody tells him or her to do and never asks questions. The same goes for those patients described as "pleasant." A "turkey" is something quite different. A turkey is a patient who asks a lot of questions, demands respect, knows his or her rights, and won't stop wanting to be a part of his or her own healing care. In other words, a smart and careful medical consumer.

Here are abbreviations you are likely to encounter in medical records, on forms or prescriptions, or overheard in hospital rooms and corridors:

a = before

aa = of each

a.c. = before meals

Ad. = to, up to

ADL = activities of daily living

ad lib. = as needed, as desired

A.F. = auricular fibrillation

agit = shake, stir

AM = morning

AMA = against medical advice

Ap. = appendicitis

Aq. = water

ASHD = arteriosclerotic heart disease

B.E. = barium enema

b.i.d. = twice a day

Bl. time = bleeding time

B.M. = bowel movement

B.M.R. = basal metabolic rate

BP = blood pressure

BRP = bathroom privileges

Bx = biopsy

C = centigrade

c = with

CA = cancer

CAD = coronary artery disease

cap(s) = capsule(s)

CBC = complete blood count

CBD = common bile duct

cc = cubic centimeter(s)

CC = chief complaint

CCU = coronary care unit

CHD = coronary heart disease or congential heart disease

CHF = congestive heart failure

Chol = cholesterol

Cl. time = clotting time

cm = centimeter

CNS = central nervous system

comp = compound

cont rem = continue the medicine

COPD = chronic obstructive pulmonary disease

CSF = cerebrospinal fluid

CV = cardiovascular

CVA = cardiovascular accident

CVP = central venous pressure

CXR = chest x-ray

d = give

D&C = dilation and curettage

D&E = dilation and evacuation

dd in d = from day to day

dec = pour off

dexter = the right

dil = dilute

disp. = dispense

div = divide

DM = diabetes mellitus

DNR = do not resuscitate

dos = dose

dur dolor = while pain lasts

D/W = dextrose in water

Dx = diagnosis

ECG or EKG = electrocardiogram

EEG = electroencephalogram

emp = as directed

ER = emergency room

ext = for external use

F = Fahrenheit

FBS = fasting blood sugar

febris = fever

FH = family history

Fx = fracture

GA = general anesthesia

garg = gargle

GB = gallbladder

GC = gonorrhea

GI = gastrointestinal

GL = glaucoma

gm = grams

"gomer"= "Get out of my emergency room" (a patient no one wants to treat)

"gork"= a brain-damaged person

gr. = grains

grad = by degrees

gravida = pregnancies

gtt = drops

GTT = glucose tolerance test

GU = genitourinary

GYN = gynecology

h = hour

Hb or Hgb = hemoglobin

HCT = hematocrit

HHD = hypertensive heart disease

HOB = head of bed

h.s. = at bedtime, before retiring

Hx = history

ICU = intensive care unit

I&D = incision and drainage

IM = intramuscular

I.M. = infectious mononucleosis

ind = daily

I&O = intake and output (measure fluids going into and out of body)

IPPB = intermittent positive pressure breathing

IV = intravenous

IVP = intravenous pyelogram

L = left

liq = liquid

LLE = left lower extremity

LLQ = left lower quadrant

LMP = last menstural period

LOL = "Little Old Lady" (a passive, unquestioning female senior citizen)

LP = lumbar puncture

LPN = licensed practitioner nurse

LUE = left upper extremity

LUQ = left upper quadrant

m = murmur

M = mix

m et n = morning and night

mg = milligrams

MI = heart attack (myocardial infarction)

ml = milliliters

mor dict = in the manner directed

M.S. = morphine sulfate

NA = nursing assistant

neg. = negative

N-G = nasogastric

no. = number

noct. = at night

non rep; nr = do not repeat

non repetat = no refill

NPO = non per os (nothing by mouth)

NS = normal saline

NSR = normal heart rate

N&V = nausea and vomiting

o = none

O_2 = oxygen

oc = oral contraceptive

OD = right eye

O.D. = once a day

OL = left eye

OOB = out of bed

OPD = outpatient department

OR = operating room

OS = left eye

OT = occupational therapy

OU = both eyes

P; $\bar{P}$ = after

Para = number of births

Path. = pathology

Pc = after meals

PE = physical examination; or pulmonary embolus

PI = present illness

pil = pill

PM = evening

p.o. = per os (by mouth)

Post. = posterior

post-op = postoperative, after the operation

PR = pulse rate; or rectally

pr = per rectum (by rectum)

prn = as needed, as often as necessary

Prog. = prognosis

pt = patient

PT = physical therapy

PTA = prior to admission

Px = prognosis

q = every

qd = once a day

qh = every hour (q4h = every four hours; q8h = every eight hours; and so on)

q.i.d. = four times a day

qn = every night

q̄od = every other day

qs = proper amount, quantity sufficient

qv = as much as desired

R = right

rbc = red blood cells

RBC = red blood cell count

rep = repeat

RHD = rheumatic heart disease

RLQ = right lower quadrant

RN = registered nurse

ROM = range of motion

RR = respiratory rate; recovery room

RT = radiation therapy

RTI = reproductive tract infection

rub = red

RUQ = right upper quadrant

Rx = prescription; or therapy

s̄ = without

S&A = sugar and acetone (a urine test)

sc = subcutaneous

scop. = scopolamine

SH = social history

SICU = surgical intensive care unit

sig = write; let it be imprinted; label; directions

sig ut dict = take as directed

sing = of each

SOB = shortness of breath

sol = solution

solv = dissolve

SOP = standard operating procedure

SOS = can repeat in emergency

ss = half

S&S = signs and symptoms

SSE = soapsuds enema

stat = right away, immediately

STD = sexually transmitted disease

STI = sexually transmitted infection

suppos = suppository

Sx = symptoms

T&A = tonsillectomy and adenoidectomy

tab = tablet

TAT = tetanus antitoxin

tere = rub

TIA = transient ischemic attacks

t.i.d. = three times a day

tinc. or tinct. = tincture

top = apply topically

TPR = temperature, pulse and respiration

Tx = treatment

ung = ointment

URI = upper respiratory infection

ut dict = as directed

UTI = urinary tract infection

VD = venereal disease

VS = vital signs

wbc = white blood cells

WBC = white blood cell count

WC = wheelchair

X = times

y.o. = year old

⇧ = increase

⬈ = increasing

⬇ = decrease

⬊ = decreasing

⇨ = leads to

⇦ = resulting from

♂ = male

♀ = female

MEDICAL LANGUAGE

As the medical world becomes more specialized and technical (and as new medical "cure" are invented yearly), medical terms seem to multiply overnight. To unlock the code, all you need is the key to translating the terms.

As a rule, these seemingly complex medical terms, derived from ancient Greek, are built from three blocks—prefixes, roots, and suffixes. They can be easily deciphered if the meanings of the blocks are known.

The following lists may help you translate the medical language you hear or read.

Prefixes

Prefixes are the blocks that sit at the front of words and generally tell "where," "if," and "how much":

a, an = not, without

ab = away from

acid = sour

ad = near (*d* changes to *c, f, g, p, s,* or *t* when it precedes roots that begin with those letters)

alb = white

amphi(i) = both, twice as much

ante = before

anti = against

ap(o) = detached

brady = slow

contra = against, counter to

cry = cold

dia = through or passing through, going apart, between, across

dys = painful, difficult

e = out from

ecto = outside of, outer, exterior

endo = within

epi = upon, on, over

erythr = red

eso = inside

exo = outside of

hemi = half

hyper = increased, excessive, above

hypo = under, below, deficient

in = not (*n* changes to *l, m,* or *r* when it precedes roots that begin with those letters)

infra = below

inter = between

intra = within

leuco, leuko = white

macro = large

mal = bad, ill, wrongful, disordered

meta = after, beyond, changing

micro = small

para = beyond, beside

peri = around

poly = many, multiple

post = after

pre = before, in front of

pseud(o) = false

re = again

retro = backward, behind

sub = under, below

super = above, beyond, over

supra = above

syn, sy, syl, sym = with, together

tachy = fast

Roots

Roots are at the center of each word. They usually indicate the affected body part:

abdomin = abdomen, stomach

adeno = gland

adip = fat

angi(o) = vessel (blood, lymph)

arteri(o) = artery

arthr(o) = joint

aur = ear

blephar = eyelid

brachi = arm

bronch = windpipe

cardi(o) = heart

cephal = head

cervic = neck

chole, cholo = bile, gall

cholecyst = gallbladder

chondr = cartilage

col(o) = colon

colpo = vagina

crani(o) = skull

cut = skin

cystido, cysto = bladder, sac, cyst

cyto = cell

dent = tooth

enter = intestine

fasci = face

gastr(o) = stomach

glyco = sugar

gnath = jaw

hema, hemato, hemo = blood

hepat(o) = liver

hyster(o) = uterus

ile, ili = intestines, lower abdomen

labi = lip

lact = milk

lapar = loin, flank, abdomen

laryng = windpipe

lipo = fat

lumbar = loin

mast = breast

meno = menstruation

ment = mind

myel = marrow

myelo = spinal cord

myo = muscle

nephro(o) = kidney

neur(o) = nerve

ocul = eye

odont = teeth

oophor = ovary

ophthalm = eye

orchii(o) = testicle

os = mouth, opening

oss, oste(o) = bone

ot(o) = ear

ov = egg

pharyng = throat

phleb = vein

pleur = rib

pneuma, pneumato, pneumo = air, gas, lung

pod = foot

procto = anus, rectum

pulmo = lung

ren = kidney

rhino = nose

salping = fallopian tube

sperm, spermato = semen

splen = spleen

staphyl = uvula

stear = fat

tact = touch

teno = tendon

thorac(o) = chest

thromb = clot, lump

tracheo = windpipe

ur = urine

ureter(o) = tube from kidney to bladder, carrying urine

urethra = tube from bladder to the exterior

vas = vessel, duct

veno = vein

vesic = bladder

Suffixes

Suffixes, the final block in the word, specify what has gone wrong with—or what will be done to—the part of the body designated by the prefix and root:

algia = pain

blast = a growth in its early stages

cele = tumor, hernia

cente = puncture

desis = fusion

dynia = pain

ectomy = excision of, surgical removal

hydr = water

itis = inflammation

lysis = freeing of

megaly = very large

oma = tumor, swelling

oscopy = looking at an organ or internal part

osis = disease, abnormal condition or process

ostomy = creation of an artificial opening

otomy = incision, cutting into

pathy = disease of, abnormality

pexy = fix, sew

plasty = reconstruct, formation of

pnea = breathing

ptosis = falling, drooping

rhage, rhagia, rrhage, rrhagis = bursting forth, bleeding

rhea, rrhea = flow, discharge

scler(osis) = hard, hardening

uria = urine (condition of, presence in)

Putting It Together

Prefix, root, and suffix come together to form medical terms, such as "endocarditis." To decode the word, just consult the lists: prefix "endo" means within; "cardio" has to do with the heart; and "itis" means inflammation. So therefore, "endocarditis" means "inflammation of the inside of the heart," a more or less accurate description of the condition

MEDICAL TESTING

Medical tests are one way a practitioner has of obtaining the information needed to provide the best medical care possible. After gathering your medical history and conducting a physical exam,

chances are the practitioner will recommend tests to help complete the diagnosis.

Medical tests can be divided into four categories: screening, diagnostic, prognostic, and monitoring. Screening is usually a simple test to determine if a particular problem is present in a person who appears healthy and has no complaints. Diagnostic tests confirm or deny a practitioner's impressions. Prognostic tests are conducted after a diagnosis has been made to gather additional information. Monitoring is done to evaluate medical treatment.

Medical tests can also be divided into two classifications: invasive and noninvasive. A test that involves penetration of the body is an invasive test. Such tests normally pose greater risks than noninvasive tests, which do not penetrate the body.

Testing can be done in the hospital, in a practitioner's office, in a laboratory or clinic or even at home, and which setting is most appropriate is determined by the type of test being performed. For example, a blood test is generally performed in a practitioner's office, while an invasive test such as a cardiac catheterization (a test of the heart function) should be done in a hospital. Blood pressure readings and other simple tests can be done in the home. Ask your practitioner about the settings where your test may be performed, and consider cost, convenience, and safety when making your decision.

Common Diagnostic Tests

The following diagnostic tests and procedures are among those most requested by medical practitioners today.

Angiogram. An x-ray picture of a blood vessel made after injecting an opaque substance or dye through a thin tube (catheter) into blood vessels to make the vessels visible on x-ray film. An angiogram of the arteries is called arteriogram; of the veins, venogram or phlebogram; of the lymph vessels, lymph-angiogram; of the heart's arteries, coronary angiogram.

Arthrogram. An x-ray picture of a joint; used to detect injury or damage.

Arthroscopy. An examination of a joint by means of a long, flexible viewing tube inserted into the joint; used to detect injury or damage.

Barium enema. X-ray pictures of the large intestine (colon) made after injecting barium sulfate into the rectum; used to locate abnormalities in the colon. Often called a lower GI (gastrointestinal) series.

Barium meal. X-ray pictures of the esophagus, stomach and duodenum (first part of the small intestine) made after the patient swallows barium sulfate on an empty stomach. Used to locate problems or abnormalities in the digestive tract. Often called an upper GI (gastrointestinal) series or a barium swallow.

Biopsy. The removal of a small portion of body tissue for microscopic analysis; often used to check growths that might be cancerous.

Bronchoscopy. An examination of the bronchi (air passages) of the lungs with a flexible, fiberoptic viewing tube that has been inserted in the throat.

Cardiac catheterization. The insertion of a thin, flexible tube (a catheter) through a vein or artery into the heart. Used to collect information about the heart's structure and performance and to inject a opaque substance (dye) so that an x-ray can be made.

Carotid or cerebral arteriogram. An x-ray picture of the blood vessels of the neck or brain; used in diagnosing stroke. See angiogram.

Cholesterol test. A sampling of the blood to determine the amount of cholesterol in the blood.

Colonoscopy. An examination of the colon with a flexible, fiberoptic viewing tube.

Complete blood cell count (CBC). An examination of blood samples to get a count of the number of red cells, white cells, and hemoglobin in the blood and to determine the percentage of red cells in the blood. Used to check for infection or screen for blood disorders.

Computerized axial tomography (CAT or CT) scan. A highly detailed picture of internal body parts constructed by a computer from hundreds of x-rays; frequently used to locate disease, tumors, or abnormalities in the selected part of the body.

Coronary angiogram. An x-ray picture of the heart's arteries. Coronary angiography is a form of cardiac catheterization.

Cystogram. An x-ray of the bladder made by inserting a thin tube through the urethra into the bladder.

Echocardiogram. An ultrasound recording of the heart's internal structures; used to locate heart valve problems or heart deformities.

Electrocardiogram (ECG or EKG). A recording of the heart muscle's activity that is collected by electrodes placed on the body. Used to detect heart damage, as after a heart attack, and to monitor the effect of certain drugs.

Electroencephalogram (EEG). A recording of the brain's electrical impulses and brain patterns that is collected by electrodes placed on the scalp. Often used to detect brain damage, diagnose epilepsy, or confirm brain death.

Electromyogram (EMG). A recording of the electrical activity of resting and contracting muscles that is collected by an electrode and a thin needle attached to the skin. Used to detect weakness, paralysis, or other problems in the muscle.

MEDICAL TESTING: QUESTIONS TO ASK

New and improved technology has greatly increased the number of medical tests available As with any surgical procedure, be sure to get a second opinion when an invasive or dangerous test is recommended. Ask your practitioner the following questions to help you make a decision about medical testing:

- Why does this test (or retest) need to be done? Find out why your practitioner is recommending a particular test or why a test needs to be done again. Was the first flawed, or is there something new that needs to be done?

- What will you be looking for in the results of these tests?

- Will the procedure be painful, and is it dangerous? If the test might lead to complications more dangerous than the condition itself, you may want to reconsider having the test.

- What are the potential risks of this test? Will they outweigh the benefits? Many tests may be dangerous or cause serious problems and side effects

- How much will it cost? Will my insurance cover the expense?

- How much time will it take?

- Where will the test be performed? While some tests are done right in the practitioner's office, others require hospitalization or are performed on an outpatient basis.

- How accurate is this test? Many procedures have a chance of a false-negative (the test does not detect a disorder that actually exists) or a false-positive (the test detects a disorder that does not exist) result. Discuss the percentage of error with your practitioner and ask if there is a more accurate option. In addition, find out how the test results are verified.

- Is this the most appropriate test? Explore your options when it comes to testing. A more comprehensive test may provide more information and cost less than a series of several specialized tests.

- What will happen if I don't have this procedure done? If your condition will not be affected by the outcome of the test, then you may want to consider if it is really necessary.

Endoscopy. The use of a hollow tube that contains a light source and a viewing lens to examine interior parts of the body. Some of the tubes are rigid for direct viewing, while others are flexible and can be "snaked" through various parts of the body. The newer flexible scopes owe their success in large part to the development and application of fiberoptics technology. Fiberoptic devices are thin, flexible tubes containing bundles of glass filaments that can transmit light around bends and curves to illuminate the inside of the body. In some cases forceps, scissors, or other tiny instruments can be threaded through channels in the scope to facilitate surgical procedures. In addition, the pictures taken by the lens of the scope can be fed to a television monitor for better viewing by practitioners.

The more common endoscopes are

1. *Arthroscope.* A fiberoptic instrument used to examine the interior of a joint, such as a knee or shoulder, by insertions through a small incision made above the joint.

2. *Bronchoscope.* An instrument inserted through the mouth to examine the lungs and bronchial tree. A rigid bronchoscope is a straight, hollow tube that permits direct viewing of the airway passages. A flexible bronchoscope uses a fiberoptic system that permits an inspection of the full bronchial system.

3. *Colonoscope.* A flexible fiberoptic instrument inserted through the anus to examine the large intestine from the anus to the cecum (the first part of the large intestine).

4. *Cystoscope.* A rigid fiberoptic instrument that is inserted through the urethra to view the urethra and bladder or to obtain urine and tissue samples.

5. *Gastroscope.* A flexible fiberoptic instrument that is inserted through the mouth or the nose to examine the upper portion of the digestive tract (esophagus, stomach, and duodenum).

6. *Laparoscope.* A thin fiberoptic instrument that is inserted through a small incision in the abdomen, usually near the navel, and is used to examine the liver, spleen, and intestines.

7. *Laryngoscope.* A thin fiberoptic instrument that is inserted through a nostril in order to view the base of the tongue, epiglottis, larynx, and vocal cords.

8. *Proctoscope.* A short (about five or six inches), rigid or flexible fiberoptic instrument that is inserted through the anus to examine the rectum.

9. *Sigmoidoscope.* A rigid or flexible instrument inserted through the anus to examine the sigmoid colon (the S-shaped portion of the colon just above the rectum). The rigid sigmoidoscope is a lighted tube about twelve inches long and one inch in diameter. The flexible sigmoidoscope employs fiberoptics and is about two feet long.

Lower gastrointestinal (GI) series. See barium enema.

Magnetic resonance imaging (MRI). A magnetic field process (instead of radiation) that produces detailed, computer-generated pictures of the body.

Mammogram. An x-ray picture of the breast; used to diagnose certain conditions, including breast cancer.

Myelogram. An x-ray picture of the fluid-filled space around the spinal cord; used to locate tumors, nerve injuries, and slipped discs.

Positron emission tomography (PET). A technique for making computer-generated images of the brain or other body organs by injecting radioactive isotopes into the body; used to locate abnormal tissue.

Spinal tap. A sampling of cerebrospinal fluid removed by a long needle from the spinal canal; used to diagnose diseases of and injuries to the brain and spinal cord, especially in suspected cases of meningitis and stroke.

Thermogram. A photograph of the surfaces of the body made by a camera with heat-sensitive film; often used to detect varicose veins and breast tumors.

Ultrasound scan. A picture of organs and structures deep inside the body made by using high-frequency sound waves.

Upper gastrointestinal (GI) series. See barium meal.

Venogram. An x-ray picture of the interior of a vein. See angiogram.

X-ray. A picture of the body's internal structures made with electromagnetic rays with a short wavelength.

OUTPATIENT PROCEDURES

As an outpatient, you arrive at the hospital's outpatient clinic, also called a freestanding ambulatory care center, at the appointed time. The staff does for you what needs to be done. Then you go home. An inpatient would stay in a hospital room at least overnight.

Today, nonsurgical outpatient treatments include procedures that once entailed expensive stays in the hospital—for example, chemotherapy. Advanced techniques and cost-containment efforts have led to increased outpatient offerings. Opting for treatment as an outpatient or electing home care—whether initially or as a method to abbreviate a hospital stay—might easily reduce one's medical bill by half.

There are clouds behind the silver lining, however. Some people use *hospital* outpatient services when they could do just as well or better with their family doctor, internist, or pediatrician. A study conducted at Brandeis University has shown that many people who use these hospital outpatient departments pay more because of higher overhead and because hospital physicians tend to order more tests.

Another outpatient clinic drawback is excessive waiting time. At least half the people in a clinic will wait for more than an hour to see a doctor, according to a study done at the New Jersey Medical School in Newark. Why? "In some cases, the doctor is unavoidably late," the researchers said. "In other instances, physician tardiness indicates a surprising disregard for patients' feelings."

The benefits of having surgery the outpatient way are more clear-cut. Time and money spent are kept to a minimum. In addition, third-party payers—the health insurance companies, such as Blue Cross/Blue Shield—encourage outpatient services.

Outpatient surgical procedures have brought convenience as well. In rural areas, consumers are now able to have procedures performed in their doctor's offices or at nearby, freestanding surgical centers instead of traveling hundreds of miles for a lengthy hospital stay. Less time is lost from work. And maybe even more significant, outpatient care is a true cost saving over inpatient care when all costs are taken into consideration.

Of course, if you do not have health insurance, same-day outpatient services make even more sense.

Checkpoints for the Potential Outpatient

Here are some things to investigate before becoming an outpatient:

- If you decide, in conjunction with your medical professional, to have the procedure done at a freestanding, walk-in surgical clinic, make sure it is a professional, properly inspected facility. Visit the

---

Outpatient Surgery Options

Since the early 1990s, more surgical procedures are done on an outpatient basis than on an inpatient basis. As of 1997, more than fifty million operations are being done in outpatient settings and fewer than thirty million operations will be performed on hospitalized consumers. Here's a breakdown of the leading categories of outpatient surgeries as of 1995.

Surgical Category	*Percentage of the Total Number of Outpatient Operations*
Ophthalmology	30.8
Plastic surgery	14.8
Gastroenterology	11.9
Gynecological	9.1
Podiatry	7.3
General surgery	6.2
Ear, nose and throat	6.1
Orthopedic	6.1
Urology	3.4
Pain block	3.0
Dental	1.1
Neurology	0.2

---

place. Look for sufficient space and privacy in the recovery room, as well as general overall cleanliness and professional ambience. Ask what you will be charged and what services are included in that charge.

Also, ask if it is an accredited ambulatory health-care facility; this isn't a critical question, but it might be an indicator of quality. The organization that accredits ambulatory facilities is Association for Ambulatory Healthcare, 9933 Lawler Avenue, Skokie, IL 60077-3702; 708-676-9610. You might want to give a call to your local department of health or your state's department of hospital facilities licensing to see if any complaints have been leveled against the clinic. Find out if the physician serving you is board-certified in the specialty practiced.

- Be aware that just about anyone can open an ambulatory facility, call it anything they want and start doing business. Most states only require that the place have a licensed physician, meet health and safety codes, and comply with a few other minimal standards. Facilities are rarely inspected and then usually on an unannounced basis.

- There is no such thing as minor surgery. Sudden emergencies can and do happen during all types of operations. Make certain that the place you choose, whether associated with a hospital or not, is located near emergency facilities—just in case.

Ten Most Frequently Performed Outpatient Procedures

Endoscopy of large intestine with or without biopsy	837,000
Extraction of lens (removal of the lens of the eye)	738,000
Insertion of prosthetic lens	588,000
Operations on male genital organs	549,000
Endoscopy of small intestine with or without biopsy	543,000
Repair of inguinal hernia	452,000
Cystoscopy with or without biopsy	473,000
Excision or destruction of lesion or tissue of skin or other subcutaneous tissue	440,000
Myringotomy with insertion of tube	340,000
Arthroscopy of knee	340,000
All outpatient procedures for men	12,331,000

Source: National Center for Health Statistics, "Ambulatory Surgery in the United States, 1994."

- Find out what happens if you do not recover completely enough to be sent home safely that same day. This is especially important if you are using a freestanding facility without hospital affiliation. Are there provisions for hospitalization, or are you on your own? Will they call an ambulance for you, or will you have to make any necessary arrangements yourself?

- Make sure ahead of time that your health insurance policy includes ambulatory-care coverage. Determine whether it recognizes the procedure you are having as one that can be performed in an outpatient facility and whether your insurance company approves of and deals with the facility you are using. Just about all health policies cover and actually encourage same-day surgery, but check it out in advance. It's your obligation, not your doctor's, to know what is covered and not covered by your insurance.

- Your decision on whether to be an inpatient or an outpatient will be based on advice you get, monetary considerations, courage, and perhaps ultimately, convenience. The quick, one-stop concept is pretty appealing if you are the kind of person who can't be bothered with an unnecessary and time-consuming layover. And you get to sleep in your own bed that same night. This is, for most of us humans, a great selling point.

SURGICAL PROCEDURES

Surgery is a serious proposition—even minor surgery has its risks. If you've been told you need surgery or if you're considering having an elective procedure done, you owe it to yourself to get all the facts, from the credentials and qualifications of the physician performing the procedure to the list of possible complications and outcomes.

Choosing a Surgeon

At some point in your life, you may need to choose a surgeon. Despite how intimidating the process may seem, it is not as difficult as you might think. The key to selecting the best surgeon for you is to be organized, patient, and persistent. You need to know as much as you possibly can about the person your select.

As with choosing a general practitioner, you need to consider the education of a surgeon. (See Choosing a Practitioner, p. 424.) Usually, a surgeon's education includes undergraduate work, medical school, and a general residency (hands-on training at a hospital or clinic under the supervision of physicians). Then, a three- to four-year surgical residency usually follows. This residency trains future surgeons and prepares them for certification examinations. Do not hesitate to ask where a surgeon was educated, where advanced training was undertaken, and how recently and where he or she has gone for continuing education.

After a surgical residency, a physician may take an examination given by a medical specialty board in order to become certified. Board certification indicates that a physician has completed a course of study in accordance with the national educational standards. It has been called a minimum standard of excellence—there are some excellent doctors without board certification, as well as some inferior doctors with it—but it is a good signs that the physician is up to date on the procedures, theories and success-failure rates in the specialty. (See Choosing a Practitioner, p. 424, and Specialists and Board Certification, p. 428, for more information on specialists.)

Top Ten Surgical Procedures for Men

According to the National Center for Health Statistics, 15.9 million procedures were performed on men in 1994. The following procedures are the ten most common invasive tests and surgeries undergone by men in that year. (The figures exclude newborn infants and, therefore, don't include circumcision—by far the most common male surgical procedure—done on some 60 percent of newborn boys in the United States.)

Procedure	Number performed
Arteriography and angiocardiography using contrast material	1,058,000
Cardiac catheterization	633,000
Respiration therapy	577,000
Diagnostic ultrasound	538,000
Computerized axial tomography	500,000
Endoscopy of small intestine with or without biopsy	409,000
Coronary artery bypass graft	363,000
Removal of coronary artery obstruction	280,000
Prostatectomy	263,000
Endoscopy of large intestine with or without biopsy	225,000

BE SURE TO ASK

Without a doubt, you should meet the surgeon you have in mind before putting your care in his or her hands. Recently, it has become quite common for people to be scheduled for surgery by one specialist without ever meeting or talking to the surgeon. Don't let this happen to you. Sit down and talk with several surgeons you are considering to talk about their credentials and the details of the procedure you're going to have. During this interview, you should ask the following:

- Are you board-certified? What specialty are you certified in and what board certifies you? (You can confirm a physician's board certification by calling the American Board of Medical Specialties at 800-776-CERT.)

- How often have you performed the procedure I require? The more frequently a surgeon performs a procedure, the better the chances that it will be a success.

- Are you in group or solo practice? If a doctor is in group practice, you may be contracting with the group and not necessarily with the doctor to whom you are speaking. If you want a particular doctor, be sure to have the group guarantee it.

- What are your fees? Don't be afraid to ask this, and have the doctor put it in writing. Today, most people need to pay something out of pocket for surgery, and some elective procedures may not be covered by insurance. Keep in mind that doctor's fees are negotiable. If you can't afford the quoted fee, negotiate a price you can afford. You'll be surprised at how easy it is to get the price down.

- What are the most common complications associated with this procedure? You want to be as well prepared as possible before surgery. If the doctor skirts the issue or says there is no possibility of complications, consider leaving. No surgery is without some possible complication. A good surgeon will go over the possibilities and give you the percentages that these complications occur. Ask any and all questions necessary to get the answers you need to make a decision.

- What is the nosocomial infection rate associated with this procedure? (Nosocomial infections are those acquired in the hospital.) Nationally, the rate is close to 10 percent. However, more than half of all infections are preventable if hospital personnel follow proper anti-infection procedures. Although it is unlikely that a hospital will release its overall figure, ask the surgeon to give you the infection rate experienced at that hospital for patients under his or her care. If the number is in the midrange of single digits, the hospital is probably doing a halfway decent job of controlling this national problem.

continues

- What are the success rates of this procedure? The success rate means more than simply surviving. Ask the surgeon what your chances are of 100 percent success—that is, regaining normal function. If less than 100 percent, have the surgeon detail what you can expect your functional level to be after you've completely recovered from the procedure. This is important because if the functional level is low, you may want to weigh it against the risk of surgery.

Keep in mind that a surgical residency and board certification are not required for an individual to be known as a surgeon. Licensed physicians can proclaim themselves to be any specialist they desire. Thus, it is essential that you question your would-be surgeon thoroughly.

You'll also need to consider the question of experience. It is assumed that surgeons become more skilled at procedures they do often, so you'll want to look for someone who is experienced in the procedure you need. However, the number of times a procedure is performed should not be the only factor used to determine skill. A practitioner at a small hospital might be very skilled in a procedure but, because of the number of patients in the area, may not have the opportunity to perform it often. In addition, a practitioner who has done a high number of a particular procedure might be performing the surgery more often than is necessary.

You can receive referrals to a surgeon from another practitioner. Other sources for referrals include a local medical society, a hospital referral service (though these usually only recommend physicians with privileges at that hospital), friends and family, and even the telephone book or newspaper advertisements. Your health insurance company may also provide referrals. In fact, health maintenance organizations (HMO) usually only cover procedures done by

specialists they contract with. If you belong to an HMO, find out its policy on referrals to specialists.

Choosing a Hospital

Where medical care is provided is as important as who provides it, and the choice of a hospital can be one of the most important decisions of all.

In some communities, the number of options may be limited, though the progress of the medical establishment has made more than one hospital available to most consumers. Your choice of a hospital may also be restricted by a managed care plan or a health maintenance organization (HMO), an insurance company that requires you use one of its practitioners and medical facilities for your care.

The various types of hospitals from which to choose include the following:

1. *Specialty hospitals.* These take care of only one kind of medical condition or one type of patient. It might admit only those patients with cancer or orthopedic problems, or only children. Specialty hospitals concentrate on a single disease or condition or type of patient, and presumably the staff becomes expert in dealing with it.

2. *General medical/surgical hospitals.* These are, in effect, a conglomeration of little specialty hospitals under one roof. Still, a general hospital occasionally sends a patient to a specialty hospital for more focused and more knowledgeable care.

3. *Community hospitals.* These are the most common type of hospital in the United States. Such hospitals may have as few as fifty beds or as many as several hundred. They point out that they are large enough to give the consumer big-time medicine, yet small enough to provide personal attention.

4. *Medical centers.* These are large institutions that are able to treat rare conditions that community hospitals might not be able to handle. These medical centers are usually affiliated with universities, and many experts are on the staffs of these hospitals. However, a medical center may not be the right choice for a consumer hoping for a relaxed and easy recuperation or personalized care.

5. *Teaching hospitals.* These hospitals train both under- and postgraduate medical students. Such hospitals range in size from a few hundred to possibly as high as a few thousand beds, and nearly all teaching hospitals have major medical school ties. Teaching hospitals offer expertise, the newest technology, and the latest, up-to-the-minute knowledge. However, keep in mind that these hospitals exist as much for education as they do for the care of the patients, with patients being used as teaching examples for the medical students, interns, and residents to work on and learn from. This form of medicine—with its teaching rounds when students, interns, and residents converge around patients' beds—is just not for everybody.

6. *Osteopathic and allopathic hospitals.* These are staffed with doctors of osteopathy, or D.O.'s, and differ little these days from the allopathic hospital (staffed with medical doctors, or M.D.'s). There are far fewer osteopathic hospitals than allopathic ones. Osteopaths and their hospitals tend to serve smaller, more rural communities than do M.D.'s and their hospitals. Some hospitals offer privileges to both D.O.'s and M.D.'s.

Anesthesia

There are three basic types of anesthesia: local, regional, and general.

Local anesthesia is used for procedures in which only a small portion of the body needs to be anesthetized for a short time (such as when you dentist uses Novocain before drilling).

Regional anesthesia is used to numb a portion of the body for up to three hours. The four types of regional anesthesia are caudal, epidural, nerve block, and spinal. Each designation refers to the regions of the body affected by the anesthesia. A caudal block is an anesthetic injected in the area below the lumbar vertebrae in the sacrum (the triangle-shaped bone between the hips). It deadens the area where it is injected. An epidural is delivered via a catheter to an area in the lower back between the lumbar vertebrae. It is a complete pain block for the abdominal region. A nerve block occurs when an anesthetic is injected into an area where main nerves are located such as the hand or foot. It differs from local anesthesia in that it "deadens" or numbs the area that the main nerve affects. Spinal anesthesia is that injected directly into the spinal fluid. It anesthetizes the region from the stomach to the toes (in other words, the lower part of your body).

General anesthesia is used to anesthetize the entire body for extended periods of time.

The Anesthesiologist

The anesthesiologist is the specialist responsible for maintaining the state of sleep you'll be in during your surgery. While an anesthesiologist may seem to be a somewhat minor member of your surgical team, this specialist actually plays a vital role. Anesthesiology is also the area in which a great deal of errors occur. Even in the most routine procedures, there is still a risk from the anesthesia.

Anesthesia in the hospital setting is usually administered by a physician (anesthesiologist) who is board-certified in anesthesiology or by a certified nurse-anesthetist who works under the supervision of an anesthesiologist. Both professionals are highly skilled with specialized training in the use and administration of anesthesia. You should find out what training and experience that individual has and ask whether the person has ever been sanctioned by the hospital or the state licensing agency.

It's important to talk with your anesthesiologist before the surgery. Most patients see their anesthesiologist only the night before the operation. He or she will slip into your room, make brief introductions, and start asking you questions about your health history. The idea is to find anything in your physical makeup that could conceivably cause trouble when you are put under: allergies, heart problems, high blood pressure, low blood pressure, and so on.

That really is not enough. To be fair to both you and the anesthesiologist, you should seek out him or her ahead of time. Ask your doctor or your surgeon to tell you who your anesthesiologist will be and ask for help in making an appointment to talk. Anesthesiologists are independent vendors and sell their expertise to many hospitals, but it is worth the effort to search for them and pin them down for even just half an hour or so. You should ask the following questions:

- Which kind of anesthesia will be used? General or local? Gas or injection? Why one and not the other? What dangers are there?

- What is the fee? (Like the surgeon's, it is also a charge separate from the hospital bill.)

- What is going to happen in the operating room and just afterward in the recovery room?

- Will he or she be there giving the anesthesia to you? Many anesthesiologists have such a large and geographically wide practice that they can't be at every operation they are responsible for. They hire help. An entirely different anesthesiologist might stand in for the person you met and talked with.

In some hospitals, anesthetists (nurses with some advanced training) often do the job instead. Your anesthesiologist may merely check in by phone from whatever other hospital he or she happens to be working in at the moment. An emergency situation could arise, one that only the anesthesiologist could handle, but he or she could be unavailable. Tell your anesthesiologist that you want him or her in the operating room with you, monitoring your progress in person, and get it in writing.

Surgical Risks

Mortality Rates

Modern medicine has come a long way since the turn of the century when surgical death rates made dying from an operation as likely as surviving one. Today, only one out of every seventy-five persons dies as a direct result of all surgery performed. (The exact rate is 1.33 percent.) The percentage of people who die during or as a direct result of an operation is termed the mortality rate.

Yet overall mortality rates are of little significance to you who must deal with one operation. Of importance to you is the mortality rate for the procedure you are contemplating and what factors increase or decrease those percentages.

The mortality rates associated with the procedure are calculated on the total number of procedures performed. For example, the procedure closed reduction and internal fixation of fracture of the femur (surgical repair of a broken leg) has a mortality rate of 3.7 percent based on 28,000 procedures studied. That translates into 1,036 deaths resulting from the procedure or one death for every twenty-seven procedures performed. The important point to consider is the percentage of deaths, rather than the actual numbers. The percentage gives you a much better perspective on what your survival chances are. Thus, in this case your chance of surviving the operation is 96.3 percent. Certain factors may raise the overall mortality rate. Depending on the procedure, age may be a factor. In other instances, other medical conditions that you might have may lower your chances of survival.

Complications

Mortality is not the only hazard facing consumers considering surgery. There is also the prospect of complications (conditions that develop as a result of the procedure), some of which may be life-threatening. The rate at which these complicating factors occurs is called the morbidity rate. It is expressed as a percentage.

While there are standard definitions of what a complication is, there are no standards for what is major, minor, or what counts as a complication. Thus, a very meticulous study of one set of practitioners that looks at every event that extends the hospital stay or increases the cost of care could report a very high complication rate, while a sloppy study that counts only events that ultimately led to a bad outcome could report a very low one. It is also well understood among medical researchers that wide variations in surgical outcomes and complications associated with specific surgical procedures are fairly routine.

Nosocomial Infections

A nosocomial infection is one you acquire while you're hospitalized, and it's especially risky for surgical patients because microbes can multiply quickly in an open wound. Studies indicate that between 5 and 10 percent of all patients develop nosocomial infections, which are often spread by hand contact and may occur as a result of direct contact between medical staff and patients. However, when hospitalized, you can protect yourself by doing the following:

- Demand that all medical and nonmedical personnel wash their hands before touching you.

- Request a room change if your roommate develops a nosocomial infection.

- Request that shaving of body hair be done the morning of surgery, not the night before. Also, find out if shaving is absolutely necessary. Some studies indicate a higher risk for infection when shaving occurs the night before surgery.

- If you have a catheter (a tube that drains a body cavity or the bladder), make sure the staff checks it regularly for proper drainage. A clogged catheter is a prime breeding ground for germs.

Iatrogenic Illnesses

Iatrogenic illnesses are doctor-caused or doctor-produced in the sense that you didn't have the condition until the doctor did something to you, such as accidentally cutting into adjacent tissue with the scalpel or failing to remove a surgical sponge.

Medications errors are another example of iatrogenic illnesses. In some hospitals, the medication error rate can run as high as 11 percent, while 2 to 3 percent is not uncommon even in the best of hospitals. Only constant vigilance by you or a family member or friend serving as an advocate can guard against potential medication errors. (See Medications, p. 449, for information on preventing medication errors in the hospital.)

SECOND OPINION

When faced with any sort of serious medical procedure or surgery, you should seek a second opinion. A second opinion is simply another practitioner's recommendation on your diagnosis and treatment—the opinion of a second, independent health-care practitioner. These opinions are then compared and taken into consideration when making a decision about medical care.

While at one time getting a second opinion was considered to be overly cautious and expensive, today many insurers insist a second opinion be sought before they will cover a procedure. Doctors themselves often initiate second opinions by referring a patient to another practitioner or specialist.

The Need for a Second Opinion

A second opinion is useful because not all doctors agree on medical problems—what they are, how to diagnose them, and how (or even whether) to treat them. And too often people simply accept the opinion of their family doctors or surgeons. At times, this may lead to a lot of pain, financial hardship, and perhaps complications and doctor-caused mishaps because of possibly unnecessary procedures—all of which could have been avoided if they'd only asked for another view on the matter in the first place.

A second opinion is vitally important when a trip to the hospital looms in your near future. Even a good doctor, convinced that the benefits of surgery outweigh more conservative and less costly treatment, can be eager to rush you into the operating room. A second opinion might confirm the original diagnosis (and perhaps the need for hospitalization), but it could also contradict the first doctor's conclusions and thus precipitate some doubt about the need for hospitalization. You may even require a third, tie-breaking opinion.

But don't limit the search for a second opinion merely to procedures that involve surgery. Many types of therapy performed in a hospital are risky or invasive, even though not surgical. Ask another doctor for assurance about the need for any procedure that concerns you.

Where to Find a Second Opinion

You should consider finding a doctor for a fair and original second opinion rather than accepting a referral from your practitioner. A lot of second-opinion doctors recommended by first-opinion doctors turn out to be far from impartial. This is true in part because surgeons are the doctors most often asked for second opinions, and they generally recommend surgery over less invasive procedures.

The other, more prevalent problem is that second-opinion doctors may be reluctant to disagree with the friend who recommended them. The truth is that doctors depend on each other for referrals, and too many nonconfirming second opinions may lead to a loss of referrals.

To find a practitioner, check *The Official ABMS Directory of Board Certified Medical Specialists* in your local library's reference section. In addition, check with your employer's benefits department or ask your insurance company to provide you with a list of physicians it uses for its second opinion program. A Medicare beneficiary may contact the local Social Security Administration office for a directory of doctors who participate in the Medicare second-opinion program.

MEDICAL RIGHTS

Informed Consent

Informed consent is, simply, the idea that you have the right to available information about your condition and about the benefits and risks of any procedures the doctors want to perform on you. The information should include side effects, possible complications, likely outcomes, alternative procedures, and information on what will happen if you decide against a procedure. Then you can make an informed decision about what is done to your body and your life before you give the go-ahead or refusal.

However, informed consent can be controversial. Many physicians and their trade organizations believe that informed consent is a nonworkable idea that obstructs quality care, while patients and consumer groups feel that informed consent is an important tool in creating a true doctor-patient partnership.

Some doctors believe that medicine is too complicated for unschooled nonphysicians to understand, but medical consumers think that doctors ought to try to simplify medical information to make it accessible to the general public. And since doctors do not get paid to talk but to perform procedures, some may consider taking time to discuss potential risks and options a loss of time and money. Also, more than a few doctors believe that, if they explain things accurately, a patient might decide not to have the test, procedure, or operation.

Many doctors also contend that patients really don't want to know everything about their conditions and upcoming procedures. They say that the fear created in a patient by hearing all the things that could go wrong is detrimental to the patient's well-being. The facts, though, paint a different picture. A survey undertaken by the President's Commission for the Study of Ethical Problems in Medicine and Biomedical and Behavioral Research found that 96 percent of patients said they wanted to know everything. That number included 85 percent who said they would even want to hear the most "dismal facts" even if one of those facts was imminent death.

Furthermore, a number of studies have shown that people who are told all the possibilities ahead of time make much better postoperative adjustments to stress and pain. Psychologist Irving Janis calls this phenomenon "emotional inoculation," in which patients can prepare themselves and even rehearse recovery scenarios.

Consent Forms

When you enter a hospital or health-care facility for a procedure, you give your informed consent by signing a consent form. This form may be a "blanket" consent form that gives the facility permission to treat your condition and applies to any and all procedures provided during your stay. Some forms may only apply to a specific procedure. Some facilities ask you to sign a consent form that includes a release against negligence on the part of the hospital or clinic or that requires you to waive your right to litigation in the event of malpractice. However, because the hospital is considered to have such a great advantage over the patient, these forms are not legally binding.

If you have not been informed to your satisfaction and/or are more than a bit unsure about giving your consent to your doctor's game plan, don't sign any form. Ask for more information. Ask about survival rates and statistical proofs of the effectiveness and safety of the procedure. (A lot of this territory should have already been covered during office visits and previous discussions.) If you are really doubtful, ask for printed materials that provide support for the route your doctor wants to take.

Also, make sure that the procedure described in the form is the same one that your doctor described to you. If it seems that the form grants permission for other procedures that you weren't aware of, don't sign the form until the point is clarified.

If you don't sign the consent form, chances are you won't be admitted to the hospital. However, you should also know that these forms aren't set in stone, and you can revise them before signing them in order to protect your rights. A hospital consent form is not the law. The form is a contract that's subject to revision, and you have the right to revise it. You also have the right to say no to anything proposed. While some hospital administrators may balk at your revisions, most will let you sign an amended form. This is because administrators usually realize that consent forms deny patients their rights and refusing to amend such a form could lead to complaints or a lawsuit.

Consent Form for a Specific Procedure

The consent form reproduced here is similar to ones used in most hospitals, give or take a few phrases and clauses. A form of this sort is a specific consent form—that is, it indicates that

Consent to Operation or Other Special Procedure

PATIENT_____ AGE_____

DATE_____ TIME_____ A.M./P.M. CONSENT OBTAINED AT _____
(i.e. physician's office, hospital, etc.)

1. I authorize the performance upon _____ of the following operation (Myself or name of patient)

or procedure_____

      (State nature and extent of operation)

to be performed at The Hospital under the direction of Dr. _____ and/or such associates and assistants as may be selected by him/her.

2. The nature and purpose of the operation, referred to in Paragraph 1 hereof and the possible alternative methods of treatment have been explained to me by Dr. _____ and to my complete satisfaction. No guarantee or assurance has been given by anyone as to the results that maybe obtained.

3. I acknowledge that I have been afforded the opportunity to ask any questions with respect to the operation and any risks or complications thereto and to set forth, in the space provided below, any limitations or restrictions with respect to this consent:

_____

_____

_____

      (If None, write "none")

4. I consent to the performance of operations, procedures and treatment in addition to or different from those now contemplated as described above, whether or not arising from presently unforeseen conditions, which the above-named doctor or his/her associates or assistants may in his/her or their judgment consider necessary or advisable in my present illness.

5. I understand that anesthesia shall be administered during this operation under the direction of the responsible physician.

6. For the purpose of advancing medical education, I consent to the admittance of observers to the operating room.

7. I consent to the disposal by hospital authorities of any tissues or parts that may be removed.

I CERTIFY THAT I HAVE READ AND FULLY UNDERSTAND THE ABOVE CONSENT, THAT THE EXPLANATIONS THEREIN REFERRED TO WERE MADE, THAT ALL BLANKS OR STATEMENTS REQUIRING INSERTION OR COMPLETION WERE FILLED IN, AND THAT INAPPLICABLE PARAGRAPHS, IF ANY, WERE STRICKEN BEFORE I SIGNED.

      Signature of Patient_____
      Signature of Witness_____
      (Witness to signature only)

When a patient is a minor or incompetent to give consent:

      Signature of person authorized
      to consent for patient_____
      Relationship to patient _____

The foregoing consent was signed in my presence, and in my opinion the person did so freely with full knowledge and understanding.
      Signature of Physician_____
      Signature of Witness _____
      (Witness to signature only)

by your signature you have agreed to the performance of a specific procedure in a specific way for which you have received adequate informational background. A different form should be completed before every procedure that you believe requires a consent contract.

Be sure that all the clauses are true and represent your beliefs before you sign the form. Be careful. The forms are filled with booby traps. If you need to alter, amend, or revise the form to fit your situation, then do so. For example, in the form shown here, you might possibly require more space to set forth your reservations than the extremely generous and expansive two lines afforded you in number 3. Or you might not go along with number 4, which, in effect, makes a mockery of the form and the entire informed consent process. You might not want your operation to be that day's surgical show, so number 6 would be something you couldn't agree to. Some forms have patients consenting to allow filming and videotaping of their operations. You might not want that. Let them know they are refused permission to do so.

Also mark down items that aren't on the form that you think must be on it before you will give your consent. For example, an important condition you might wish to add is that you will not consent to the operation unless it is performed by your surgeon. You do not consent to a colleague, resident, or intern doing the operation for the first time while your surgeon acts as a teacher/observer.

Don't be rushed into signing the form. Give it a few good thinks and enough time to tailor it to your specific situation. If you don't understand something on the consent form, request that somebody from the administrator's office or the hospital's legal department clarify the form or parts of it for you.

Informed consent is not and should not be a piece of paper, but a process, a partnership of information-sharing and trust between doctor and patient.

MEDICAL RECORDS

A medical record is composed of your medical history, including conditions, diagnoses, medical complaints, practitioner's comments, laboratory results, x-rays, and descriptions of procedures and treatments. Keeping track of your medical record can be very worthwhile; it can provide information needed to make a future diagnosis, help resolve conflict with an insurance c ompany, and keep help you track of allergies you have and medications you use. It's also helpful to keep a record in case you move or change doctors.

Yet very few men keep medical records. Most assume that such records are kept by their physician, dentist, or optometrist and that they'll be accurate and easy to obtain if need be. However, this is not always the case.

Access to Medical Records

Requesting and receiving copies of your medical records from health-care professionals should be a relatively easy process, yet many people find it a struggle. The process is complicated by a patchwork of confusing state laws, court decisions, and health department regulations.

Only twenty-five states have some form of legislation that permits direct access to them. These states are

Alaska	Minnesota
Arkansas	Montana
California	Nevada
Colorado	New Hampshire
Connecticut	New Jersey

Florida   New York
Georgia   Oklahoma
Hawaii   South Dakota
Indiana   South Carolina
Louisiana   Virginia
Maryland   Washington
Michigan   West Virginia
                 Wisconsin

In Maine, Massachusetts, and Texas, physicians have the option of providing a summary of the patient's records in place of the entire record.

In all of the states not included on the list, there are no laws governing access to medical records. But keep in mind that no state has a law restricting access to medical records. This means that there is nothing to preclude your ask-

HOW TO REQUEST YOUR MEDICAL RECORD

As with any administrative request, knowing the formalities and going about the request in the proper way help guarantee the best outcome. The following procedure may be used to access medical records:

- Contact the practitioner or facility that has your records and ask about their general procedures for releasing records. If your state is one of those with access laws, let the contact person at the office or facility know that you know your rights of access. Some office personnel claim that it is illegal for you to have copies of your records. When this happens, ask what specific state law prohibits access. Remember that there is no state where it is illegal to obtain copies of your medical record.

- Always put your request in writing. This documents your efforts and is proof that you are working through normal channels. Include your name, address, patient identification number (if known), and the specific entry or file that you want. Indicate your willingness to pay reasonable copying fees (anything less than fifty cents a page).

- If your initial request is denied by the office manager or records administrator, ask him or her to put the denial in writing. Also ask for the reasons you are being denied access to your records—for example, state law, health department regulation, or office policy. Then ask for the statue number or specific regulation.

- Learn about any appeals process that permits you to resubmit your request for specific parts of your record.

- Contact the hospital patient representative if you are having problems obtaining hospital records. To may wish to consider asking a physician who is your ally to request copies of your records on your behalf.

- When all else fails, contact a lawyer familiar with your state's laws. You may be able to obtain a court order from a magistrate or civil court judge if you can show good cause for needing your medical records.

ing a practitioner or facility for copies of your records. In fact, you should do so.

Federal Laws on Access

The federal Privacy Act and Freedom of Information Act guarantees access to medical records from federal hospitals. This includes military hospital, Veterans Administration hospitals, and prison hospitals. If you are in active duty, write to the hospital at your post or a previous duty station. Retirees and those who are no longer in active duty should write to the National Archives Record Center, 9700 Page, St. Louis, MO 63132. Be sure to include your military identification number, branch of service and dates of service.

Medical Information Bureau

You may never have heard of the Medical Information Bureau (MIB), but it has heard of you. In fact, it probably knows more about you and your health than you can imagine. How is this possible, you ask? If you have ever completed an insurance company application form, you know that these companies want to know a lot about your present and past medical history. And most people comply and answer the many detailed questions. The chances are excellent that the information you provided on the application found its way to the MIB.

Because insurance companies rely on the information stored at the MIB to determine whether or not they will insure you, it is very important that your file is accurate. In the past, your right to inspect your file was limited to all nonmedical information, the names of insurance companies that reported information to the MIB, and the names of insurance companies the received a copy of the information in your file

within the six months preceding your request. If you wanted medical information, you needed to ask a cooperative physician to request the information for you.

However, the MIB now discloses medical information to consumers. A copy of the information is available for a fee of $8. Write to the MIB and ask for a copy of the form "Request for Disclosure of MIB Record Information": Medical Information Bureau, P.O. Box 105, Essex Station, Boston, MA 02112; 617-426-366.

HEALTH INSURANCE

Nothing in health care is more confusing than health insurance. Today, more than ever before, insurance is a profusion of terms and options, some of which were never heard of a decade ago. Fee-for-service plans, managed care plans, Medicare, and Medicaid are just four types of insurance that can create havoc in the mind of an average consumer.

Traditional Fee-for-Service Plans

There are three types of traditional indemnity insurance: hospital insurance, medical/surgical insurance, and major medical insurance. With these forms of insurance, the providers of medical care are paid on a fee-for-service basis, meaning they are reimbursed for the services they provide. The reimbursements are determined by the "usual, customary and reasonable (UCR) rate"—a charge for medical care that is consistent with the going rate for that service in that geographical area.

A consumer can determine what services are covered—or are not covered—by an the insurance company by reading its schedule of benefits, which lists the services a policy will cover or the maximum amounts payable for certain conditions.

1. *Hospital insurance.* This form of insurance covers the use of inpatient and outpatient facilities. It has limits on certain aspects such as on the number of days of hospitalization or on the total number of dollars that can be spent. Services that are not covered will be stated in the schedule of benefits. Most hospital insurance plans require a policyholder to pay an initial deductible (usually $100 to $500, depending on the plan) before the insurance company will pay for care. After that initial deductible is met, the plan usually pays for all approved expenses.

2. *Medical/surgical insurance.* This covers, as you may expect, both medical treatment and surgical treatment. Doctors' visits to the hospital, some office visits leading up to hospitalization or surgery, medications, x-rays, anesthesia, and laboratory tests are covered by the medical portion. The costs for surgical procedures, a surgical team, anesthesiologist, and some procedures performed in a doctor's office are covered by the surgical portion. There may be a dollar limit on the benefits payable. This form of insurance is commonly provided with hospital insurance.

3. *Major medical insurance.* Most medical and surgical expenses associated with serious illness are covered by major medical insurance. This form of insurance doesn't cover preventive care, though it provides extended coverage for hospital and medical services. After an initial deductible is met, the insurance company pays a certain percentage of expenses while the consumer pays the remaining percentage (called a coinsurance). The insurance company, for example, may pay 80 percent, while you would pay 20 percent out of pocket.

Some companies also offer stop-loss provisions. This ensures that you will not pay further once out-of-pocket expenses reach a certain amount, for example, $1,000. After that amount has been reached, the policy covers 100 percent of expenses up to a maximum limit.

If the practitioner who provides the care is not a participating provider with your insurance company, you may have to pay the difference between what the provider charges and what the insurance plan reimburses. This is called balance billing. If you negotiate, some physicians will accept the reimbursement as payment in full or will lower their fee to accommodate you.

4. *Comprehensive insurance.* Comprehensive insurance is a plan that combines these three types of insurance in one policy. As with major medical insurance, there is usually a deductible and a coinsurance up to a stop-loss limit. A lifetime benefit for such a plan may be $1 to $5 million.

These plans cover all services, with a few exceptions, from any practitioner. At times, certain procedures and services (such as hospitalization) must be preapproved in order to be covered.

Managed Care

In a managed care system of health-care delivery, an individual is required to seek care from those practitioners and facilities who are approved by the company. In addition, those practitioners and facilities are required to accept the fee offered by the company as payment-in-full. In this way, balance billing is eliminated. There are many different forms of managed care, as well as a number of options. Some choices include health maintenance organizations, preferred provider organizations, and health maintenance organizations with point-of-service plans.

1. *Health maintenance organizations (HMOs).*
   In an HMO, individuals pay a fixed monthly premium. In return, comprehensive medical care within a system of HMO-approved physicians and facilities is provided. Members of an HMO must choose a single primary-care physician from the list of approved doctors. This physician then acts as a gatekeeper, providing medical care and referrals to specialists as needed. An individual must go through this physician for all medical care. For each HMO patient a physician cares for, the physician receives a fixed monthly payment.

All but a small portion of medical care is prepaid in an HMO. Physician's fees and services, hospital fees, surgical fees, outpatient surgery, home health care, nursing home services, and routine checkups and immunizations are covered. Patients may be responsible for a copayment, a set amount charged regardless of the cost of the services. A typical copayment is $5 to $10.

The limited choice of physicians is thought to be a drawback of HMOs. If care is sought from a practitioner who is not within the HMO system, those services may not be covered. If the HMO offers a point-of-service option (discussed below), those services may be partially covered.

2. *Preferred provider organizations (PPOs).* A PPO is very similar to an HMO. However, in this system, patients are not required to use a specific practitioner or go through that practitioner for referrals. Instead, care is covered as long as members choose practitioners from the panel of physicians provided by the PPO. Again, services may not be covered or may only be partially covered if provided by a physician outside of the approved panel.

3. *Point-of-service plans (POSs).* A POS is an option for those in an HMO or PPO that offers an choice for those who wish to seek care from physicians outside the company's network. In a POS, an individual chooses a primary-care physician, but can seek care elsewhere at any time. However, out-of-network care, as it's called, is subject to additional fees and higher copayments. Self-referral to a specialist—even a specialist within the network—may be considered an out-of-network service.

ERISA and COBRA

The Employment Retirement Income Security Act of 1974—ERISA—is another aspect of insurance to consider. The act is a set of laws that regulate how employers administer health insurance benefits. ERISA requires that employees are provided with all information and documents about their health benefits, and it requires that employers pay all claims made by beneficiaries. An appeal and a written explanation must be submitted if a claim is denied.

The Consolidated Omnibus Budget Reconciliation Act of 1986—COBRA—gives employees the option of temporarily continuing their health insurance after leaving their employer in a number of circumstances—for example, if they are fired or laid off or if they quit. The act gives people the opportunity to maintain coverage, for example, until they find another job or become eligible for coverage by a different insurance company.

COBRA applies to termination of employment, death, divorce or legal separation, reduction of hours, eligibility for Medicare, and loss of independent status by a child. Under COBRA, the employee pays the premiums for the insurance. It is offered for thirty-six months for widows, divorced spouses, spouses of Medicare-eligible employees, and dependent children. It is offered for eighteen months for employees with reduced hours or for those who have been fired.

In 1996, the Health Insurance Portability and Accountability Act, also known as the Kassebaum-Kennedy Bill, was put into place to help people gain access to continued health care if they lose or change their jobs. The law prohibits insurers from denying coverage to people genetically predisposed to particular illnesses and victims of domestic abuse. It bars insurers for imposing a waiting period of more than twelve months before covering preexisting conditions and also guarantees that insurance companies cannot deny coverage to companies with fewer than fifty employees. The measures help those who might previously have been denied coverage to obtain health insurance.

Medicaid

Created in 1965, Medicaid is a joint federal and state health insurance plan that benefits low-income individuals, including the aged, blind, disabled, pregnant women, adults with dependent children, and children under the age of six. States can also decide to offer coverage to other groups, such as residents of long-term-care facilities.

According to Medicaid law, a basic list of services must be included in any state Medicaid program. These services include the following:

- Inpatient hospital services

- Outpatient hospital services

- Physician services

- Medical and surgical services of dentists

- Laboratory and x-ray services

- Nursing home services for those 21 and over

- Home health care for persons eligible for nursing home services

- Family planning services and supplies

- Rural health clinic services

- Federally qualified health center services

- Nurse-midwife services

- Services of certified pediatric or family nurse practitioners

- Early and periodic screening, diagnostic and treatment services for children under 21, and treatment for conditions identified in screening

- Assurance of availability of necessary transportation

Again, states have the option of offering up to thirty-two additional services—for example, physical therapy, dental services, eyeglasses, and chiropractic services.

Local welfare offices can provide information on eligibility for Medicaid and the services offered in your state. To determine eligibility for Medicaid, an application must be submitted to the state welfare department. The state then determines if an individual meets the criteria for the program.

In some states, managed care programs are being offered to Medicaid recipients. With a Medicaid HMO, the state pays a monthly premium to a private HMO, which then takes on the individual as a member. The HMO option is designed to give individuals easier access to health care by guaranteeing them access to network providers, as many practitioners are reluctant to accept Medicaid assignment. It also helps to reduce state spending on insurance. As with any HMO, those who enroll in a Medicaid HMO are limited to the list of approved providers only.

Medicare

Individuals age 65 and older, as well as those who are permanently or totally disabled and those with end-stage renal disease (kidney disease), are covered by Medicare, the federal insurance plan.

Medicare has two parts: part A and part B. Part A of Medicare is free to those who are eligible. It is similar to hospital insurance, covering (with limitations) hospital stays and care in a skilled nursing home or by a home health agency. Part B covers doctor fees, outpatient hospital services, and medical supplies and services. As of 1997, part B coverage cost $43.80 per month. Policies that supplement Medicare, known as "Medigap" policies, are available to cover costs that Medicare does not. Those who are over 65 who are not eligible for Medicare may be able to purchase part A coverage for a monthly premium.

Medicare HMOs are also an option for Medicare beneficiaries and retiring employees over 65 who were already members of an HMO. HMO coverage takes the place of Medicare benefits and is required to provide all the basic Medicare services. Some Medicare HMO also provide some additional services. These services may include hearing aids, eyeglasses, rehabilitation services, and prescription drugs. However, to receive the extra services, beneficiaries may be required to pay a monthly premium in addition to what they may already be paying for Medicare coverage.

Medicare Eligibility

To be eligible for Medicare you must be a citizen of the United States (by birth or naturalization) or an alien admitted for permanent residence who has lived in the United States for at least five years.

Also, individuals must be entitled to payments under the Social Security or the Railroad Retirement Act, which, in turn, means that they must have fulfilled a work requirement. This means that they must have worked for at least forty quarters—or a total of ten years—in jobs covered under the Social Security Act.

A person can also be covered based on the record of someone who is covered. For example, spouses are eligible if they are age 65 or older and if their spouse is insured; widows and widowers are covered if they were married for more than one year prior to the death of the spouse; and divorced persons are eligible if they were married to the spouse for at least ten years and have not remarried.

SHOPPING TIPS

Do not buy more insurance than you need for yourself and your family. Duplicate policies only mean duplicate premium expenses. And if you make a claim against both insurance companies, don't expect to collect twice. The companies will invoke the coordination of benefits clause in your plan and only pay up to their contractual obligations.

- Check the rating of the insurance company to determine its financial condition. Companies such as A.M. Best, Duff & Phelps, Moody's, and Standard & Poor rate insurance companies, according to their financial stability and ability to pay claims. (Check your library for publications by these companies.)

- Check with your state's insurance department to determine if a particular company is authorized to sell its policies in your state. Also check on the particular plan to determine if it has been approved for sale by the insurance commissioner.

- Make sure the salesperson clearly explains the policy's schedule of benefits, and you fully understand the contract. This includes waiting periods, exclusions, periods of noncoverage, and preexisting conditions. (The time to discover a services isn't covered is *before* you sign the contract, not *after*.)

- Don't purchase a policy with excessively high deductibles and stop-loss limit. Individual deductibles of $2,500 to $3,000 and family deductibles of up to $5,000 may cost you more in out-of-pocket expenses than they return in benefits. Shop for a stop-loss limit under $5,000.

- Purchase group insurance if at all possible. Group plans are generally less expensive and in some cases may offer more complete coverage than individual plans. (Join a social, fraternal, or alumni group if it will help you purchase insurance at lower rates.)

- Consider joining a health maintenance organization (HMO) if one in your area has an open enrollment period. You may discover that you get twice the coverage for the same amount of premium and lower deductibles and copayments. (In some cases, you may not have any deductible or copayment with an HMO.)

- Always answer the insurance application as honestly as you can. Incomplete answers could leave you open to having your insurance policy canceled, thereby making it more difficult for you to purchase subsequent insurance.

- Always pay your premium by a check made out to the company, not the salesperson. Also inquire about any discount for paying your premiums on an annual basis. (The next best thing is to pay quarterly.)

continues

> • Always take advantage of the thirty-day "free-look" period offered by your insurance company. If, before the thirty days have expired, you discover that the policy is not right for you or your family, you may return it and receive a full refund of your premium.

Medicare Enrollment

To enroll in Medicare, you must take action when you turn 65. You can apply anytime within three months before your 65th birthday and three months after. If you apply within this "personal enrollment period," your Medicare coverage will begin on your 65th birthday. If you apply later than this, your coverage will begin on the date of application, not on your 65th birthday. Questions can be directed to the Social Security Administration at 800-772-1213.

Those who are already being covered by Social Security or Railroad Retirement benefits when they turn 65 are automatically enrolled in part A of Medicare and must apply to enroll in part B. Those who apply for Social Security after they turn 65 are asked to apply for Medicare at the same time.

A card and notification of Medicare coverage will be sent three to four months before a person's 65th birthday. A person who is covered does not need a Medicare card in order to be covered; the hospital can bill using the Social Security number if the card is not available.

Choosing a Practitioner

Not every practitioner accepts every form of insurance, so it's important to find out what your practitioner's policy is on coverage. Most practitioners will accept coverage (meaning they act as participating providers) from large insurance companies, such as Blue Cross/Blue Shield. However, smaller companies may not be widely accepted.

To maximize your coverage, you can check with your insurance company for a list of doctors in your area that will accept that form of insurance. If you have Medicare, check with the local Social Security office for participating physicians. Medicaid recipients can ask at the state welfare office for a list.

Once you've determined your practitioner does accept your insurance, make sure that he or she accepts the company's reimbursement as payment-in-full. Reimbursement is the key word. At times, the amount offered as payment by an insurance company is less than what the doctor charges for that service. If this occurs, the balance must be paid by the patient (balance billing). To avoid surprises, find out up front what the charges for care will be. If the insurance company's payment will be less than the fee, ask your doctor to accept the reimbursement as payment-in-full—some practitioners will agree to this arrangement. You can also try to negotiate the price of the service with the physician in order to lower the amount you will have to pay out-of-pocket.

For more information:

Health Insurance Association of America
555 13th St., N.W., Suite 600
Washington, DC 20004-1660
202-824-1600

GLOSSARY OF INSURANCE TERMS

Just as the medical profession has its specialized language, insurance companies also often fall back on a system of cumbersome codes that often only insiders understand. Here, in straight-forward language, are the meanings of common health insurance terms.

Accumulation period. The number of days during which the insured person must incur eligible medical expenses at least equal to the deductible in order to receive a benefit.

Allocated benefits. Benefits for which the maximum amount payable for specific services is itemized in the insurance contract.

Ambulatory benefits. Benefits available to an insured person for health-care services received while not confined to a hospital bed as an inpatient—for example, outpatient care, emergency room care, home health care, or preadmission testing.

Ambulatory surgical center. A medical facility that performs outpatient surgical procedures.

Application. A signed statement of facts that an insurance company uses to decide whether to sell a person a policy.

Assignment. An agreement in which the insured person instructs the insurance company to pay the hospital, doctor, or medical supplier directly for services received and at the payment rate established by the insurer.

Benefits. The amount of money or services an insurance company will pay or provide under the provisions of the policy.

Cancellation. The termination of a policy before it would normally expire.

Claim. A notification by an insured person or his or her doctor or hospital to the insurance company stating that the person received a medical service and is requesting payment in accordance with the policy.

COBRA. The Consolidated Omnibus Reconciliation Act of 1985 that requires employers to offer continuation of group-health insurance coverage to certain employees and dependents for eighteen to thirty-six months after they leave their companies' employ.

Coinsurance/copayment. A cost-sharing requirement in many health insurance policies in which the insured person assumes a portion or percentage of the costs of covered services. The most common cost-sharing provision has the person responsible for 20 percent of covered expenses while the insurer pays the remaining 80 percent.

Conditionally renewable clause. A provision that permits a policyholder to renew a policy up to a certain age limit (such as 65) providing all conditions of the insurance contract have been met.

Conversion clause. A provision in a group policy that provides the insured person with the opportunity to purchase individual coverage in the event the group policy is terminated.

Coordination of benefits. A practice insurance companies use to avoid duplication of payment when a person is covered by more than one policy.

Covered expense. A medical expense that an insured person incurs and the insurance company agrees to pay.

Custodial care facility. A facility that provides around-the-clock room and board to aged or handicapped persons who require personal care, supervision, or assistance in daily activity.

Deductible. The amount the policyholder must pay before an insurance plan pays for any portion of the cost.

Disability insurance. Insurance that pays the insured person a portion of an insured person's salary when the person is sick or injured and unable to work.

Disease-specific insurance. Insurance that provides benefits should a specific illness such as cancer, heart disease, poliomyelitis, encephalitis, or spinal meningitis develop.

Effective date. The date insurance begins; the first day a person can file a claim and have benefits paid.

Eligibility. Determination of whether an applicant qualifies for coverage for health care rendered.

Employer mandate. A requirement that employers provide or arrange health insurance coverage for employees. Typically, such proposals require coverage of workers' families, too.

Exclusions. Specific conditions or circumstances under which a policy will not provide benefits. The specific services excluded from a policy may be found in the policy's schedule of benefits.

Explanation of benefits. A statement from an insurance company itemizing the medical services an insured person received and the amount of insurance coverage provided for each service.

Fee for service. An arrangement under which doctors or other health-care providers are paid separately for each service they perform. Some economists say this method of payment may give doctors an incentive to provide more services than they need.

First-dollar coverage. A policy with no deductible that covers the first dollar of expenses.

Free look. A period of time—usually ten to thirty days—during which a person may return the policy and receive a full refund of any premium paid.

Grace period. A period of time (usually thirty or thirty-one days) after the date a premium is due

during which the policy remains in force and the premium may still be paid without penalty.

Group insurance. Insurance, usually issued through employers and unions, that covers a group of persons.

Guaranteed renewable clause. A provision that guarantees the policyholder the right to renew as long as premiums are paid on time. While the insurance is in force, the company cannot raise the premium unless all policyholders have their premiums raised at the same time.

Health insurance purchasing cooperative (HIPC). An entity that buys insurance coverage and medical care for a large number of people, including employees of small businesses.

Health maintenance organization (HMO). An prepaid group health plan, which provides a range of services in return for fixed monthly premiums.

Home health care. Care rendered in a patient's home such as nursing services, therapy or medications.

Hospital insurance. Insurance that covers costs of hospital care resulting from injury or illness.

Indemnity benefits. A fixed-dollar payment for a specific health care service such as $100 a day for hospitalization. Should the cost of care be more than the policy pays, the insured person is responsible for the difference.

Indemnity policy. Insurance that pays a specified amount of money each day or week that the insured person is in the hospital and that pays a set amount for medical and surgical procedures.

Individual insurance. A policy that is purchased by an individual and that is not part of a group plan. The policy covers the individual and, usually, that person's dependents.

Individual practice association (IPA). A prepaid health-care plan that is offered to groups of people by physicians in private practice.

Inpatient. Someone who is officially admitted and occupies a hospital room while receiving hospital care, including room, board, and general nursing care.

Inside limit. A provision that limits insurance payment for any type of service, regardless of the actual cost of the service.

Intermediate care facility. A facility that provides health care and services to persons who do not require the care and services of a hospital or a skilled nursing facility.

Lapsed policy. An insurance policy that has been canceled for nonpayment of premiums.

Level of care. The type and intensity of treatment necessary to adequately and efficiently treat an illness or condition.

Major medical insurance. Insurance that offsets the large expenses of a severe and prolonged illness or injury.

Managed care. A method of delivering, supervising, and coordinating health care, often through health maintenance organizations and other networks of doctors and hospitals. The purpose is to eliminate inappropriate services, control costs, and assure access to effective treatments.

Managed competition. A health policy that combines free-market forces with government regulation. Large groups of consumers and businesses buy health care from organized networks of doctors and hospitals, which are supposed to compete by offering low prices and high quality.

Medicaid. A government program that provides assistance to the poor.

Medical-surgical insurance. Insurance that covers some of fees of physicians and surgeons for care provided in the hospital, office, or home and covers part of the cost of laboratory tests performed outside the hospital.

Medicare. The government's medical insurance program for people age 65 and older, those who are permanently and totally disabled, and those with end-stage renal disease (kidney disease that required dialysis or a transplant).

Medicare-approved amount. A dollar figure approved by Medicare that will be either the "usual and customary charge," the prevailing charge or the actual charge (whichever is lowest) and is the amount Medicare pays the doctor.

Medicare assignment. An agreement by a physician or medical provider to accept the Medicare-approved amount as payment in full for services rendered to a Medicare beneficiary.

Optionally renewable clause. A provision that gives an insurance company the right to cancel the coverage at any anniversary or, in some cases, at any premium due date. However, the company may not cancel the coverage between such dates.

Outpatient. Someone who is not officially admitted as an inpatient to a hospital but receives hospital care (for example, laboratory work and x-rays) without occupying a hospital bed or receiving room, board, or general nursing care.

Period of noncoverage. Provisions that specify periods when the insurance contract is not in force.

Policy. The legal document issued by the insurance company to the policyholder that outlines the conditions and terms of the insurance. Also called the contract.

Policy limit. The maximum benefits an insurance company will pay under a particular policy.

Preexisting condition. An injury occurring, disease contracted, or physical/mental condition that existed prior to issuance of a health insurance policy. Usually, benefits will not be paid for services related to preexisting conditions, although many insurance companies cover these conditions after a certain waiting period.

Preferred provider organization (PPO). An organization of doctors and hospitals that provides medical services to groups of people at discounted rates. Members of the groups agree to use only the "preferred" providers.

Premium. The amount paid—monthly, quarterly, semiannually, or annually—to purchase insurance and keep it in force.

Prepaid plan. A plan that provides medical services to a group of persons who pay for the services in advance in the form of a monthly fee. Health maintenance organizations and individual practice associations are prepaid plans.

Provider. A term used to describe doctors, nurses, hospitals, pharmacists, and anyone else who provides health care.

Renewal clause. A clause that indicates the provisions under which the policy may or may not be renewed. Since many individual health insurance policies are written for a limited time, usually one year, they must be renewed at the end of each term. The provisions most often encountered are

1. *Guaranteed renewable.* The company guarantees a person's right to renew a policy to a specific age, commonly 65. A guaranteed renewable policy may also have a guaranteed premium which will not be raised during the term of the policy.

2. *Conditionally renewable.* The policy may be renewed until the person reaches a certain age, usually 65, provided the person has complied with the other conditions of the policy.

3. *Optionally renewable.* The company may decline to renew the policy on the anniversary date.

Rider. A document that amends the policy. It may increase or decrease benefits, waive the condition of coverage, or in any other way amend the original contract.

Schedule of benefits. The list of medical services that a particular insurance policy will cover or the maximum amounts payable for certain conditions.

Skilled nursing facility (SNF). A facility that provides skilled nursing care and related services for patients who require inpatient medical or nursing care.

Stop-loss provision. A provision that limits an insured person's out-of-pocket expenses to a set amount, after which the insurance policy pays all expenses up to the plan's maximum benefits.

Surgical schedule. A list of cash allowances that are payable for various types of surgery, with maximum allowances based upon the severity of the operation.

Tax cap. A limit on federal tax breaks for health insurance. The term can apply to employers or employees or both.

Third-party payer. An organization (such as an insurance company) that reimburses medical-care providers (such as hospitals and medical practitioners) for services provided to policyholders.

Usual, customary, and reasonable. A charge for medical care that is consistent with the going rate for identical or similar services in the same geographic area.

Waiting period. The length of time an employee must wait from his or her date of employment or application for insurance coverage to the date his or her insurance goes into effect.

Worker's compensation insurance. An insurance program, usually established by the state, that provides benefits to employees who are injured in the course of their employment.

DEPARTMENT OF VETERANS AFFAIRS

The Department of Veterans Affairs (VA) is the successor to the Veterans Administration, an independent agency, and was made the fourteenth cabinet department in 1989. The Department of Veterans Affairs, whose central office is in Washington, D.C., is headed by the Secretary of Veterans Affairs and is made up of several suborganizations, which include the National Cemetery System, the Veterans Benefits Administration and the Veterans Health Administration. Higher officials of the VA are appointed by the president of the United States and are also subject to Senate approval.

The VA ensures medical and hospital services as well as various types of benefits for veterans and their families. Benefits include health care (medical centers, nursing home care units, and outpatient clinics), life insurance plans and centers, education assistance, rehabilitation concerning vocations, compensation for military service (for disabilities and in cases of death), and pension payments.

Veterans Health Administration

The Veterans Health Administration, the largest health-care system in the United States, operates 173 medical centers with fifty-one thousand beds, 391 outpatient centers, 131 nursing homes, 39 residential living centers, and numerous community and outreach clinics. Each year, the VA treats nearly a million patients in VA hospitals, seventy-nine thousand in nursing homes, and twenty-five thousand in residential living centers. There are approximately 27.5 million visits to VA outpatient centers. Total spending for medical care in the Veterans Health Administration was $16.7 billion in 1996.

The VA is also associated with more than 159 medical and dental schools. It is estimated that more than half of the practicing physicians in the United States have trained in VA facilities.

Eligibility

Veterans of all military, naval, and air service are eligible for benefits from the Department of Veterans Affairs. To be eligible for medical services from the Veterans Health Administration, however, certain service-connected criteria must be met. Veterans can write, call, or visit any regional VA office near them at 800-827-1000 for information concerning their eligibility for benefits. Veterans may also obtain information and application forms from local veteran organizations and from the American Red Cross.

Restrictions and exact conditions of eligibility apply. Veterans who were discharged dishonorably cannot receive care. In addition, veterans can be treated in VA medical centers only for those medical conditions incurred while in active service. Veterans with service-connected disabilities can receive different benefits, according to their disability ratings (a medical determination as to the extent of disability and expressed as a percentage such as 100 percent, 70 percent, or 50 percent disabled).

Hospital and Outpatient Care

Hospital care and some outpatient care can be obtained by any veteran who has sustained a service-connected disability and whose condition originated or was aggravated during active service.

Eligibility for hospital care is divided into category 1 and category 2. Category 1 veterans are veterans who receive a pension; veterans who are eligible for Medicaid; veterans exposed to ionizing radiation (atom bomb tests), environmental hazards in the Persian Gulf and Agent Orange in Vietnam; former prisoners of war; veterans of World War I or earlier conflicts; and other low-income veterans. Veterans who do not fit into category 1 may receive benefits if they agree to make a copayment, that is, pay a percentage of their care. Such veterans fall into category 2.

Nursing Home Care

Veterans who have sustained a service-connected disability or whose condition originated or was aggravated during active service have first priority for nursing home care. Eligible veterans include those exposed to herbicides in Vietnam; veterans exposed to ionizing radiation; veterans with a condition relating to environmental exposure in the Persian Gulf; former prisoners of var; veterans on VA pension or eligible for Medicaid; and Veterans of the Mexican Border period or World War I. Other veterans may be eligible upon assessment of income.

Residential medical care may be provided to low-income veterans who require long-term rehabilitative or maintenance care but minimal medical care.

Dental Services

Complete dental care is provided for veterans with service-connected dental disabilities, prisoners of war (for six months or more), or veterans who have service-connected disabilities rated at 100 percent. Dental care (dental examination and one-time dental treatment) is available to a veteran who has had at least 180 days of service and who has a dental condition that developed or was aggravated during active service and existed at the time of discharge.

Pharmacy Services

Prescription medications are available free to veterans receiving medication for treatment of a service-related condition; veterans with a disability rating of 50 percent or more; and low-income veterans. Prescription medications for other veterans is available for a small copayment.

Other Benefits and Allowances

Other services provided by the VA include registry programs and treatment for veterans exposed to ionizing radiation, Agent Orange or environmental hazards in the Gulf War. Some veterans are eligible for travel expenses to receive VA medical care. Alcohol and drug dependence treatment programs as well as prosthetic services and services for blind veterans are also available, including talking books, tapes, guide dogs, and electronic and mechanical aids.

Readjustment services are available for veterans who have difficulty adjusting to civilian life or who suffer from post-traumatic stress disorder, a condition in which the veteran suffers flashbacks, nightmares, and anxiety after exposure to traumatic conditions.

Other health-related benefits for veterans include health insurance programs, burial benefits, and death benefits. The VA offers several insurance plans: plans specifically tailored to World War I veterans, World War II veterans, Korean conflict veterans, service-disabled veterans, and World War II/Korean conflict veterans with service-connected or nonservice connected disabilities.

Also available, among various other group insurance programs, is a group life insurance that covers reservists, National Guard members, and ROTC members. The VA also provides burial benefits, such as reimbursement for burial expenses, a burial allowance, a burial flag, optional interment in a national cemetery, and a headstone or marker. These benefits are provided for the surviving spouse and children of war veterans or veterans who died in a VA medical facility or who were entitled to VA compensation or pension. Death benefits of certain veterans also extend to the surviving spouse and children: educational assistance and compensation is available to family members.

For more information:

Veterans Affairs Department
810 Vermont Ave., N.W.
Washington, DC 20420
800-827-1000
800-829-4833 (TDD)
http://www.va.gov

Veterans Affairs Department
Persian Gulf Helpline
800-PGW-VETS

Benefits, Compensation, Insurance and Pensions

*American Legion National Organization
1608 K St., N.W.
Washington, DC 20006
202-861-2711

*American Red Cross
Military/Social Services
18th and D Sts., N.W.
Washington, DC 20006
202-639-3586

*Army and Air Force Mutual Aid Association
Fort Meyer
Arlington, VA 22211
800-336-4538
703-522-3060

*Disabled American Veterans
807 Maine Ave., S.W.
Washington, DC 20024
202-554-3501

 * Private veterans-services organizations that assist the veteran with claims for benefits

Suggested Reading

AIDS/HIV

Alyson, Sasha, ed. *You Can Do Something About AIDS.* Boston: The Stop AIDS Project, 1990.

American Foundation for AIDS Research. *The AIDS/HIV Treatment Directory.* New York: The Foundation, 1995.

Edison, Ted. *The AIDS Caregiver's Handbook.* New York: St. Martin's, 1993.

Faison, Brenda S., and Laila Moustafa, ed. *AIDS Handbook: A Complete Guide to Education and Awareness.* Durham, NC: Designbase, 1991.

Ford, Michael Thomas. *100 Questions and Answers About AIDS: What You Need to Know Now.* New York: William Morrow and Co., 1993.

Hombs, Mary Ellen. *AIDS: Crisis in America: A Reference Handbook.* Santa Barbara, CA: ABC-Clio, 1992.

Schwartzberg, Steven S. *The Crisis of Meaning: How Gay Men Are Making Sense of AIDS.* New York: Oxford University Press, 1996.

Aging

Beers, Mark, Steven Urice, and Claire Zion, ed. *Aging in Good Health: A Complete Essential Medical Guide for Men and Women Over 50 and Their Families.* New York: Pocket Books, 1992.

Cirino, Linda D. *On Your Own Terms: The Senior's Guide to an Independent Life.* New York: Hearst Books, 1995.

Men's Health Books Staff, Doug Dollemore, and Mark Giuliucci. *Age Erasers for Men: Hundreds of Fast and Easy Ways to Beat the Years.* Emmaus, PA: Rodale Press, 1994.

Alcoholism

Al-Anon Family Group Headquarters. *How Al-Anon Works for Families and Friends of Alcoholics.* Virgina Beach, VA: Al-Anon Family Group Headquarters, 1995.

Alcoholics Anonymous World Services Staff. Alcoholics Anonymous: The Story of How Many Thousands of Men and Women Have Recovered From Alcoholism. New York: Alcoholics Anonymous World Services, 1986.

Kaufman, Edward. *Help at Last: A Complete Guide to Coping with Chemically Dependent Men.* Palm Beach Gardens, FL: Gardner Press, 1991.

Allergies

Novick, Nelson L. *You Can Do Something About Your Allergies.* New York: Macmillan, 1994.

Rothfeld, Glenn S., and Suzanne LeVert. *Natural Medicine for Allergies: The Best Alternative Methods for Quick Relief.* Emmaus, PA: Rodale Press, 1996.

Consumer Reports Books, eds., et al. *Allergies: A Complete Guide to Diagnosis, Treatment and Daily Management.* Yonkers, NY: Consumer Reports Books, 1992.

Alzheimer's Disease

Aronson, Miriam K., Ed.D., ed., and Alzheimer's Disease and Related Disorders Association. *Understanding Alzheimer's Disease.* New York: Charles Scribner's Sons, 1988.

Bair, Frank E., ed. *Alzheimer's, Stroke and 29 other Neurological Disorders Sourcebook.* Detroit: Omnigraphics, 1993.

Hay, Jennifer. *Alzheimer's and Dementia: Questions You Have...Answers You Need.* Allentown, PA: People's Medical Society, 1996.

Mace, Nancy L., M.A., and Peter V. Rabins, M.D., M.P.H. *The 36-Hour Day: A Family Guide to Caring for Persons with Alzheimer's Disease, Related Dementing Illnesses and Memory Loss Later in Life.* Rev. ed. Baltimore, MD: Johns Hopkins University Press, 1991.

Powell Lenore S., Ed.D., and Katie Courtice. *Alzheimer's Disease: A Guide for Families.* Rev. ed. Reading, MA: Addison-Wesley, 1993.

Arthritis

Arthritis Foundation Staff. *250 Tips for Making Life with Arthritis Easier.* Marietta, GA: Longstreet Press, 1997.

Arthritis Foundation Staff. *The Arthritis Foundation's Answers to All Your Questions.* Marietta, GA: Longstreet Press, 1997.

Childers, Norman F. *Arthritis—A Diet to Stop It: The Nightshades, Aging and Ill Health.* Gainesville, FL: Horticultural Publications, 1986.

Cook, Allan, ed. *The Arthritis Soucebook.* Detroit: Omnigraphics, 1997.

Ford, Norman D. *18 Natural Ways to Stop Arthritis Now.* New Canaan, CT: Keats, 1997.

Hawk, John K. *The Arthritis Encyclopedia.* New York: Facts on File, 1997.

Irving, Ann F., Ann Kushner, Irving Kushner, and the Arthritis Foundation Staff. *Understanding Arthritis.* New York: Macmillan, 1997.

Moyer, Ellen. *Arthritis: Questions You Have...Answers You Need.* Allentown, PA: People's Medical Society, 1997.

Sobel, Dava, and Arthur C. Klein. *Arthritis: What Works.* New York: St. Martin's, 1992.

Back Pain

Bonati, Alfred O., M.D., and Shirley Linde, Ph.D. *No More Back Pain.* New York: Pharos Books, 1991.

Inlander, Charles B., and Porter Shimer. *Backache: 51 Ways to Relieve the Pain.* New York: Walker and Co., 1997.

Levin-Gervasi, Stephanie. *The Back Pain Sourcebook: Everything You Need to Know.* Los Angeles: Lowell House, 1996.

McIlwain, Harris H. *Winning With Back Pain: How to Beat Back Pain and Take Control of Your Life.* New York: John Wiley and Sons, 1997.

Miller, Robert H., and Christine A. Opie. *Back Pain Relief: The Ultimate Guide.* Santa Barbara, CA: Capra Press, 1997.

Rothfeld, Glenn S., and Suzanne LeVert. *Natural Medicine for Back Pain.* New York: Macmillan, 1996.

Salmans, Sandra. *Back Pain: Questions You Have...Answers You Need.* Allentown, PA: People's Medical Society, 1995.

Birth Defects and Genetic Diseases

Gormley, Myra Vanderpool. *Family Diseases: Are You at Risk?* Baltimore: Genealogical Publishing, 1989.

Nightingale, Elena O., and Melissa Goodman. *Before Birth: Prenatal Testing for Genetic Disease.* Cambridge, MA: Harvard University Press, 1990.

Profet, Margie. *Protecting Your Baby-to-Be: Preventing Birth Defects in the First Trimester.* Reading, MA: Addison-Wesley, 1995.

Cancer

Altman, Roberta, and Michael J. Sarg., M.D. *The Cancer Dictionary.* New York: Facts on File, 1992.

Bruning, Nancy. *Coping With Chemotherapy.* New York: Ballantine, 1993.

Evans, Richard A. *Making the Right Choice: Treatment Options in Cancer Surgery.* Garden City Park, NY: Avery Publishing Group, 1995.

Murphy, Gerald P., M.D., Lois B. Morris, and Dianne Lange. *The American Cancer Society's Informed Decisions: The Complete Book of Cancer Diagnosis, Treatment and Recovery.* New York: Viking, 1997.

Walters, Richard. *Options: The Alternative Cancer Therapy Book.* Garden City Park, NY: Avery Publishing Group, 1993.

Winawer, Sidney J., M.D., and Moshe Shike, M.D. *Cancer Free: The Comprehensive Prevention Program.* New York: Simon and Schuster, 1995.

Breast Cancer

Colmore, Perry. *Living With Breast Cancer: 39 Women and 1 Man Speak Candidly About Surviving Breast Cancer.* Andover, MA: Andover Townsman, 1997.

Murcia, Andy. *Man to Man: When the Woman You Love Has Breast Cancer.* New York: St. Martin's, 1990.

Prostate Cancer

Bostwick, David. *The American Cancer Society's Prostate Cancer: What Every Man and His Family Needs to Know.* New York: Random House, 1996.

Korda, Michael. *Man to Man: Surviving Prostate Cancer.* New York: Random House, 1996.

Morra, Marion, and Eve Potts. *The Prostate Cancer Answer Book: An Unbiased Guide to Treatment Choices.* New York: Avon, 1996.

Oesterling, Joseph E., and Mark A. Moyad. *The ABC's of Prostate Cancer: A Book That Could Save Your Life.* Landham, MD: Madison Books, 1996.

Phillips, Robert H., Ph.D. *Coping with Prostate Cancer.* Garden City Park, NY: Avery Publishing Group, 1994.

Salmans, Sandra. *Prostate: Questions You Have...Answers You Need.* Allentown, PA: People's Medical Society, 1996.

Walsh, Patrick. *The Prostate: A Guide for Men and the Women Who Love Them.* New York: Warner Books, 1997.

Skin Cancer

Robins, Perry. *Play It Safe in the Sun.* New York: Skin Cancer Foundation, 1994.

Robins, Perry, and Maritza Perez. *Understanding Melanoma: What You Need to Know.* New York: Skin Cancer Foundation, 1996.

Cholesterol

Moyer, Ellen. *Cholesterol and Triglycerides: Questions You Have...Answers You Need.* Allentown, PA: People's Medical Society, 1995.

Chronic Fatigue Syndrome

Bell, David S. *The Doctor's Guide to Chronic Fatigue Syndrome: Understanding, Treating and Living With Chronic Fatigue Immune Dysfunction Syndrome.* Reading, MA: Addison-Wesley, 1995.

Berne, Katrina. *Running on Empty: The Complete Guide to Chronic Fatigue Syndrome.* Alameda, CA: Hunter House, 1995.

Feiden, Karyn. *Hope and Help for the Chronic Fatigue Syndrome: The Official Book of the CFS/CFIDS Network.* Englewood Cliffs, NJ: Prentice Hall, 1990.

Johnson, Hillary. *Osler's Web.* New York: Crown, 1996.

Colds and Flu

Davenport, Penny. *Colds and Flu, The Natural Way.* Rockport, MA: Element Books, 1995.

Inlander, Charles B., and Cynthia K. Moran. *77 Ways to Beat Colds and Flu.* New York: Waler and Co., 1994.

Complementary Medicine

Albright, Peter, M.D. *The Complete Book of Complementary Therapies.* Allentown, PA: People's Medical Society, 1997.

Bonk, Melinda, ed. *Alternative Medicine Yellow Pages.* Puyallup, WA: Future Medicine Publishing, 1994.

Bradford, Nikki, ed. *The Hamlyn Encyclopedia of Complementary Health.* London: Hamlyn, 1996.

Burton Goldberg Group. *Alternative Medicine: The Definitive Guide.* Fife, WA: Future Medicine Publishing, 1994.

Acupuncture

Chang, Stephen. *The Complete Book of Acupuncture.* Berkeley, CA: Celestial Arts Publishing, 1995.

Fleischman, Gary F. *Acupuncture: Everything You Always Wanted to Know (But Were Afraid to Ask).* Barrytown, NY: Barrytown, 1995.

Acupressure

Bauer, Cathryn. *Acupressure for Everybody: Gentle, Effective Relief for More Than 100 Common Ailments.* New York: Henry Holt and Co., 1991.

Herbal Therapy

Green, James. *Male Herbal.* Freedom, CA: The Crossing Press, 1991.

Puotinen, C.J. *Herbs for Men's Health: A Keats Good Herb Guide.* New Canaan, CT: Keats, 1997.

Homeopathy

Hammond, Christopher. *The Complete Family Guide to Homeopathy: An Encyclopedia of Safe and Effective Remedies.* New York: Viking/Penguin, 1996.

Weiner, Michael. *The Complete Book of Homeopathy.* New York: Fine Communications, 1997.

Massage Therapy

DePaoli, Carlo. *The Healing Touch of Massage.* New York: Sterling Publishing, 1995.

Feltman, John, ed. *Hands-On Healing: Massage Remedies for Hundreds of Health Problems.* New York: Random House, 1995.

LaCroix, Nitya. *Erotic Massage: Simple, Sensuous Techniques for Enhancing Sexual Pleasure.* San Francisco: Harper San Francisco, 1994.

McGilvery, Carole. *Step by Step Massage: A Guide to Massage Techniques for Health, Relaxation and Vitality.* New York: Smithmark Publications, 1994.

Contraception

Hatcher, Robert, et al. *Contraceptive Technology.* New York: Irvington Publishers, 1994.

Winikoff, Beverly, M.D., M.P.H., Suzanne Wymelenberg, and Consumer Reports Books, eds. *The Contraceptive Handbook: A Guide to Safe and Effective Choices.* Yonkers, NY: Consumer Reports Books, 1992.

Death and Dying

Colen, B.D. *The Essential Guide to a Living Will: How to Protect Your Right to Refuse Medical Treatment.* Englewood Cliffs, NJ: Prentice Hall, 1991.

Barnett, Terry H. *Living Wills and More: Everything You Need to Ensure That All Your Medical Wishes Are Followed.* New York: John Wiley and Sons, 1992.

Burnell, George M. *Final Choices: To Live or to Die in An Age of Medical Technology.* New York: Plenum Publishing, 1993.

Kubler-Ross, Elisabeth. *On Death and Dying: What the Dying Have to Teach Doctors, Nurses, Clergy and Their Own Families.* New York: Macmillan, 1969.

Volkan, Vanik D., and Elizabeth Zintl. *Life after Loss: The Lessons of Grief.* New York: Scribner, 1994.

Wong, Mary M., ed. *The National Directory of Bereavement Support Groups and Services, 1996 edition.* Forest Hills, NY: ADM Publishing, 1996.

Dentists and Dental Care

Latell, Jack K., D.S., Andrew Kaplan, D.M.D., and Gray Williams, Jr. *The Mount Sinai Medical Center Family Guide to Dental Health.* New York: Macmillan, 1991.

Stay, Flora Parsa, D.D.S. *The Complete Book of Dental Remedies.* Garden City Park, NY: Avery Publishing Group, 1996.

Depression

Chan, Connie. *If It Runs in Your Family: Depression.* New York: Bantam Books, 1993.

Engler, Jack, and Daniel Goleman. *The Consumer's Guide to Psychotherapy.* New York: Simon and Schuster, 1992.

Klein, Donald F., and Paul H. Wender. *Understanding Depression.* New York: Oxford University Press, 1993.

Real, Terrence. *I Don't Want to Talk About It: Overcoming the Secret Legacy of Male Depression.* New York: Scribner's Reference, 1997.

Rosenthal, Norman E. *Winter Blues.* New York: Guilford Press, 1993.

Salmans, Sandra. *Depression: Questions You Have...Answers You Need.* Allentown, PA: People's Medical Society, 1995.

Diabetes

Biermann, June, and Barbara Toohey. *The Diabetic's Total Health Book.* New York: Jeremy Tarcher, 1992.

Brisco, Paula. *Diabetes: Questions You Have...Answers You Need.* Allentown, PA: People's Medical Society, 1993.

Krall, Leo P., M.D., and Richard S. Beaser, M.D. *Joslin Diabetes Manual.* 12th ed. Philadelphia: Lea and Febiger, 1989.

Lodewick, Peter, June Biermann, and Barbara Toohey. *The Diabetic Man: A Guide to Health and Success in All Areas of Your Life.* Los Angeles: Lowell House, 1996.

Diet and Nutrition

Brendenberg, Jeff, Alisa Bauman, and Men's Health Books Editors. *Food Smart: A Man's Plan to Fuel Up for Peak Performance.* Emmaus, PA: Rodale Press, 1996.

Garrison, Robert H., Jr., M.A., R.Ph., and Elizabeth Somer, M.A., R.D. *The Nutrition Desk Reference.* New Canaan, CT: Keats, 1990.

Gittleman, Ann Louise. *Super Nutrition for Men and the Women Who Love Them.* New York: Evans and Co., 1996.

Drug Abuse

Dodd, David. *Playing It Straight: Personal Conversations on Recovery, Transformation and Success.* Deerfield Beach, FL: Health Communications, 1996.

Fanning, Patrick, and John O'Neill. *The Addiction Workbook: A Step-by-Step Guide to Quitting Alcohol and Drugs.* Oakland, CA: New Harbinger Publications, 1996.

Eating Disorders

Costin, Carolyn. *The Eating Disorders Sourcebook: Everything You Need to Know About Anorexia, Bulimia and Other Eating Disorders.* Los Angeles: Lowell House, 1996.

Haslam, David. *Bulimia: A Guide for Sufferers and Their Families.* Newton, MA: Butterworth-Heinemann, 1996.

Krasnow, Michael. *My Life as a Male Anorexic.* Binghamton, NY: Haworth Press, 1996.

Emergency Care and First Aid

The American Medical Association. *AMA Handbook of First Aid and Emergency Care.* Rev. ed. New York: Random House, 1990.

American Red Cross, and Kathleen A. Handal. *The American Red Cross First Aid and Safety Handbook.* New York: Little, Brown and Co., 1992.

Mayell, Mark, and Natural Health Magazine, eds. *The Natural Health First Aid Guide: The Definitive Handbook of Natural Remedies for Treating Minor Emergencies.* New York: Pocket Books, 1994.

Eye Conditions

Salmans, Sandra. *Your Eyes: Questions You Have...Answers You Need.* Allentown, PA: People's Medical Society, 1996.

Shulman, Julius. *Cataracts.* New York: St. Martin's, 1995.

Zinn, Walter J., and Herbert Solomon. *The Complete Guide to Eyecare, Eyeglasses and Contact Lenses.* 4th ed. Hollywood, FL: Lifetime Books, 1996.

Gay Health Care

Eliason, Michele. *Who Cares? Health Issues for Lesbian, Gay and Bisexual Persons.* New York: National League of Nursing, 1996.

Peterson, K. Jean, ed. *Health Care for Lesbians and Gay Men: Confronting Homophobia and Heterosexism.* Binghamton, NY: Harrington Park Press, 1996.

Shernoff, Michael, ed. *Sourcebook on Lesbian/Gay Health Care.* Washington, D.C.: National Lesbian/Gay Health Foundation, 1988.

Hair Loss

Bruning, Nancy P. *What You Can Do About Chronic Hair Loss.* New York: Dell, 1993.

Peters, Ken, David Stuss, and Nick Wadell. *Hair Loss Prevention Through Natural Remedies: A Prescription for Healthier Hair.* Santa Rosa, CA: Atrium Publishers Group, 1996.

Sudlick, Neil S., Donalde R. Richardson, and Consumer Reports Books. *Your Hair: How to Keep It: Treatment and Prevention of Hair Loss for Men and Women.* Yonkers, NY: Consumer Reports Books, 1992.

Headaches

American Council for Headache Education. *Migraine, The Complete Guide.* New York: Dell, 1994.

Burks, Susan L. *Managing Your Migraine: A Migraine Sufferer's Practical Guide.* Totowa, NJ: Humana Press, 1994.

Rapoport, Alan, and Fred Sheftell. *Conquering Headache: An Illustrated Guide to Understanding and Control of Headache.* Chicago: Login Publishers Consortium, 1995.

Hearing Disorders

Hay, Jennifer. *Hearing Loss: Questions You Have...Answers You Need.* Allentown, PA: People's Medical Society, 1994.

Tannenhaus, Nora. *What You Can Do About Hearing Loss.* New York: Dell, 1993.

Vernick, David M., M.D., and Constance Grzelka. *The Hearing Loss Handbook.* Yonkers, NY: Consumer Reports Books, 1993.

Heart Disease and Hypertension

Jones, Paul, M.D., and Angela Mitchell. *The Black Health Library Guide to Heart Disease and Hypertension.* New York: Henry Holt and Co., 1993.

Karpman, Harold L. *Preventing Silent Heart Disease: Detecting and Preventing America's Number-One Killer.* New York: Crown, 1989.

Ornish, Dean, M.D. *Dr. Dean Ornish's Program for Reversing Heart Disease.* New York: Random House, 1990.

People's Medical Society. *Your Heart: Questions You Have...Answers You Need.* Allentown, PA: People's Medical Society, 1996.

Prevention Magazine Staff, eds. *Lower Your Blood Pressure: Controlling Your Blood Pressure Without Drugs.* Stamford, CT: Longmeadow Press, 1991.

Simon, Harvey B., M.D. *Conquering Heart Disease: New Ways to Live Well Without Drugs and Surgery.* Boston: Little, Brown and Co., 1994.

Incontinence

Vierck, Elizabeth. *Seven Steps to Normal Bladder Control: Simple, Practical Tips and Techniques for Staying Dry.* Gig Harbor, WA: Harbor Press, 1997.

Infertility

Comhaire, F.H., ed. *Male Infertility.* London: Chapman and Hall, 1995.

Friedeman, Joyce S. *How to Become Your Own Best Infertility Counselor.* Fort Thomas, KY: Jolance Press, 1995.

Harkness, Carla. *The Infertility Book: A Comprehensive Medical and Emotional Guide.* Berkeley, CA: Celestial Arts, 1992.

Johnson, Patricia Irvin. *Taking Charge of Infertility.* Indianapolis, IN: Perspective Press, 1994.

Mason, Mary-Claire. *Male Infertility: Men Talking.* New York: Routledge, 1993.

Insurance

Inlander, Charles B. *Getting the Most for Your Medical Dollar.* New York: Wings Books, 1993.

Inlander, Charles B., and Michael A. Donio. *Medicare Made Easy: Everything You Need to Know to Make Medicare Work for You.* Allentown, PA: People's Medical Society, 1997.

Long-Term Care

Boyer, Niel J. *A Complete Guide to Long-Term-Care Insurance.* Westport, CT.: Practical Legal Publications, 1990.

Cassel, Edythe J. *The Continuing Care Retirement Community: A Guidebook for Consumers.* Washington, D.C.: American Association of Homes and Services for the Aging, published annually.

The Directory of Nursing Homes. Baltimore, MD: HCIA, published annually.

The Directory of Retirement Facilities. Baltimore, MD: HCIA, published annually.

Falk, Ursula A. *On Our Own: Independent Living for Older Persons.* Buffalo, NY: Prometheus Books, 1990.

Matthews, Joseph. *Beat the Nursing Home Trap: A Consumer's Guide to Choosing and Financing Long-Term Care*. 2nd ed. Berkeley, CA: Nolo Press, 1993.

National Directory for Eldercare Information and Referral. Washington, D.C.: National Association of Area Agencies on Aging, published annually.

Malpractice

Bartone, John C. *Consumer's Reference Book and Index Concerning Medical Malpractice*. Annandale, Va.: ABBE Publisher's Association of Washington, D.C., 1996.

Male Menopause

Braverman, Eric. *Male Menopause*. New Canaan, CT: Keats, 1997.

Cherniske, Stephen A. *The DHEA Breakthrough*. New York: Ballantine, 1997.

Hallberg, Edmund C. *The Grey Itch: The Male Menopause Syndrome*. Loomis, CA: Ombudsman Press, 1977.

Hill, Aubrey. *Viropause: The Male Menopause: Emotional and Physical Changes Midlife Men Experience*. Far Hills, NJ: New Horizon Press, 1993.

Ley, Beth M. *DHEA: Unlocking the Secrets to the Fountain of Youth*. Aliso Viejo, CA: BL Publishing, 1995.

Sahelian, Ray, M.D. *DHEA: A Practical Guide*. Garden City Park, NY: Avery Publishing Group, 1996.

Medical Records

People's Medical Society. *Your Complete Medical Record*. Allentown, PA: People's Medical Society, 1993.

Medical Rights

Annas, George J. *The Rights of Patients*. Carbondale, IL: Southern Illinois University Press, 1989.

Inlander, Charles B., and Eugene I. Pavalon. *Your Medical Rights: How to Become an Empowered Consumer*. Allentown, PA: People's Medical Society, 1990.

Medical Testing

Ferguson, Tom, M.D., and David Sobel, M.D. *The Patient's Guide to Medical Tests*. New York: Summit Books, 1985.

Pinckney, Cathey, and Edward Pinckney. *The Patient's Guide to Medical Tests*. 3rd ed. New York: Facts on File, 1987.

Medications

Mosby's Complete Drug Reference. 7th ed. Saint Louis, MO: Mosby, 1997.

The Physician's Desk Reference. Montvale, NJ: Medical Economic Data, 1996.

Graedon, Joe, and Teresa Graedon, Ph.D. *The People's Guide to Deadly Drug Interactions*. New York: St. Martin's, 1995.

Long, James W., M.D., and James J. Rybacki, Pharm.D. *The Essential Guide to Prescription Drugs*. New York: HarperCollins, 1994.

Melatonin

Pierpaoli, Walter, and William Regelson. *The Melatonin Miracle: Nature's Age-Reversing, Disease-Fighting, Sex-Enhancing Hormone*. New York: Pocket Books, 1996.

Reiter, Russel J., and Jo Robinson. *The Melatonin Revolution: Your Body's Natural Wonder Drug*. New York: Bantam, 1995.

Salhelian, Ray, M.D. *Melatonin: Nature's Sleeping Pill.* Marina Del Rey, CA: Be Happier Press, 1995.

Men's Health

Bauman, Alisa, Brian Paul Kaufman, and Men's Health Books, eds. *Symptom Solver: Understanding and Treating the Most Common Male Health Concerns.* Emmaus, PA: Rodale Press, 1997.

Caine, K. Winston, Perry Garfinkel, and Mens' Health Books, eds. *The Male Body: An Owner's Manual: The Ultimate Head-to-Toe Guide for Staying Healthy and Fit for Life.* Emmaus, PA: Rodale Press, 1996.

Dashe, Alfred M. *The Man's Health Sourcebook.* Los Angeles: Lowell House, 1996.

Consumer Reports Books, eds., and Allen B. Weisse. *The Man's Guide to Good Health.* Yonkers, NY: Consumer Reports Books, 1991.

Men's Fitness Magazine, and Kevin Cobb. *Men's Fitness Magazine's Complete Guide to Health and Well-Being.* New York: HarperCollins, 1996.

Reed, James N. *The Black Man's Guide to Good Health: Essential Advice for the Special Concerns of African-American Men.* New York: Berkeley Publishing Group, 1994.

Oppenheim, Michael, M.D. *The Man's Health Book.* Englewood Cliffs, NJ: Prentice Hall, 1994.

Wertheimer, Neil. *Total Health for Men: How to Prevent and Treat the Health Problems That Trouble Men Most.* Emmaus, PA: Rodale Press, 1995.

On-Line Health

Ferguson, Tom, M.D. *Health Online.* Reading, MA: Addison-Wesley, 1996.

Goldstein, Douglas, and Joyce Flory. *The Online Consumer Guide to Healthcare and Wellness.* Burr Ridge, IL: Irwin Professional Publishing, 1996.

Ryer, Jeanne C. *HealthNet: Your Essential Resource for the Most Up-to-Date Medical Information Online.* New York: John Wiley and Sons, 1996.

Wolff, Michael. *Net Doctor: Your Guide to Health and Medical Resources Online.* New York: Random House, 1996.

Osteoporosis

Bonnick, Sydney L. *The Osteoporosis Handbook.* 2nd ed. Dallas, TX: Taylor Publishing, 1997.

Jacobwitz, Ruth S. *About Osteoporosis.* New York: William Morrow and Co., 1996.

Physical Fitness

American Heart Association. *The Healthy Heart Walking Book: A Complete Program for a Lifetime of Fitness.* New York: Macmillan, 1995.

Brechle, Thomas R., and Roger W. Earle. *Fitness Weight Training.* Champaign, IL: Human Kinetics, 1994.

Golden, Manine and Mark Hopr. *Stretches: Simple Exercises to Make You Limber.* Kansas City, MO: Andres and McMeel, 1997.

Read, Malcolm, M.D., and Paul Wade. *What to Do When It Hurts: Self-Diagnosis and Rehabilitation of Common Aches and Pains.* Allentown, PA: People's Medical Society, 1996.

Sprague, Ken. *Sports Strength: Strength Training Routines to Improve Power, Speed and Flexibility for Virtually Every Sport.* New York: Berkely Publishers Group, 1993.

Whitmore, Jack H., and David C. Costhill. *Physiology of Sport and Exercise.* Champaign, IL: Human Kinetics, 1994.

Practitioners

American Medical Association Directory of Physicians in the United States. 34th ed. Chicago: American Medical Association, 1995.

Leeds, Dorothy, and Jon M. Strauss, M.D. *Smart Questions to Ask Your Doctor.* New York: HarperCollins, 1992.

McCall, Timothy B., M.D. *Examining Your Doctor: A Patient's Guide to Avoiding Harmful Medical Care.* Secaucus, NJ: Carol Publishing Group, 1996.

Sribnick, Richard L., M.D., and Wayne B. Sribnick, M.D. *Smart Patient, Good Medicine: Working with Your Doctor to Get the Best Medical Care.* New York: Walker and Co., 1994.

Board Certification

Boyden, Karen, ed. *Medical and Health Information Directory, 1996–97.* 8th ed. Detroit: Gale Research, 1996.

The Official ABMS Directory of Board Certified Medical Specialists, 1997. 29th ed. New Providence, NH: Marquis Who's Who, 1996.

Pregnancy

Inch, Sally. *Birthrights: What Every Parent Should Know About Birth in Hospitals.* New York: Pantheon, 1984.

Kitzinger, Sheila. *Homebirth and Other Alternatives to Hospitals.* London: Dorling-Kindersley, 1991.

Korte, Diana, and Roberta Scaer. *A Good Birth, A Safe Birth: Choosing and Having the Childbirth Experience that You Want.* 3rd rev. ed. Boston: Harvard Common Press, 1992.

Prostate Disease

Gelbard, Martin, M.D., and William Bentley. *Solving Prostate Problems.* New York: Fireside, 1995.

Salmans, Sandra. *Prostate: Questions You Have...Answers You Need.* Allentown, PA: People's Medical Society, 1996.

Relaxation Therapies

Sutcliffe, Jenny. *The Complete Book of Relaxation Therapies.* Allentown, PA: People's Medical Society, 1991.

Repetitive Motion Injuries

Tannenhaus, Nora. *Relief from Carpal Tunnel Syndrome and Other Repetitive Motion Disorders.* New York: Dell, 1991.

Self-Care

Powell, Don R., Ph.D. *Self-Care: Your Family Guide to Symptoms and How to Treat Them.* Allentown, PA: People's Medical Society, 1996.

Prevention Magazine, eds. *The Doctors Book of Home Remedies.* Emmaus, PA: Rodale Press, 1990.

Sexual Development

Madaras, Lynda, and Dane Saavedra. *The What's Happening to My Body? Book for Boys.* New York: Newmarket Press, 1984.

McCoy, Kathy, Ph. D, and Charles Wibbelsman, MD. *The New Teenage Body Book.* Rev. ed. New York: Putnam Publishing, 1992.

Sexual Dysfunction

MacKenzie, Bruce and Eileen, and Linda Christie. *It's Not All in Your Head: A Couple's Guide to Overcoming Impotence.* New York: Henry Holt and Co., 1991.

Morgenstern, Steven. *Overcoming Impotence: Doctor's Guide to Regaining Sexual Vitality.* 2nd ed. Englewood Cliffs, NJ: Prentice Hall, 1994.

Sexuality

Bechtel, Stefan, and Laurence Roy Stains. *Sex: A Man's Guide.* Emmaus, PA: Rodale Press, 1996.

Comfort, Alex, M.D., D.Sc. *The New Joy of Sex.* New York: Crown Publishers, 1991.

Westheimer, Ruth K., Ed.D. *Dr. Ruth's Encyclopedia of Sex.* New York: Continuum, 1994.

Sexually Transmitted Infections

Ebel, Charles. *Managing Herpes[md]How to Live and Cope with a Chronic STD.* Research Triangle Park, NC: American Social Health Association, 1994.

Sleep Disorders

Inlander, Charles B., and Cynthia K. Moran. *67 Ways to Good Sleep.* New York: Walker and Co., 1995.

Johnson, T. Scott, M.D., and Jerry Halberstadt. *Phantom of the Night.* Cambridge, MA: New Technology Publications, 1995.

Lipman, Derek S., M.D. *Stop Your Husband from Snoring.* Emmaus, PA: Rodale Press, 1990.

Pascualy, Ralph, M.D., and Sally Warren Soest. *Snoring and Sleep Apnea: Personal and Family Guide to Diagnosis and Treatment.* New York: Raven Press, 1994.

Skin

Schorr, Lia. *Lia Schorr's Skin Care Guide for Men.* Englewood Cliffs, NJ: Prentice Hall, 1985.

Wesley-Hosford, Zia. *The Complete Guide to Skin Care for Men.* San Diego, C: Harcourt Brace and Co., 1987.

Smoking

Maximin, Anita, and Lori Stevic-Rust. *The Stop Smoking Workbook.* Oakland, CA: New Harbinger Publications, 1996.

Stress

Chichester. *Stress Blaster.* New York: St. Martin's, 1997.

Inlander, Charles B., and Cynthia K. Moran. *Stress: 63 Ways to Relieve Tension and Stay Healthy.* New York: Walker and Co., 1996.

Witkin, George. *The Male Stress Syndrome: How to Become Stresswise in the 90s.* 2nd ed. New York: Newmarket Press, 1994.

Stroke

Ancowitz, Arthur, M.D. *The Stroke Book: One-on-One Advice About Stroke Prevention, Management and Rehabilitation.* New York: William Morrow and Co.: 1993.

Caplan, Louis R., M.D., Mark L. Dyken, M.D., and J. Donald Easton, M.D. *The American Heart Association Family Guide to Stroke Treatment, Recovery and Prevention.* New York: Times Books, 1994.

Frye-Pierson, Janice, R.N., B.S.N., CNRN, and James F. Toole, M.D. *Stroke: A Guide for Patient and Family.* New York: Raven Press, 1987.

Hay, Jennifer. *Stroke: Questions You Have...Answers You Need.* Allentown, PA: People's Medical Society, 1995.

Singleton, Lafayette, M.D., and Kirk Johnson. *The Black Health Library Guide to Stroke.* New York: Henry Holt and Co., 1993.

Surgery

Huddleston, Peggy. *Prepare for Surgery, Heal Faster: A Guide of Mind-Body Techniques.* Cambridge, MA: Angel River Press, 1996.

Inlander, Charles B., and Ed Weiner. *Take This Book to the Hospital With You.* Allentown, PA: People's Medical Society, 1997.

Inlander, Charles B. *Good Operations—Bad Operations.* New York: Viking Press, 1991.

McCabe, John. *Surgery Electives: What to Know Before the Doctor Operates.* Santa Monica, CA: Carmania Books, 1994.

Philipott-Howard, John, and Mark Casewell. *Hospital Infection Control: Policies and Practical Procedures.* Philadelphia: W. B. Saunders, 1994.

Urinary Tract Conditions

Seal, G. Mark. *A Patient's Guide to Urology: Plumbing Problems in Layman's Terms.* Toledo, OH: High Oaks Publishing, 1995.

Vasectomy

AVSC Staff, and William M. Moss. *Contraceptive Surgery for Men and Women.* 2nd ed. Durant, OK: Essential Medical Informatin Systems, 1991.

Gonzales, Betty. *No-Scalpel Vasectomy: An Illustrated Guide for Surgeons.* New York: AVSC International, 1994.

Vitamins and Minerals

Hendler, Sheldon Saul, M.D., Ph.D. *The Doctor's Vitamin and Mineral Encyclopedia.* New York: Simon and Schuster, 1990.

Moyer, Ellen. *Vitamins and Minerals: Questions You Have...Answers You Need.* Allentown, PA: People's Medical Society, 1993.

Weight Reduction

Jensen, R.M., and Diane Parker, ed. *Balance: The Wellness and Weight Control Primer for Men.* San Jose, CA: R and E Publishers, 1993.

Shaevitz, Morton H. *Lean and Mean: The No-Hassle, Life-Extending Weight Loss Program for Men.* New York: Berkeley Publishers Group, 1994.

Index